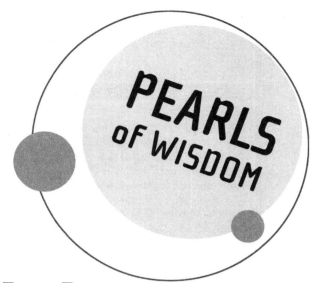

PEARLS of WISDOM

Anesthesiology
BOARD REVIEW
Third Edition

J. Sudharma Ranasinghe, MD, FFARCSI

Kerri M. Wahl, MD

Eric A. Harris, MD, MBA

David A. Lubarsky, MD, MBA

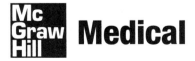
McGraw Hill **Medical**

New York   Chicago   San Francisco   Lisbon   London   Madrid   Mexico City
Milan   New Delhi   San Juan   Seoul   Singapore   Sydney   Toronto

Anesthesiology Board Review: Pearls of Wisdom, Third Edition

1 2 3 4 5 6 7 8 9 0   QDB/QDB   16 15 14 13 12

ISBN 978-0-07-176145-1
MHID 0-07-176145-4

Notice

Medicine is an ever-changing science. As new research and clinical experience broaden our knowledge, changes in treatment and drug therapy are required. The authors and the publisher of this work have checked with sources believed to be reliable in their efforts to provide information that is complete and generally in accord with the standards accepted at the time of publication. However, in view of the possibility of human error or changes in medical sciences, neither the authors nor the publisher nor any other party who has been involved in the preparation or publication of this work warrants that the information contained herein is in every respect accurate or complete, and they disclaim all responsibility for any errors or omissions or for the results obtained from use of the information contained in this work. Readers are encouraged to confirm the information contained herein with other sources. For example and in particular, readers are advised to check the product information sheet included in the package of each drug they plan to administer to be certain that the information contained in this work is accurate and that changes have not been made in the recommended dose or in the contraindications for administration. This recommendation is of particular importance in connection with new or infrequently used drugs.

This book was set in Adobe Garamond by Thomson Digital.
The editors were Kirsten Funk, Catherine A. Johnson, and Peter J. Boyle.
The production supervisor was Sherri Souffrance.
Project management was provided by Kunal Mehrotra, Thomson Digital.
Quad/Graphics Dubuque was printer and binder.

This book is printed on acid-free paper.

Library of Congress Cataloging-in-Publication Data

Anesthesiology board review. — 3rd ed. / Sudharma Ranasinghe ... [et al.].
   p. ; cm. — (Pearls of wisdom)
 Includes bibliographical references and index.
   ISBN 978-0-07-176145-1 (pbk. : alk. paper) — ISBN 0-07-176145-4 (pbk. : alk. paper)
 I. Ranasinghe, Sudharma. II. Series: Pearls of wisdom.
 [DNLM: 1. Anesthesia—Examination Questions. 2. Anesthesiology—methods—Examination Questions.
3. Anesthetics—Examination Questions. WO 218.2]

 617.9'60076—dc23

                                          2012016229

McGraw-Hill books are available at special quantity discounts to use as premiums and sales promotions, or for use in corporate training programs. To contact a representative, please e-mail us at bulksales@mcgraw-hill.com.

DEDICATION

Dedicated to two great departments of anesthesiology at the University of Miami and Duke University Medical Center who made this all possible.

J. Sudharma Ranasinghe
Kerri M. Wahl
Eric A. Harris
David A. Lubarsky

CONTENTS

CONTRIBUTORS

Swapna Chaudhuri, MD, PhD
Professor and Assistant Chair, Administration
Department of Anesthesiology
Texas Tech University Health Sciences Center
Lubbock, Texas

ENT Surgery

Christian Diez, MD
Assistant Professor
Department of Anesthesiology
Miller School of Medicine
University of Miami
Miami, Florida

Cardiopulmonary Resuscitation

John B. Eck, MD
Associate Professor, Anesthesiology and Pediatrics
Department of Anesthesiology
Duke University Medical Center
Durham, North Carolina

Pediatric Anesthesia
Neonatal Anesthesia

Eric A. Harris, MD, MBA
Associate Professor
Department of Anesthesiology
Miller School of Medicine
University of Miami
Miami, Florida

Clinical Pharmacology
Geriatric Patients
Outpatient Surgery
Preoperative Evaluation
Pharmacogenetics
Vascular Surgery

Jennifer Hochman Cohn, MD
Assistant Professor of Clinical Anesthesiology
University of Miami
Miller School of Medicine
Divison of Obstetric Anesthesia
Miami, Florida

Acid Base, Fluids, and Electrolytes
GI Disorders and Obesity
Peripheral Nerve Blocks

Allison Lee, MD
Assistant Professor of Clinical Anesthesiology
University of Miami
Miller School of Medicine
Miami, Florida

Allergic Reactions
Genitourinary and Renal Surgery
Hypothermia

David A. Lubarsky, MD, MBA
Chairman
Department of Anesthesiology
Miller School of Medicine
University of Miami
Miami, Florida

Vinaya Manmohansingh, MD
Assistant Professor
Department of Anesthesiology
Miller School of Medicine
University of Miami
Miami, Florida

Postoperative Recovery and Outcome

Timothy E. Miller, MB, ChB
Assistant Professor of Anesthesiology
Department of Anesthesiology
Duke University Medical Center
Durham, North Carolina

Anesthesia and the Liver
Transplant Surgery

Nicholas Nedeff, MD
Assistant Professor
Department of Anesthesiology
Miller School of Medicine
University of Miami
Miami, Florida

Anesthesia Risks/Standards/Billing

Chaturani T. Ranasinghe, MD
Assistant Professor
Department of Anesthesiology
Center for the Study and Treatment of Pain
NYU Langone Medical Center
New York, New York

Chronic Pain Management

J. Sudharma Ranasinghe, MD, FFARCSI
Professor of Clinical Anesthesiology
University of Miami
Miller School of Medicine
Chief of Obstetric Anesthesia
Jackson Memorial Medical Center
Miami, Florida

Autonomic Pharmacology and Physiology
Blood Therapy
Caudal, Epidural and Spinal Anesthesia
Electrical and Fire Safety in the Operating Room
Hemostasis
Inhalation Agents
Local Anesthetics
Machines
Muscle Relaxants
Neurosurgery
Nonopioid Intravenous Anesthetics
Obstetrics
Opioids and Substance Abuse
Patient Monitors
Respiratory Physiology and Anesthesia
Statistics

Aaron J. Sandler, MD, PhD
Assistant Professor of Anesthesiology
Department of Anesthesiology
Duke University Medical Center
Durham, North Carolina

Patient Positioning

Todd Smaka, MD
Assistant Professor
Department of Anesthesiology
Miller School of Medicine
University of Miami
Miami, Florida

Thoracic Surgery

Robert Thiele, MD
Fellow, Critical Care Anesthesiology
Department of Anesthesiology
Duke University Medical Center
Durham, North Carolina

Critical Care Medicine

Kerri M. Wahl, MD
Professor
Director, Abdominal Transplantation
Department of Anesthesiology
Duke University Medical Center
Durham, North Carolina

Endocrine
Airway and Intubation
Orthopedic Surgery

Jimmy Windsor, MD
Director, Congenital Cardiac Anesthesiology
University of Miami
Miller School of Medicine
Miami, Florida

Cardiac Physiology and Surgery

Christopher C. Young, MD
Associate Professor of Anesthesiology
Assistant Professor of Surgery
Section Chief, Critical Care Medicine
Department of Anesthesiology
Duke University Medical Center
Durham, North Carolina

Aspiration Pneumonitis
Critical Care Medicine

PREFACE

The ABA has abandoned K-type questions. To that we say, "Good riddance!" In a book like ours, it is the answers, not the format of the questions, that make the book. Therefore, no matter what the ABA does, the simple question/answer format here will serve you well!

Anesthesiology Board Review: Pearls of Wisdom, now in its third edition, has proven itself as the best preparation immediately before the exam. Hundreds of questions have been garnered from across the nation and from multiple institutions and contributors. The questions found here have only the correct answer. Read it, remember it, and score well!

New to this edition is the inclusion of new chapters on important topics such as vascular surgery and electrical safety in the OR. Also new is the addition of key terms to help you in your studying. These terms frequently appear in the board exams and will help you identify concepts that need further review. These key terms can be found at the end of each chapter.

As anyone will tell you, reviewing board review books doesn't make you smart, and just knowing the answers in this book does *not* guarantee a good board exam score. If you read something, and do not understand the answer, or are not sure about a related topic that pops into your mind, *look it up*!

Neither this tome nor its humble authors are substitutes for Barash, Stoelting, and Miller. Our book is a quick pre-boards review and was edited for that purpose; their textbooks are for the acquisition of knowledge. So use their books when you need a more complete understanding.

Good luck!

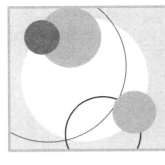

Acid Base, Fluids, and Electrolytes

For a long time it seemed to me that life was about to begin — real life. But there was always some obstacle in the way, something to be gotten through first, some unfinished business, time still to be served, a debt to be paid. At last it dawned on me that these obstacles were my life. This perspective has helped me to see there is no way to happiness. Happiness is the way. So treasure every moment you have and remember that time waits for no one. Happiness is a journey, not a destination.

Souza

○ **What is the most common underlying disorder in respiratory acidosis?**

Alveolar hypoventilation leading to hypercarbia.

○ **What ABG results would you expect to see in acute respiratory acidosis?**

In respiratory disorders, pH and $PaCO_2$ are inversely related. The pH decreases 0.05–0.08 for each 10 mm Hg increase in PCO_2. In the acute stage, bicarbonate would increase in compensation only 0.8 mmol/L for each 10 mm Hg increase in PCO_2.

○ **How does apnea affect $PaCO_2$?**

$PaCO_2$ increases by 6 mm Hg in the first minute of apnea and then increases by 3 mm Hg for each minute thereafter.

○ **List compensatory mechanisms for respiratory acidosis.**

Augmented ventilatory drive occurs via feedback to the brain and the medullary respiratory control center, mediated by central and carotid body chemoreceptors. Metabolic buffering through decreased hepatic HCO_3 uptake and shift of HCO_3 from red blood cells to plasma, carbonate release from bone, and decreased urea and lactic acid production (which utilizes HCO_3). Acutely HCO_3 increases 0.8 mmol/L for each 10 mm Hg of CO_2 greater than 40.

Long-term increase in $PaCO_2$ induces renal compensation with decreased chloride and phosphate reabsorption, increased HCO_3 reabsorption, and increased H^+ secretion. Chronically, HCO_3 increases 5 mmol/L for each 10 mm Hg of $PaCO_2$ greater than 40.

○ **What ABG results would you expect to see in acute metabolic alkalosis?**

In a metabolic alkalosis state, you would expect a pH >7.44. The bicarbonate level on ABG is normally approximately 1 mEq/L less than the total CO_2 on a simultaneously drawn serum electrolyte panel. If either the HCO_3^- level on ABG or CO_2 on electrolyte panel exceeds 24 or 25 mEq/L, respectively, by >4 mEq/L, either a primary or metabolic acidosis is present [Barash et al., 2009].

1

○ **What is the acute respiratory compensatory response to metabolic alkalosis?**

Reflex alveolar hypoventilation. $PaCO_2$ increases 0.5–0.6 mm Hg per 1 mEq increase in bicarbonate. If compensation is occurring, the last two digits of the pH should approximate $HCO_3^- + 15$. Respiratory compensation will rarely allow for a $PaCO_2$ above 55 mm Hg [Barash et al., 2009]. Eventually, the kidneys will tend to excrete more bicarbonate (chronic compensatory response).

○ **What is the acute respiratory compensatory response to metabolic acidosis?**

Reflex alveolar hyperventilation. $PaCO_2$ decreases 1.2 mm Hg per 1 mEq decrease in bicarbonate. Respiratory compensation will occur to a minimal CO_2 of 10–15 mm Hg. $PaCO_2$ should approximate $[HCO_3^-] \times 1.5 + 8$. The last two digits of the pH should also approximate $HCO_3^- + 15$ [Barash et al., 2009].

○ **What happens to the $PaCO_2$ and the PaO_2 in a patient with a high fever?**

In general, increases in temperature will cause the $PaCO_2$ and P_AO_2 to increase. As the temperature of a solution increases, more molecules will enter the gas phase, thus increasing the partial pressure of each gas. Gas solubility is inversely proportional to temperature.

○ **What are two common and clinically relevant causes of metabolic alkalosis?**

Loss of gastric fluid (vomiting and nasogastric suctioning) and loss of acidic urine secondary to diuretic therapy (thiazides, furosemide, and ethacrynic acid). Both are associated with NaCl deficiency and extracellular fluid depletion, and are often described as chloride-sensitive.

○ **What is the mechanism by which hypovolemia results in metabolic alkalosis?**

Under the influence of the renin–angiotensin system, aldosterone causes the kidney to reabsorb sodium and secrete potassium and hydrogen ions (to restore extracellular fluid volume). Hypokalemia will augment further hydrogen ion secretion and bicarbonate reabsorption, maintaining the metabolic alkalosis.

○ **Metabolic alkalosis is frequently associated with what volume status change?**

Hypovolemia from marked loss of sodium.

○ **What are the two main forms of metabolic acidosis?**

Anion gap and non-anion gap metabolic acidosis.

○ **How do you calculate the anion gap?**

The anion gap measures the difference in charge between the naturally occurring cations and anions.

It is calculated using the equation: $(Na^+ + K^+) - (Cl^- + HCO_3^-)$. A normal anion gap ranges from 8 to 16. However, patients who are hypoalbuminemic or hypophosphatemic may have a normal calculated gap in the face of unmeasured anions. Consequently, a corrected anion gap equation exists [Miller, 2010]:

Corrected anion gap = Calculated anion gap + 2.5(normal albumin [g/dL] − observed albumin [g/dL]).

○ **What are the most common causes of anion gap metabolic acidosis?**

A common pneumonic used to remember causes of anion gap metabolic acidosis is "MUDPILES," which includes *m*ethanol/*m*annitol, *u*remia, *d*iabetic ketoacidosis, *p*araldehyde, *i*sopropyl alcohol, *l*actic acidosis, *e*thanol/*e*thylene glycol/*e*thyl ether, and *s*alicylates.

○ **In the surgical patient, metabolic acidosis is frequently caused by circulatory failure and accumulation of lactic acid. What is the appropriate treatment?**

The most important goal is to maintain adequate tissue perfusion and oxygenation. Volume resuscitation with fluid or blood and maintenance of cardiac output should be the initial therapy. If the arterial pH is less than 7.20, increasing controlled ventilation and administration of sodium bicarbonate to pH = 7.20 to 7.30 may be necessary. When the arterial pH decreases below 7.00, the circulatory system becomes refractory to sympathomimetics. Sodium bicarbonate administration can be used to enhance response to drug therapy. It should not be utilized as a sole treatment modality [Miller, 2010]. Impairment of liver function will compound the metabolic acidosis secondary to failure to metabolize lactate to bicarbonate.

○ **What acid–base disturbance would you expect to find in COPD?**

It will depend on whether the primary problem is bronchitis (blue bloater) or emphysema (pink puffer). Bronchitic patients have severely deranged matching of ventilation and perfusion, which results in severe hypoxemia and hypercarbia. Under stable conditions the body will adjust to this respiratory acidosis with a compensatory metabolic alkalosis. Emphysematous patients are better able to maintain V/Q matching as lung tissue and vasculature are equally destroyed. ABGs typically show mild hypoxemia and minimal CO_2 retention, as patients are able to maintain a normal CO_2 by increasing their minute ventilation. As the disease progresses CO_2 will be retained and the ABGs will resemble those of a patient with bronchitis.

○ **What effect does alkalosis has on serum potassium, serum calcium, and shifting of the oxygen hemoglobin dissociation curve?**

Alkalosis causes a decrease in serum potassium and ionized calcium and a left shift in the oxygen hemoglobin dissociation curve.

○ **What causes a right shift in the oxygen hemoglobin dissociation curve?**

A right shift in the oxygen hemoglobin dissociation curve means oxygen is more easily released from hemoglobin to tissues (increased $P50$). Causes include acidosis, increased carbon dioxide, increased temperature, and increased 2,3-DPG.

○ **What causes a left shift in the oxygen hemoglobin dissociation curve?**

A left shift means oxygen is less easily released to tissues. Causes include alkalosis, decreased temperature, decreased 2,3-DPG, and abnormal forms of hemoglobin (fetal hemoglobin, methemoglobin, carboxyhemoglobin, and hemoglobin S).

○ **What are the factors affecting blood oxygen content?**

The amount of oxygen in blood depends mainly on the hemoglobin concentration (Hb) and hemoglobin saturation (SaO_2) at a given PaO_2, with a small contribution from dissolved O_2:

Oxygen content = CaO_2 = (Hb × SaO_2 × 1.34 mL/dL blood) + (0.003 mL O_2/dL blood/mm Hg × PaO_2).

○ **How much oxygen is dissolved in blood and under what conditions is this significant?**

Only 0.003 mL of O_2 per mm Hg PO_2 is dissolved in 100 cm^3 of plasma. At normal levels of hemoglobin this contribution is insignificant, but this situation changes in severely anemic patients. In a patient with Hb of 5.0 g/dL placed on supplemental O_2 with a PO_2 of 500 mm Hg, 1.5 mL of O_2 is dissolved in each deciliter, accounting for 18% of total oxygen content (normal 1.4–1.9%).

○ **What is the oxygen–hemoglobin dissociation curve and *P*50?**

The Hb–O_2 dissociation curve is the sigmoidal relationship of the partial pressure of oxygen and the saturation of hemoglobin. The *P*50 (26–27 mm Hg under normal physiologic conditions) is the PO_2 that yields a hemoglobin saturation of 50% and defines the affinity of hemoglobin for oxygen.

○ **How do changes in the hematocrit affect oxygen transport?**

Total oxygen delivery is the product of arterial oxygen content and cardiac output: $DO_2 = CaO_2 \times CO$. The arterial oxygen content is dependent on P_AO_2 (P_AO_2 = Alveolar partial pressure of oxygen) and hemoglobin concentration. Deficiencies in oxygen delivery may be due to a low P_AO_2 (V/Q mismatch, impaired diffusion of O_2 into blood), a low hemoglobin concentration, or reduced cardiac output (including distribution of blood to tissues and O_2 extraction). In patients with chronic severe anemia compensatory mechanisms to increase oxygen delivery include increase in cardiac output (increase in heart rate and reduction in blood viscosity) and increased extraction (resulting in a lower mixed venous oxygen saturation).

○ **What information is necessary for the accurate interpretation of a blood gas sample?**

Source (arterial vs. venous), temperature of the sample (body, room air, or stored on ice), ventilator settings, the FiO_2 at which the sample was drawn, and age of the patient. Also, consider when the sample was drawn.

○ **What happens to the PaO₂ and PaCO₂ in an arterial blood gas sample that has an air bubble trapped in the syringe?**

In general, the blood values move to equilibrate with the air bubble values. This means blood PaO_2 will tend to move toward 150 mm Hg (value in air at atmospheric pressure), increasing or decreasing to achieve that. The $PaCO_2$ will tend to decrease moving toward 0. Air has negligible CO_2 and the typical blood gas sample has some value higher than this for $PaCO_2$, so with equilibration the $PaCO_2$ in the sample will tend to decrease.

○ **What is the effect of temperature on blood gas analysis?**

The PO_2 measurement performed with a blood gas electrode at 37°C gives an overestimate if the patient is hypothermic and an underestimate if the patient is febrile. The percentage of error is greatest for venous values (PO_2 values <100 mm Hg) and if the patient's temperature is 20°C. Conventionally, blood gas analysis is done at 37°C. Warming a blood gas sample will decrease gas solubility (PO_2 and PCO_2) and elevate blood gas tension. The reverse is true for cooling a blood sample. Several algorithms exist for temperature correction (to the patient's temperature), such that the true partial pressure can be calculated. In hypothermic patients, the pH should be maintained close to 7.4, which would keep the corrected pH in the alkalotic range.

○ **Where must you sample blood to measure mixed venous oxygen saturation?**

MVO_2 saturation is measured in the pulmonary artery. A true mixed venous blood sample measures venous drainage from the inferior vena cava, superior vena cava, and right heart.

○ **Why is mixed venous oxygen sampling so important?**

It represents the overall balance between oxygen consumption and oxygen delivery and therefore provides a critical assessment of tissue oxygen metabolism.

○ **What is the normal mixed venous oxygen tension (PvO₂) and saturation?**

Normal mixed venous oxygen tension (PvO_2) is 35–45 mm Hg, corresponding to a mixed venous oxygen saturation of 65–75%. It is higher under general anesthesia.

○ **What factors affect SvO₂ (mixed venous oxygen saturation)?**

SvO_2 varies directly with cardiac output, hemoglobin, and arterial saturation and inversely with oxygen consumption. The normal SvO_2 is 75%. When the SvO_2 is less than 30%, tissue oxygen balance is compromised and anaerobic metabolism ensues.

○ **What factors cause a low mixed venous oxygen?**

Both an increase in oxygen consumption and tissue extraction as seen in febrile and hypermetabolic states can lead to a low mixed venous oxygen if a compensatory increase in O_2 delivery does not occur. Decreased O_2 delivery (hypoxia, low cardiac output, and decreased hemoglobin concentration) also leads to a low mixed venous oxygen level if tissue utilization remains constant. Lowering of hemoglobin saturation and a right shift of the oxygen hemoglobin dissociation curve will also tend to decrease mixed venous oxygen tension.

○ **What causes a high mixed venous oxygen?**

Increased cardiac output, decreased oxygen consumption (hypothermia), impaired tissue uptake (cyanide poisoning), or a severe left shift of the oxygen hemoglobin dissociation curve all cause increased mixed venous oxygen saturation. A sampling error from a wedged PA catheter, a left-to-right intracardiac shunt, or sepsis should be considered.

○ **Given that total body water (TBW) is about 60% of body weight, what percentage of body weight is intracellular, extracellular, interstitial, and intravascular?**

Intracellular volume (ICV) constitutes 40% of TBW and includes red cell volume.

Extracellular volume (ECV) represents the remaining 20% of TBW.

ECV is composed of plasma volume and interstitial volume. Plasma volume comprises 1/5th (~5% of TBW) of the ECV, the remaining 4/5th (~15% of TBW) of which is interstitial volume.

○ **Should TBW estimates be increased or decreased in obese patients?**

Decreased by 20–30% on a per kg basis. Estimates are lower as a result of decreased lean body mass.

○ **How does ascites fluid accumulate?**

The difference in the colloid osmotic pressure (COP) and hydrostatic pressure between plasma and the interstitial fluid helps maintain the intravascular volume. Usually the plasma oncotic pressure is 20 mm Hg more than interstitial fluid.

The Starling equation represents the pressure gradients that exist across capillary membrane, which is responsible for the net fluid movement:

$$\text{Fluid movement} = k[(P_c + \pi_i) - (P_i + \pi_c)],$$

where k is the capillary filtration constant, P_c is the capillary hydrostatic pressure, P_i is the interstitial hydrostatic pressure, π_c is the capillary COP, and π_i is the interstitial COP.

Edema = excess fluid in the interstitial space (transudate/exudate).

Ascites is excess fluid in the peritoneal cavity that accumulates due to increased capillary hydrostatic pressure, increased permeability, decreased intravascular protein (colloid pressure <11 mm Hg), or due to obstruction to lymph flow. Example: cirrhosis, malignancy, or cardiac failure.

○ **What are the physiologic responses to blood loss?**

The decrease in blood volume leads to arteriolar constriction. Venous pressure falls and the capillary pressure decreases. This causes net movement of interstitial fluid into the capillaries. The circulating blood volume is restored in about 12–72 hours. Preformed albumin moves into circulation from extravascular stores. The hematocrit may not fall for several hours. The peak reticulocyte count increase occurs in 10 days. The red blood cell count is restored in about 4–8 weeks.

○ **What is Bainbridge reflex?**

The Bainbridge reflex, also called the atrial reflex, is increase in heart rate due to increase in central venous pressure.

○ **What is normal plasma osmolality?**

Normal plasma osmolality is 280–295 mOsm/kg.

○ **How is osmolality calculated?**

$$\text{Plasma osmolality (mOsm/kg)} = \text{Na}^+ \text{ (mEq/L)} \times 2 + \frac{\text{glucose (mg/dL)}}{18} + \frac{\text{BUN (mg/dL)}}{2.8}$$
$$+ \frac{\text{any solute (mg/dL)}}{(\text{molecular weight of the solute})/10}.$$

○ **Give an example of hyperosmolar coma?**

Hyperosmolar nonketotic coma and is seen in type II diabetes.

Hyperglycemic diuresis causes dehydration and hyperosmolality.

Sever hyperglycemia may lead to factitious hyponatremia. (This is dilutional hyponatremia. High osmotic gradient causes water to move from ICF to ECF.)

Each 100 mg/dL increase in plasma glucose lowers plasma sodium by 1.6 mEq/L.

Ketoacidosis is not a feature because enough insulin is available to prevent ketone body formation.

○ **Which hormones regulate serum osmolality?**

Water and sodium reabsorption in the kidney are influenced by hormonal factors: ADH, atrial natriuretic peptide (ANP), and aldosterone. Sodium concentration is the primary determinant of plasma osmolality. Plasma hypertonicity stimulates ADH release, which enhances water reabsorption in the collecting ducts. ANP, which is released in response to atrial stretch, has vasodilatory effects and increases excretion of sodium and water. Aldosterone causes sodium reabsorption in the distal renal tubules.

○ **What is the relationship between serum sodium concentration and water balance?**

Generally, due to renal mechanisms: hypernatremia means "too little free water" rather than "too much sodium"; hyponatremia means "too much free water" rather than "too little sodium."

○ **How is urine osmolality calculated?**

$$\text{Urine osmolality (mOsm/kg)} = 2 \times (\text{urinary sodium [mEq/L]} + \text{urinary potassium [mEq/L]})$$
$$+ \frac{\text{urine urea nitrogen (mg/dL)}}{2.8}.$$

○ **Loss of free water may cause hypernatremia. What are normal insensible losses? How does temperature affect insensible losses?**

Insensible loss averages 700 cm^3 per day of a total 2,300 cm^3 daily loss of water. High temperature increases water loss as sweat – 100–1,400 cm^3. Other insensible losses remain unchanged.

○ **What tests indicate that the kidney is conserving sodium?**

1. Urine sodium (<20 mEq/L)
2. Fractional excretion of Na^+ <1% of creatinine clearance

○ **What is the sodium concentration of the following frequently used intravenous fluids?**

Normal saline (0.9% NS) – 154 mEq/L.

Half-normal saline (0.45% NS) – 77 mEq/L.

Three percent saline – 513 mEq/L.

Lactated Ringer's (LR) – 130 mEq/L.

Five percent dextrose (D5W) – 0.

○ **What are the effects of infusion of LR solution?**

LR is a balanced salt solution with electrolyte composition similar to extracellular fluid: Na 130 mmol/L, Cl 110 mmol/L, K 4–5 mmol/L, Ca 2 mmol/L, and lactate 28 mmol/mL, 275 mOsmol/L, pH 6.2. Ringer's solution was developed by Sydney Ringer in 1880. In the 1930s Alexis Hartmann added lactate to act as a buffer, which hydrates to carbonic acid and finally CO_2. LR solution contains calcium (2 mmol/L) and in a 1:1 ratio will clot blood at room temperature and 37°C. LR is used to provide maintenance water and electrolytes and for IV resuscitation.

○ **What causes the metabolic acidosis seen with large-volume IV infusion of normal saline?**

Saline solutions are nonphysiologic due to the level of chloride significantly greater than plasma (154 mmol, as compared with 98–102 mmol), lack of potassium, calcium, and magnesium that are present in normal plasma, and the lack of bicarbonate buffer. The mechanism for the acid–base disturbance has been described as a "dilutional hyperchloremic acidosis" (plasma expansion and dilutional reduction of bicarbonate) or more recently Stewart's physicochemical theory where hyperchloremia reduces the strong-ion difference (SID) leading to acidosis through dissociation of water to maintain electrochemical neutrality.

○ **What is the SID?**

The SID is the net charge balance of all strong cations (Na, K, Ca, and Mg) and strong anions (Cl and lactate). The normal SID is 40–49 mEq/L. SID determines (along with CO_2 and weak acids) what the plasma hydrogen ion concentration will be. The electrochemical forces generating the SID determine water dissociation, and therefore the hydrogen ion concentration required to balance plasma ionic charges. The net result always has to be a plasma ionic charge equal to zero (electrochemical neutrality). An increase in plasma chloride ion concentration will result in a decrease in SID, leading to an increased hydrogen ion concentration, and acidosis.

○ **What are the possible adverse effects of hyperchloremia following normal saline infusion?**

Metabolic acidosis, derangement in coagulation with increased bleeding, renal vasoconstriction with a decrease in glomerular filtration rate and renal blood flow, and increased postoperative nausea and vomiting (gut hypoperfusion or splanchnic vasoconstriction).

○   **How can resuscitation with crystalloids lead to coagulopathy?**

Crystalloids lack oxygen-carrying capacity and are devoid of both red blood cell mass and coagulation factors. With ongoing resuscitation, a dilutional coagulopathy can occur [Barash et al., 2009].

○   **What are the differences between crystalloid and colloid solutions?**

Crystalloids are fluids that contain water and electrolytes, which are grouped as balanced, hypertonic, and hypotonic solutions. Colloids contain a high-molecular-weight solute (albumin or starch) that will not pass through an intact capillary membrane, thus generating a COP. Colloid solutions are 1:1 volume expanders. Replacement requirements using crystalloids have traditionally been believed to be 3- or 4-fold the volume of blood lost, due to crystalloid's distribution in a ratio 1:4 like extracellular fluid, leaving only 20% in the IV space. However, evidence from recent randomized controlled trials (RCTs) reveals crystalloid resuscitation volumes less than 2-fold the volume of colloids will achieve comparable end points to colloids [Hartog et al., 2011. See reference on page 522].

The most commonly used crystalloid solutions are normal saline, LR solution, Isolyte, Normosol, and Plasma-Lyte. The most common colloids are 5% and 25% albumin, 6% hetastarch (Hextend or Hespan), pentastarch, and dextrans in 6% and 10% concentrations.

○   **Are colloids more effective plasma expanders than crystalloids?**

1.   Achievement of hemodynamic goals: It seems hemodynamic changes by colloids are immediate effects that do not last long and do not lead to improved clinical outcomes in comparison with crystalloids.

      Proof: SAFE trial compared albumin with crystalloid in ICU patients (7,000 patients); VISEP study included >500 patients with sepsis; Wills study included children (>120 patients).
      • All showed that it is safe to resuscitate only with crystalloid.

2.   Edema formation (extravascular lung water and pulmonary edema): There is no difference between crystalloids and colloids.
      Aggressive overresuscitation is bad with both. Positive fluid balance may be a strong prognostic risk factor for death.
      Albumin may be harmful in some situations such as traumatic brain injury (higher 28-day mortality in SAFE study).

3.   All synthetic colloids carry inherent risk of anaphylactic reactions, coagulopathy, and renal impairment – mechanism not fully understood (osmotic nephrosis?).

○   **In what patient population does colloid administration improve mortality?**

Albumin has been associated with decreased renal failure and decreased mortality among several subsets of hypoalbuminemic patients, mainly those suffering from severe sepsis, extensive burns, and spontaneous bacterial peritonitis patients [Miller, 2010]. In patients with cirrhosis *and* spontaneous bacterial peritonitis, albumin 1.5 g/kg IV given at the time of diagnosis followed by 1.0 g/kg IV on day 3 reduces long-term mortality by 46% [Miller, 2010]. The VISEP trial (2008), a two-by-two factorial trial comparing strict with conventional glucose control as well as LR with low-molecular-weight hydroxyethyl starch (HES) in severe sepsis, randomized 537 patients prior to being stopped early [Brunkhorst., et al., 2008. See reference on page 522]. As compared with LR solution, HES administration was associated with higher rates of acute renal failure and renal replacement therapy in this European study from SEPnet.

In the Australian SAFE trial (2004), which randomized 6,997 critically ill patients to albumin or saline, there was no difference in mortality. In traumatic brain injury, fluid resuscitation with albumin was associated with higher mortality rates compared with saline [The SAFE Study 2007. See reference on page 522].

○ **What is the effect of hetastarch on coagulation?**

Synthetic colloids prolong partial thromboplastin time and reduce factor VIII:C and vWF levels up to 50–80% when used in doses of 1–1.5 L. Hetastarch also decreases expression and subsequent activation of glycoprotein IIb/IIIa, thereby interfering with platelet adhesion and clot formation [Kozek-Langnecker, 2005. See reference on page 522]. At recommended doses, up to 20 mL/kg, interference with crossmatching is minimal. Bleeding and allergic reactions are more frequently seen in doses above 20–25 mL/kg [Miller, 2010].

○ **What are symptoms of hypernatremia?**

Dehydration of brain cells causes lethargy or mental status changes proceeding to coma, seizures, and death. Acute and severe hypernatremia may precipitate intracranial hemorrhage. Additional signs and symptoms include thirst, shock, myoclonus, muscle tremor, rigidity, increased intravascular fluid volume, peripheral edema, and pleural effusion.

○ **What are the major causes of hypernatremia?**

Diabetes insipidus (DI; central and nephrogenic).

Insensible losses (burns, sweating).

Osmotic diuresis (mannitol, hyperglycemia).

Hypertonic fluid administration.

○ **Describe the EKG changes associated with hyponatremia.**

At sodium levels below 115 mEq/L, one can see QRS widening and ST elevation.

○ **Describe the clinical manifestations of hyponatremia.**

Serious symptoms of hyponatremia seen at Na^+ <125 mEq/L are mainly CNS-related secondary to cellular water intoxication. Serious neurological manifestations are seen at Na^+ <120 mEq/L. Symptoms include weakness, lethargy, muscle cramps, abdominal cramps, confusion, anorexia, nausea, vomiting, headache, delirium, seizures, and coma. Hyponatremia with increased intravascular volume can cause pulmonary edema, hypertension, and congestive heart failure, especially at Na^+ <100 mEq/L. Chronic hyponatremia may be asymptomatic until the serum sodium concentration drops below 115 mEq/L. Chronic changes are partially compensated; acute changes are much more dramatic.

○ **How fast should hyponatremia be corrected?**

No faster than 0.5–1.0 mEq of Na^+/(L h) using normal saline in patients with decreased total body sodium content. Initial goal is to correct the plasma sodium to 130 mEq/L. Water restriction is the treatment in hyponatremic patients with normal or increased total body sodium. If the patient is symptomatic (coma, seizures), the sodium level is corrected with a combination of hypertonic saline 3%, fluid restriction, and/or furosemide, until symptoms resolve, and then slowly thereafter.

○ **Describe the consequences of excessively rapid sodium replacement in hyponatremia.**

Central pontine myelinolysis consisting of quadriplegia, dysarthria, and dysphasia. In general, one should not replete the sodium much faster than it was lost.

○ **If hypertonic saline 3% is used for correction of hyponatremia, how is the replacement volume calculated?**

$$Na^+ \text{ deficit} = \text{total body weight} \times (\text{desired } [Na^+] - \text{present } [Na^+]).$$

$$\text{TBW} = \text{weight (kg)} \times 0.60.$$

$$\text{Salt replacement} = (130 - \text{actual serum sodium}) \times \text{TBW}.$$

$$\text{Volume of hypertonic saline (L)} = \frac{\text{salt replacement}}{\text{sodium content of 3\% saline}}.$$

Sodium content of 3% saline is 513 mEq/L.

For the calculation of salt replacement 130 mEq/L or the lowest serum sodium level reached until the patient becomes asymptomatic may be used. Goal rate of correction = 0.6–1.0 mEq/L/h to a sodium concentration of 130 mEq/L. Half the deficit should be replaced over the first 8 hours and the remainder over 1–3 days, if symptoms remit.

○ **How is plasma sodium concentration interpreted in the presence of hyperglycemia?**

High glucose concentration draws water out of cells and dilutes sodium in plasma. For every 100 mg/dL of glucose above 200 mg/dL, serum sodium is decreased by 1.6 mEq/L.

○ **What is "pseudohyponatremia?"**

Pseudohyponatremia, also called isotonic hyponatremia, is a laboratory artifact in the presence of severe hyperproteinemia or hyperlipidemia. Plasma sodium concentration is normal. Dilution of the measurement sample produces an artificially low sodium measurement by flame photometry. Hyperosmolality resulting from non-sodium molecules (glucose, mannitol) results in water shifting from the intracellular space to dilute the extracellular sodium concentration.

○ **Urine sodium levels below what value may distinguish extrarenal from renal sodium losses contributing to hyponatremia?**

Urinary sodium concentration less than 20 mEq/L implies extrarenal sodium loss.

○ **DI implies what tonicity of urine and plasma (hypertonic or hypotonic)?**

DI is characterized by dilute urine with hypertonic plasma osmolality. This condition may be caused by decreased synthesis or secretion of ADH (central DI) or renal organ unresponsiveness (nephrogenic DI).

○ **Describe the ECG effects of hypokalemia.**

Progressive flattening of the T wave, increasingly prominent U wave, increased amplitude of the P wave, prolongation of the PR interval and ST-segment depression, cardiac arrhythmia in the presence of digitalis toxicity, and AV block. Hypokalemia prolongs membrane repolarization and can lead to a long QT syndrome, TdP, and ventricular fibrillation [Miller, 2010].

○ **Describe the EKG changes frequently associated with hyperkalemia.**

Hyperkalemia: mild elevations of 6–7 mEq/L can lead to narrowed and peaked T waves with shortening of the QT interval. This progresses to a widened QRS and prolonged PR intervals, flattened P waves, and possible second- or third-degree AV block. With continued severe hyperkalemia, sine-wave ventricular flutter or asystole may occur [Miller, 2010].

○ **What are the clinical manifestations of hyperkalemia?**

Hyperkalemia leads to depolarization of cell membranes. Patients present with neuromuscular weakness that may progress to flaccid paralysis and hypoventilation. Alterations in the cardiac conduction system secondary to enhanced membrane depolarization and increased automaticity predispose to dysrhythmias [Miller, 2010].

○ **What is the treatment for acute hyperkalemia?**

The therapeutic goals are to lower serum potassium concentration, correct hypotension, and prevent arrhythmias.

Physiologic antagonists: 500 mg calcium chloride or 1 g calcium gluconate is enough to temporarily stabilize the heart (cardiac membrane stabilization) from the effects of hyperkalemia and is indicated in the presence of peaked T waves. The effects are immediate.

Shift K^+ from plasma back into the cell: intravenous glucose (25–50 g dextrose, or 1–2 amps D50) plus 5–10 U regular insulin will reduce serum potassium levels within 10–20 minutes, and the effects last 4–6 hours.

Hyperventilation, inhaled β-agonists, and, in the past, bicarbonate (1 mEq/kg, or 1–2 amps in a typical adult) were recommended; however, keep in mind that bicarbonate rarely helps, and furthermore binds Ca^{2+}, which may be counterproductive.

Increase excretion: diuretics (furosemide, 20–40 mg IV), resin exchange (Kayexalate), dialysis, and aldosterone agonists (fludrocortisone).

○ **What are the clinical manifestations of hypokalemia?**

Symptoms usually occur at potassium concentrations below 3.0 mEq/L. They include mental status changes, fatigue, muscle weakness and myalgias, hypoventilation (respiratory muscle weakness), and eventually complete paralysis. Smooth muscles may also be affected and present as paralytic ileus. Cardiovascular effects include dysrhythmias, hypotension, and myocardial dysfunction.

○ **How do changes in pH affect serum potassium?**

Plasma potassium concentration changes 0.6 mEq/L per 0.1 change in arterial pH (range 0.2–1.2 mEq/L per 0.1 U change), that is, if pH decreases from 7.4 to 7.3, serum potassium increases from 5.5 to 6.5 mEq/L (respiratory or metabolic acidosis).

During alkalosis, plasma potassium concentration decreases. During acidosis, plasma potassium concentration increases.

○ **What factors produce intercompartmental shifts of potassium?**

Extracellular pH, insulin, catecholamines, plasma osmolality, and possibly hypothermia.

○ **How do you maintain perioperative potassium (K^+) homeostasis?**

Total body potassium is approximately 40–50 mEq/kg. Mostly intracellular.

The kidneys are the principal organ in K homeostasis. Aldosterone, ADH, and glucocorticoids increase K secretion and catecholamines decrease renal secretion.

Acute hypokalemia can be managed by KCl infusions. Hyperkalemia is managed by calcium gluconate IV, sodium bicarbonate, and glucose–insulin mixtures.

Epinephrine and beta-2 agonists decrease serum K^+ concentrations by redistribution.

○ **What is the major cause of extrarenal potassium depletion?**

Decreased potassium levels are always either renal or gastrointestinal. The most common cause of renal potassium depletion is related to diuretic therapy or enhanced mineralocorticoid activity. GI losses are secondary to vomiting, nasogastric suctioning, or diarrhea.

○ **List medications that may cause hyperkalemia.**

1. Error, due to sample lysis
2. Internal potassium balance (extracellular shift):
   - Succinylcholine
   - Digitalis
   - Nonselective beta-blockers
   - Antibiotics
3. External potassium balance (decreased renal excretion):
   - Nonsteroidal anti-inflammatory drugs: impair renin and aldosterone secretion
   - Angiotensin-converting enzyme inhibitors: block angiotensin II–mediated aldosterone biosynthesis
   - Heparin: inhibits adrenal steroidogenesis
   - Spironolactone: blocks renal mineralocorticoid receptor
   - Triamterene, amiloride: aldosterone-independent defects in tubular potassium secretion

○ **How does magnesium depletion affect potassium?**

Magnesium depletion is associated with renal potassium wasting and hypocalcemia.

○ **How would you estimate the deficit in total body potassium in a patient with plasma potassium of 3 mEq/L? Or 2 mEq/L?**

A decrease in serum potassium from 4 to 3 mEq/L corresponds to a 100–200 mEq decrement in total body potassium in a normal adult. Each additional fall of 1 mEq/L in serum potassium represents an additional deficit of 200–400 mEq.

○ **At what preoperative serum potassium levels would you not proceed with surgery?**

Although all patients undergoing elective surgery should have normal serum potassium levels, delaying surgery is not recommended if the serum potassium level is *above* 2.8 mEq/L *or below* 5.9 mEq/L, if the cause of the potassium imbalance is known, and if the patient is in otherwise optimal condition.

The range of safe potassium levels has changed over the years as more data have become available on the safety of preoperative hypokalemia and the dangers of replacing potassium in a hospital environment. Potassium-depleted myocardium is unusually sensitive to digoxin, calcium, and, most important, potassium [Barash et al., 2009].

None of the studies have shown increased morbidity or mortality under anesthesia with a potassium level of more than 2.6 mEq/L.

○ **At what preoperative serum sodium levels would you not proceed with surgery?**

For elective surgery lower limit of serum sodium is 131 mEq/L. All patients undergoing surgery should have serum sodium concentrations of less than 150 mEq/L before anesthesia.

○ **What is the effect of nondepolarizing neuromuscular blocking agents on plasma potassium concentration?**

Nondepolarizing muscular blocking agents do not affect plasma potassium levels. However, when succinylcholine depolarizes muscle that has been previously traumatized or denervated, myoneural receptors proliferate over the cell membrane, and a depolarizing drug binding to the increased numbers of receptors can produce large increases in serum potassium. This can cause life-threatening arrhythmias and cardiac arrest.

○ **Describe the EKG abnormalities associated with hypercalcemia and hypocalcemia.**

Hypercalcemia: shortened Q-T interval (shortened ST segment).

Hypocalcemia: prolonged Q-T interval (prolongation of ST segment), leading to heart block.

○ **What are the clinical manifestations of hypercalcemia?**

Clinical symptoms are typically not seen with mildly elevated plasma calcium levels. Manifestations of hypercalcemia become more evident with levels higher than 14 mg/100 mL. Symptoms include altered mental status, lethargy, depression, nausea/vomiting, anorexia, constipation, abdominal, flank and bone pain, polydipsia, polyuria, renal calculi, and alterations in the cardiac conduction system [Miller, 2010].

○ **Describe the medical therapy for severe hypercalcemia.**

Maximize renal calcium excretion with normal saline infusion containing 20–30 mEq/L K^+ and furosemide to promote a diuresis of 200–300 cm^3/h. Careful monitoring of potassium and magnesium is required. Additional therapy options include pamidronate, calcitonin, steroids, mithramycin, and dialysis.

○ **What are the clinical manifestations of hypocalcemia?**

Mental status changes, confusion, seizures, laryngospasm, perioral and extremity paresthesias, hypotension, arrhythmias, hyperreflexia, and tetany as evidenced by a positive Chvostek sign (facial spasms elicited by tapping of the facial nerve at the angle of the mandible) and Trousseau sign (carpopedal spasm elicited by inflating a blood pressure cuff above the systolic blood pressure for several minutes) [Miller, 2010; Barash et al., 2009].

○ **Describe the EKG abnormalities associated with hypermagnesemia.**

Magnesium depresses cardiac conduction, leading to prolonged PR intervals and widened QRS complexes [Miller, 2010].

○ **What are the clinical manifestations of hypermagnesemia?**

Normal serum magnesium concentration ranges from 1.7 to 2.4 mg/dL. Side effects of hypermagnesemia include sedation, muscle weakness, hypotension, mild tachycardia or bradycardia, chest pain or tightness, blurred vision, nausea/vomiting, hypoventilation, and rarely pulmonary.

Elevated magnesium levels potentiate the effect of both depolarizing and nondepolarizing muscle relaxants and local anesthetics. Loss of deep tendon reflexes occurs at levels beyond 10–12 mg/dL. Respiratory arrest and coma occur at levels above 15–20 mg/dL and asystole can occur when levels exceed 20–25 mg/dL [Chestnut et al., 2009; Miller, 2010].

○ **What is the treatment for hypermagnesemia?**

Magnesium is a competitive antagonist of calcium and regulates calcium access into cell membranes and at the motor end plate. Treatment of magnesium toxicity includes prompt discontinuation of magnesium infusions and intravenous administration of calcium gluconate 1 g or calcium chloride 500 mg. Support of respiratory function may require temporary intubation and mechanical ventilation [Miller, 2010].

○ **What are the clinical manifestations of hypomagnesemia?**

Central nervous system irritability, seizures, hyperreflexia, skeletal muscle spasm, and ventricular arrhythmias [Miller, 2010].

Key Terms

ABGs in compensated respiratory acidosis
ABGs in respiratory acidosis/metabolic alkalosis
Acid–base management
Acidosis: anion gap differential diagnosis
Ascites formation and Starling equation
Bainbridge reflex
Blood O_2 transport
Crystalloid resuscitation: coagulopathy
Determinants of mixed venous O_2
Drugs causing hyperkalemia and treatment
ECG effects of hypocalcemia
ECG in hypermagnesemia
Fluid resuscitation: crystalloid versus colloid
Hetastarch: platelet function and coagulation
Hyperkalemia: angiotensin receptor
Hypermagnesemia: treatment

Hyperosmolar coma
Hypokalemia: ECG effects
Hyponatremia: causes
Hypoxia: effect on CO_2 response
Intravascular: extravascular volume ratio
Magnesium: complications
Metabolic acidosis and normal saline
Mixed venous O_2 physiology
Oxygen delivery versus PaO_2
Oxygen–Hb dissociation curve shift
Oxygen saturation versus PaO_2
$P50$ of hemoglobin: factors influencing
Peripheral O_2 delivery
Renal compensation in respiratory alkalosis
Respiratory compensation in metabolic alkalosis
Severe hyponatremia: treatment

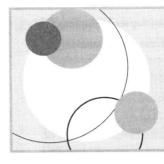

Airway and Intubation

When you reach the end of your rope, tie a knot in it and hang on.
Thomas Jefferson

○ **What is the most common cause of upper airway obstruction?**

Tongue and jaw relaxation occluding the posterior oropharynx.

○ **What are the perioperative complications of laryngoscopy?**

Mechanical complications include possible trauma to eyes, neck, jaw, teeth, lips, mouth, tongue, and pharyngeal and laryngeal structures. Others include hypotension, hypertension, increased intracranial pressure, arrhythmias, bradycardia, laryngospasm, bronchospasm, aspiration, tube misplacement in the stomach or mainstem bronchus, as well as failed intubation.

○ **What are the main indications for endotracheal intubation?**

To address insufficient respiratory effort (ventilation) and inadequate airway patency, protect the airway (mental status, integrity of reflexes, hemodynamic stability), improve oxygenation, or tracheal toilet.

○ **Does tracheal intubation prevent aspiration?**

Not absolutely. Microaspiration can still occur.

○ **What is the recommended inflation pressure of endotracheal tube cuffs?**

The cuff pressure should be less than 25–35 mm Hg (capillary perfusion pressure of tracheal mucosa); otherwise tracheal mucosal damage may occur, including possible necrosis.

○ **What is the incidence of "sore throat" after endotracheal intubation?**

Incidence 45–70% [Loeser et al., 1976. See reference on page 522].

○ **What is the incidence of laryngeal injury after short-term intubation?**

The overall incidence is 6.2% [Peppard et al., 1983. See reference on page 522]. The most common complication is hematoma of the vocal cords (4.5%). Mucosal laceration occurs in approximately 1 in 1,000 intubations. Perforation of the trachea is a rare complication usually occurring with the use of a stylet and forceful passage. Subcutaneous emphysema should prompt investigation.

○ **What is the cause of hoarseness after endotracheal intubation lasting more than 7 days?**

Pressure of the endotracheal tube on the recurrent laryngeal nerve between the thyroid lamina and arytenoid cartilage. Hoarseness lasting more than 7 days is rare.

○ **List the common causes of postextubation stridor.**

Stridor results from an extrathoracic obstruction (laryngeal edema) and produces inspiratory wheezing. Common causes of postextubation strider include too large of an endotracheal tube, trauma from laryngoscopy and/or intubation, excessive coughing or bucking on the tube, neck manipulation during surgery, and a current or recent upper respiratory infection. Bilateral recurrent laryngeal nerve injury due to excessive cuff pressure may also cause respiratory distress and obstruction.

○ **What is the treatment of postextubation stridor?**

Warmed, humidified oxygen, nebulized racemic epinephrine, and steroids.

○ **What maneuver should be performed during tracheal intubation in a patient with a full stomach?**

Sellick maneuver (cricoid pressure).

○ **Is cricoid pressure effective in the presence of a nasogastric tube?**

Yes.

○ **What is the correct position of the tip of the endotracheal tube?**

Approximately 4 cm above the carina.

○ **What are two contraindications to nasotracheal intubation?**

Maxillofacial trauma (basilar skull fracture) and coagulopathy.

○ **What is the most common complication of nasotracheal intubation?**

Epistaxis.

○ **How is transtracheal needle jet insufflation performed?**

A #14 or #16 gauge plastic cannula is inserted through the cricothyroid membrane and directed distally into the trachea. The cannula should be connected to a high-pressure oxygen source (i.e., 50 psi) with a low compliance circuit (fresh gas outlet and oxygen flush valve or pipeline O_2) using a 5 mm ETT adaptor piece with oxygen tubing and a three-way stopcock. Oxygen is delivered in intermittent bursts of 1 second on and 4 seconds off. Insertion of an oropharyngeal airway will allow passive exhalation of insufflated oxygen.

○ **How long can a patient be supported with needle jet insufflation until an airway can be secured?**

Approximately 45–60 minutes. $PaCO_2$ increases by 6 mm Hg in the first minute of apnea and then increases by 3 mm Hg for each minute thereafter.

○ **What limits this form of surgical airway?**

Hypercapnia, due to inadequate ventilation.

○ **When is an emergency cricothyroidotomy indicated?**

When ventilation by mask or LMA is not adequate, intubation is unsuccessful and emergency noninvasive airway ventilation attempts fail.

○ **Describe the anatomy of cricothyroidotomy.**

Cricothyroidotomy is performed to establish an emergency airway.

The cricothyroid membrane covers the cricothyroid space located in the anterior neck between the thyroid cartilage superiorly and the cricoid cartilage inferiorly. The membrane is typically 10 mm in height and 8 mm in width and lies directly underneath the skin and a thin facial layer. It can be identified 1–1.5 fingerbreadth below the laryngeal prominence (Adam's apple). It is often crossed horizontally in the upper third by the left and right superior cricothyroid arteries.

Because of the course of veins and arteries and its proximity to the vocal folds, any incision or needle puncture to the cricothyroid membrane should be made in its inferior third directed posteriorly.

○ **Describe the technique of cricothyroidotomy.**

Specialized percutaneous cricothyroidotomy systems are available.

Patient positioned supine; head midline or extended on the neck. Using aseptic precautions, cricothyroid membrane is localized and local anesthetic infiltrated. A 1–1.5 cm vertical incision of the skin only is made over the lower third of the cricothyroid membrane. Aiming 45° caudad, a percutaneous puncture of the subcutaneous tissue and cricothyroid membrane is made with the 18 gauge needle catheter assembly and syringe.

After air is aspirated, catheter is advanced to the trachea. After inserting guidewire through the catheter, catheter is removed and the tracheal cannula, fitted internally with a dilator, is advanced over the wire. Skin incision needs to be extended and the dilator and wire are removed once the cannula–dilator has been fully inserted.

○ **Emergency cricothyroidotomy is performed with a #11 blade between which cartilages?**

Thyroid and cricoid cartilages.

○ **When may emergency tracheostomy be performed instead of emergency cricothyroidotomy?**

In pediatric patients, where cricothyroidotomy is generally contraindicated. Because of the smaller size and greater soft tissue compliance of the pediatric airway, the cricoid cartilage plays a major role in maintaining patency of the tracheal lumen. An injury to this structure could be disastrous.

○ **What is the narrowest part of the respiratory tract in children?**

The inferior ring portion of the cricoid cartilage.

○ **According to Poiseuille's law, if the radius of the conducting airway is reduced from 4 to 3 mm, resistance to airflow will increase by how much?**

Sixteen-fold.

○ **The funnel-shaped narrowing of the glottis and subglottic airway commonly known as "steeple sign" is observed in what type of extrathoracic airway obstruction?**

Croup or laryngotracheobronchitis.

○ **What is the effective dose of intravenous lidocaine able to partially blunt the cardiovascular response to intubation?**

1.5 mg/kg.

○ **How long does it take for preoxygenation to achieve 96% denitrogenation of the lungs?**

In patients breathing 100% oxygen it will take 3–4 minutes. Preoxygenation will enable apnea without hypoxemia for 3–5 minutes in patients with a normal FRC and oxygen consumption.

○ **What is the minimal time required for preoxygenation before induction of general anesthesia for cesarean section?**

Three minutes.

○ **What is the minimal time required for four deep breaths of oxygen before induction of general anesthesia for cesarean section?**

About 30 seconds. These must be vital capacity breaths to effectively accomplish denitrogenation. Pregnant patients have a reduced FRC, increased oxygen consumption, and therefore will desaturate very quickly, despite adequate preoxygenation.

○ **What is the time to spontaneous ventilation after thiopental and succinylcholine?**

It has been shown that rapid sequence induction using succinylcholine dose of 0.5–0.6 mg/kg IV results in rapid-onset intubation conditions that were similar to 1.0 mg/kg (50–60 seconds for excellent intubation conditions). However, the patients who received 0.5–0.6 mg/kg had a significantly shorter time to recovery of spontaneous respirations (mean 3.5–4 minutes) than patients who received 1 mg/kg (6.2 minutes). This indicates that 0.5–0.6 mg/kg may be a safer dose than 1 mg/kg in patients requiring rapid sequence intubation, since it allows the potential for more rapid resumption of spontaneous respiration in patients at risk for a "can't intubate, can't ventilate" scenario [Miller, 2010].

○ **In which clinical situations is the use of retrograde intubation or a lightwand considered a better choice than fiber-optic bronchoscopy for assisting endotracheal intubation?**

Bleeding in the oral cavity.

○ **What is the maximum safe dose of lidocaine for topical anesthesia of the airway?**

4.5 mg/kg, not to exceed a total of 300 mg. Reduce dosage for children, elderly, and acutely ill.

○ **Is the use of an LMA contraindicated in a scenario of failed intubation and impossible mask ventilation if the patient is at increased risk for aspiration of gastric contents?**

No. The use of an LMA may be lifesaving in this situation. Hypoxemia, not aspiration, is the major risk for this patient.

○ **What is the reported incidence of downfolding of the epiglottis during insertion of the LMA in adults?**

Ten percent [Brimacombe et al., 2002. See reference on page 522].

○ **Which are the only "fail-safe" signs for the correct placement of an endotracheal tube?**

Persistence of appropriate levels of end-tidal carbon dioxide is the only one. In the unlikely situation where capnography is unavailable, visualization of the tube passing through the cords and fiber-optic confirmation of tracheal rings and the carina distal to the tip of the endotracheal tube.

○ **Is rapid sequence induction appropriate in a patient with a full stomach suffering from Ludwig's angina?**

No. Rapid sequence induction may lead to a catastrophic loss of the airway due to the inability to intubate and ventilate the patient. Safer options are an awake fiber-optic intubation, awake blind nasal intubation, and elective tracheostomy.

○ **Are there any differences in oxygenation and ventilation between endotracheal intubation and the Combitube?**

Yes. With the Combitube, the $PaCO_2$ is higher. The PaO_2 is also greater due to the physiologic "PEEP" maintained by the vocal cords.

○ **What should be done immediately after a failed intubation and inadequate two-handed mask ventilation?**

An LMA should be inserted immediately and placement confirmed with detection of exhaled CO_2. [ASA difficult airway algorithm, 2003. See reference on page 522].

○ **What is the most effective external laryngeal maneuver that can achieve a better direct laryngoscopic view of the vocal cords?**

Backward, upward, and rightward pressure (BURP) on the cricoid cartilage.

○ **What is the failure rate of intubation using a lightwand?**

1% of cases [Hung et al., 1995. See reference on page 522].

○ **What are the appropriate sizes of LMA and fiber-optic bronchoscope for patients weighing 10–20 kg?**

Number 2 LMA and 3.5 mm bronchoscope.

○ **What are the choices of LMA and fiber-optic bronchoscope for an average sized adult patient?**

Number 4 LMA and 5 mm bronchoscope.

○ **In an intubated patient, hypoxemia, bronchospasm, atelectasis, and coughing are all signs of what?**

Right mainstem intubation.

○ **What are the intubation criteria for patients with burns?**

Four standard "P" criteria for intubation: patency of airway, protect against aspiration, pulmonary toilet, and positive-pressure ventilation.

Airway burns are most likely to occur in patients with severe facial burns, intraoral, nasal, or pharyngeal burns, or burns suffered in an enclosed-space fire or explosion. Due to the risk of airway edema, hypoxemia, carbon monoxide, and cyanide toxicity, early elective intubation should be strongly considered in all patients. Direct heat injury caused by inhalation of air heated to 150°C or higher produces immediate injury to the airway mucosa resulting in edema, erythema, and ulceration above the vocal cords. Edema causing upper airway obstruction may not occur for 12–18 hours. Deep face burns may cause edema with obstruction or distortion of the airway, decreased clearance of secretions, and impaired protection of the airway with aspiration.

○ **What are the key considerations for evaluation of the potentially difficult airway?**

Use the mnemonic LEMON as an airway assessment tool.

- *Look* at the patient's airway and history for detection of medical, surgical, or anesthetic factors that may indicate the presence of a difficult airway.
- *Evaluate* the airway using the 3–3–2 rule: normal mouth opening is three fingerbreaths; mental to hyoid bone distance (mandibular dimension) is three fingerbreaths; thyroid cartilage notch is two fingerbreaths below the hyoid bone.
- *Mallampati* score assignment.
- *Obstruction* of the airway should be detected.
- *Neck* mobility should be determined.

○ **Which is the only abductor muscle of the vocal cords?**

The posterior cricoarytenoid muscle.

○ **Which is the only muscle of the larynx supplied by the superior laryngeal nerve?**

The cricothyroid muscle.

○ **How do you diagnose unilateral vocal cord paralysis?**

Flexible endoscopy in the awake patient with inspection of vocal cords.

○ **What are the three principal cranial nerves innervating the airway?**

Trigeminal (nasopharynx), glossopharyngeal (pharynx, tonsillar pillars, soft palate, and posterior third of the tongue), and vagus nerves (mucosa from the epiglottis to distal airways: superior and recurrent laryngeal nerves).

The superior laryngeal branch of the vagus nerve supplies sensation above the vocal cords and function of the cricothyroid muscle (tension of the vocal cords) and a portion of the transverse arytenoid muscle. The recurrent laryngeal nerve provides innervation to all remaining intrinsic laryngeal muscles and sensation below the vocal cords.

○ **What are the effects of laryngeal nerve palsy?**

Resulting position of the vocal cords depends on whether unilateral/bilateral recurrent nerve or external branch of superior laryngeal is damaged or not.

○ **What sequelae result from superior laryngeal nerve injury?**

Superior laryngeal nerve injury would cause loss of sensation above the vocal cords and decreased ability to shorten and adduct the true vocal cords. This results in decreased vocalization ability (bilateral palsy causes hoarseness and tiring of voice) and a reduction in upper airway protective reflexes.

○ **What are the effects of unilateral recurrent laryngeal nerve damage?**

Cord on the injured side assumes a paramedian position because the unopposed ipsilateral cricothyroid muscle adducts the cord toward the injured side.

If the external branch of superior laryngeal nerve is also damaged, the true vocal cords will be more medial and less tense. Voice is weak and hoarse and risk of aspiration increases.

Eventually, the muscles compensate somewhat and the vocal cords become more medially positioned.

○ **What is the position of the vocal cords when bilateral recurrent laryngeal nerve paralysis occurs?**

Both vocal cords lie within 2–3 mm of the midline in the adducted position. Voice is of limited strength, but good quality. Airway is often inadequate; stridor and dyspnea may occur with modest exertion. Life-threatening obstruction may occur with infection and edema of vocal cords.

Recurrent laryngeal nerve courses around the subclavian artery on the right side, and aorta on the left. It may be injured during thyroid and cervical spine surgery.

○ **T/F: Placing local anesthetic-soaked cotton pledgets into the pyriform fossae will block the internal branch of the superior laryngeal nerve.**

True. An alternate technique includes direct infiltration (2 mL of local anesthetic) at the level of the thyrohyoid membrane inferior to the greater cornu of the hyoid bone. The superior laryngeal nerve innervates the base of the tongue, posterior surface of the epiglottis, aryepiglottic fold, and the arytenoids. Blockade is usually inadequate as a solo technique for awake intubation.

○ **Which nerve provides sensory innervation of the pharynx?**

Glossopharyngeal nerve.

○ **T/F: The laryngeal skeleton consists of 10 cartilages.**

False. The laryngeal skeleton consists of nine cartilages: three single (thyroid, cricoid, and epiglottic) and three paired (arytenoid, corniculate, and cuneiform). The hyoid bone is not part of the larynx.

○ **What are the most common disorders associated with atlantoaxial instability?**

Rheumatoid arthritis, achondroplasia, ankylosing spondylitis, and Down syndrome (occurs less frequently than atlantooccipital instability, 10–20% vs. 60%).

○ **Is atlantoaxial instability more likely in the pediatric population?**

Yes, the pediatric patient has several predisposing factors including a disproportionally large head, immature cervical musculature, ligamentous laxity, and wedge-shaped cervical vertebrae. This makes children especially prone to C1–C2 subluxation. Extreme rotation and extension should be avoided.

○ **What is at the top of your differential diagnosis if 8 hours after general endotracheal anesthesia, the mother of a 4-year-old with Down syndrome reports the child cannot ambulate?**

Cervical spinal cord injury secondary to ligamentous laxity and subluxation at the atlantoaxial joint (C1–C2) may occur with laryngoscopy or positioning of the head for central line placement. The incidence of atlantoaxial dislocation is 20% in Down syndrome patients and most are asymptomatic, which accounts for the recommendation of routine screening at age 5 years or before participation in the Special Olympics.

○ **During intubation using direct laryngoscopy and a Macintosh blade, the most cervical motion occurs at which level between the occiput and C5?**

Occipitoatlantal and atlantoaxial joints.

○ **What is the course of preoperative evaluation if you highly suspect atlantoaxial subluxation?**

The "Down series" consists of flexion, extension, and neutral lateral radiographs of the cervical spine. If atlantoaxial instability exists (5 mm or greater distance between the posterior and inferior aspects of the anterior area of the atlas and adjacent surface of the odontoid process), further evaluation with CT and myelography is indicated. Through-the-mouth odontoid views may also be helpful.

○ **What are the high-risk perioperative periods for inducing atlantoaxial subluxation in children with Down syndrome?**

The high-risk perioperative periods for flexion–extension as well as rotation include laryngoscopy and tracheal intubation, mask ventilation, positioning (central line placement), transport, tracheal suctioning, and radiograph plate placements.

○ **During a laparoscopic cholecystectomy, 10 minutes after CO_2 insufflation of the peritoneal cavity, the peak airway pressure measured from the endotracheal tube increases from 30 to 45 cm H_2O and the pulse oximetry reading decreases to 88% on 100% oxygen. Air entry could not be heard in the left lung. What is the most likely diagnosis?**

Right endobronchial intubation. Other considerations include pneumothorax, bronchial obstruction by mucus plug or cuff herniation, and severe bronchospasm.

○ **Immediately following extubation a patient develops inspiratory stridor, tracheal tug, and paradoxical movement of the chest and abdomen. What is the diagnosis and management?**

Laryngospasm. Management includes suctioning the oropharynx, applying a jaw thrust maneuver, inserting an oral or nasal airway, and positive-pressure ventilation with 100% oxygen (or PEEP). The condition is usually self-limiting and may be triggered when the vocal cords or the area of the trachea below the cords detects the entry of water, mucus, blood, or other substance. Severe cases may require deepening the level of anesthesia (propofol 0.5 mg/kg, or lidocaine 100 mg IV, or inhalational agent). If this technique fails and the patient desaturates (SpO_2 <85%), a small dose of succinylcholine (20–40 mg IV) followed by mask ventilation or reintubation is needed.

○ **What is laryngospasm?**

A reflex prolonged closure of the glottis mediated by the superior laryngeal nerve. The muscles most involved are the lateral cricoarytenoid and the thyroarytenoids (adductors of the glottis) and the cricothyroid (a tensor of the vocal cords).

○ **Give several examples of stimuli capable of provoking laryngospasm.**

Presence of bloody secretions or vomitus in the airway, visceral pain, chemical irritation of laryngeal or pharyngeal mucosa, and tracheal intubation or extubation during inappropriate depth of anesthesia.

○ **What drug might you give prior to the extubation to decrease the chance of laryngospasm?**

Lidocaine IV or injected down the endotracheal tube.

○ **How does postobstructive pulmonary edema (POPE) or negative pressure pulmonary edema occur?**

There are two recognized types of POPE.

Type I may be associated with any cause of acute airway obstruction (e.g., postextubation laryngospasm). The pathogenesis of POPE I is multifactorial.

Most likely, forced inspiration against a closed glottis causes large negative intrapleural and transpulmonary pressure gradients promoting transudation of edema fluid from the pulmonary capillaries into the interstitium.

Type II develops after surgical relief of chronic upper airway obstruction in patients otherwise not at risk for pulmonary edema (i.e., post-tonsillectomy/adenoidectomy). POPE II results from sudden removal of PEEP produced by the obstructing lesion, which leads to interstitial fluid transudation and pulmonary edema.

Causes include vigorous spontaneous ventilation against an obstructed airway (upper airway mass, laryngospasm, infection, inflammation, edema, vocal cord paralysis, strangulation), rapid reexpansion of lung, or vigorous pleural suctioning (thoracentesis, chest tube).

○ **The first sign of negative pressure pulmonary edema following relief of upper airway obstruction is hypoxemia. What is the treatment?**

Supportive respiratory care.

Supplementary oxygen, trial of CPAP or pressure support, inhaled beta-agonist, diuresis, and in severe cases re-intubation.

○ **What is the pathophysiology of POPE?**

Movement of fluid into the alveoli is a balance between the hydrostatic pressure in the pulmonary vasculature and the intramural pressure in the alveoli.

With upper airway obstruction, the patient may continue to make forceful inspiratory efforts against a closed glottis creating negative intrathoracic pressures. The negative intrapleural pressure and a complex of attendant cardiac events shift this balance to favor extravasation of fluid out of the pulmonary vessels. Negative intrapleural pressure causes increased flow into the right side of the heart. The right ventricle bulges into the left ventricle impairing its emptying. At the same time there is marked sympathetic discharge that increases the pulmonary vascular resistance. Together these increase the hydrostatic pressure in the pulmonary vasculature, leading to a positive transmural pressure. Venous return is increased, cardiac output is decreased, and fluid transudates into the alveolar spaces.

○ **If proper treatment is instituted, what is the usual course of POPE?**

A chest radiograph shows bilateral pulmonary edema. This usually resolves spontaneously within 24 hours, but diuretics and CPAP ventilation may be used to assist in resolution. Other causes of pulmonary edema or hemoptysis should be considered and ruled out.

○   **Emergency surgery, patient with a full stomach, and potassium level 6.0 mEq/L. What is your choice of muscle relaxant for a rapid sequence induction?**

Rocuronium 1–1.2 mg/kg IV. Nondepolarizing blocker with a slightly longer onset of action (60–75 seconds) than succinylcholine (45–60 seconds).

Intubating conditions with rocuronium are satisfactory and similar to those observed after succinylcholine, 60–90 seconds after rocuronium 0.6 mg/kg IV (0.6 mg is 2 × ED95). It also depends on what other drugs were administered with rocuronium. In the vast majority of patients receiving alfentanil 15 μg/kg, followed by propofol 2.0 mg/kg, and rocuronium 0.45 mg/kg, good to excellent conditions for intubation will be present 75–90 seconds after the completion of drug administration. The intermediate duration of action associated with an intubating dose of rocuronium provides adequate surgical relaxation for most outpatient cases [Perry et al., 2002. See reference on page 522].

Key Terms

Airway anesthesia: anatomy
Airway assessment: coexisting disease
Airway evaluation
Airway innervation/laryngeal innervation
Atlantoaxial instability: causes
Cricothyroidotomy: anatomy
Difficult airway algorithm
Difficult airway: management
Endobronchial intubation
Laryngeal anatomy
Laryngospasm mechanism/complication
Laryngospasm: pulmonary edema

Laryngospasm: treatment options
Nasal fiber-optic intubation
Obesity: airway evaluation
Pharynx: sensory innervation
Postextubation stridor: causes/treatment
Rapid induction: shortest onset
Rheumatoid arthritis: complications
Superior laryngeal nerve block: anatomy
Time to spontaneous ventilation after thiopental/ succinylcholine
Tracheal innervation

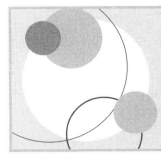

Allergic Reactions

You see things; and you say "why?" but I dream things that never were; and I say "why not?"
George Bernard Shaw

○ **What symptoms do prostaglandins produce?**

Prostaglandins are arachidonic acid derivatives produced via the cyclooxygenase pathway. They are mediators of the inflammatory response. Symptoms produced include bronchoconstriction, systemic hypotension (secondary to peripheral vasodilation), increased capillary permeability, and coronary vasospasm. Prostaglandins E_1 and E_2 produce bronchodilation, inhibit histamine release, and produce vasodilation of the peripheral, coronary, and pulmonary circulations. Prostaglandins E_1, E_2, and $F_{2\alpha}$ have uterotonic effects. Common adverse effects include flu-like symptoms, pyrexia, flushing, headache, vomiting, and diarrhea.

○ **What is the definition of *atopy* and what is the significance of this diagnosis?**

Atopy or *atopic syndrome* is a tendency to allergic sensitization, which appears to have a genetic predisposition. Patients exhibit multiple symptoms and signs of allergy such as asthma, allergic rhinitis, conjunctivitis, urticaria, eczema, and multiple drug allergies. They may give a history of anaphylaxis or positive skin prick test or other test, which signifies sensitivity to a substance. Atopic patients appear to have a much higher risk of latex allergy and anaphylactic or anaphylactoid reactions during anesthesia.

○ **Early signs of anaphylaxis that can be seen in the awake patient include what?**

Flushing, urticaria (hives), itching, dizziness or decreased level of consciousness, dyspnea, and/or bronchospasm.

○ **Signs of anaphylaxis that may be seen in patients undergoing general anesthesia include what?**

Cardiac, respiratory, or cutaneous manifestations including tachycardia, hypotension, arrhythmia; bronchospasm, increase in peak airway pressures, hypoxemia, laryngeal or pulmonary edema; flushing, rash, or hives.
Hypotension may be the only sign of anaphylaxis under general anesthesia.

○ **What is the most likely cause of death from anaphylaxis [Bochner et al., 1991. See reference on page 522]?**

Cardiovascular collapse. Inability to intubate, ventilate, or oxygenate due to upper airway edema, bronchospasm, pulmonary edema, or any combination of the above also places the nonintubated patient at risk.

○   **What is the differential diagnosis following a suspected anaphylactic episode?**

A vasovagal reaction may be confused with anaphylaxis in the awake patient. The patient may become diaphoretic, nauseated, and presyncopal; however, itching, flushing, urticaria, wheezing, or cyanosis will not occur.

Under general anesthesia, the differential diagnosis includes anesthetic agents, with their associated hemodynamic effects, septic shock, hypotension from other causes, cardiac arrhythmia, myocardial infarction, pulmonary thromboembolism, fat embolism or venous air embolism, bronchospasm, pneumothorax, and pulmonary edema.

○   **What is the mainstay of treatment for anaphylaxis?**

Epinephrine.

○   **What are the beneficial effects of epinephrine during anaphylaxis?**

Alpha-1-adrenergic-mediated vasoconstriction mitigates angioedema, relieving upper airway obstruction; shock is prevented by increasing peripheral vascular resistance. Beta-1 adrenergic stimulation produces positive chronotropic and inotropic effects, while beta-2 stimulation produces bronchodilation. Beta-adrenergic effects also increase cyclic adenosine monophosphate (cAMP), leading to lowered release of histamine, tryptase, and other inflammatory mediators from basophils and mast cells.

The clinical effects of epinephrine are dose-dependent. *Beta-adrenergic* effects occur at lower doses and *alpha-adrenergic* effects predominate at doses greater than 10 μg/min.

○   **Describe the initial treatment protocol for intraoperative anaphylaxis?**

Stop the administration of the expected allergen. If the allergen has been given IM or SQ, place a tourniquet above the injection site and consider injecting a small dose (0.2 mg) of epinephrine at the site to reduce uptake of the allergen into the intravascular space.

Maintain the airway and administer 100% oxygen. Support oxygenation and ventilation.

Intubate the patient if an endotracheal tube is not already in place.

Discontinue all anesthetic agents because they are cardiovascular depressants. Remember that inhalational agents are not appropriate bronchodilators during anaphylaxis and that halothane also sensitizes the heart to catecholamines, leading to arrhythmias.

Rapid intravenous volume administration should be started. Several liters of fluid may be needed. Large volume deficits occur secondary to massive increases in vascular permeability.

Epinephrine administration is the mainstay and should be given promptly. An infusion titrated to clinical effect is less dangerous than the 1 mg bolus typically used in cardiac arrest, which can lead to unwanted side effects.

Inform the surgeons and prepare to terminate the surgery if possible. Check for drugs injected or instilled into a body cavity.

○   **What is the best route of administration of epinephrine therapy during anaphylaxis?**

Intramuscular injection into the mid-anterolateral thigh is suggested to be the preferred route of administration as skeletal muscle vasodilation promotes rapid absorption. This is in contrast to the subcutaneous route where localized vasoconstriction delays absorption.

Clinical consensus for intramuscular administration is a dose of 0.01 mg/kg of a 1 mg/mL (1:1,000) solution to a maximum of 0.5 mg in an adult or 0.3 mg in a child. Studies show prompt administration is essential to survival. The dose may be repeated every 5–15 minutes as needed.

IV administration is controversial in the community setting. Securing IV access may be difficult in the patient in shock and there is no clear consensus on dosing. In the perioperative setting, IV dosing is dictated by the severity of reaction. For Grade I reactions (cutaneous–mucous signs), epinephrine is not required. Titrated boluses of 10–20 μg may be necessary for Grade II reactions (hypotension, tachycardia, dyspnea, gastrointestinal disturbances); 100–200 μg boluses are required for Grade III reactions and this may need to be repeated every 1–2 minutes or followed by an infusion of 1–4 μg/min. Cardiac arrest requires resuscitation with high-dose epinephrine. A commonly used schedule is 1–3 mg over 3 minutes and 3–5 mg over 3 minutes, followed by an infusion of 4–10 μg/min.

Patients receiving beta-blocker therapy may not respond to treatment with epinephrine. Anaphylaxis may be especially severe. Beta-receptor blockade may result in unopposed alpha-adrenergic stimulation and vagotonic effects, which can lead to augmented release of inflammatory mediators. Particularly severe anaphylaxis is also associated with ACE inhibitor therapy.

Side effects include pallor, tremor, anxiety, palpitations, headache, and dizziness. Overdose may lead to pulmonary edema and hypertension.

○ **Describe the second line of treatment of anaphylaxis.**

The second-line treatment of anaphylaxis involves the administration of the H_1 antagonist diphenhydramine 50 mg IV; the use of H_2 blocking agents such as ranitidine or cimetidine is controversial.

Epinephrine infusion at 0.05–0.1 μg/(kg min) is used for persistent hypotension. Fluid and volume status should be managed aggressively to compensate for large fluid shifts. Invasive arterial and venous catheters are useful for monitoring, infusion of vasoactive drugs, and blood sampling.

Inhaled beta-2 agonists are used to treat bronchospasm. The airway should be evaluated for persistent laryngeal edema. Corticosteroids are given early and continued over the following 24 hours to prevent delayed reactions; the onset of effects is seen in 4–6 hours. Hydrocortisone is the preferred agent due to rapid onset and response in alleviating respiratory symptoms.

In the absence of any identifiable causes, latex allergy should be considered and all latex products removed from contact with the patient. Close observation should be continued for at least 24 hours and the airway reevaluated prior to extubation.

○ **How long does it take for signs of anaphylaxis to occur after contact with an allergen?**

Signs and symptoms of anaphylaxis usually occur within minutes, particularly after IV injection, with the majority occurring within 1 hour of exposure. Symptoms may reappear 6–8 hours after the initial anaphylactic manifestations have resolved (biphasic reaction) and have been reported as long as 72 hours after the initial event.

○ **What medication is most commonly responsible for anaphylactic reactions?**

Anaphylactoid reactions are most commonly seen with intravenous contrast media (incidence of 5–8%).

○ **What is the prophylaxis for IV contrast allergy?**

Use of H1 antihistamines (diphenhydramine 50 mg orally 1 hour before) and corticosteroids (methylprednisolone 32 mg orally 12 and 2 hours before or prednisone 50 mg orally 13, 7, and 1 hour before) is supported by the available trials that have examined treatments to prevent anaphylactoid reactions to radiological contrast media [Delaney et al., 2006. See reference on page 522]. H_2 receptor blockers (cimetidine 300 mg 1 hour before or ranitidine 50 mg orally 1 hour before) also may be used.

O **A patient tells you that he is allergic to penicillin. What is the reported incidence of penicillin allergy, and what is the true incidence of fatal anaphylactic reaction?**

Ten to 20% of hospitalized patients claim to be allergic to penicillin. The incidence of fatal reactions occurs in 0.002% of penicillin-treated cases, or 375 deaths per year in the United States.

O **Is there really cross-reactivity between penicillins and cephalosporins?**

Yes, but the exact incidence is not known and is likely small, around 5%. Penicillins are the most allergenic of all drugs with allergic reactions noted in 1–10% of patients. They possess a dicyclic nucleus that consists of a thiazolidine ring connected to a beta-lactam ring. Cephalosporins also share a beta-lactam ring so allergy to one may potentially cause cross-reactivity to the other. In practice, patients with histories of penicillin allergy have a minimally increased incidence of reactions to cephalosporins. It is concluded that it is safe to administer cephalosporin antimicrobials to the penicillin-allergic patient. However, some recommend caution in administering a cephalosporin to any patient with a history of a severe immediate allergic reaction to the penicillins.

O **T/F: Does premedication prevent anaphylaxis?**

False! Premedication may decrease the risk or the severity of the overall response, but anaphylaxis can still occur. Pretreatment with diphenhydramine, cimetidine (or ranitidine), and corticosteroids for 24 hours prior to exposure is still practiced. Routine premedication with histamine receptor blocking agents is still controversial.

High-risk patients who are likely to benefit most from prophylaxis with H_1 and H_2 receptor blocking agents include those with a history of adverse drug reactions and allergies, patients undergoing procedures with a high incidence of histamine release (such as during extracorporeal circulation), and patients in poor physical condition (such as those with significant heart disease). Also at high risk are patients who are at increased risk of complications from vigorous hydration and reduced response to drug therapies. Premedication may mask and even delay a diagnosis of anaphylaxis occurring under general anesthesia.

O **Which patients are at increased risk for latex allergy?**

Patients with the following:
- Chronic exposure to latex-based products (including health care workers – especially with a history of eczema)
- Atopy or multiple allergies
- Allergies to bananas, avocados, chestnuts, kiwi, or mangos
- History of intolerance to latex-based products (balloons, condoms)
- History of intraoperative anaphylaxis of uncertain etiology
- Spina bifida
- Previous urologic reconstructive surgery
- History of multiple surgical procedures
- History of spinal cord trauma
- Rubber industry workers

O **What is meant by latex precautions?**

"Latex precautions" indicate that no obvious allergy exists but that the use of latex should be avoided. Special precautions should be taken with patients at risk of developing latex allergy. These include children with spina bifida or genitourinary anomalies, necessitating multiple reconstructive surgeries and exposure to rubber urethral catheters.

○ **Identify commonly used objects from the operating room that contain latex.**

Commonly used objects in the operating room that contain latex include gloves, bite blocks, nasal airways, red rubber endotracheal tubes, reservoir bags on breathing circuits, urinary catheters, IV injection ports, stoppers on medication vials, Penrose-type tourniquets, syringe plungers, BP cuff tubing, stethoscope tubing, elastic bandages, and some types of adhesive tape.

○ **How does one know if a piece of OR equipment contains latex?**

Latex-containing products must be labeled as such by the manufacturer.

○ **T/F: PVC tracheal tubes and laryngeal mask airways are safe to use in latex-allergic patients.**

True. These two types of airway management equipment do not contain latex.

○ **What is the most effective way to manage a patient with a history of latex allergy?**

All latex-containing materials should be identified and removed from the environment. A *latex allergy kit* with alternative latex-free equipment for substitution should be created and immediately available for use. Epinephrine should be immediately available.

○ **Can you have an anaphylactic reaction to corticosteroids and antihistamines?**

Although extremely rare, anaphylactic reactions to some commonly used corticosteroid preparations and antihistamines have occurred and positive skin tests were subsequently noted. As a rule, *any medication* can cause an anaphylactic reaction.

○ **How should a patient be monitored after an anaphylactic reaction?**

Patients should be closely observed for at least 24 hours, preferably in an intensive care setting. Symptoms of anaphylaxis can recur during that period. Vasopressor support should be weaned and eventually discontinued as tolerated. Frequent evaluations should be performed in order to identify late-appearing sequelae from shock and the resuscitation process.

○ **T/F: Appropriate management of laryngeal edema seen in patients with hereditary angioedema includes epinephrine, antihistamines, and steroids.**

False. The symptomatology mimics anaphylaxis but is recalcitrant to epinephrine, antihistamines, or steroids. Hereditary angioedema is characterized by an absence of C1 esterase inhibitor in the plasma (uncontrolled activation of the complement system) with resultant episodic painless edema of the skin (face and limbs) and mucous membranes (respiratory and gastrointestinal tract) from release of vasoactive mediators that increase vascular permeability. Preoperative prophylaxis includes danazol (anabolic steroid), transfusion of FFP, or purified preparation of C1 esterase inhibitor. Long-term prophylaxis treatments include antifibrinolytic therapy and anabolic steroids. During an acute attack no specific treatment is reliably effective. The airway must be secured with an endotracheal tube.

○ **What is the definition of an anaphylactoid reaction?**

An anaphylactoid reaction is clinically indistinguishable from an anaphylactic reaction but is without an immunologic basis (non-IgE). It has been suggested by some experts that the term should no longer be used. During anaphylaxis, IgE antibodies produced from a prior exposure cross-link with the allergen, triggering the release of chemical mediators from mast cells and basophils. Anaphylactoid reactions are chemotoxic processes, the triggering agent resulting in the direct activation of complement and histamine release and degranulation of mast cells and basophils.

○ **Can you differentiate between anaphylactic and anaphylactoid reactions clinically?**

No. They are clinically indistinguishable. Both are equally life threatening and can result in major cardiovascular, pulmonary, and dermatologic responses.

○ **An otherwise healthy patient presents for knee arthroscopy. One gram of cefazolin is given preoperatively. General anesthesia is induced with midazolam, sodium thiopental, fentanyl, and vecuronium. The patient unexpectedly arrests on induction. What is wrong?**

The most likely cause is an allergic reaction to intravenously administered drugs (antibiotics, muscle relaxants > thiobarbiturates > opiates). Other causes of hypotension (such as hypovolemia unmasked by thiopental) should be considered in the differential diagnosis. High doses of fentanyl and vecuronium have been associated with vagotonic bradycardic arrest.

○ **What lab test can aid in making the diagnosis of allergic reaction in the OR?**

Serum tryptase. Tryptase is found in mast cells along with histamine and has a half-life of 2–3 hours, aiding in diagnosis.

○ **Which classes of anesthetic drugs are most likely responsible for allergic reactions intraoperatively?**

Muscle relaxants, especially succinylcholine	69.2%
Latex	12.1%
Antibiotics	8%

○ **Why do muscle relaxants so frequently result in anaphylaxis and allergic reactions?**

Nondepolarizing muscle relaxants contain either quaternary or tertiary ammonium ions to which patients frequently develop IgE antibodies. It is hypothesized that females, who more commonly have reactions to these medications, do so because of prior exposure to ammonium compounds in cosmetics and other products. Benzylisoquinolinium compounds (atracurium, mivacurium) are more likely to cause anaphylactic reactions than their aminosteroid counterparts (vecuronium, rocuronium, pancuronium). Patients may develop cross-reactivity between muscle relaxants so it is best to choose an agent from another class if there is a history of allergy. Patients may be sensitized for up to 30 years after exposure.

○ **Is there a cross-reactivity between latex allergy and food allergy?**

Between 21% and 58% of patients with natural rubber latex (NRL) allergy have food allergies. NRL allergy precedes the food allergies in most patients; however, the converse may also be seen. In addition, there may be simultaneous onset or the range of food hypersensitivities may increase over time.

Cross-reactivity between latex and certain foods began being reported in the early 1990s, with associations found to bananas and chestnuts. The condition has been described as "latex-fruit syndrome." Using radioallergosorbent test (RAST) inhibition assays and immunoblotting techniques, several fruit allergens have been identified that cross-react with NRL. A group of plant defense-related proteins, class I chitinases, are thought to be responsible.

The most frequent associations of NRL allergy have been made with banana, avocado, kiwi, and chestnut. Certain studies also make an association with potato, tomato, and shellfish allergy. Less frequent and less significant associations include papaya, pineapple, passion fruit, mango, fig, nuts (almond, hazelnut), stone fruits (peach, cherry, apricot), melon, and apple; also guava, fish, carrot, pear, strawberry, peanut, pepper, grape, coconut, oregano, sage, dill, condurango bark, milk, spinach, beet, loquat, and lychee.

○ **How do you diagnose perioperative allergic reactions?**

The severity of allergic reactions has been classified according to a four-step grading scale. Grade I allergic reactions manifest as cutaneous–mucous signs (erythema, urticaria, angioedema). Grade II features include mild cutaneous–mucous features that may be associated with cardiovascular and/or respiratory signs. Cardiovascular signs may include tachycardia, bradycardia, arrhythmias, and hypotension. Grade III reactions feature cardiovascular collapse that may or may not be associated with cutaneous–mucous signs and/or bronchospasm. Grade IV is full-blown cardiac arrest.

After the event, further diagnostic evidence is based on elevated blood histamine levels, which may be increased 30 minutes to 2 hours after the reaction. Serum tryptase levels are elevated and blood may be drawn between 15 and 60 minutes for Grade I and II reactions and within 30 minutes to 2 hours for Grade III and IV reactions. In certain cases, IgE assays are available; leukocyte histamine release test may also be useful for reactions to neuromuscular blocking agents. Skin testing is considered to be the gold standard method of diagnosis.

Key Terms

Anaphylaxis: epinephrine treatment
Anaphylaxis treatment
Latex allergy: foods
Latex allergy treatment

Operating room equipment containing latex
Penicillin–cephalosporin cross-sensitivity
Perioperative allergic reactions: diagnosis
Prophylaxis: IV contrast allergy

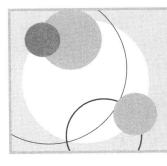

Anesthesia Risks/ Standards/Billing

One cannot refuse to eat just because there is a chance of being choked.
Chinese Proverb

○ **What is the death rate from general anesthesia in patients with an American Society of Anesthesiologists (ASA) class I or II?**

Approximately 1 in 200,000–500,000 [Lagasse et al., 2002. See reference on page 522].

○ **What is the incidence of brain damage resulting from anesthesia?**

Based on closed claims data, the incidence of brain damage is about 9%. There were 867 claims for permanent brain damage out of 8,954 since 1970. The percentage has remained the same from 1990 to 2007 [Cheney et al., 2006. See reference on page 522].

○ **Is the incidence of brain damage different based on the anesthetic technique?**

No, there is no significant difference. The incidence of brain damage ranges from 8% to 10% regardless of anesthetic technique.

○ **What are the most common complications based on closed claims data?**

Death (26%), nerve injury (22%), and brain damage (9%).

○ **According to the National Practitioner Data Bank (NPDB) Annual Report, what was the average medical malpractice payment for physicians in 2003?**

For physicians, which accounted for 80.4% of reports of malpractice payments by health care professionals, the median payment was $160,000 (obstetrics $290,000) and mean payment $294,814.

○ **What is root cause analysis (RCA)?**

A systematic approach used to evaluate an event with the purpose of determining the cause in order to make changes to decrease the chances of the event recurring. RCA is used by many different fields and uses many different techniques; therefore, the overall goal and guiding principles are similar but many forms of RCA exist.

○ **What is the RCA process designed to do?**

To answer three basic questions: What happened? Why did it happen? What can be done to prevent it from happening again?

○ **What are some general principles of RCA?**

1. The primary aim is to identify the root cause of a problem and prevent or minimize it from recurring.
2. RCA must be done systematically and findings must be backed up by documented evidence.
3. There may be more than one root cause.
4. All solutions should be identified, with the preferred solution chosen being the one that is most effective, simplest, and of lowest cost.
5. Identification of root causes is dependent on the way the event or problem is defined.
6. A time line and a sequence of events need to be established for effective analysis.
7. RCA helps to change culture from reactive to proactive, by analyzing events that have occurred in order to prevent recurrence.
8. RCA is often seen as a threat to many cultures and is often met with resistance.

○ **What are the general steps for an effective RCA?**

Identify an event or problem. Gather data and evidence and construct a time line. Identify root causes. Identify solution that will eliminate or decrease the risk of recurrence. Come to a consensus agreement for solutions to implement. Implement the changes and evaluate them for effectiveness.

○ **What is the incidence of awareness following general anesthesia?**

Data published in 2004 from a multicenter trial of 19,575 patients reported that the incidence of awareness with recall after surgery under general anesthesia was 0.13% (1.3 patients per 1,000) [Sebel et al., 2004. See reference on page 522].

○ **What is the incidence of intraoperative awareness due to equipment malfunction?**

Nine percent of claims were attributed to light anesthesia due to vaporizer or ventilator malfunction.

○ **What are some risk factors for intraoperative awareness?**

Cardiac surgery was involved in 23% of claims compared with other claims involving general anesthesia, which accounted for 6%. In most cases the patients were female. Patient hypotension and inability to tolerate sufficient anesthetic made up 11% of recall claims.

○ **What is the difference between the following practice parameters: standards, guidelines, and advisories?**

Practice standards are rules or the minimum requirements for clinical practice. In general, they represent accepted principles for sound patient management. They may be modified only under unusual circumstances.

Practice guidelines describe a basic management strategy or a range of basic management strategies. Guidelines are recommendations developed systematically to assist in decision making regarding patient care. They are supported by analysis of the current literature and by a synthesis of expert opinion. They may be adopted, modified, or rejected according to clinical needs and constraints. Practice guidelines are not intended as standards or absolute requirements and are not intended to replace local institutional polices.

Practice advisories are intended to assist decision making in areas of patient care where scientific evidence is insufficient. Advisories provide a synthesis and analysis of expert opinion. They may be adopted, modified, or rejected according to clinical needs and constraints.

○ **Is the following practice parameter a standard, guideline, or an advisory? "An anesthesiologist shall be responsible for determining the medical status of the patient, developing a plan of anesthesia care and acquainting the patient or the responsible adult with the proposed plan."**

A standard.

○ **Is the following practice parameter a standard, guideline, or an advisory? "No routine laboratory or diagnostic screening test is necessary for the preanesthetic evaluation of patients. Preoperative tests may be ordered, required, or performed on a selective basis for purposes of guiding or optimizing perioperative management."**

An advisory.

○ **The ASA practice parameter on preoperative fasting states that the minimum fasting period for drinking nonhuman milk is how many hours?**

Six hours.

○ **Is the above practice parameter a standard, guideline, or advisory?**

A guideline.

○ **What are ASA statements?**

Statements are the opinions, beliefs, and best medical judgments of the House of Delegates. They are not subjected to the same level of review as ASA standards or guidelines. The decision whether to implement some, none, or all ASA statements should be based on the judgment of anesthesiologist.

○ **What are the ASA guidelines for the administration of sedation by nonanesthesiologists?**

The ASA published guidelines in 2002 to offer suggestions to practitioners providing sedation. The following points are included in their analysis:

- The clinician should be familiar with aspects of the patient's medical history that might affect sedation, such as preexisting medical and surgical conditions, time of last oral intake, allergies, current medications, tobacco, alcohol, or drug use, and issues that arose during previous attempts at sedation.
- Informed consent for sedation must be given, including a discussion of benefits, risks, and alternatives.
- Vital signs must be monitored and recorded by a designated person other than the practitioner performing the procedure. Pulse oximetry, heart rate and rhythm, blood pressure (taken at intervals of at least every 5 minutes), measurement of ventilation (by watching chest rise, auscultation, or end-tidal CO_2), and monitoring response to verbal, tactile, or painful stimuli must be monitored.
- Oxygen must be available and should be administered routinely during deep sedation.
- Emergency equipment and drugs must be immediately available, including reversal agents for benzodiazepines and narcotics. At least one practitioner present must be familiar with these drugs, and possess the skills to open an airway and provide bag–mask ventilation if needed. A practitioner certified in ACLS should be available (within 5 minutes) during moderate sedation, and should be present in the room during deep sedation.
- Intravenous access must be maintained throughout the procedure.
- Patients receiving propofol, barbiturates, or ketamine must be treated with all of the precautions given to a patient receiving deep sedation, even if the intended level of sedation is light or moderate.
- Following the procedure, the patient must be monitored in an appropriately staffed recovery facility.

○ **What should be done if you suspect a coworker is impaired?**

The physician should be reported to the person's supervisor, such as a residency program director in the case of a resident or the chief of the anesthesia group, rather than law enforcement authorities. This is because the primary concern is treatment, not punishment of the physician.

○ **What are the goals of an impaired physician referral program?**

The goals are to assist the physician in recovery from addiction, protect the confidentiality of both the impaired physician and the reporting physician, and assist the impaired physician to successfully return to work. Success rates for physicians returning to work having completed an impaired physician program are estimated at greater than 70%.

○ **What are the Joint Commission anesthetic standards regarding moderate sedation?**

Moderate sedation is considered an anesthetic and therefore requires a preanesthetic and a postanesthetic assessment.

○ **What are the Joint Commission standards for administering anesthesia?**

Anesthesia can be administered by the following, provided that it is in accordance with hospital policies and state law: an anesthesiologist, an MD or DO other than an anesthesiologist, a doctor of dental surgery or dental medicine, a podiatrist, a CRNA under the supervision of an anesthesiologist or operating physician except in opt-out states, an AA under the supervision of an anesthesiologist, or a resident in an approved educational program.

○ **A patient with multiple sclerosis (MS) presents for left total knee replacement. What is your preference for choice of anesthesia?**

General anesthesia is usually preferred to regional anesthesia (RA). MS is not an absolute contraindication to RA, but postoperative exacerbation of the disease due to stress, pain, or temperature elevation (an increase of 0.5°C may completely block conduction in demyelinated nerve fibers) may be confused with presumed residual effects of RA. Epidural is recommended rather than spinal anesthesia, which has been reported to cause exacerbation of the disease. Epidural and other regional techniques appear to have no adverse effect.

○ **A surgical patient is concerned about his risk of death due to anesthesia. What would you tell him?**

Numerous recent studies suggest that the risk of death from anesthesia is between 1 in 10,000 and 1 in 200,000. Far more important to perioperative morbidity and mortality are the patient's comorbidity and surgery risk factors.

○ **What are the most common causes of anesthesia-related death?**

Sixty percent of anesthesia-related deaths and 90% of anesthesia-related brain damage are caused by embarrassment of the respiratory system.

Ninety percent of cases are still deemed associated with operator error. The top five errors are overdose, wrong choice of anesthetic agent, inadequate preparation, inadequate crisis management, and inadequate postoperative management.

○ **You are performing a general anesthetic and suddenly the power fails. After a few long moments, the lights come back on, but only some of the electrical equipment is working. What should you do?**

You are probably on emergency power. Electrical receptacles that are backed up on emergency power are red and all essential equipment should be plugged into these receptacles. You should finish the case expediently, and expect further power interruption. Do not start any elective cases on emergency power. You may consider changing your anesthetic technique to total intravenous anesthesia (hypnotic, narcotic, amnesic, and muscle relaxant) and may need to manually ventilate the patient, preferably on 100% oxygen without using the anesthesia machine.

○ **What is the definition of time unit in anesthesia billing?**

The anesthesia claim is calculated as follows: base units (value assigned by the American Society of Anesthesiology to each procedure/surgery) plus time units (which starts when the anesthesia practitioner begins to prepare the patient for anesthesia services in the operating room or an equivalent area and ends when the anesthesia practitioner is no longer providing anesthesia services to the patient) plus special units (modifying units such as age of patient, medical condition, etc.).

○ **T/F: Anesthesia time begins when the anesthesiologist begins to prepare the patient for the induction of anesthesia in the operating room and requires the continuous presence.**

True.

○ **T/F: Anesthesia start and stop time must be reported in actual minutes.**

True.

○ **T/F: Most insurance carriers allow one time unit for each 15-minute interval, or fraction thereof, starting from the time the physician begins to prepare the patient for induction and ending when the patient is placed under postoperative supervision and the anesthesiologist is no longer in personal attendance.**

True.

○ **Which services are paid as part of the "base units" and should not be billed separately?**

Transporting, positioning, prepping, and draping of the patient

Placement of external devices necessary for cardiac monitoring, oximetry, temperature, EEG, etc.

Placement of peripheral intravenous lines necessary for fluid and medication administration

Placement of an airway

Placement of nasogastric or orogastric tube

Intraoperative interpretation of monitored functions

Interpretation of lab determinations

Nerve stimulation for determination of level of paralysis or localization of nerve

Insertion of urinary bladder catheter Blood sampling

○ **T/F: The preoperative examination time is included as part of the base units and should not be included in the anesthesia time.**

True.

○ **T/F: Preoperative examination must be done within 48 hours prior to the surgery.**

True.

○ **T/F: Placement of arterial, central venous, and pulmonary artery catheters and TEE (excluding heart cases) are not included in the base units.**

True.

○ **Certain procedures are billed as a flat-fee service with a specific CPT code. There is no time associated with these charges. What are these procedures?**

Arterial lines, CVPs, Swan–Ganz catheters, blocks for pain management, and TEE.

○ **Can you bill for cancelled surgery prior to induction?**

Yes, it can be billed with the appropriate E&M code. Reason for cancelled surgery should be properly documented in the patient's chart.

○ **When can you bill for postoperative pain service?**

Postoperative pain service can be billed separately if two conditions are met:

1. It must be done outside of anesthesia time.

2. Surgeon must document in the medical record that the care is being referred to the anesthesia provider.

Key Terms

Adverse outcomes in anesthesia: frequency
Anesthesia mortality: causes
Closed claims: brain damage
Federal regulation agencies: ORs
Intraoperative awareness: equipment malfunction
Intraoperative awareness: risk factors

Joint Commission: anesthetic standards
Physician impairment referral
Practice guidelines versus standards
Root cause analysis: essential elements
Time unit definition

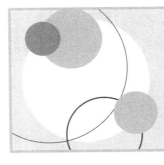

Anesthesia and the Liver

Whoever undertakes to set himself up as judge in the field of truth and knowledge
is shipwrecked by the laughter of the gods.
Albert Einstein

○ **What is the blood supply of the liver?**

The liver receives 20–25% of the cardiac output and contains 10–15% of the total blood volume. Seventy-five percent of the blood supply is derived from the portal vein and 25% from the hepatic artery. The hepatic oxygen supply, however, is derived approximately 50% from each.

○ **How does anesthesia affect liver blood flow?**

It depends on the type of anesthesia. Regional anesthesia has minimal effects on liver blood flow unless accompanied by hypotension. General anesthesia uniformly decreases liver blood flow by approximately 20–30%.

○ **What factors reduce liver blood flow during anesthesia?**

Hypoxemia, hypocarbia, hypercarbia, hypovolemia, hypotension, and sympathetic stimulation. Surgical manipulation in the right upper quadrant can reduce hepatic blood flow up to 60% from sympathetic activation or direct compression of the vena cava and splanchnic vessels. Pneumoperitoneum significantly decreases hepatic blood flow during laparoscopic cholecystectomy compared with small incision gallbladder surgery. Patient positioning, mode of ventilation (positive pressure ventilation, PEEP, hyperventilation), and use of inhalational agents above 1 MAC may reduce liver blood flow.

○ **What are the effects of CO_2 on the liver blood flow?**

Hypocapnia decreases hepatic arterial blood flow. Hypercapnia increases portal vein blood flow (due to splanchnic vasoconstriction) and overall total hepatic blood flow, while decreasing hepatic artery flow.

○ **What are the most common causes of hepatomegaly?**

- Apparent – low-lying diaphragm
- Cirrhosis – early
- Inflammation – hepatitis and abscesses
- Metabolic – fatty liver, amyloid, and glycogen storage disorders
- Tumors – primary and secondary carcinoma, leukemias, and lymphomas
- Venous congestion – heart failure and hepatic vein occlusion
- Biliary obstruction – particularly extrahepatic

○   **What are the cardiovascular implications of alcoholic liver disease during anesthesia?**

Overt or subclinical cardiomyopathy and ventricular arrhythmias.

○   **What are the typical hemodynamic changes seen in cirrhosis?**

- Hyperdynamic circulation (low systemic vascular resistance, compensatory increase in cardiac output, low-to-normal mean arterial pressure, mild tachycardia).
- Central hypovolemia (total body volume is increased; effective arterial blood volume is decreased).
- Hyporesponsiveness to vasopressor therapy.
- Flow-dependent oxygen consumption.
- Changes in the hepatic and splanchnic vasculature (portal hypertension, portal-systemic shunting, decreased hepatic blood flow).
- Increase in mixed venous oxygen saturation.
- Pulmonary arteriovenous anastomoses result in arteriovenous shunting and oxygen desaturation (hepatopulmonary syndrome [HPS]).

○   **What are the typical arterial blood gases seen in cirrhosis?**

Mild to moderate hypoxemia and respiratory alkalosis.

○   **What electrolyte changes are seen in patients with chronic liver disease?**

Typically, hyponatremia due to retention of water and impaired handling of sodium by the kidneys and hypokalemic metabolic alkalosis. Hypophosphatemia, hypocalcemia, and hypomagnesemia are also seen.

○   **Why are patients with fulminant hepatic failure prone to hypoglycemia?**

Hypoglycemia is common due to failure of gluconeogenesis, insufficient insulin degradation, and depletion of glycogen stores in the liver.

○   **Is regional anesthesia contraindicated in patients with chronic liver disease?**

Coagulopathy and portal hypertension may contraindicate the use of regional anesthesia. Peripheral nerve blocks may pose less risk than a spinal or epidural technique if the nerve sheaths are located in a manually compressible space.

○   **Would you decrease the dose of local anesthetics in patients with liver disease?**

In theory, ester local anesthetics (procaine, chloroprocaine) can have a prolonged duration of action due to a decrease in plasma pseudocholinesterase levels. Amide local anesthetic (lidocaine, bupivacaine, ropivacaine) doses need to be reduced due to decreased intrinsic clearance.

○   **A patient with massive ascites is scheduled for surgery requiring general anesthesia. How would you secure the airway?**

By rapid sequence induction with cricoid pressure (or awake intubation). Increase in intra-abdominal pressure due to moderate or massive ascites and gastric and intestinal hypomotility increases the risk of aspiration.

○ **A cirrhotic patient develops prolonged apnea after succinylcholine. What are the causes?**

Slightly prolonged duration of apnea is expected following succinylcholine in patients with liver disease due to a decrease in synthesis of pseudocholinesterase. Duration of longer than 10 minutes should alert one to the possibility of other causes.

○ **What drugs have a prolonged effect in pseudocholinesterase-deficient patients?**

Succinylcholine, mivacurium, ester local anesthetics (possibly), and trimethaphan.

○ **A cirrhotic patient undergoing portacaval shunt surgery has profuse surgical bleeding. Transfusion of red cells and fresh frozen plasma is in progress. The patient is hypotensive despite adequate replacement of intravascular volume. What is the most likely cause?**

Myocardial depression and peripheral vasodilation due to acute hypocalcemia from citrate toxicity, as citrate binds calcium. Citrate phosphate dextrose adenine (CPDA-1) is an anticoagulant preservative in blood. Citrate levels are high following rapid blood infusion (>1.5–2 mL/kg/min) and/or decreased metabolism due to hypothermia and/or states of absent or reduced liver blood flow. Ionized calcium levels <0.56 mEq/L are likely to be associated with hypotension.

○ **What is the cause of coagulopathy in advanced liver failure?**

Multifactorial:

1. Vitamin K deficiency – impaired storage or absorption.
2. Impaired synthesis of coagulation factors (all except factor VIII).
3. Splenic sequestration of platelets (if chronic alcoholic, there may be bone marrow suppression).
4. Low-grade DIC. The liver clears fibrin degradation products, so accumulated FDPs inhibit platelet aggregation and normal cross-linking of fibrin monomers.

○ **Which are the vitamin K–dependent coagulation factors?**

Factors II, VII, IX, and X, and proteins C, S, and Z.

○ **How do you manage coagulopathy in patients scheduled for major surgery?**

This includes administration of vitamin K (lack of response within 24 hours with prothrombin time [PT] ratio still >1.5 implies severe liver disease), FFP to correct PT within 3 seconds of normal or INR <1.5, cryoprecipitate for fibrinogen levels below 100 mg/dL, and transfusion of platelets to levels above 100,000/μL or transfusion threshold of 50,000/μL. Desmopressin may be efficacious. PT is the best prognostic indicator for recovery of liver function and may be very resistant to attempted normalization with factor replacement therapy.

○ **Can recombinant factor VIIa be used in the treatment of bleeding in liver disease?**

rFVIIa has been used safely to treat patients with acute hepatic trauma, bleeding after liver biopsy, bleeding from chronic liver disease with cirrhosis, and after liver transplantation. It is however only effective if there are adequate levels of platelets and fibrinogen.

○ **A cirrhotic patient undergoing surgery for portacaval shunt is bleeding intraoperatively, in spite of administration of FFP, cryoprecipitate, and platelets. What is your differential diagnosis?**

Suspect primary fibrinolysis and/or portal hypertension with excessive filling pressures. This may be demonstrated by thromboelastography or other laboratory tests and measurement of central filling pressures or stroke volume.

○ **What drugs are available to treat primary fibrinolysis in patients with liver disease?**

Epsilon-aminocaproic acid (EACA) or tranexamic acid.

○ **Is intraoperative administration of vitamin K indicated in a bleeding patient?**

Although peak effects may take as long as 24 hours, beneficial effects may be observed within hours after IM administration.

○ **How does severe parenchymal liver disease and biliary disease impair blood coagulation?**

The clotting factors V, VII, IX, and X, prothrombin, and fibrinogen are all dependent on the liver for synthesis. Parenchymal liver disease causes impaired formation of coagulation factors, fibrinolytic proteins and their inhibitors, as well as defective hepatic clearance of activated fibrinolytic factors (tissue plasminogen activator). Thrombocytopenia and platelet dysfunction are also contributory. Biliary obstruction may decrease vitamin K absorption due to the absence of bile salts. In early stage cholestatic liver disease there may be TEG evidence of hypercoagulability due to increased levels of fibrinogen and preservation of platelet counts and function.

○ **Is DDAVP effective during intraoperative bleeding in cirrhotic patients?**

DDAVP may improve hemostasis by increasing factor VIII and von Willebrand factor levels. Desmopressin can cause hypotension, hyponatremia, and increased platelet adhesiveness.

○ **Would you use halothane in a cirrhotic patient?**

Question of academic interest only as halothane use in the United States has become obsolete! Halothane is not contraindicated, but it should be avoided. It is accompanied by the most prominent decrease in hepatic blood flow and oxygen supply and has the greatest incidence of postoperative hepatitis of all available inhaled anesthetic agents, due to its high degree of metabolism (halothane > sevoflurane > enflurane > isoflurane > desflurane). Anesthesia-induced hepatitis can occur on an immunologic basis with exposure to halothane, but this finding is rare and there is no evidence that cirrhosis is a predisposing factor.

○ **Is cisatracurium the drug of choice for neuromuscular blockade in patients with liver disease?**

Cisatracurium is ideal for muscle relaxation, being an intermediate-acting drug relatively independent of renal or hepatic function for elimination.

○ **Which muscle relaxants are largely eliminated by the liver?**

Vecuronium and rocuronium.

○ **What are the considerations if you choose to use pancuronium or vecuronium in patients with liver disease?**

The initial dose is increased due to increased volume of distribution. Repeated dosing is dictated by elimination pathways: pancuronium has prolonged elimination; vecuronium <0.15 mg/kg, the kinetics and duration of action are unaltered.

○ **What drugs are effective if spasm of the sphincter of Oddi is suspected?**

Atropine, glucagon, naloxone, and nitroglycerin.

○ **What are the hemodynamic consequences of IVC cross-clamping?**

Clamping of the inferior vena cava decreases venous return, which results in a decrease in preload and cardiac output, often >50%. This leads to hypotension, which causes a compensatory increase in SVR and heart rate.

○ **What plasma proteins are synthesized by the liver?**

All plasma proteins except factor VIII, von Willebrand factor, and gamma globulins. Under normal conditions albumin makes up 60% of total serum proteins.

○ **What are the principal physiologic functions of albumin?**

Albumin maintains normal plasma oncotic pressure and is the peripheral binding and transport protein for a large number of drugs. A serum albumin <2.5 g/dL will clinically impact colloid oncotic pressure, placing the patient at risk for increased third-space fluid shifts (edema and ascites) and significant alterations in protein–drug binding.

○ **What is the half-life of albumin in plasma?**

The half-life of albumin is 20 days. Consequently, albumin levels will be normal in acute fulminant liver failure. Exogenous albumin lasts about 4 hours.

○ **List the major factors contributing to postoperative liver failure.**

Patients with preexisting liver disease, massive blood transfusion, hepatic oxygen deprivation (hypoxemia, anemia, decreased arterial pressure or cardiac output, and decreased hepatic blood flow), septicemia, and drug toxicity.

○ **What are the commonest causes of postoperative jaundice?**

- Prehepatic – overproduction of bilirubin from hemolysis, excessive bleeding, or resolving hematoma
- Intrahepatic – ischemia from hepatic hypoperfusion and drug-induced liver injury
- Posthepatic – retained common bile duct stone and intraoperative hepatobiliary injury

In reality, often multifactorial and difficult to diagnose. High AST/ALT is supportive of ischemia.

○ **What factors are responsible for altered drug pharmacokinetics in patients with advanced liver disease?**

Impaired hepatocyte function (P450 cytochrome biotransformation, transport processes, or biliary excretion), reduced hepatic blood flow, changes in free fraction of protein-bound drugs, and altered volume of distribution.

○ **What are the best laboratory tests for evaluation of liver function?**

Parenchymal damage with failure of synthetic function:

- Prothrombin (PT)
- Albumin
- Aminotransferases: ALT (alanine) is the gold standard biomarker for hepatocellular injury
- AST (aspartate)

Cholestasis of obstructive liver disease:

- Bilirubin (total, conjugated, and unconjugated)
- Alkaline phosphate

Due to the liver's large functional reserve, routine laboratory values may be normal in the presence of significant underlying disease.

○ **What are the causes of an abnormal alkaline phosphatase?**

Mild elevations in ALP occur in around 10% of the population and can be normal. High ALP comes from either the liver (cholestasis, fatty liver, hepatitis, liver tumor/metastasis, drugs) or bone (increased turnover – Paget's disease, bone metastases), and needs to be investigated.

○ **Preoperative assessment of a patient scheduled for elective surgery is unremarkable except for an unexpected elevation in transaminase levels. What is the correct plan of action?**

Patients with asymptomatic mild elevations in transaminase levels (less than ×2 normal) may undergo surgery without any increased risk of adverse outcome. Levels higher than this need further investigation including viral hepatitis, recreational drug use, and ETOH screening.

○ **T/F: The perioperative mortality associated with acute hepatitis is the same in cases of acute viral hepatitis as those with acute alcoholic hepatitis.**

False. The surgical mortality rate in patients with alcoholic hepatitis is believed to be worse, in some series approaching 100%. The diagnosis is likely if the AST/ALT ratio exceeds 2:1.

○ **In acute viral hepatitis, what is the first sign of acute liver failure?**

Coagulopathy and elevation of PT/INR.

○ **What are the risk factors associated with perioperative complications in cirrhotic patients?**

Male gender, high Child–Pugh score, ascites, cirrhosis other than primary biliary cirrhosis (especially cryptogenic cirrhosis), elevated serum creatinine, chronic obstructive pulmonary disease, preoperative infection, upper GI bleeding, ASA III or IV, high surgical severity score, surgery of the respiratory system, and intraoperative hypotension.

○ **What liver function tests are most predictive of outcome following surgery in patients with chronic liver disease?**

Laboratory evaluation of liver function is complicated by the liver's large functional reserve; routine laboratory values may be normal in the presence of significant underlying disease. Those that loosely reflect liver function include PT, albumin, bilirubin, and serum ammonia level.

Child's scoring system is a predictive scoring index to stratify mortality risk in patients having hepatobiliary surgery.

Child-Pugh Scoring System

	Group		
	A	**B**	**C**
Serum bilirubin (mg/dL)	<2	2–3	>3
Serum albumin (g/dL)	>3.5	3–3.5	<3
Ascites	None	Easily controlled	Poorly controlled
Encephalopathy	None	Minimal	Advanced
Nutrition	Excellent	Good	Poor

Using this method, mortality rates of 10%, 31%, and 76% were identified in Child's class A, B, and C, respectively. The Pugh modification replaces nutrition with PT prolongation (A: 1–4 seconds; B: 5–6 seconds; C: >6 seconds). In patients with primary biliary cirrhosis, the bilirubin limits are increased in each category.

○ **Describe a patient with Child's classification C of liver disease.**

Bilirubin >3 mg/dL (PBC and PSC patients >10 mg/dL), albumin <2.8 g/dL, tense ascites, advanced encephalopathy (Grade III–IV), poor nutrition, and surgical risk mortality rate 50–80%. The Pugh modification replaces nutrition with PT prolongation: Child-Pugh group C: – PT >6 seconds over control or INR >2.3.

○ **Describe a Child's C patient with cirrhosis according to the Child–Turcotte–Pugh (CPT) scoring system.**

Measure	2 points	3 points
Total bilirubin (mg/dL)	2–3	>3
Serum albumin (g/L)	28–35	<28
INR	1.71–2.2	>2.2
Ascites	Mild	Severe
Encephalopathy	I–II	III–IV (or refractory)

Child's group C patient will have 10–15 points on the CPT scoring system. One-year survival 45%; 2-year survival 35%. For primary sclerosing cholangitis or primary biliary cirrhosis the upper limit for bilirubin for 2 points is 10 mg/dL.

○ **T/F: The odds ratio for perioperative mortality after cholecystectomy in patients with cirrhosis compared with that in patients without liver disease is 8.5.**

True. Liver disease markedly increases the risk of perioperative death (odds ratio 8.47; 95% confidence interval 6.34–11.33).

○ **What is a transjugular intrahepatic portosystemic shunt (TIPS)?**

A TIPS is a percutaneous interventional radiologic procedure that creates a connection (using an expandable metallic stent or Gore endoprosthesis) within the liver between the portal and systemic circulations. A TIPS is placed to reduce portal pressure in patients with complications related to portal hypertension, primarily acute or recurrent/refractory variceal bleeding that cannot be successfully controlled by conventional medical treatment. Unproven but promising indications include refractory ascites, hepatorenal syndrome, hepatic hydrothorax, and hepatic venous outflow obstruction (Budd–Chiari syndrome). TIPS reduces portal venous pressure by approximately 50%.

○ **What is the most accurate predictive scoring system for survival in adult patients undergoing a TIPS procedure or those listed and waiting for liver transplantation?**

Model for end-stage liver disease (MELD).

○ **What is the MELD score?**

The MELD is a scoring system for assessing the severity of chronic liver disease. It was initially developed to predict death within 3 months of surgery in patients who had undergone a TIPS procedure and was subsequently found to be useful in determining prognosis and prioritizing for receipt of a liver transplant. MELD uses the patient's values for serum bilirubin, serum creatinine, and the INR to predict 3-month mortality. A Child's C is equivalent to a MELD of 14, with a 6% predicted 90-day mortality rate.

○ **Would you rather have a MELD score of 25 or 10?**

MELD is a scoring system for assessing the severity of chronic liver disease. A maximum MELD score is 40. In interpreting the MELD score in hospitalized patients, the predicted 3-month mortality: MELD is <9 (1.9% mortality), 10–19 (6% mortality), 20–29 (20% mortality), 30–39 (52.6% mortality), and 40 (71.3% mortality). MELD–UNOS modification also includes the question, "has the patient had dialysis twice in the past week?" If the patient is dialysis dependent, the MELD score is increased. The score is also adjusted for patients who are hyponatremic, MELD-Na. MELD scoring has been used as an index for predicting 90-day mortality in alcoholic hepatitis and postoperative mortality in cirrhotic patients.

○ **How does the pediatric model to predict survival in patients with end-stage liver disease differ from MELD?**

Pediatric end-stage liver disease (PELD) score is calculated on the basis of age <1 year, albumin, bilirubin, INR, and growth failure <2 standard deviations.

○ **What is the Pringle maneuver?**

Interruption of hepatic vascular inflow by temporary occlusion of the portal triad (hepatic artery, portal vein, and bile duct). The liver will tolerate 60 minutes of continuous vascular occlusion and 120 minutes of intermittent accumulated ischemia time.

○ **Which zone of hepatocytes surrounding a terminal afferent blood vessel is at risk for ischemia?**

Zone 3.

○ **What is a Phase I reaction?**

Functionalization reaction (90% oxidation) in the cytochrome P450 system or to a lesser extent mixed-function oxidases subject to enzyme induction, tolerance, and competitive reactions. Susceptible to impairment due to disease; located in the ischemia-susceptible zone 3.

○ **What is the first-pass effect?**

Clearance of drugs with a high ratio of hepatic extraction dependent on liver blood flow (lidocaine, morphine, verapamil, labetalol, and propranolol).

○ **What is the best choice for general anesthesia in the cirrhotic patient?**

Propofol, succinylcholine, fentanyl, cisatracurium, oxygen, and isoflurane (some prefer desflurane) – these drugs do not have altered pharmacodynamics in the cirrhotic, due to either termination of action via redistribution or metabolism that is not liver based. Avoid a reduction in hepatic blood flow due to hypotension, excessive sympathetic activation, or high mean airway pressure. Maintain $PaCO_2$ 35–40 mm Hg. Enlist a strategy for renal protection.

○ **Following exposure to hepatitis C virus through a needle stick, what is the likelihood of becoming infected and what are the CDC guidelines for laboratory testing?**

The average incidence of anti-HCV seroconversion after unintentional needle stick from an HCV-positive source is 1.8%.

Testing for anti-HCV includes use of an antibody screening assay, and for screening test-positive results, a more specific supplemental assay. The only tests approved by the US FDA for screening of HCV infection are those that measure anti-HCV (HCV EIA) and CIA. Supplemental testing with a more specific assay (recombinant immunoblot assay [RIBA] for anti-HCV) prevents reporting false-positive results. HCV RNA using gene amplification techniques (nucleic acid test [NAT] for HCV RNA PCR) can be detected in serum or plasma within 1–2 weeks after exposure to the virus and weeks before the onset of ALT elevations or anti-HCV appears. A negative test requires RIBA for anti-HCV prior to reporting results. The incubation period for HCV is 2 weeks to 6 months.

○ **In a case of accidental needle stick injury, which situations are considered serious exposures?**

- Exposure to a large amount of blood.
- Blood came in contact with cuts or open sores on the skin.
- Blood was visible on a needle that stuck someone.
- Exposure to blood from someone who has a high viral load.

○ **What is the recommended postexposure prophylaxis for a health care worker (HCW) following accidental needle stick injury?**

In the case of HIV, there is a 0.3% risk of seroconversion following a needle stick injury and 0.09% risk in mucous membrane exposure.

The exposure site should be washed with soap and water.

The risk of seroconversion should be assessed by contacting experts for advise (occupational health office).

In the case of HIV, postexposure prophylaxis should be taken within 1 hour for best results (reduce seroconversion rate by 80%) or should be taken within 36 hours at least.

Treatment with two or three antiretrovirals (ARVs) such as AZT, 3TC, and Viread should be continued for 4 weeks, if tolerated. For the less serious exposures, two drugs may be adequate (AZT and 3TC). The HCW should have HIV antibody testing by enzyme immunoassay (baseline testing and follow-up testing at 6 weeks, 12 weeks, and 6 months) [Landowitz and Currier, 2009. See reference on page 522].

The risk of seroconversion for hepatitis B following a needle stick injury is about 30%. The HCW exposed to hepatitis B virus and not known to be immune should be tested for HBsAg.

If previously vaccinated but not tested for anti-HBsAg in the past 24 months, should be tested for immunity because the duration of protection is unknown (10% or more will not achieve protective titers after vaccination).

If inadequate (<10 mIU/mL), hepatitis B immunoglobulin ×1 and vaccine booster should be given.

If clearly susceptible to hepatitis B (serious occupational exposure), hepatitis B hyperimmunoglobulin and recombinant hepatitis B vaccine should be given.

For hepatitis C, there is no effective postexposure prophylaxis or therapy. Immunoglobulin is not recommended. Follow-up testing is done for hepatitis C and liver function tests. Fifty percent may progress to chronic liver disease and significant number may develop cirrhosis and hepatocellular cancer.

○ **Should you test the source patient?**

After obtaining consent, the source patient should be tested as follows.

If unknown HIV status:

- Rapid ELISA (results in 5–30 minutes). If positive test, confirm with Western blot.
- Testing for HBsAg.
- ELISA for antibodies against HCV.

If the source patient is at risk for recent HIV (seroconversion may take 2–12 weeks), NAT should be considered.

○ **Provide an interpretation of the following hepatitis B serologic testing results: HbsAg positive, anti-HBc positive, HBV-DNA positive, and HbeAg positive.**

Results indicate a persistent infection: replicative (excludes the patient from eligibility for liver transplantation in most centers).

○ **What are the consequences of hepatic enzyme induction?**

Exposure to many compounds stimulates microsomal xenobiotic-metabolizing activity in the liver through an increase in the cellular amount of RNA coding for the specific enzyme. Clinical effects are apparent when the rate-controlling step of drug detoxification or elimination is affected or with the formation of toxic intermediates.

Key Terms

Abnormal alkaline phosphatase: causes
Cholestasis: coagulopathy treatment
Factor VII: hemostatic function in liver disease
Hepatic dysfunction: diagnosis
Hepatic protein synthesis
Hepatic synthesis capacity: diagnosis
Hepatic synthesis impairment: diagnosis
Hepatitis B: needle stick treatment
Hepatitis C: lab sign of infection
Hepatitis: diagnosis

Hepatomegaly: causes
Liver failure: CV changes
Liver function tests
Mortality risk: cirrhosis
Needle stick injury management
Postoperative hepatic dysfunction risk factors
Postoperative jaundice: causes
Postoperative jaundice: differential diagnosis
Synthetic hepatic function: prothrombin time (PT)
Tests of hepatocellular disease

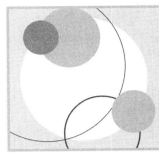

Aspiration Pneumonitis

Most people die of a sort of creeping common sense, and discover when it is too late that the only things one never regrets are one's mistakes.
Oscar Wilde

○ **What factors characterize an aspirate?**

Particulate or liquid (secretions, blood, gastric fluid, bile), size, foodstuffs, pH, and infected or noninfected.

○ **Classically, what volume and pH of aspirate are critical in causing a significant problem (Mendelson's syndrome) after gastric fluid aspiration?**

Greater than 0.4 mL/kg (25 mL) of gastric contents with a pH of 2.5 or less.

○ **What can happen to volume status and wedge pressure after a severe aspiration?**

Pulmonary capillary wedge pressure and volume status can actually decrease after severe pulmonary aspiration due to loss of fluid through pulmonary capillaries. This can cause significant hypotension.

○ **What are the radiographic manifestations of acid aspiration?**

Varied. May be new bilateral diffuse infiltrates, irregular "patchy" bronchopneumonic pattern, or lobar infiltrates in the posterior segments of the upper lobes and the superior segment of the lower lobes.

○ **Are the chest x-ray findings of aspiration immediate or delayed in onset?**

They may be delayed up to 6–12 hours, in some cases. Look first at the right lower lobe, where findings will be most common, for evidence of infiltration, pneumonia, atelectasis, pulmonary edema, and fulminant chemical pneumonitis.

○ **What features of the chest x-ray help distinguish aspiration pneumonitis from cardiac failure?**

While diffuse bilateral infiltrates and pulmonary edema may be present in both scenarios, acute cardiac enlargement and pulmonary venous congestion suggest a primary cardiac cause.

○ **What patients are at increased risk of aspiration?**

According to Sakai et al., 4-year retrospective review, the incidence of perioperative pulmonary aspiration is 1 of 7103, with morbidity 1 of 16,573 and mortality 1 of 99,441. [Sakai et al., 2006. See reference on page 522]. The majority of pulmonary aspirations occur during laryngoscopy and tracheal extubation. Risk factors include pregnancy, gastric contents of increased volume or acidity, increased intragastric pressure, decreased tone of the lower esophageal sphincter (LES), gastroesophageal reflux, ASA III or IV status, emergency surgery, inadequate muscle relaxation or difficulty during laryngoscopy, impaired laryngeal reflexes, decreased mental status, full stomach, large amounts of gas in the stomach, alcohol intoxication, and ineffective cricoid pressure.

○ **What is the primary treatment for gastric aspiration?**

A stepwise approach using suction, analysis of arterial blood gases for pH and oxygenation, aggressive and early ventilatory support, adequate fluid resuscitation, and bronchoscopy for large particulate aspiration is recommended.

○ **Does a nasogastric (NG) tube reduce the likelihood of gastric aspiration?**

No, the presence of an NG tube does not reduce chances of gastric aspiration. In fact, reflux of stomach contents into the esophagus can increase due to the NG tube stenting open the LES, thereby increasing aspiration risk.

○ **How can you reduce the risk of aspiration?**

Give metoclopramide to stimulate gastric emptying (assuming no intestinal obstruction); increase gastric fluid pH with H_2 antagonists and nonparticulate antacids. Consider rapid sequence intubation with effective cricoid pressure and a cuffed endotracheal tube, awake intubation, or regional anesthesia avoiding heavy sedation. Delay nonemergent surgery greater than 6 hours. NG suctioning prior to extubation (when the patient is expected to have regained protective laryngeal reflexes) is prudent.

○ **What is the mechanism of action of metoclopramide (Reglan)?**

Metoclopramide is a gastrointestinal stimulant and antiemetic agent possibly decreasing aspiration. It increases LES pressure, decreases pyloric pressure, and speeds gastric emptying (decreases the gastric residual volume).

It is not the most efficacious agent as a prophylactic antiemetic.

○ **What are the effects of metoclopramide on the GI system?**

Metoclopramide is an enteric- and centrally acting dopamine receptor (D2) antagonist with some indirect enteric cholinergic agonist activity. It acts as an antiemetic centrally (at the chemoreceptor trigger zone) and is effective in improving foregut motility. LES pressure is increased, while duodenal and pyloric tones are relaxed. These effects combine to accelerate GI gastric emptying and increase coordination of antral, duodenal, and pyloric contractions. Metoclopramide has little effect on gastric, pancreatic, or biliary secretions or on colonic motility.

○ **What other drugs are known to affect GI system motility?**

Motility is enhanced by drugs that increase parasympathetic activity.

Therefore, muscarinic receptor agonists such as bethanechol, as well as drugs that increase acetylcholine concentration (neostigmine, edrophonium), all enhance GI motility. GI motility is notably slowed by the administration of opioids, as well as sympathomimetic drugs.

○ **What is the mechanism of action of ranitidine? (Zantac?)**

It is a competitive inhibitor of H_2 receptors, and thereby blocks secretion of hydrogen ions in the stomach. This effectively increases gastric pH and decreases gastric volume. The decrease in gastric volume occurs over hours.

○ **What is the duration of metoclopramide? Ranitidine?**

Metoclopramide duration is 1–2 hours; ranitidine duration is 8 hours.

○ **Liquids pass from stomach to duodenum in less than 2 hours. How long does it take for solids to pass from the stomach to duodenum?**

Up to 12 hours.

○ **What may delay gastric emptying?**

Idiopathic gastroparesis remains the most common cause of delayed gastric emptying. Diabetes mellitus, anorexia nervosa, gastric surgery, gastric outlet obstruction, obesity, stress from pain or anxiety, neurologic disorders, disease involving the gastric wall or nerves, drugs such as opioids, and pregnancy. Long bone fractures are associated with incomplete gastric emptying for up to 24 hours.

○ **Which drugs will increase and decrease LES tone?**

Increase:

Protein meal

Coffee contains a protein that increases LES pressure

Bethanechol (Urecholine)

Metoclopramide (Reglan)

Antacids

Alpha-adrenergic agents

Decrease:

Alcohol

Chocolate

Essence of peppermint

Smoking

Fatty foods

Beta-adrenergic agents

Estrogen and progesterone

Caffeine decreases LES pressure

Calcium channel blockers

Diazepam

Barbiturates

○ **Where is the vomiting center located?**

Medulla.

○ **T/F: NG and gastric tubes increase the risk of aspiration.**

True.

○ **T/F: Aspiration of blood usually results in a more benign syndrome than acid aspiration.**

True. The immediate postaspiration phase is usually characterized by tachycardia and tachypnea, much like acid aspiration; however, the symptoms of blood aspiration generally resolve rapidly and without sequelae.

○ **T/F: Adults are more likely to aspirate into the right mainstem bronchus.**

True. Over the age of 15 years.

○ **Complete upper airway obstruction by a foreign body is treated by which maneuver?**

Heimlich – subdiaphragmatic abdominal thrusts and backslaps.

○ **What are possible complications of the Heimlich maneuver?**

Rib fractures, ruptured viscera, pneumomediastinum, regurgitation (and aspiration), and retinal detachment.

○ **What is the procedure of choice for lower airway foreign body aspiration?**

Rigid bronchoscopy. Fiber-optic bronchoscopy is an alternative procedure in adults, not in children. If bronchoscopy, postural drainage, chest physical therapy, and bronchodilators fail, surgical removal may be required.

○ **What are common radiographic findings in foreign body aspiration?**

Normal chest-xray and atelectasis or infiltrates distal to the obstruction, obstructive lobar segmental overinflation in a ball-valve obstruction, and visualization of the foreign body.

○ **What are the common directly toxic (noninfected) respiratory tract aspirates?**

Gastric and small bowel contents, alcohol, hydrocarbons, mineral oil, and animal and vegetable fats. All of these produce an inflammatory response and pneumonia. Gastric contents are the most common offender.

○ **T/F: Vomiting should not be induced in an individual suspected of having ingested a toxic hydrocarbon (e.g., kerosene, gasoline, turpentine, lighter fluid)?**

True. In most cases, the risk of aspiration of the hydrocarbon contraindicates induced vomiting, particularly when an altered level of consciousness is present; gastric lavage with endotracheal intubation should be performed if there is a question regarding adequacy of airway protection.

○ **What is the antibiotic choice for gastric acid aspiration?**

None. Antibiotics should not be given prophylactically, unless there is evidence of intestinal obstruction or fecal aspiration. Treatment is on the basis of positive culture results.

○ **What is the role of corticosteroids in gastric acid aspiration?**

None. Steroids can impair wound healing.

○ **What is the main priority in treating gastric acid aspiration?**

Maintenance of pulmonary oxygenation.

Tracheal suctioning, intubation, ventilation, and positive end-expiratory pressure (PEEP) may be required. Prophylactic PEEP is not effective in preventing progression of the process. Patients with clinically apparent pulmonary aspiration who do not develop symptoms within 2 hours are unlikely to have significant respiratory sequelae.

○ **What outcomes occur in patients who do not rapidly resolve gastric acid aspiration pneumonitis?**

Adult respiratory distress syndrome (ARDS), bacterial superinfection, or progressive respiratory failure and death.

○ **Under what circumstances are antibiotics used in aspiration treatment?**

Aspiration of infected material, intestinal obstruction, immune compromised host, and evidence of bacterial superinfection after a noninfected aspirate (new fever, infiltrates, or purulence after the initial 2–3 days). Later findings may include necrotizing consolidation and abscess formation.

○ **What is the predominant oropharyngeal flora in outpatients?**

Anaerobes, which are responsible for nosocomial pneumonia.

○ **What is the antibiotic of choice for outpatient acquired infectious aspiration pneumonia?**

Clindamycin, high-dose penicillin, or augmentin (amoxicillin and clavulanate).

○ **T/F: Aspiration of liquid gastric contents with pH greater than 2.5 produces no clinical consequences.**

False. Hypoxemia, bronchospasm, and atelectasis may develop but usually resolve within 24 hours.

○ **What are the consequences of aspirating small (nonobstructing) food particles?**

Inflammation and hypoxemia, which may result in chronic bronchiolitis or granulomatosis.

○ **What is the priority treatment of near drowning?**

Correction of asphyxia and hypothermia.

○ **What are the indications for intubation and ventilation after near drowning?**

Apnea, pulselessness, altered mental status, severe hypoxemia, and respiratory acidosis.

○ **T/F: The presence of a cuffed endotracheal tube makes aspiration pneumonia an unlikely cause of new pulmonary infiltrates.**

False. Silent aspiration previously undetected may occur prior to or after endotracheal intubation.

○ **T/F: Retrospective reviews indicate that antibiotic therapy for aspiration pneumonia will hasten the resolution of pulmonary infiltrates.**

False.

○ **With aspiration pneumonia presenting as a lobar infiltrate, which sites are the most common?**

Right lower lobe as most aspirations occur in the supine position, and the right lower lobe has the most gravity-dependent position.

○ **What strategies can reduce the risk of aspiration in ICU patients?**

Elevation of head of bed >30°, maintain blood glucose levels <150 mg/dL, minimize use of drugs that alter level of consciousness (e.g., benzodiazepines) or delay gastric emptying (e.g., opioids), initiate a bowel regimen to reduce ileus (consider prokinetic agents), and early ambulation.

○ **What surgical interventions can reduce the incidence of chronic aspiration?**

Nissen fundoplication can significantly reduce the incidence of chronic aspiration episodes, particularly in children. Gastrostomy tube placement alone is not adequate prevention for chronic aspiration.

Key Terms

Acid aspiration pneumonitis: diagnosis
Drugs affecting lower esophageal sphincter (LES) tone
Gastric emptying drugs
Gastric fluid pH: drug affecting
H_2 blockers: onset time

Metoclopramide: GI effects
Perioperative gastric aspiration: management
Prevention of passive regurgitation
Pulmonary aspiration: management

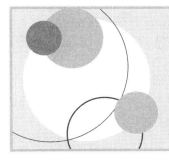

Autonomic Pharmacology and Physiology

If winning isn't everything, why do they keep score?
Vince Lombardi

○ **What is a commonly used α₂-agonist for treating hypertension and its mechanism?**

Clonidine. α_2-Agonists act at the presynaptic membrane to inhibit further release of catecholamines. This is a classic feedback mechanism. The sympatholytic effect results in a decrease in sympathetic outflow from the CNS medullary pressor centers, reducing activity in peripheral sympathetic neurons without affecting baroreceptor reflexes.

○ **Describe the anesthetic implications of clonidine as a premedication.**

Clonidine is a centrally acting, selective, partial alpha 2 agonist (220:1, alpha2: alpha1). Its use as an oral premedication (5 μg/kg) has the following effects:

1. Blunting of reflex tachycardia due to direct laryngoscopy.
2. Decrease in intraoperative cardiovascular lability.
3. Decrease in plasma catecholamine concentrations.
4. Decrease in the MAC of inhaled agents.
5. Decrease in perioperative myocardial ischemic episodes in patients with CAD.
6. Augmentation of pressor responses to ephedrine.
7. Secretory glands: inhibition of salivary, tracheobronchial, lacrimal, digestive, and exocrine sweat gland secretions.

○ **Describe rebound hypertension caused by abrupt withdrawal of clonidine.**

Rebound hypertension may occur but is symptomatic in only 5–20% of patients. It is more likely to occur after abrupt withdrawal of clonidine in patients who had been receiving doses exceeding 1.2 mg per day or if clonidine therapy is discontinued before or at the same time as concurrent beta-adrenergic blocking agent therapy. The clinical features may include nervousness, tachycardia, diaphoresis, abdominal pain, and headache followed by hypertension.

○ **Which two classes of hypertensive medications cause withdrawal hypertension and should not be stopped prior to a patient having surgery?**

β-Blockers and clonidine.

Withdrawal of both is associated with rebound hypertension and myocardial ischemia. Calcium channel blockers can cause coronary spasm when stopped abruptly. All antihypertensive medications should be continued until the day of surgery with the possible exception of diuretics (depletion of intravascular volume) and ACE inhibitors (hypotension with induction). Note that withdrawal hypertension may occur with many different antihypertensive drugs including reserpine, hydralazine, guanethidine, methyldopa, and hydrochlorothiazide.

○ **Should beta-blockers be continued throughout the perioperative period?**

Yes. Beta-adrenergic antagonists decrease myocardial oxygen demand by decreasing heart rate and cardiac contractility. Abrupt withdrawal of beta-blockers may result in rebound increases in heart rate and blood pressure in patients with coronary artery disease causing ischemia, infarction, or ventricular arrhythmias. Outcomes may be improved in those at high risk of ischemia by adequate preoperative and postoperative beta-blockade.

○ **How are acetylcholine and esmolol metabolized?**

Acetylcholine is hydrolyzed by acetylcholinesterase (tissue esterase or true esterase). Esmolol is metabolized by red blood cell esterases. These two enzymes are distinct from plasma esterase or pseudocholinesterase, whose function is not known but which is known to break down succinylcholine.

○ **Where is the site of action of bronchodilators?**

There are two types of bronchodilators:

Anticholinergic drugs: They act via acetyl choline antagonism at the muscarinic receptors.

β_2 receptor agonists: These drugs act on the β_2 receptor, increasing intracellular c-AMP concentration in the bronchial smooth muscle which leads to decreased Ca influx and consequent relaxation.

○ **Metoprolol is a selective β_1 antagonist. Why is it that in large doses metoprolol increases airway resistance?**

Selectivity is relative and dose-related. At large doses, β_2 receptors are also blocked causing bronchoconstriction.

○ **Compare the action of albuterol with ipratropium.**

Albuterol is a selective beta 2 agonist causing smooth muscle relaxation by increasing cyclic AMP intracellularly in the smooth muscle of the respiratory tract.

Ipratropium acts by blocking the muscarinic receptors in the bronchial smooth muscle and causes bronchodilation.

The combination of both agents causes better bronchodilation as compared with any of them used alone.

The side effects also differ based on the mechanism of action.

Beta-adrenergic bronchodilators may decrease serum potassium concentrations, especially when the recommended dose is exceeded, and can cause EKG changes such as flattened T waves, prolongation of the QT_c interval, and ST segment depression.

Ipratropium can cause an acute attack of glaucoma or condition may be exacerbated if ipratropium-containing inhalation aerosol is sprayed directly into the eyes. In addition, it may lead to urinary retention.

○ **A patient with a history of CAD and bronchospasm presents with supraventricular tachycardia (SVT). What would be a reasonable medication to give?**

Verapamil, digoxin, or beta-blockers.

(However, these drugs slow AV nodal conduction but may increase conduction along the accessory pathway. Therefore, they should not be used in wide QRS complex SVT due to WPW syndrome.)

Adenosine is the drug of choice for terminating SVT but contraindicated in patients with asthma and those taking dipyridamole.

○ **What are the effects of catecholamines on the cardiovascular system?**

Catecholamines principally affect the heart via the activation of β-receptors; activation of β-1 and β-2 receptors has a positive chronotropic effect, while β-1 stimulation also adds a positive inotropic effect. With respect to the vasculature, α-1 and α-2 stimulation results in vasoconstriction, while β-2 stimulation causes vasodilation. Dopamine's effects on the CV system depend on its dosage. Low-dose dopamine (2–5 μg/(kg min)) results in blood vessel relaxation via the D-1 receptor. This is especially pronounced in the renal and mesenteric vascular beds. Higher doses (5–10 μg/(kg min)) result in positive inotropic and chronotropic cardiac effects via stimulation of the β-1 receptor. High-dose dopamine (10–20 μg/(kg min)) results in vasoconstriction via α-1 receptor stimulation.

○ **What is the presumed mechanism of adrenergic denervation hypersensitivity?**

No signal is sensed after denervation, so cells respond by putting out more receptors to "catch" a signal. In the transplanted heart, surgical denervation of the postganglionic sympathetic nerves results in upregulation of beta-adrenergic receptors and downregulation of muscarinic receptors. Increased beta-adrenergic receptor density and adenylate cyclase stimulation account for the augmented chronotropic response to catecholamine stimulation.

○ **What are the side effects of beta agonist drugs?**

Beta$_1$ agonists: tachycardia, arrhythmias, hypertension, and hypotension at higher doses.

Beta$_2$ agonists: fine tremor of the hands, restlessness, nervousness, and headache are common. They can also cause flushing and palpitations. Rarely: arrhythmia, hypokalemia, hyperglycemia, muscle cramps, nausea and vomiting, and allergic reactions. Elderly are at increased risk.

○ **Norepinephrine (Levophed) is being infused through a peripheral IV, and extravasation is noted, with blanching of the skin. What should be done?**

The area should be infiltrated with phentolamine 5–10 mg in 10 cm^3 saline to minimize the risk of skin necrosis. Phentolamine antagonizes undesirable alpha stimulation. Administration of norepinephrine should be restricted to central venous access.

○ **A patient was brought to the OR with dopamine running into a peripheral IV. The patient is complaining of intense pain at the IV site. Diagnosis and initial management?**

Infiltration of the IV and extravasation of dopamine into skin or subcutaneous tissues, such as norepinephrine, produces intense local vasoconstriction that should be treated by local infiltration of phentolamine. IV should be discontinued immediately.

○ **During an epidural C-section, the patient complains of severe nausea. Diagnosis?**

The nausea may be due to hypotension from sympathetic blockade, anxiety, exteriorization of the uterus or mesenteric traction, and pain from insufficient sensory block height.

○ **Following a reversal of neuromuscular blockade with atropine–neostigmine, a patient becomes restless and combative. Diagnosis?**

Hypoxia and/or hypercarbia.

Then consider the possibility that atropine can enter the CNS and produce a central anticholinergic syndrome ("mad as a hatter"). Physostigmine, a tertiary amino anticholinesterase, can be used to treat this syndrome.

○ **What are the main divisions of the autonomic nervous system and where are they located?**

Sympathetic and parasympathetic divisions. The sympathetic nervous system (SNS) originates from the thoracolumbar region of the spinal cord (T1 to L2,3) with preganglionic fibers synapsing in ganglia that are distant from effector organs. The parasympathetic, or craniosacral, nervous system has cranial outflows from cranial nerves III, VII, IX, and X and sacral branches that converge to form the pelvic nerves. The ganglia are proximal to or within the innervated organ.

Preganglionic neuron cell bodies (of both sympathetic and parasympathetic systems) are located in the intermediolateral horn of the spinal cord.

○ **What is the sympathetic chain?**

It is a ganglionated nerve chain extending from the base of skull to the coccyx, lying 2–3 cm lateral to the vertebral column. Inferiorly, the two chains unite and terminate on the anterior surface of the coccyx.

○ **How does the SNS innervate its end organs?**

Efferents exit the cord in the anterior nerve roots and travel a short distance into the ventral white rami, where they synapse in the paired paravertebral ganglia. Long postganglionic unmyelinated nerves leave via the gray rami, reenter the spinal nerve, and innervate the target organs.

○ **How does the parasympathetic nervous system innervate its end organs?**

The craniosacral outflow tracts extend out as long preganglionic fibers that synapse at ganglia that are near the effector organs. Short postganglionic fibers make the terminal connections to elicit the end-organ response.

○ **What are the neurotransmitters of the SNS and parasympathetic nervous system?**

Acetylcholine is used as the preganglionic neurotransmitter at the level of the ganglia in both the SNS and parasympathetic nervous system. It is also the postganglionic neurotransmitter of the parasympathetic nervous system. Norepinephrine is used in the postganglionic fibers of the SNS, except for those fibers which innervate sweat glands, which use acetylcholine.

○ **What are the subtypes of cholinergic receptors and where are they found?**

There are two main types of receptors that bind acetylcholine: nicotinic and muscarinic. Nicotinic receptors have two major subtypes: those found in the ganglia of the autonomic nervous system and those located at the neuromuscular junctions. Muscarinic receptors are also divided into the M_1 type, which are primarily in the ganglia and central nervous system, and the M_2 type located mainly on peripheral visceral organs.

○ **What are the effects of muscarinic receptor antagonism?**

Cardiac: tachycardia.

Bronchial: bronchodilation and drying of secretions.

GI tract: smooth muscle relaxation and slowing of peristalsis.

GU tract: lowering of bladder tone and increase of sphincter tone.

Eye: mydriasis.

○ **Compare the anticholinergic drugs glycopyrrolate and atropine.**

	Atropine	*Glycopyrrolate*
Sedation	+	0
Antisialagogue	+	+ +
Tachycardia	+ + +	+ +
Smooth muscle relaxation	+ +	+ +
Mydriasis	0	+
Prevention of motion sickness	0	+
Reduction of gastric acid secretion	+	+

○ **Describe the mechanism of action of glycopyrrolate.**

Glycopyrrolate is a quaternary ammonium compound, which causes competitive antagonism of acetylcholine at the muscarinic receptors sites. It acts on all three subtypes M1, M2, and M3. These postganglionic receptor sites are present in the autonomic effector cells of the smooth muscle, cardiac muscle, sinoatrial and atrioventricular nodes, and exocrine glands.

○ **What is the advantage of using glycopyrrolate as an anticholinergic medication versus atropine?**

Glycopyrrolate does not cross the blood–brain barrier (no central anticholinergic syndrome possible) and it has a longer duration of action than atropine (6–8 hours, with 2 hours of vagolytic activity). Onset of action is better matched with neostigmine compared with atropine, avoiding the initial tachycardia and arrhythmia seen with neostigmine–atropine.

○ **A patient appears to be disoriented after receiving atropine for treatment of bradycardia. What is the diagnosis and treatment?**

Immediately rule out causes secondary to neurologic or metabolic disorders (hypotension, hypoxemia, hypercarbia, acidosis, hypoglycemia, and electrolyte disorders). Atropine can cross the blood–brain barrier and cause CNS symptoms in relatively large doses (1–2 mg). Physostigmine is an anticholinesterase that penetrates the blood–brain barrier and may reverse the CNS effect of atropine.

○ **What is the mechanism of sedation with scopolamine?**

Scopolamine crosses the blood–brain barrier and depresses the reticular activating system, producing sedation. Paradoxical restlessness and delirium are possible. Other properties include antisialagogue, amnesia, prevention of motion sickness, and minimal effect on heart rate.

○ **Describe the features of anticholinergic syndrome and its treatment.**

Scopolamine and to a lesser degree atropine enter the CNS and can cause this syndrome.

Symptoms range from restlessness and hallucinations to somnolence and unconsciousness. Presumably these effects are due to antagonism of central effects of acetylcholine.

Physostigmine 15–60 μg/kg IV is a specific treatment. Edrophonium, pyridostigmine, and neostigmine are not effective due to their inability to cross into the CNS.

○ **Describe the pharmacology of physostigmine.**

Mechanism of action: antagonizes action of anticholinergics, which block the postsynaptic receptor sites of acetylcholine, by reversibly inhibiting the destruction of acetylcholine by acetylcholinesterase, thereby increasing the concentration of acetylcholine at sites of cholinergic transmission. Since physostigmine is a lipid-soluble tertiary amine, which (unlike the quaternary amines neostigmine and pyridostigmine) can cross the blood–brain barrier, it acts against both central and peripheral anticholinergic effects. Easily penetrates the blood–brain barrier. Rapidly hydrolyzed by cholinesterases. Time to peak effect: 20–30 minutes IM or within 5 minutes IV. Duration of action and elimination: 30–60 minutes. Largely destroyed in the body by hydrolysis, with very small amounts eliminated in urine.

○ **Describe the treatment of a cholinergic crisis.**

Atropine 35–70 μg/kg IV every 3–10 minutes until the muscarinic symptoms improve.

Pralidoxime may be used to improve muscle weakness that results from an overdose of neostigmine and pyridostigmine used to treat myasthenia gravis. Dosing: 1–2 g IV, and then 250 mg IV every 5 minutes. Supportive therapy for respiratory insufficiency may be needed.

○ **What happens to acetylcholine after it binds to its various types of receptors?**

Acetylcholine is hydrolyzed by acetylcholinesterase at cholinergic synapses and to a lesser extent pseudocholinesterase to acetate and choline. Choline is taken back up by the neuron and reused while acetate diffuses away and is eliminated.

○ **Where is acetylcholinesterase or "true cholinesterase" synthesized?**

It is a membrane-bound enzyme that is synthesized in the Golgi apparatus of neuronal cell bodies and red blood cells.

○ **Where is plasma cholinesterase or pseudocholinesterase synthesized?**

This is a soluble enzyme that is synthesized in the liver and circulates in the blood.

○ **What is the interaction between SNS and parasympathetic nervous system?**

Most organs are innervated by both divisions of the autonomic nervous system. In general, each gets to antagonize the other in creating an end-organ response. This allows for tighter regulation of organ function and homeostasis.

○ **What is dysautonomia?**

Autonomic dysfunction due to generalized, segmental, or focal disorders of the central or peripheral nervous system. The most serious anesthetic risk is orthostatic hypotension. Dysautonomic crises triggered by stress are characterized by hypertension, tachycardia, abdominal pain, diaphoresis, and vomiting.

○ **What causes dysautonomia?**

Congenital, familial, or acquired (infectious states, drugs, or trauma). Each may lead to different signs or symptoms, depending on the location and degree of autonomic dysfunction. It can be seen in patients with diabetes mellitus, Parkinson disease, cystic fibrosis, Riley–Day syndrome, Shy–Drager, amyloidosis, Guillain–Barré, and spinal cord injuries.

○ **What is spinal shock?**

Acute high spinal cord injury (commonly at C5–6) with mechanical disruption of SNS outflow from T1 to L2 producing loss of sensation, flaccid paralysis, and loss of spinal reflexes below the level of injury. Diminished sympathetic activity results in hypotension and bradycardia secondary to vasodilatation, decreased preload (after an initial massive increase), and unopposed vagal activity.

○ **What is the duration of spinal shock?**

Symptoms may resolve within 72 hours or persist for 6–8 weeks, or longer.

○ **Can succinylcholine be used in a patient with spinal shock?**

It is safe within the first 24 hours of spinal trauma. After that, the possibility of developing life-threatening hyperkalemia increases secondary to the proliferation of extrajunctional acetylcholine receptors. If unsure of the time of injury, rocuronium may be a good alternative for securing the airway.

○ **What is autonomic hyperreflexia?**

Following the period of spinal shock, there is a gradual return of spinal reflexes. Lacking any descending central regulatory control, the SNS becomes overreactive to external stimuli, either cutaneous or visceral. This may begin as early as a few weeks or as long as 2 years after the injury to the spinal cord and is common with transection at T5 or above, and unusual with injuries below T10.

○ **What are the signs of autonomic hyperreflexia?**

With spinal cord lesions at T6 or higher, interruption of normal descending inhibitory impulses allows cutaneous or visceral stimulation below the transection to induce unopposed hyperactive sympathetic discharge (vasoconstriction and hypertension) with baroreceptor-mediated reflex bradycardia and vasodilatation above. Other symptoms include visceral and muscle spasm, sweating, piloerection, and uncontrolled motor activity below the level of the lesion. Extreme elevations in blood pressure (due to the fact that more than half the sympathetic system is unmodulated below the lesion and activated) can lead to retinal or cerebral hemorrhage, convulsions, or coma [Colachis and Clincot, 1997. See reference on page 522].

○ **What is the treatment for autonomic hyperreflexia?**

Prevention of the stimulus or pharmacological intervention. First, eliminate the predisposing factor, if possible, which is usually surgical manipulation by incision or bladder distention. Treatment for hypertension includes esmolol, labetalol, nitroglycerin, or nitroprusside in the form of boluses or infusions. Other agents that have been used are ganglionic blockers, such as trimethaphan or alpha-adrenergic antagonists, such as phentolamine or phenoxybenzamine.

○ **What are the anesthetic options for patients with a history of autonomic hyperreflexia?**

General and regional techniques can offer adequate levels of anesthesia to prevent sympathetic hyperreflexia. Regional anesthesia eliminates noxious signals from the lower sacral nerve roots, thereby preventing the reflex. Some suggest that a spinal approach is better than epidural, especially with bladder distention in urologic procedures, as there may be sparing of the sacral roots with epidural anesthesia. With general anesthesia, the depth of anesthesia is more important than the choice of agent. However, one must always be prepared to treat a hypertensive crisis.

○ **What are the signs of autonomic dysfunction in patients with diabetes mellitus?**

Diabetic autonomic neuropathy primarily involves the heart and GI tract. Clinical signs include orthostatic hypotension, hypertension, painless myocardial ischemia, diminished baroreceptor and cardiac reflexes, resting tachycardia, and gastroparesis.

○ **What are the anesthetic concerns regarding the autonomic nervous system in patients with Guillain–Barré syndrome?**

Guillain–Barré syndrome is an acute demyelinating polyneuropathy characterized by ascending motor paralysis areflexia and variable paresthesias. These patients tend to have exaggerated hypotensive and hypertensive responses and cardiac dysrhythmias (atrial tachycardia or fibrillation), which are often unresponsive to carotid massage suggestive of hypoactive vagal innervation. Observation of the EKG and invasive hemodynamic monitoring may be prudent during positioning and other surgical anesthetic stimuli. Pharyngeal muscle weakness is also a concern for airway protection and may necessitate postoperative ventilation.

○ **What is the precursor of norepinephrine synthesis?**

Tyrosine.

○ **What is the rate-controlling step in the synthesis of norepinephrine?**

Conversion of tyrosine to DOPA, a step controlled by the enzyme tyrosine hydroxylase.

○ **What are the precursors of epinephrine?**

Epinephrine is produced by the conversion of phenylalanine (phenylalanine hydroxylase) to tyrosine, tyrosine (tyrosine hydroxylase) to DOPA, DOPA (DOPA decarboxylase) to dopamine, dopamine (dopamine β-hydroxylase) to norepinephrine, and finally norepinephrine (phenylethanolamine-*N*-methyltransferase [PNMT]) to epinephrine.

○ **Where is norepinephrine converted to epinephrine?**

In the adrenal medulla, and to a limited extent in the brain. PNMT methylates NE to epinephrine.

○ **How is norepinephrine and epinephrine release by the adrenal medulla regulated differently from that of the neurotransmitter?**

The adrenal medulla is homologous to sympathetic ganglia. Cholinergic preganglionic fibers of the SNS release acetylcholine and stimulate the adrenal medulla to release catecholamines. Stimuli include hypotension, hypothermia, hypoglycemia, hypercapnia, hypoxemia, fear, and pain. Norepinephrine is the adrenergic neurotransmitter of the SNS that is released by postganglionic fibers at end-organ tissues (heart, smooth muscle, and glands).

○ **Biosynthesis of NE in sympathetic nerve terminals involves what intermediaries?**

Tyrosine, DOPA, and dopamine.

○ **Once dopamine is formed in the cytoplasm of the sympathetic nerve terminal, what happens to it?**

Dopamine is taken up into the storage vesicles in the sympathetic nerve terminal where it is converted to norepinephrine by dopamine-β-hydroxylase.

○ **Name two drugs that block the reuptake of norepinephrine causing an enhanced response to catecholamines?**

Cocaine and tricyclic antidepressants.

○ **A parkinsonian patient requires urgent coronary artery bypass graft surgery while he is taking selegiline (selective inhibitor of monoamine oxidase [MAO] type B). Should the patient stop taking MAO inhibitors (MAOIs) prior to surgery?**

Although earlier recommendation was to discontinue these drugs 14 days prior to surgery, it is shown that anesthesia can be safely administered in patients treated with MAOIs [Stoelting's Co-existing Disease, 2008].

However, indirect-acting sympathomimetics and meperidine must be avoided in these patients to prevent an exaggerated response and hyperpyrexia, respectively.

○ **What are MAO type A and B?**

MAOIs act by inhibition of the metabolic breakdown of norepinephrine, serotonin, or dopamine by the MAO enzyme. MAO type A preferentially deaminates serotonin and norepinephrine and also selectively dopamine. MAO type B metabolizes dopamine, phenylethylamine, and various trace amines. MAOIs can be divided into reversible and irreversible types. Irreversible inhibitors (e.g., selegiline, phenelzine, tranylcypromine) take 1–4 weeks after cessation for the enzyme to regain its activity. Therefore, for the surgical perspective, earlier recommendation was a period of discontinuation of 2 weeks of the irreversible blockade MAO for its restoration. On the other hand, reversible MAOI (e.g., moclobemide) has a half-life of only 1–3 hours.

○ **Describe the interaction of MAOIs and opioids.**

MAO is the enzyme responsible for deamination of monoamines such as serotonin, dopamine, norepinephrine, and epinephrine. MAOIs irreversibly complex with the enzyme and as a result the monoamine concentration increases in the CNS. Administration of opioids, especially meperidine, can lead to (Type 1) excitatory response (hyperpyrexia, agitation, skeletal muscle rigidity, and headache) or a (Type 2) depressive response (hypotension, depression of ventilation, and coma). Derivatives of meperidine (fentanyl, sufentanil, and alfentanil) have been associated with similar adverse reactions, although the incidence is much smaller. The opioid effects of morphine may be potentiated but it is not associated with the above effects.

Meperidine, pentazocine, and dextromethorphan block presynaptic reuptake of serotonin and potentiate development of serotonin syndrome.

○ **How might a hypertensive crisis be avoided in patients taking MAOIs?**

A hypertensive crisis may be avoided by refraining from foods containing tyramine or medications that cause the presynaptic release of endogenous catecholamines (exaggerated responses to vasopressors and sympathetic stimulation). Direct-acting vasopressors are first-line therapy. Sympathomimetic agents to avoid include ketamine, pancuronium, ephedrine, and epinephrine-containing solutions. Meperidine can cause hyperthermia, seizures, and coma.

Hazardous interactions may be seen with both reversible and irreversible MAOIs.

Decreased presynaptic metabolism of catecholamines and serotonin by MAOIs may be responsible for hemodynamic instability, hyperpyrexia, and death when these patients are exposed to stress and anesthesia. Indirectly acting sympathomimetics (amphetamine, ephedrine, metaraminol) produce epinephrine-related hypertensive crisis. Directly acting sympathomimetics (norepinephrine, epinephrine, isoprenaline) are regarded as safe.

○ **How should you conduct general anesthesia in these patients?**

Avoid meperidine (hyperpyrexic coma) and indirect-acting sympathomimetic drugs (hypertensive crisis). Anticipate hemodynamic instability. If an adverse drug reaction occurs, convert from a narcotic-based anesthetic to a volatile anesthetic technique with postoperative sedative infusion. All patients are considered to be at some level of risk. "MAOI-safe" surgery recommends use of morphine and fentanyl.

MAOI also causes inhibition of hepatic microsomal enzymes, leading to accumulation of free narcotics and CNS depression. Therefore, use morphine and fentanyl with close observation.

○ **Is neuraxial anesthesia safe in patients taking MAOIs?**

Epidural and intrathecal anesthesia result in a blockade of sympathetic system. Therefore, there is a potential for this type of anesthetics to produce hypotension and consequent need for vasopressors. Therefore, some anesthesiologists may favor general anesthesia. If vasopressors are needed, direct-acting drugs such as phenylephrine are recommended at reduced doses to minimize exaggerated hypertensive response as seen in these patients.

The addition of epinephrine to local anesthetic solutions should probably be avoided.

○ **What are some sympathetic agonists with alpha effects?**

Phenylephrine has predominantly alpha 1 agonist activity (high doses may stimulate alpha 2 and beta receptors). The primary effect is peripheral vasoconstriction with rise in systemic vascular resistance and arterial blood pressure. Reflex bradycardia can reduce cardiac output. Direct vasoconstrictive effect on the coronary arteries increases coronary blood flow.

Methyldopa is an example of alpha 2 agonist with a central action. This results in decrease in sympathetic tone and fall in peripheral vascular resistance.

Clonidine is another alpha 2 agonist used for antihypertensive and negative chronotropic effect.

Clonidine also decreases anesthetic and analgesic requirement and causes sedation and anxiolysis. During regional anesthesia clonidine prolongs the duration of nerve block. The other benefits include decreased postoperative shivering, inhibition of opioid-induced muscle rigidity, and attenuation of opioid withdrawal syndrome. Side effects of clonidine are bradycardia, hypotension, dry mouth, respiratory depression, and sedation.

○ **What are some sympathetic agonists with alpha and beta effects?**

Both ephedrine and epinephrine stimulate alpha 1, beta 1, and beta 2 receptors. The cardiovascular effects are increase in blood pressure, heart rate, contractility, and cardiac output. Both cause bronchodilation. However, there are important differences between the two drugs. Since ephedrine is a noncatecholamine (like phenylephrine) it has a longer duration, is much less potent, has direct and indirect effects, and causes stimulation of central nervous system (increases MAC).

Norepinephrine causes direct alpha stimulation and beta 1 activity. In the absence of beta 2 activity it causes intense (arterial and venous) vasoconstriction. Extravasation therefore can cause tissue necrosis.

○ **What are beta-adrenergic effects?**

The stimulation of beta 1 receptors located in the heart causes positive chronotropic (increased heart rate), dromotropic (increased conduction), and inotropic (increased contractility).

The stimulation of beta 2 receptors that are primarily located in smooth muscles and gland cells causes relaxation of smooth muscle. This results in bronchodilation, vasodilation, and relaxation of the uterus, bladder, and gut.

Beta 2 receptor activation also causes glycogenolysis, lipolysis, gluconeogenesis, and insulin release. Activation of sodium potassium pump by beta 2 agonist drives potassium intracellularly and can induce hypokalemia.

Beta 3 receptors are found in the gall bladder and brain adipose tissue. They may play role in lipolysis and thermogenesis in brown fat.

○ **What type of receptors does norepinephrine bind?**

Norepinephrine binds both types of adrenergic receptors: α_1 and $\beta_1 > \beta_2$.

○ **What happens to norepinephrine after it binds to alpha 1 and beta-adrenergic receptors?**

There are several mechanisms for terminating the action of norepinephrine. The majority is taken up into the nerve ending and re-stored in synaptic vesicles to be re-released or deaminated by MAO. Uptake by non-neuronal tissues or metabolism by MAO and/or COMT in the blood, liver, and kidney also occurs, to a limited extent.

○ **A patient on isoproterenol 3 μg/kg/min is hypotensive. Why?**

Isoproterenol is a pure beta-adrenergic agonist. The β_2-vasodilating effect reduces systemic vascular resistance and diastolic blood pressure. Recommended infusion rate is 2–10 mcg/min to clinical response. A dose of 3 μg/kg/min is too high.

○ **Why is the administration of beta-agonists relatively ineffective in the treatment of chronic congestive heart failure?**

Tolerance or downregulation of cardiac beta-receptors.

○ **T/F: Administration of epinephrine is contraindicated in patients taking β-1 adrenergic blocking drugs (cardioselective).**

False. Unopposed α-responses with the administration of epinephrine is a potential problem in patients taking nonselective beta-blockers, but it is not contraindicated.

○ **What are the hemodynamic effects of alpha-blockers?**

Alpha-blockers act by preventing adrenergic activity. An example of an alpha-blocker is phentolamine.

Alpha 1 antagonism and direct smooth muscle relaxation causes peripheral vasodilation and decrease in blood pressure. The drop in blood pressure provokes reflex tachycardia. This tachycardia is augmented by blockade of alpha 2 receptors in the heart since alpha 2 blockade promotes release of norepinephrine by eliminating negative feedback.

The degree of the response to alpha agonist depends on the degree of existing sympathetic tone.

○ **A newborn of a mother treated with propranolol for hyperthyroidism during pregnancy is diagnosed with bradycardia and hypoglycemia. What is the most likely explanation?**

Beta antagonists can cross the placenta and cause these symptoms in the fetus, especially toward the end of the third trimester. Nonselective beta-blockers decrease glycogenolysis that ordinarily occurs in response to the release of epinephrine during hypoglycemia.

○ **Do beta-adrenergic blockers affect plasma potassium concentration?**

Beta-adrenergic blockers inhibit the uptake of potassium into skeletal muscle; therefore, the plasma concentration of potassium is increased.

○ **Describe carotid sinus innervation and effects of carotid sinus stimulation.**

Baroreceptors (pressure sensors) located in the aortic arch and the carotid sinuses react to alterations in stretch caused by blood pressure leading to alterations in heart rate.

Increase in mean arterial pressure (MAP) stretches the walls of the carotid sinus. This stretch increases the firing rate of sensory fibers in the carotid sinus nerve (glossopharyngeal), which informs the vasomotor center that MAP is above 100 mm Hg (or SBP > 170 mm Hg), which seems to be the body's set point for MAP. The vasomotor center responds by increasing the firing rate of cardiac vagal fibers and decreasing the firing rate of cardiac sympathetic fibers, so that heart rate and contractility are decreased. Simultaneously, the vasomotor center will decrease the firing rate of sympathetic vasoconstrictor fibers to the arterioles so that peripheral resistance falls. All these changes will act to reduce arterial pressure.

○ **Which anesthetic agents will depress the normal baroreceptor activity?**

All volatile anesthetic agents depress normal baroreceptor response. However, isoflurane, desflurane, and sevoflurane appear to have the least effect while halothane blocks the baroreceptor activity.

Propofol also suppress baroreceptor activity. Heart rate does not change significantly after an induction dose because propofol may reset or inhibit the baroreflex, reducing the response to hypotension.

Key Terms

Albuterol versus ipratropium pharmacology

Autonomic hyperreflexia/pathophysiology/signs/
  anesthetic technique

Autonomic nervous system: anatomy

Autonomic neurotransmitters

Baroreceptor: anesthetic effects

Beta stimulation pharmacodynamics

Beta-adrenergic effects

Bronchomotor tone: catecholamines

Cardiovascular pharmacology: catecholamines

Carotid sinus innervation

Central anticholinergic syndrome: treatment

Clonidine withdrawal

Hemodynamic effects of alpha-blockers

Hyperreflexia: anesthetic considerations

Ipratropium: mechanism of action

Mechanism of action of glycopyrrolate

Mechanism of epinephrine hyperglycemia

Neurotransmitter receptors

Oral clonidine: MAC effect

Parasympathetic physiology

Physostigmine pharmacology

Rebound hypertension: causative drugs

Scopolamine reversal

Subarachnoid block and autonomic hyperreflexia

Sympathetic agonists: alpha versus beta

Sympathetic nervous system transmitters

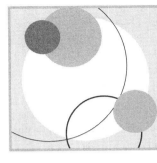

Blood Therapy

What lies behind us and what lies before us are small matters compared to what lies within us.
Ralph Waldo Emerson

○ **What is a massive transfusion?**

Massive transfusion is defined as the transfusion of blood approximately equal to the total body blood volume within 24 hours. In a normal adult, this is approximately 10 Units.

○ **What are potential problems with massive blood transfusion?**

Hypothermia, thrombocytopenia, hypokalemia, hyperkalemia, dilution of clotting factors, acidosis, ARDS, pulmonary edema, hypocalcemia, and hypomagnesemia due to citrate intoxication, hepatitis, or other infectious diseases.

○ **What is the most common complication of massive transfusion?**

The traditional answer: dilutional thrombocytopenia. In current practice, this may not be true when packed red blood cells (PRBCs) are used for massive transfusion. It has been shown that coagulation factors (fresh frozen plasma [FFP]) are necessary after ≥12 U and patients who received 20 or more PRBCs require platelet therapy.

○ **Which clotting factors are most likely to be decreased as a result of massive transfusion?**

Factors V and fibrinogen. With the use of **PRBCs**, fibrinogen levels decrease significantly in contrast to the use of whole blood, in which fibrinogen levels remain unchanged unless DIC is present. Factor VIII is probably stored in endothelial cells and released during surgical stress.

○ **What causes coagulopathy in massively transfused patients?**

Multifactorial etiology: dilutional thrombocytopenia, depletion of coagulation factors (V, VIII, and fibrinogen), and DIC. Risk factors include the volume of blood given and the duration of hypotension and hypoperfusion. Hemolytic transfusion reaction also causes coagulopathy and should be considered [Boliger et al., 2010. See reference on page 523].

○ **How should dilutional coagulopathy from massive packed cell transfusion be treated?**

During massive transfusions of PRBCs, patients receive only a small residual plasma volume (50 mL), which contains clotting factors. Investigations of patients receiving large-volume isovolemic transfusions suggest that clinically significant dilution of fibrinogen; factors II, V, and VIII; and platelets will occur after volume exchange

67

of approximately 140%, 200–230%, and 230% (1.4, 2, 2.3 blood volumes), respectively. Resuscitation from hypovolemia will result in reaching these thresholds at smaller percentage volume exchanges. Treatments includes cryoprecipitate (fibrinogen), FFP (clotting factors), and platelet transfusions [Barash et al., 2009, Miller, 2010].

○ **What is a type and screen and how is it performed?**

Type and screen is ABO–Rh typing and antibody screening. ABO typing is performed by testing red blood cells (RBCs) for A and B antigens, and the serum for A and B antibodies. Recipient serum is mixed with commercially prepared type O RBCs and incubated. If no agglutination is observed, the screen is negative. If the screen is positive, serum is tested using selected reagent RBCs to identify the antibodies present.

○ **What should be done if the type and screen report indicates screen positive?**

The blood bank performs an antibody identification, and sets aside 2 RBC U that lack the corresponding antigens. This is done in advance of surgery.

○ **What are the three phases of type and crossmatch of blood?**

Immediate phase, incubation phase, and antiglobulin phase.

1. The first phase combines recipient serum and donor cells to test ABO group compatibility at room temperature. It also identifies MN, P, and Lewis incompatibilities. This phase takes approximately 5 minutes.
2. The second phase incubates the products from the first in albumin at 37°C, enhancing incomplete antibodies. This phase primarily detects antibodies in the Rh system.
3. The last phase is the indirect antiglobulin test. Antiglobulin serum is added to the previously incubated test tubes. This phase aids in the detection of incomplete antibodies in Rh, Kell, Duffy, and Kidd systems.

○ **What is the incompatibility risk of typed blood, screened blood, and fully crossmatched blood?**

The risk of incompatibility of ABO/Rh-compatible blood is 0.1–0.2% (99.8% *safe*) if the patient has never been transfused. The risk increases to 1.0% if the patient has had a previous transfusion. Adding a negative antibody screen decreases the risk to 0.06% (99.94% *safe*). Fully crossmatched blood should carry a risk less than 0.05% (99.95% *safe*) [Miller, 2010].

○ **What is the most common blood group? What percentage of the population is Rh positive?**

The most common blood group is type O. Forty-five percent of Caucasians, 49% of American blacks, 79% of American Indians, and 40% of Asians are blood type O. Approximately 85% of the population is Rh positive and 15% Rh negative [Barash et al., 2009].

○ **List three ways of collecting autologous blood for transfusion.**

Predonation of the patient's blood days or weeks prior to surgery, *intraoperative isovolemic hemodilution* using blood withdrawal and simultaneous volume replacement with cell-free substitutes, or *perioperative blood salvage* during and immediately after surgery.

○ **What are the relative contraindications to autologous blood donation?**

Severe aortic stenosis, severe left main coronary artery disease, anemia, recent myocardial infarction or unstable angina, hypertrophic cardiomyopathy, active bacterial infection, or low blood volume (weight <100 lb).

○ **Describe the process of intraoperative autotransfusion.**

Intraoperative autotransfusion is defined as the reinfusion of patient blood salvaged during the operation. Red "cell savers" collect and anticoagulate the salvaged blood with citrate or heparin as it leaves the surgical field, filter to remove debris and clots, wash with saline, and concentrate RBCs by centrifugation, and the concentrate is then reinfused to the patient suspended in saline in aliquots of 125–225 mL with an Hct of 45–65%.

○ **What are the potential complications of intraoperative blood salvage (IBS)?**

Cost, contamination, removal of essential blood components (clotting factors and platelets), and air embolism.

  a. Reinfusion of materials that might remain after the washing process such as fat, microaggregates, air, red cell stroma, free hemoglobin, heparin, bacteria, tumor, and debris from a contaminated surgical field.

  b. Massive air embolism has been reported. Direct return of blood to the patient from the cell saver device and the use of pressure infusor devices applied to the collected blood bags are not recommended.

  c. Dilutional coagulopathy is associated with large-volume IBS because washing removes clotting factors and most of the platelets. DIC-like coagulopathy has also been reported especially with the older cell saver devices.

○ **What is acute normovolemic hemodilution (ANH)?**

This is a point-of-care method of autologous blood procurement.

The term ANH refers to the removal of blood from a surgical patient immediately before or just after induction of anesthesia (1–1.5 L, to a hematocrit of 27–33%), and replacement with asanguinous fluid to maintain normovolemia. The removed blood is stored in a CPD bag at room temperature up to 6 hours to preserve platelet function and later reinfused. ANH is employed to reduce the need for allogeneic blood and to avoid potential transfusion-associated complications. An additional potential advantage of ANH is improvement in tissue perfusion as a result of decreased viscosity.

The presence of malignancy or wound infection may contraindicate blood recovery during surgery (cell saver), but not ANH.

○ **What is the rationale for acute hemodilution?**

During surgery, the patient will lose blood at a lower hematocrit and the fresh whole blood withdrawn immediately prior to surgery will be available for reinfusion. This procedure may reduce total red cell volume loss, enhance the maximum allowable blood loss before blood transfusion, as well as reduce the need for transfusion of allogeneic blood.

○ **In isovolemic hemodilution, what mechanisms serve to maintain oxygen delivery?**

Increase in cardiac output (CO), redistribution of blood flow to organs with greater oxygen requirements, increased oxygen extraction, and decreased hemoglobin oxygen affinity.

○ **What is the effect of normovolemic hemodilution to a hematocrit of 28% from 41% on heart rate, blood pressure, and CO in healthy elderly patients?**

In healthy elderly patients, with normovolemic hemodilution, the hematocrit is reduced from 41% to 28%, stroke volume increases with heart rate, and blood pressure remains unchanged. Venous return, right atrial pressure, and CO are increased secondary to decreased viscosity and systemic vascular resistance and increased contractility. There is a reduction in oxygen delivery as a result of the failure to fully compensate for the lowered oxygen-carrying capacity by an increased CO. Oxygen delivery is maximum in the hematocrit range of 35–45%.

○ **What is the primary reason for increase in CO with isovolemic hemodilution?**

Anemia must be fairly severe (hemoglobin <7 g/dL) before CO increases. The rise in CO is related mainly to a decrease in blood viscosity and enhanced sympathetic stimulation. As hematocrit decreases, a reduction in blood viscosity causes a decrease in peripheral vascular resistance and increase in stroke volume (increased venomotor tone and venous return), so that CO rises without an increase in blood pressure.

○ **What happens to the oxygen transport during hemodilution?**

Over a wide range of hematocrits (usually between 30% and 45%), isovolemic hemodilution is self-correcting. The decrease in the oxygen-carrying capacity of the blood due to decreased RBCs is matched by improvement in oxygen transport due to improved blood flow to the tissues. Decreasing hematocrit from 40% to 20% decreases the viscosity by 50%.

○ **What is the cardiovascular effect of acute anemia in an otherwise healthy patient?**

Basic CO can rise 5-fold to maintain oxygen delivery. As plasma volume increases, the hematocrit decreases (euvolemia is achieved without RBC transfusion), resulting in reduction in blood viscosity and peripheral vascular resistance. Heart rate does not increase in the absence of hypovolemia. Redistribution of blood flow to the heart and brain occurs with increased tissue oxygen extraction.

○ **A patient's oxygen delivery is impaired by severe anemia. What are the compensatory mechanisms?**

Oxygen delivery is determined by arterial oxygen content and CO. In severe anemia, arterial oxygen content (normally 20 mL O_2/dL blood with hemoglobin 15 g/dL) is decreased. The compensatory mechanisms in anemia are to increase CO and tissue oxygen extraction.

○ **How does a healthy heart compensate for anemia during hemodilution?**

By redistribution of blood flow to the coronary circulation. Under basal conditions the heart already has a high extraction ratio (ER; between 50–70% and 30% in most other tissues).

○ **What is ER (Extraction Ratio)?**

The ER defines what fraction of the total oxygen delivered is consumed or extracted by the tissues; ER = oxygen consumption/oxygen delivery. In healthy resting adults the overall ER of oxygen from capillary blood is about 25%, but may increase to 70–80% during maximal exercise in well-trained athletes.

○ **What is the relationship between oxygen extraction ratio (O_2ER) and anemia?**

As the hematocrit decreases below normal, there is a decrease in systemic oxygen delivery, but the O_2ER increases, which helps maintain a constant oxygen uptake in the tissues. The point at which the compensatory increase in oxygen extraction begins to fail corresponds to an oxygen ER of 0.5 (50%). Many institutions use this value as a transfusion trigger, when this information is available.

○ **What is the reason for decreased hemoglobin oxygen affinity in anemia?**

Increased 2,3-diphosphoglycerate. In chronic anemia, increased oxygen extraction by tissues produces increased concentration of deoxyhemoglobin in the RBC, which stimulates the production of 2,3-DPG and lowers the affinity of hemoglobin A for oxygen.

○ **Which data may be useful in determining a RBC transfusion threshold?**

CO, arterial and mixed venous oxygen, and the whole-body ER.

○ **What are indicators of inadequate oxygen delivery to tissues?**

Although total oxygen delivery (DO_2) and oxygen uptake (VO_2) can be directly measured, they cannot be measured at the tissue or cellular level. Inadequate oxygen delivery to tissues produces hypoperfusion, ischemia, and evidence of anaerobic metabolism. Clinical indicators are hypotension, decreased urine output, and altered mental status, which are nonspecific and late developing. Laboratory indicators include acidosis, worsening base deficit, anion gap, and lactate levels. Gastric tonometry (measuring CO_2/pH) can be used as a measure of oxygen debt in the splanchnic circulation. The tongue has also been used as a site of measurement where elevations in sublingual CO_2 represent potential hypoperfusion.

○ **What values may indicate significantly impaired oxygen delivery?**

There is no safe level of mixed venous oxygen, but acutely ill patients are at risk when SvO_2 <0.60–0.65 and oxygen extraction exceeds 65–75%. Reduction of total oxygen consumption <50% baseline indicates significantly impaired oxygen delivery. Blood lactate concentration is an unreliable indicator of tissue hypoxia.

○ **What happens once the critical threshold for hemoglobin is reached during hemodilution?**

According to the studies, at Hct of 10% and a whole-body ER of approximately 50%, no further increase in oxygen consumption (VO_2) occurs; the tissue converts to anaerobic metabolism, which leads to metabolic acidosis and hemodynamic instability. Death occurs due to high output failure with severe tissue hypoxia.

○ **What is "critical oxygen delivery?"**

Oxygen consumption is usually independent of delivery due to compensatory increased extraction. Critical oxygen delivery is the point at which oxygen delivery is no longer capable of supporting cellular respiration because extraction exceeds a critical threshold, and oxygen consumption becomes directly proportional to oxygen delivery. Progressive lactic acidosis results from cellular hypoxia.

○ **What is the formula to calculate oxygen delivery?**

Tissue oxygen delivery (DO_2) is the product of blood flow and arterial oxygen content, and at the whole-body level represented by the product of CO and the arterial oxygen content. $DO_2 = CO [(Hb \times 1.39) SaO_2 + 0.003 PaO_2]$, where CO is the cardiac output, Hb is the hemoglobin, SaO_2 is the arterial oxygen saturation, and PaO_2 is the partial pressure of oxygen in arterial blood.

○ **How can you estimate the volume of blood to be removed preoperatively when you are using the normovolemic hemodilution/autotransfusion technique to reduce the loss of red cells intraoperatively?**

The volume can be calculated according to the following formula: $V = EBV(\{HCT_{original} - Hct_{final}\}/Hct_{average})$, where V is the volume to be removed and EBV is the estimated blood volume (65 mL/kg multiplied by weight [kg]).

○ **What is the normal blood volume in adults, children, infants, and neonates?**

Adults 70 (men 75 and women 65); children 75; infants 80; full-term neonates 85 (mL/kg).

○ **According to the CDC-RBC panel, what are the indications for perioperative RBC transfusion?**

The Consensus Development Conference-RBC panel (September 1984) concluded that the sole indication for erythrocyte transfusion was to increase oxygen-carrying capacity. In a healthy individual, an Hgb of 7 or greater was considered safe, and an Hgb of 10 appropriate for those with compromised critical organs.

Association of Anaesthetists of Great Britain and Ireland (June 2008) – guidelines for transfusion of red cells:

1. A hemoglobin concentration of 8–10 g/dL is a safe level even for patients with significant cardiorespiratory disease.

2. A hemoglobin concentration <7 g/dL is a strong indication for transfusion.

3. When the hemoglobin concentration decreases to 5 g/dL, transfusion will become essential.

In summary, the use of a single hemoglobin "trigger" of 10 g/dL of hemoglobin for surgical transfusion is no longer recommended. One must consider all physiologic and surgical factors that place the patient at risk for complications of inadequate oxygenation. Those without compromised critical organ blood flow can be transfused at an Hgb of 6–7 g/dL. Prolonged times with an Hgb <5 g/dL are associated with poor outcomes [Practice Guidelines for Perioperative Blood Transfusion and Adjuvant Therapies Anesthesiology, 2006. See reference on page 523].

○ **How can you calculate maximum allowable blood loss?**

An estimate of allowable blood loss can be calculated by using EBV, initial hematocrit, and desired ending hematocrit. Blood loss = EBV × {Hct(initial) − Hct(final)}/Hct(average). The calculation assumes euvolemia is maintained.

○ **What is the difference in volume and components between FFP and cryoprecipitate?**

The main difference is that cryoprecipitate has much more fibrinogen. FFP (225 mL) contains 1 U/mL of all procoagulants and 3–4 mg/mL of fibrinogen. A single donor unit of cryoprecipitate (10 mL) contains 80–145 U of factor VIII, 250 mg of fibrinogen, von Willebrand factor, factor XIII, and fibronectin.

○ **How is FFP prepared?**

After removal of RBCs from the whole blood, remaining platelet-rich plasma (PRP) is further centrifuged to separate the platelets from the plasma. The remaining plasma contains all the blood coagulation factors, fibrinogen, and other plasma proteins. The plasma is frozen within 6 hours of donation to prevent inactivation of temperature-sensitive coagulation factors V and VIII.

○ **How is FFP administered?**

Prior to the administration of FFP, it must be thawed in a water bath at 30–37°C with agitation, which takes approximately 30 minutes. After thawing, the units of FFP are stored at 1–6°C and must be transfused within 24 hours. FFP should be administered through a component administration set with a 170-μm filter.

○ **What are the indications for administration of FFP?**

According to the updated report by the ASA Task Force on Perioperative Blood Transfusion and Adjuvant Therapies (2006), FFP transfusion is indicated for:

1. Correction of excessive microvascular bleeding (coagulopathy) in the presence of PT >1.5 times normal, INR >2.0, or aPTT >2 times normal

2. Correction of coagulopathy secondary to transfusion of more than one blood volume when PT/INR or aPTT cannot be obtained in a timely fashion

3. Urgent reversal of warfarin therapy

4. Correction of known coagulation deficiencies for which specific concentrates are not available

5. Heparin resistance (antithrombin III deficiency) in a patient requiring heparin

FFP is given to achieve a minimum of 30% plasma factor concentration.

○ **How is cryoprecipitate prepared and administered?**

Cryoprecipitate is prepared from a unit of FFP. It is the cold-insoluble white precipitate that forms when a bag of FFP is thawed at 1–6°C. This cold-insoluble material is removed following centrifugation and immediately frozen at −18°C and can be stored for up to 1 year.

Cryoprecipitate must be transfused rapidly and within 4–6 hours of thawing if given to replace factor VIII levels. Units are usually pooled and should be given through a 170-μm component filter.

○ **What are the indications for cryoprecipitate administration?**

According to the updated report by the ASA Task Force on Perioperative Blood Transfusion and Adjuvant Therapies (2006), cryoprecipitate transfusion is indicated for:

1. When the fibrinogen concentration is <80–100 mg/dL in the presence of microvascular bleeding

2. To correct excessive microvascular bleeding in massively transfused patients when fibrinogen concentration cannot be measured in a timely fashion

3. Patients with congenital fibrinogen deficiencies

○ **What is the difference between high- and intermediate-purity factor VIII concentrates? What are the indications for transfusing them?**

The intermediate-purity concentrate contains significant therapeutic quantities of the von Willebrand component of factor VIII, whereas the high-purity preparations contain principally the hemophilia A component of factor VIII (VIII-C). Intermediate-purity factor VIII concentrates are preferred for von Willebrand disease and recombinant or highly purified factor VIII concentrate for hemophilia A.

○ **How is platelet concentrate prepared and how many platelets are in a platelet transfusion?**

Platelet concentrate is prepared from whole blood within 8 hours of collection. After the collection of approximately 500 mL of whole blood into collection bags containing citrate-based anticoagulant preservative solution, the blood is centrifuged. Following centrifugation, the Platelet Rich Plasma (PRP) is separated into an attached empty satellite bag. This PRP is centrifuged again and separated into 1 U of platelet concentrate and 1 U of plasma. Each unit of platelets contains approximately 5.5×10^{10} platelets in 50–70 mL of plasma. An adult dose pack of platelets contains 6–7 U of platelet concentrate.

○ **How are platelet pheresis units ("single donor") prepared?**

Platelet pheresis units are obtained by performing apheresis on volunteer donors. During this procedure, large volumes of donor blood are processed into extracorporeal circuit and centrifuged to separate the components. The red cells and plasma are returned to the donor. From a single donor, the equivalent of 5–8 U is obtained and suspended in a volume 200–400 mL of plasma.

○ **How are platelets administered?**

Both platelets and platelets pheresis may be stored at room temperature (20–24°C) for up to 5 days with continuous gentle agitation to prevent platelet aggregation. Platelets can be infused through a platelet or standard component administration set with a 170-μm filter. Microaggregate filters (20–24 μm) should not be used because they will remove most of the platelets.

○ **Is it necessary to administer ABO-specific platelets?**

The administration of ABO-specific platelets is not required because platelet concentrates contain few RBCs (where ABO antigens are expressed). However, the administration of pooled platelet components of various ABO types can transfuse plasma containing anti-A and/or anti-B, resulting in human leukocyte antigen (HLA) antibody formation.

○ **What are the indications for platelet transfusion?**

Correction of a deficiency in either platelet number (thrombocytopenia) or platelet function in patients at risk for bleeding or with evidence of clinically significant bleeding.

Perioperative factors to consider for the transfusion of platelets for a borderline platelet count of 50–100,000/dL include the type of surgery, anticipated and actual blood loss, extent of microvascular bleeding, presence of medications (aspirin), and disorders known to affect platelet function or coagulation (uremia).

The prophylactic administration of platelets is not recommended in patients with chronic thrombocytopenia caused by increased platelet destruction (idiopathic thrombocytopenic purpura). Prophylactic platelet transfusion is rarely indicated when the count is >100,000/dL and is usually indicated perioperatively when the count is below 50,000/dL. Spontaneous bleeding may occur with counts <20,000/dL.

○ **How much does the transfusion of 1 U of platelets increase the platelet count?**

In an adult, 1 U of platelet concentrate generally increases the platelet count by approximately 5,000–8,000/mm^3.

○ **Should the PRBCs be diluted before administration to ensure rapid infusion?**

When additive solutions such as Adsol® are used, no dilution is necessary. For PRBCs stored in preservatives in which the hematocrit may be as high as 70–80%, 60–100 mL of 0.9% saline can be added to facilitate rapid infusion and minimize hemolysis. Although the infusion flow rate of the diluted unit and total volume infused will be increased compared with the undiluted state, the time required for transfusion of 90% of the red cell mass is unchanged.

○ **Which solutions are considered "incompatible" with PRBCs?**

Lactated Ringer's (theoretical clot formation due to calcium) and 5% dextrose in water or 0.2% saline and plasmanate (hemolysis).

○ **What is the potassium load with transfusion?**

The extracellular concentration of potassium in stored blood steadily increases with time. The amount of potassium transfused is typically <4 mEq/U. Transfusion rates exceeding 100 mL/min may predispose to hyperkalemia (and hypocalcemia).

○ **Does a massive transfusion produce hyperkalemia?**

Except with patients in whom blood replacement fails to restore perfusion and reverse the acidosis, hyperkalemia rarely occurs in a massive transfusion. There is a progressive fall in the serum potassium levels in a massive transfusion, and this fall is related to the volume transfused. Hypokalemia is commonly encountered perioperatively due to citrate metabolism to bicarbonate producing a metabolic alkalosis and intracellular shifts of potassium.

○ **What is the incidence of posttransfusion hepatitis from any cause?**

Negligible, and probably warrants a case report. Eighty-five percent of posttransfusion hepatitis from infective agents is caused by hepatitis C virus. Prior to 1990, there were no screening tests for HCV. The rate of posttransfusion HCV infection has since decreased from 8% to 10% to less than 1 chance per 2 million U of blood or blood products transfused [Dodd, 2007. See reference on page 523].

The incidence of hepatitis B (HBV) transmission is estimated to be 1 in 205,000. Hepatitis A, for which there is no carrier state, is rarely seen in association with transfusion (1 in 10^6). With the use of nucleic acid technology (NAT) window period is reduced to 12 days for hepatitis C and 10 days for HIV. For hepatitis B, NAT is not yet available and therefore using hepatitis B surface antigen (HbsAg) as the screening test, the window period is 59 days.

○ **What is the incidence of HIV-1 transmission from transfusion?**

With the use of NAT the window of infectivity, which is the time from being infected to a positive test result, has decreased to 10 days. The incidence of HIV transmission has decreased to less than 1 chance per 2 million U of blood or blood products transfused [Dodd, 2007. See reference on page 523].

○ **A patient being seen for her preoperative evaluation prior to knee surgery would like to donate her own blood. Her surgery is in 2 days. Recommendations?**

The most practical schedule for obtaining more than 1 U of autologous blood is to draw units at weekly intervals for 3 weeks, preferably having the last unit withdrawn 1 week and no fewer than 72 hours prior to surgery. Donation 2 days prior to surgery is extremely unlikely to affect homologous blood transfusion requirements.

○ **Should FFP be used to neutralize heparin?**

FFP is contraindicated to neutralize heparin. It is a source of antithrombin III and transfusion could instead potentiate the action of heparin. Heparin resistance may result from low antithrombin III, which is increased with FFP transfusion.

○ **If there is a greater than 40% probability of transfusing a patient during surgery, what would be the appropriate preoperative order to Transfusion Services?**

Type and crossmatch. ABO group and Rh type of the patient are determined, an antibody screening test is performed, and compatible units of blood are made available before surgery.

○ **When would it be appropriate to require preoperative type and screen blood orders?**

If there is only a modest possibility of transfusion (<10%), and in cases with possible blood loss where the patient is multiparous or has had a prior transfusion (indicating possible difficulty crossmatching in an emergency). ABO group and Rh type of a patient are determined and a screening test is performed on a patient's serum for "unexpected" red cell alloantibodies. The screening test takes 30–120 minutes to complete and remains valid for 72 hours. If the antibody screen is negative, fully crossmatched blood can be available within 15–30 minutes.

○ **Compare the following terms: "type and hold," "type and screen," and "type and cross."**

Type and hold: ABO and Rh types are determined.

Type and screen: ABO and Rh types are determined. Additionally, the patient's serum is screened against group O donor RBCs with known antigens that will react with antibodies that are commonly implicated in hemolytic transfusion reactions.

Type and cross: type and screen plus a crossmatch. Crossmatching involves adding the patient's serum to actual donor RBCs to detect antigen/antibody reactions.

○ **What is the difference between the whole blood lost by the patient and stored whole blood for transfusion?**

In stored whole blood, platelet function is 5% of normal after 48 hours of storage at 4°C. There is also progressive loss of factors V and VIII to 15% and 50% of normal, respectively, after 21 days of storage.

○ **Is stored blood acidic or basic? What happens with transfusion?**

Stored CPDA-1 blood is acidic with a pH between 6.6 and 6.9. Citrate in the anticoagulant and erythrocyte metabolism producing lactate and CO_2 contribute to the acidity. With adequate tissue perfusion, citrate and lactate are metabolized to bicarbonate with transfusion.

○ **Describe the storage defect in blood.**

↓ pH due to RBC conversion of glucose to lactate

↓ 2,3-DPG

↓ ATP

↓ Glucose

↑ Plasma potassium, ammonia, and hemoglobin

↑ Ionized phosphate with ↓ 2,3-DPG

WBC and platelet function lost after 24/48 hours

↓ Labile clotting factors (V, VIII)

○ **One of the complications of massive transfusion is citrate toxicity. How is citrate metabolized?**

Citrate is metabolized by the liver. Adults with hepatic dysfunction or hypothermia or those with a transfusion rate greater than 1 U of blood every 5 minutes are at risk. The signs of citrate intoxication are those of acute hypocalcemia, as citrate binds calcium.

○ **What is citrate toxicity?**

Citrate is an anticoagulant used in stored blood products. It binds ionized calcium, causing acute ionized hypocalcemia, that is, muscle tremors, hypotension, decreased CO, myocardial irritability, and ventricular fibrillation. Usually depression of CO occurs at calcium level of 0.7–0.8 mg/dL; coagulopathy only at 0.1–0.2 mg/dL. Treatment is the administration of exogenous calcium. Citrate also binds ionized magnesium; consider hypomagnesemia, especially for dysrhythmia (torsades de pointes).

○ **Should you routinely administer calcium salts IV to prevent hypocalcemia during blood transfusions?**

No, calcium administration is rarely necessary. Citrate is metabolized efficiently by the liver, and decreased ionized calcium levels should not occur unless the rate of transfusion exceeds 1 mL/kg/min or about 1 U of blood per 5 minutes in an adult. Risk factors include impaired liver function, hypoperfusion, and hypothermia. Low ionized calcium levels do not correct readily; giving IV calcium salts in doses is generally recommended (1 g), but calcium levels return toward normal when hemodynamic status improves. Therefore, even in patients with low-output states, the emphasis should be placed on correcting the underlying disorder.

○ **A Jehovah's Witness is to undergo D&C. The surgeon discussed the possibility of hemorrhage with the patient, but the patient refused transfusion based on her religious belief. During the procedure, the bleeding becomes life-threatening and the patient subsequently expires. Is the surgeon liable for the patient's death?**

If the bleeding occurred within the standards of care, the surgeon would not be liable. The patient's refusal to accept transfusion does not protect the surgeon from liability for any negligent action that may have necessitated transfusion.

○ **Is hepatitis a risk factor when albumin is given?**

No. Albumin is a blood-derived colloid and is freed of hepatitis and other viruses by heating after chemical stabilization of the protein.

○ **Blood is routinely screened for which infectious agents?**

- Hepatitis C antibody and nucleic acid test (NAT) for HCV RNA
- Antibody to hepatitis B core antigen (anti-HBc) and HBsag
- Antibody to HIV-1 and NAT for HIV 1 RNA
- Antibody to HIV-2
- Antibody to HTLV I/II
- Serologic test for syphilis
- NAT for West Nile virus RNA

○ **What laboratory tests have been recently introduced to detect HIV, hepatitis A, hepatitis B, and hepatitis C?**

Gold standard for HIV antibody since 1985: standard enzyme immunoassay (EIA) and Western blot testing. Most people will develop detectable antibody within 2–8 weeks (average 25 days). Testing detects antigens from viral envelope of HIV-1 (gp 41, gp 120, gp 160) and HIV-2 (gp 36) and core antigen (p24).

New rapid point-of-care testing includes HIV-1 antibody in urine and OraQuick Rapid HIV-1 Antibody Test for oral fluid (swab upper and lower outer gums) and plasma. New generation of tests: nucleic acid antigen test (NAT) procedure reduces the window period of HIV from 16 to 10 days.

Detection methods for acute hepatitis A, B, and C:

A: IgM anti-HAV positive

B: IgM anti-HBc positive or HBsAg positive

C: nucleic acid testing for HCV RNA

○ **Is there any role for prophylactic FFP and platelets with RBC transfusion?**

More data suggest there is no role for prophylaxis (e.g., 2 U FFP for every 10 U RBC transfused).

Transfusion of blood components should ideally be guided by laboratory evidence of coagulopathy or clinical evidence of bleeding. After two blood volumes of blood loss, FFP is usually required.

However, recent studies indicate better outcome with early transfusion when major bleeding is expected with FFP:RBC ratio of 1:1 [Boliger et al., 2010. See reference on page 523].

○ **Which blood products should be filtered?**

All blood products should be filtered through a 170-μm filter to remove small clots and debris. Smaller pore filters can be used to filter microaggregates in patients with a history of febrile transfusion reaction.

Leukocyte-depleting filters should be used to prevent alloimmunization in susceptible patients.

○ **What is hydroxyethyl starch?**

Hydroxyethyl starch (hetastarch) is a synthetic colloid solution available as a 6% solution in 0.9% sodium chloride or lactated Ringer's for volume expansion. It has been reported to affect coagulation by decreasing factor VIII:C levels and interfering with clot formation by direct movement of hetastarch molecules into the fibrin clot. It is recommended that dosage be less than 20 mL/kg to minimize difficulties with crossmatching and bleeding.

○ **What is the significance of pulmonary edema in the transfused patient?**

The most common cause of pulmonary edema after transfusion is cardiogenic, due to fluid overload, with or without left ventricular dysfunction. Rarely transfusion can provoke a noncardiogenic pulmonary edema due to transfusion-related lung injury, massive transfusion, or gram-negative sepsis.

○ **What are the main types of blood transfusion reactions? Which is the most common?**

Febrile nonhemolytic reaction, hemolytic or delayed hemolytic reaction, and allergic-urticarial-type reaction. Febrile nonhemolytic reaction is the most common. Most of the serious transfusion reactions are immunologically mediated.

○ **What is the cause and incidence of febrile reactions to blood?**

The febrile reaction is the most common mild transfusion reaction and occurs in 1–3% of transfusions. It is caused by alloantibodies (leukoagglutinins) to white blood cell platelets or other donor plasma antigens.

Fever is presumably caused by pyrogens liberated from lysed cells. It occurs more commonly in previously transfused patients. Bacterial contamination of platelets or gram-negative sepsis may produce similar findings.

○ **What is the treatment for febrile nonhemolytic reaction?**

Acetaminophen, NSAIDs, antihistamines, and leukodepleted blood products.

○ **What is transfusion-related acute lung injury (TRALI)?**

TRALI is a form of noncardiac pulmonary edema most commonly occurring within hours of transfusion of whole blood, PRBCs, and FFP. Antibodies to leukocytes, usually of donor origin, are identified in the majority of cases. This reaction should be suspected in any patient who develops dyspnea, hypotension, and fever with bilateral pulmonary edema after a transfusion in which volume overload or cardiac dysfunction is unlikely. Symptoms usually resolve within 96 hours in response to oxygen, mechanical ventilation, and fluid support to maintain blood pressure and CO. The syndrome is fatal in 5% of cases [Hendrickson and Hillyer, 2009. See reference on page 523].

○ **What are the anticipated benefits of prestorage leukoreduction of donor blood?**

1. Decreased transmission of variant Creutzfeldt–Jakob disease (vCJD or mad cow disease), cytomegalovirus (CMV)
2. Decreased leukocyte-induced immunomodulation and other leukocyte-induced transfusion reactions
3. Decreased postoperative mortality

○ **If you need to transfuse blood in an immunosuppressed patient, what are your instructions to Transfusion Services?**

Ask the blood bank for irradiated leukodepleted blood. Removing leukocytes prevents graft versus host disease by suppressing lymphocytic mitotic activity and irradiation prevents the transmission of CMV.

Viable lymphocytes in the transfused blood can damage tissues in the immunodeficient recipient if a response develops against the patient's HLA antigens. Irradiation of red cell, granulocyte, and platelet transfusions inactivates lymphocytes.

○ **What causes immediate hemolytic transfusion reactions?**

This is usually due to ABO incompatibility but may also be due to Kell, Kidd, Lewis, and Duffy antigens. When incompatible blood is administered, antibodies (anti-A or anti-B IgG or IgM antibodies) and complement in the recipient's plasma attack the corresponding antigens on donor RBCs. The resulting hemolysis may take place in the intravascular space (most catastrophic) and/or in the extravascular space.

○ **What are the signs and symptoms of a hemolytic transfusion reaction?**

During general anesthesia, hypotension, hemoglobinuria, and diffuse bleeding. Oliguria may develop due to renal failure. Clinical manifestations in an awake patient may include fever, chills, nausea, vomiting, diarrhea, and rigors. The patient becomes hypotensive and tachycardic, restless, flushed, and dyspneic (histamine). Chest, flank, and back pain result from diffuse intravascular occlusion by agglutinated RBCs.

○ **How do you manage a hemolytic transfusion reaction?**

If a reaction is suspected, the transfusion should be stopped immediately. Notify Transfusion Services and send blood samples for compatibility testing. Management has four main objectives: (1) maintenance of systemic blood pressure (volume, pressors, inotropes, detect hyperkalemia), (2) preservation of renal function (fluid, mannitol, diuretics to promote urine output), (3) prevention of DIC (prevent stasis and hypoperfusion by avoiding hypotension and supporting CO), and (4) treatment of bronchospasm.

○ **How do you maintain urine output in the patient with a hemolytic transfusion reaction?**

Intravenous fluids, mannitol, furosemide, and alkalinize the urine with sodium bicarbonate.

○ **If a patient is receiving blood and has a potential hemolytic transfusion reaction, what should you do if he or she still needs blood?**

Stop the blood transfusion. Confirm the diagnosis of major transfusion reaction, repeat donor and recipient blood types, and avoid further transfusions unless absolutely necessary. If you must continue to transfuse, consider universal donor blood (O Rh negative PRBCs) as an error might have occurred in the typing.

○ **What tests are indicated to establish the diagnosis of hemolytic transfusion reaction?**

1. Direct antiglobulin (Coombs) test – examines recipients' RBCs for the presence of surface immunoglobulins and complement.
2. Serum haptoglobin level, plasma and urine hemoglobin, and bilirubin indicate hemolysis.
3. Repeat crossmatch with recipient and donor blood.

Also send lab studies to check for DIC (fibrinogen, PT, PTT, and platelets). Return unused blood to Transfusion Services for repeat compatibility testing. Perform analysis of urine for hemoglobinuria.

○ **If a patient experiences a fever with or without chills during blood transfusion, what is the differential diagnosis?**

Fever occurs in 0.1–1% of transfusions and must be considered an ominous sign [Barash et al., 2009].

- Febrile nonhemolytic reactions due to leukocyte antibodies can be treated with acetaminophen. Typically a temperature increase of more than 1°C occurs within 4 hours of blood transfusion and for most patients is unpleasant but temporary.
- Bacterial contamination of blood products (especially platelets).
- Acute hemolytic transfusion reaction.
- Administration of thrombocytes as a result of antibodies against thrombocytes or cytokines in the product.

○ **What is the purpose of compatibility testing prior to blood transfusion?**

These tests are designed to prevent lethal antigen–antibody interactions between donor and recipient blood.

○ **A patient is brought into the emergency room exsanguinating from blood loss. There is not enough time for complete compatibility testing. What is the first choice for blood products?**

The first choice is to transfuse type-specific, partially crossmatched blood. This incomplete crossmatch takes 1–5 minutes and is accomplished by adding the patient's serum to donor RBCs at room temperature, centrifuging it, and then looking for macroscopic agglutination (confirms no clerical or laboratory errors). ABO–Rh typing alone results in a 99.8% chance of a compatible transfusion. The addition of an antibody screen increases the safety to 99.94%, and a complete crossmatch increases this to 99.95%.

○ **What is the second preference?**

Type-specific uncrossmatched blood.

○ **What is the last option?**

O negative PRBCs.

○ **A trauma patient is being transfused with type O Rh-negative blood and has already been given 8 U. Type-specific blood for the patient is now available. Should you switch?**

If more than 2 U of type O Rh-negative uncrossmatched whole blood has been administered, the blood bank must determine that transfused anti-A and anti-B antibodies have fallen to levels that permit transfusion of type-specific blood. There is a risk of a major transfusion reaction if the patient has received enough anti-A or anti-B antibodies in type-O blood to cause hemolysis if A, B, or AB blood is subsequently given. It takes significantly more PRBC units to potentially transfuse enough plasma containing anti-A and anti-B antibodies to prevent switching to type-specific blood.

○ **What are the three dominant causes of transfusion-related fatalities in the United States?**

1. Bacterial contamination (especially with platelets, which is stored at room temperature)

2. TRALI (a white cell–related transfusion reaction)

3. Mistransfusion (ABO mismatch)

FDA reported that the death rates due to hemolytic transfusion reactions alone are more than twice that due to all infectious hazards of blood transfusion combined [Hendrickson and Hillver, 2009. See reference on page 523].

○ **How do perfluorochemicals (PFCs) transport oxygen?**

PFCs are chemically inert liquids in which the solubility for oxygen is nearly 20 times that of water. Since PFCs transport oxygen by simple solubility, the oxygen-carrying capacity is directly proportional to the percentage of PFCs in the blood stream and to the partial pressure of oxygen inspired. Direct diffusion of oxygen is off-loaded to peripheral tissues.

○   **What are the limitations of PFCs?**

(a) Short plasma half-life of 12 hours, (b) require a high inspired oxygen, that is, 400 mm Hg or greater of partial pressure, (c) completely immiscible with water and must be prepared as an emulsion, (d) costly, (e) rapidly removed from the circulation and retained in the reticuloendothelial system for about 1 week, and (f) can be used only in a single, low dosage in humans.

Key Terms

Anemia: compensatory mechanisms
Arterial O_2 content and O_2 consumption (VO_2)
Blood bank type and screen
Blood loss physiologic response
Blood transfusion: mismatch
Blood type compatibility
Calcium chelation: transfusion
Citrate intoxication: signs/diagnosis/treatment
Cryoprecipitate: fibrinogen content
Determinants of O_2 delivery
Direct antiglobulin: diagnosis of hemolytic reaction
Effect of storage on RBCs/stored blood characteristics
Etiology of delayed transfusion reaction and treatment
Euvolemic anemia: physiology
Febrile transfusion reaction mechanism/causes
FFP: indications
FFP: warfarin reversal
FVIII concentrate: indications
Hemolysis: bilirubin levels
Hemolytic transfusion reaction treatment
Inadequate O_2 delivery indicators

Indication for cryoprecipitate treatment
Isovolemic hemodilution compensation
Leukoreduction: viral transmission
Low viscosity improves blood flow
Massive transfusion and coagulopathy
Massive transfusion hypocalcemia
Maximum ABL calculation
O_2 delivery physiology
Oxygen delivery index determinants
Oxygen transport: Hct and viscosity/quantitative aspects
Positive type and screen management
Red cell substitutes, PFC problems
Refusal of blood transfusion
TRALI: mechanism and treatment
Transfusion: bacterial sepsis
Transfusion mortality: causes
Transfusion reactions: allergic
Transfusion reactions: hemolytic
Transfusion reactions: types
Uncrossmatched blood transfusion

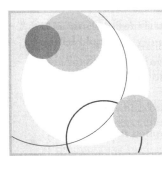

Cardiac Physiology and Surgery

It is not the brains that matter most, but that which guides them — the character,
the heart, generous qualities, progressive ideas.
Fyodor Dostoyevsky

○ **What is normal coronary artery anatomy?**

The right coronary artery arises from a point superior to the right coronary cusp of the aortic valve and then travels in the right atrioventricular (AV) groove, giving off branches along its path to the sinoatrial node, right ventricle, and part of the inferior wall of the left ventricle. The right coronary artery is the source of the posterior descending artery (PDA) in 70% of hearts. The left coronary artery arises from a point superior to the left coronary cusp of the aortic valve, and then divides into the left circumflex artery (which gives rise to the PDA in 20% of hearts) and the left anterior descending (LAD) artery. The LAD supplies most of the anteroseptal and anterior and part of anterolateral wall of the left ventricle. Both the right and left coronary arteries give rise to the PDA in 10% of hearts (codominance).

○ **What is the definition of coronary artery dominance?**

Dominance is defined by the source of the PDA, which is usually 70% right (right coronary artery), 10% balanced, and 20% left (left circumflex artery).

○ **What is the blood supply to the AV node?**

In the majority of the population (approximately 85%) the AV node is supplied by the right coronary artery. The majority of the remaining population is supplied by the circumflex artery.

○ **What do you see when the pericardium is first opened during cardiac surgery?**

Normal anterior cardiac surface anatomy is dominated by the right ventricle. The right atrium is located just to the right and superior to the right ventricle. The main trunk of the pulmonary artery arises from the right ventricle and is located to the left of the ascending aorta and the right pulmonary artery is posterior to the ascending aorta. The right coronary artery is normally anterior to the left coronary artery and is more vulnerable to the air embolism during the course of aortic cannulation and decannulation. The left coronary artery arises from the aorta and courses posterior to the main pulmonary artery trunk on the surface of the heart. The left atrium is the most posterior structure of the heart (and thus cannot be seen) and is adjacent to the esophagus, allowing for high-resolution images of the mitral valve during performance of a transesophageal echocardiogram.

○   **What are the sources of noncoronary collateral flow (NCCF)?**

NCCF to the heart is supplied from noncoronary routes such as mediastinal, pericardial, and bronchial collateral channels, through pericardial reflections surrounding pulmonary and systemic veins, as well as from the vasa vasorum along major blood vessels. The NCCF functions as supplemental feeding arteries during myocardial ischemia. Abnormal sources include a left superior pulmonary vein that drains into the coronary sinus and right heart, patent ductus arteriosus or a systemic to pulmonary artery shunt, anomalous systemic venous drainage into the left heart, and aortic regurgitation.

○   **T/F: The number of beta$_1$ receptors per unit area of the sarcolemma is fixed.**

False. Beta$_1$ receptors can increase and decrease in various disease states. These changes are called *upregulation* or *downregulation* of receptor density. In addition, the receptors can be desensitized or "internalized" by chemical changes, making them unavailable for signal transmission.

○   **Name four beta-agonist inotropic drugs.**

Dopamine, dobutamine, norepinephrine, and epinephrine.

○   **What is the law of Laplace?**

The Laplace equation states: wall tension $= P \times R/2h$, where P is the intraventricular pressure (dynes/cm^2), R is the inner radius (cm), and h is the wall thickness.

It is a simplified equation that describes the factors governing wall stress in the left ventricular chamber. According to Laplace, wall tension equals the pressure within a chamber multiplied by the radius of the chamber, divided by twice the chamber's wall thickness. When the heart dilates or fills to high pressures, wall tension increases, the LV must work harder, and myocardial oxygen demand increases.

○   **What is the New York Heart Association (NYHA) functional status classification of heart failure?**

Class I: Usual activity causes no limitations on functional status. Usual activity does not cause symptoms such as angina, dyspnea, fatigue, or palpitations.

Class II: No symptoms at rest, but usual activity can cause symptoms such as angina, dyspnea, fatigue, and palpitations.

Class III: No symptoms at rest, but less than usual activity can cause symptoms such as angina, dyspnea, fatigue, and palpitations.

Class IV: Symptoms of heart failure at rest (angina, dyspnea, fatigue, and palpitations). If any physical effort is tried, the symptoms can become even worse.

○   **What factors contribute to *myocardial oxygen supply and demand*?**

The myocardium accounts for 11% of the total body oxygen consumption, but the coronary circulation receives only 4% of the cardiac output (CO). *Myocardial oxygen supply* consists of arterial oxygen content and coronary blood flow (coronary artery diameter × coronary perfusion pressure). Heart rate, wall tension, and contractility contribute to *myocardial oxygen demand.* Supply and demand determine myocardial oxygen balance. Myocardial ischemia occurs when supply is not adequate to satisfy demand due to a multitude of reasons such as acute and/or chronic coronary blockage, sepsis, dysrhythmia, etc. It is usually predominantly subendocardial.

○ **T/F: Sinus tachycardia is associated with an increased thromboembolic risk.**

False. Sinus tachycardia is an increase in the normal heart rate to >100 bpm. It usually represents a normal physiologic response to exercise or high adrenergic states, and rarely represents the presence of organic heart disease. Persistent sinus tachycardia may suggest an underlying cause such as infection, hyperthyroidism, anemia, and hypercarbia from many causes. As the synchrony between the atria and ventricle is maintained, there are seldom any hemodynamic changes. (Decreased LV filling may be seen with very high atrial rates.)

○ **What is the relationship between CO and mixed venous oxygen content (CvO_2) in the Fick equation?**

CO (L/min) = VO_2 (oxygen consumption)/$CaO_2 - CvO_2$, where CaO_2 is the arterial oxygen content and CvO_2 is the mixed venous oxygen content. (This assumes no intracardiac shunt is present.)

○ **What are the determinants of myocardial oxygen supply?**

Myocardial oxygen supply is calculated as the product of arterial oxygen content and the coronary blood flow.

○ **What are the variables affecting left ventricular filling in normal subjects?**

Age is the major independent factor affecting LV filling in normal subjects. Other variables include gender, heart rate, systolic and diastolic blood pressure, aortic root and left atrial dimensions, left ventricular mass index, and left ventricular shortening fraction.

○ **Is there any morbidity associated with a junctional rhythm?**

Hypotension is the primary issue. Junctional tachycardia leads to a loss of the atrial contribution to ventricular filling. In a younger person where the atrial *kick* is less important than passive filling, the effects of a junctional rhythm may not be as significant. However, as diastolic dysfunction becomes more prominent, the hemodynamic effects of junctional rhythms are more pronounced, due to the loss of coordinated atrial contraction. Junctional rhythms may take the form of a tachycardia or an escape rhythm during significant bradycardia or high-grade AV block. The morbidity is usually related to the underlying cause. Junctional tachycardia is often a symptom of digitalis toxicity, recent cardiac surgery for valve replacement, or acute MI. Junctional bradycardia is symptomatic of increased vagal tone or the presence of sinus node disease (sick sinus syndrome or complete heart block).

○ **What is the effect of pressors on preload?**

In the normal heart, RV preload is determined by venous return, which is dependent on venous tone, blood volume, heart rate, gravity, and the changes in pleural pressure generated during ventilation. LV preload is dependent on RV preload, atrial contraction, ventricular compliance, and pulmonary vascular resistance. Pressors can increase or decrease preload depending on their relative effects on vascular resistance, heart rate, and CO.

○ **What are the main determinants of myocardial oxygen consumption (MVO_2)?**

Ventricular wall tension, preload (left ventricular end-diastolic volume [LVEDV]), afterload (systemic vascular resistance [SVR]), contractility (dP/dT), and heart rate.

○ **What are the key features of coronary blood flow and coronary perfusion pressure?**

Flow is tightly coupled to oxygen demand. When oxygen consumption increases (normally 8–10 mL O_2/(min 100 g)), there is an increase in coronary blood flow that is nearly proportionate to the increase in MVO_2. The myocardium has the highest A-VO_2 gradient of a vital organ (10–13 mL/100 mL). Autoregulation occurs between 60 and 200 mm Hg perfusion pressure. Mediators for autoregulation of coronary blood flow include adenosine and nitric oxide. Sympathetic activation results in coronary vasodilatation and increased coronary flow due to increased metabolic activity (increased heart rate and contractility) despite direct vasoconstrictor effects mediated by α_1-adrenoceptors.

Flow in the left coronary artery is pulsatile in nature. Flow is lower during systole with isovolumetric contraction and ejection than during diastole; therefore, the endocardium is more susceptible to ischemia, especially at lower perfusion pressure. Coronary blood flow through the right coronary endures during systole and diastole because extravascular compression is less and the right ventricular intracavitary pressures are lower. Tachycardia limits flow in diastole, which is significant in patient with coronary artery disease (CAD) with limited reserve.

Coronary blood flow is proportional to coronary perfusion pressure divided by coronary vascular resistance. Coronary perfusion pressure is determined primarily by the aortic diastolic pressure and coronary vascular resistance that is determined primarily by end-diastolic ventricular pressure, external compressive forces, and metabolic, endothelial, and neural factors that regulate intrinsic coronary tone via autoregulation.

○ **What is the mean arterial pressure (MAP)?**

MAP is calculated from the systolic and diastolic pressures as diastolic pressure + 1/3(systolic pressure − diastolic pressure). Most physicians agree that the MAP should be maintained between 60 and 70 mm Hg to ensure adequate perfusion of vital organs. Another formula is (systolic + 2 × diastolic)/3.

○ **What are the adverse effects of nitroglycerin (NTG)?**

Headache, hypotension, methemoglobinemia, and hypoxemia due to V/Q mismatch.

○ **What is the mechanism of NTG in the treatment of myocardial ischemia?**

1. Venous dilation: NTG reduces preload (thereby decreasing intramyocardial wall tension and intraventricular work), reduces left ventricular filling pressure (decreasing myocardial oxygen demand and ischemia), and increases CO in congestive heart failure (CHF) with little or no detrimental change in normal hearts.

2. Arterial dilation: NTG dilates large coronary arteries, antagonizes vasospasm, increases coronary collateral blood flow, and decreases SVR.

○ **What are the clinical findings frequently associated with a right ventricular infarct?**

Second- or third-degree AV block requiring inotropic, chronotropic, or pacemaker support, elevated jugular venous pressure, and an inability to tolerate preload reduction (especially NTG or morphine administration).

○ **What are the phases of the left ventricular cardiac cycle?**

Isovolumic contraction: The first part of the cycle involves myocardial contraction prior to the opening of the aortic valve. Due to shortening of myofibrils, there is a rise in the left ventricular intracavitary pressure causing the mitral valve to close, but ejection has not occurred yet.

Ejection phase: This is the period that occurs after the intracavitary pressure has risen to the level that exceeds that of the aorta. Once this occurs, the aortic valve opens, allowing the expulsion of blood into the aorta. The ejection of blood continues until the intracavitary pressure falls below the aortic pressure.

Isovolumic relaxation: This is a period marked by the closure of the aortic valve and a rapid decline in the intracavitary pressure as the myofibrils relax. This is the period immediately prior to the opening of the mitral valve.

Diastolic filling: Once the left ventricular intracavitary pressure has fallen to a level below the pressure of the left atrium, the mitral valve opens, allowing the left ventricular volume to increase. The cycle then begins again.

○ **What is the relationship between ventricular pressure and volume?**

The pressure and volume relationship of the ventricle is a measure of its compliance. Simultaneous measurement of pressure and volume yields a loop that looks somewhat like a square, with pressure on the y-axis and volume on the x-axis. In a normally compliant heart with normally working valves, the opening of the mitral valve marks the point when the volume of the ventricle rises with diastolic filling. The line along the x-axis moves toward the right as the ventricular volume ascends with little change in pressure. After mitral valve closure and the beginning of isovolumic contraction, movement along the x-axis stops because the rise in ventricular volume stops. This marks the beginning of isovolumetric contraction. A steep rise in intracavitary ventricular pressure and steep movement of the line along the y-axis occurs until aortic valve opening. At the opening of the aortic valve and ejection of ventricular volume, there is a simultaneous decrease in ventricular volume. Therefore, a movement of the line to the left along the x-axis and a simultaneous and a gentler rise in ventricular pressure and thus movement of the line upward along the y-axis as well occurs. This yields a line that slopes left and gently upward until aortic valve closure. Then since all of the volume has been ejected, there is no more movement along the x-axis. The steep decrease in ventricular pressure with isovolumic relaxation causes a movement of the line steeply down the y-axis to bring it back to the point where we began with mitral valve opening.

Chronic aortic regurgitation causes a volume overload of the left ventricle. This causes the entire pressure–volume loop to shift to the right along the x-axis to represent the dramatic increases in ventricular volume. The loop appears wider (along the x-axis) because the shifts in ventricular volume are wider. In contrast, aortic stenosis will shift the ventricular pressures upward, showing more dramatic rises and falls in ventricular pressure during isovolumic contraction and relaxation.

○ **What differentiates LV versus RV increased function?**

The LV is a pressure pump that increases strength of contraction while the RV is thinner walled and responds more to volume changes. The right ventricle is also very sensitive to acute rises in pulmonary artery pressure, such as an acute pulmonary embolism. The right heart is able to adapt to slower, more insidious changes in pulmonary artery pressure. The right ventricle is able to hypertrophy in order to handle extra pressure work.

○ **What is the mortality of perioperative myocardial reinfarction?**

The reported mortality from reinfarction after noncardiac surgery is 50–70%, based on old studies.

○ **A patient had an MI 2 months ago. What is his cardiovascular risk with subsequent elective surgery?**

Traditionally, it was thought that the rate of perioperative myocardial infarction rate in patients who have had an MI within 3 months of surgery is 30%, decreasing to 5% by 6 months. More recent studies suggest the risk is highly variable, depending on the amount of myocardium still at risk for ischemia, and the nature of the previous infarct (nontransmural has a higher reinfarction rate). According to recent studies, after an MI, 6 weeks is considered the time of high risk for a perioperative cardiac event, because it is the mean healing time of the infarcted lesion. The period from 6 weeks to 3 months is of intermediate risk. More than 3 months is required for cases complicated with arrhythmias and ventricular dysfunction [Antman et al., 2008. See reference on page 523].

○ **A patient is to have lower extremity revascularization surgery. What is the risk of CAD?**

Less than 10% of vascular surgery patients have normal coronary arteries, and more than 50% have advanced or severe CAD.

○ **In a patient with ischemic heart disease, why is tachycardia potentially more likely to precipitate ischemia than hypertension?**

Hypertension will increase myocardial oxygen demand, but it will also increase myocardial oxygen supply by increasing coronary perfusion pressure and perfusion time (if the heart rate reflexively slows). Tachycardia increases myocardial oxygen demand and decreases myocardial oxygen supply by decreasing diastolic coronary perfusion time.

○ **What markers are used for the laboratory diagnosis of myocardial infarction?**

No marker is completely sensitive and specific for myocardial infarction. Timing is important, as well as correlation with the patient's symptoms and EKG findings. Creatine kinase (total: mostly found in skeletal muscle) and creatine kinase-MB fraction (15–40% of isoenzyme CK in cardiac muscle is MB, with <2% in skeletal muscle) are routinely monitored. CK-MB rises in serum within 2–8 hours of onset of infarction, peaks for 12 hours, and then falls over the next 1–3 days. The cardiac index is the ratio of CK to CK-MB and is a sensitive indicator of myocardial injury. CK-MB isoforms 1 and 2 can also be measured electrophoretically, but this is labor intensive, with false positives in patients with CHF.

Troponins I and T are highly specific for myocardial injury. They begin to increase following MI within 3–12 hours, and remain elevated 5–9 days for troponin I and up to 2 weeks for troponin T. Measuring the rise in myoglobin may help in determining the size of the myocardial infarction. LDH begins to rise 12–24 hours after the event, peaks in 2–3 days, and gradually dissipates in 5–14 days. With myocardial injury isoenzyme-1 is greater in concentration than isoenzyme-2, which is inverse to the normal relationship.

○ **What are the EKG signs of right ventricular infarction?**

A routine 12-lead EKG may not be very helpful. Inferior ischemic changes accompanied by ST depression in lead V1, V2, or V3 or ST elevation in lead III greater than that in lead II may be suggestive. A more common method of assessing RV infarction is the 15-lead EKG with elevated ST segments of 1 mm or more in at least one of the leads V4R, V5R, or V6R. Presence of Q or inverted T waves is not considered an indicator of ischemia or infarction.

○ **Discuss the EKG diagnosis of myocardial ischemia.**

EKG findings depend on the duration (acute vs. evolving/chronic), extent (transmural vs. subendocardial), and localization (anterior vs. inferior-posterior) of ischemia or infarction. EKG abnormalities (ST segment, T or Q waves, or left bundle branch block) may indicate myocardial ischemia within 90 minutes of onset of symptoms, with serial EKGs more diagnostic than a single tracing. Transmural ischemia is seen with ST elevation and sometimes tall positive T waves; the overlying leads of an area of subendocardial ischemia show ST-segment depression and ST elevation in lead aVR. Severe ischemia or MI can occur with slight or even absent ST–T changes.

○ **A patient scheduled for vascular surgery has evidence of myocardium at risk for ischemia on preoperative diagnostic imaging studies. How can you decrease the risk of perioperative ischemia and atrial fibrillation?**

Prophylactic beta-blockade at least 7 days in advance of moderate-to-high risk surgery, titrating the patient's heart rate to 60–70 bpm. Postoperatively narcotics and additional beta-blockers should be given to reach a target heart rate of 80 bpm. This is a class 1 recommendation from the American College of Cardiology/American Heart Association guidelines. [2009 ACCF/AHA Focused Update on Perioperative Beta Blockade. See reference on page 523; ACC/AHA 2007 Guidelines on Perioperative Cardiovascular Evaluation and Care for Noncardiac Surgery. See reference on page 523]

○ **Immediately following aortic cross-clamp you notice ST depression. What hemodynamic factors have led to this myocardial ischemia?**

Sudden dramatic increase in afterload prevents ventricular emptying and produces a sudden increase in preload, wall tension, and subendocardial myocardial oxygen demand.

○ **How does pulmonary artery catheterization produce hemoptysis?**

Pulmonary artery rupture, aneurysm formation, or pulmonary infarction.

○ **What is the risk of pulmonary artery rupture using a PA catheter?**

Estimated in 0.2% of patients, associated with a 50% mortality rate. Rupture of the pulmonary artery usually occurs if the PA catheter balloon is overinflated while in the wedged position.

○ **What are the major cardiovascular causes of hemoptysis?**

1. Pulmonary hypertension (Eisenmenger complex, mitral stenosis, primary recurrent pulmonary emboli)
2. Pulmonary artery rupture
3. Arteriovenous malformations
4. Left ventricular failure with pulmonary edema

○ **What hemodynamic information is available from cardiac catheterization data?**

CO, cardiac index, right-sided pressures (atrium, ventricle, and pulmonary artery), pulmonary capillary wedge pressure, and calculations of different types of vascular resistance (total pulmonary vascular resistance, SVR). Calculation of valve orifice area and detection and measurement of intracardiac and extracardiac shunts are also reported.

Right heart catheterization is also the gold standard diagnosis of pulmonary hypertension. At sea level normal mean pulmonary artery pressures are between 12 and 16 mm Hg and pulmonary hypertension is present when the mean pulmonary artery pressure exceeds 25 mm Hg. During cardiac catheterization a patient may also be given increasing concentrations of oxygen and nitric oxide to test the reactivity of the pulmonary vascular bed.

○ **Describe the vasodilator medications available for the treatment of primary pulmonary hypertension (PPH) [Leuchte, 2004. See reference on page 523; Siobal 2007. See reference on page 523].**

PPH is a syndrome characterized by pulmonary hypertension in the absence of sufficient underlying heart or lung disease. Vasodilators improve survival in these patients and act as a bridge to heart lung or lung transplant surgery in these patients.

1. Inhaled nitric oxide (INO): Endogenous NO is released by endothelial cells when stimulated by acetylcholine. In vascular smooth muscle cells, NO stimulates soluble guanylate cyclase and converts guanosine triphosphate to cyclic guanosine monophosphate (cGMP). In turn, protein kinases mediate a cGMP-induced decrease in intracellular calcium and produce relaxation and vasodilation. Inhaled NO gas diffuses rapidly across the alveolar–capillary membrane into the vascular smooth muscle and mediates relaxation (short duration).
2. Nitric oxide donors: Sodium nitroprusside (SNP) and nitroglycerine (NTG). However, prolonged exposure to SNP can cause cyanide toxicity. Both SNP and NTG can cause methemoglobinemia.

3. Prostacyclins: In vascular smooth muscle cells, prostacyclins stimulate soluble adenylate cyclase and convert adenosine triphosphate to cyclic adenosine monophosphate (cAMP). In turn, protein kinases mediate a cAMP-induced decrease in intracellular calcium and produce relaxation and vasodilation. Prostaglandin I-2 and prostaglandin E-1 are both potent pulmonary vasodilators and inhibitors of platelet aggregation. Aerosol delivery of prostacyclins offers the advantage of avoiding some of the systemic effects of intravenous, subcutaneous, and oral administration.

4. Phosphodiesterase inhibitors: For example, sildenafil, a phosphodiesterase type 5 inhibitor. Phosphodiesterases are enzymes that inactivate cGMP and cAMP. Use of phosphodiesterase inhibitors prevents the breakdown of cGMP and cAMP in vascular smooth muscle cells and augments or prolongs the vasodilator signaling pathways of both NO and prostacyclin.

5. Endothelin receptor antagonists.

6. Calcium antagonists such as nifedipine or diltiazem (verapamil not recommended due to negative inotropic effects). Calcium channel blockers inhibit the influx of calcium ions into smooth muscle cells and therefore cause relaxation and vasodilation. The major adverse effects are due to decreased CO secondary to negative inotropic effect, diminished systemic blood pressure, and salt and water retention [Siobal, 2007. See reference on page 523].

○ **What is the best assessment technique to measure LV preload?**

LVEDV has traditionally been measured with a pulmonary artery catheter as LVEDP, assuming that LVEDP is equal to LA pressure, which is equal to wedge pressure. Other monitors measure stroke volume, maximum acceleration (contractility), and left ventricular ejection time (LVET) as a measure of preload status.

○ **What is the conventional TEE view for detection of intraoperative myocardial ischemia?**

The transgastric short-axis view at midpapillary level is most commonly employed for ischemia detection. A satisfactory alternate is the four-chamber view, switching intermittently to the long axis.

○ **Describe the wall motion abnormalities on TEE views during ischemia.**

During normal systole, the endocardial surfaces of the LV move toward a central point and the LV wall thickness increases. If function is reduced, one or more areas of LV will not move properly or the wall thickness will not increase, and may in fact become thinner. Ventricular regional wall motion abnormalities (RWMA) may be the most sensitive indicator available of ischemia and are better than electrocardiogram (ECG) changes at predicting the progression to myocardial infarction.

However, all segmental wall motion abnormalities are not indicative of ischemia. Abnormalities can also occur secondary to preexisting disease (e.g., prior myocardial infarction, myocarditis, rare infiltrative disease) or confounding intraoperative events (e.g., myocardial stunning after cardiopulmonary bypass [CPB]). Chronic RWMA are usually due to prior infarction.

The severity of RWMA can be classified into three categories:

Hypokinesis (reduced – mild, moderate, and severe)

Akinesis (no wall motion)

Dyskinesis (paradoxical wall motion)

LV myocardium is supplied by three major arteries – LAD, LCA, and RCA.

The *ventricular short-axis mid-view at papillary muscle level* (TEE at the lower esophageal/transgastric level looking up at the L ventricle) contains all three blood supplies from the major arteries. In this view, functions in the posterior and lateral segments indicate perfusion by the left circumflex artery; anterior and anteroseptal segments indicate perfusion by the LAD artery; midseptal and inferior segments indicate perfusion by the right coronary artery [Memtsoudis et al., 2006. See reference on page 523].

○ **Describe the advantages of TEE evaluation in mitral regurgitation (MR).**

TEE evaluations answer some of the questions, when the MR is severe requiring surgery. One of the questions is feasibility of performing repair versus replacement. Repair avoids morbidity associated with prosthesis and long-term anticoagulation. Mitral disease localized to the posterior leaflet or to a focal portion of the anterior leaflet is most amenable to repair. Conversely, heavy calcified valve requires replacement.

Agreement of the location of MR with TEE and direct surgical observation is excellent. TEE confirms enlargement of left atrium (>4 cm) and eccentric hypertrophy of the left ventricle. Left atrium will be akinetic if atrial fibrillation is present. Color flow examination of the mitral valve establishes the pattern of disturbed flow caused by regurgitation across the mitral valve and localizes the site of regurgitation, but provides only a semiquantitative estimate of the severity. The pulmonic vein flow pattern is one measure that has been used to grade MR. If severe MR is present, the left atrial pressure may exceed the pulmonary vein pressure during systole, resulting in reversal of the S wave. The severity of MR is very dependent on afterload. If moderate MR is present, the afterload should be increased and the severity is reassessed.

○ **Describe the TEE findings of MR associated with myocardial infarction and sudden hemodynamic collapse.**

Rupture of the posteromedial papillary muscle (accounting for 90% of papillary muscle ruptures), a wide gap in mitral coaptation, and eccentric significant MR swirling in the left atrium with a large flow convergence.

○ **What are the factors that affect left-to-right shunt in patients with VSD?**

When the VSD is more than 50% of the area of the aortic root, the RV and LV pressures will equalize. The determining factor at this point for the amount of left-to-right shunting becomes the relative systemic and pulmonary vascular resistances. Muscular ventricular septal defects become smaller during systole, allowing less shunting. Symptoms with VSD usually start with a QP:QS ratio of 2.5:1 or more. A combination of ASD and VSD will increase left-to-right shunting at the ventricular level. Aortic stenosis, aortic insufficiency, mitral stenosis, and pulmonary stenosis will also influence the shunt flow.

○ **What are the categories of congenital heart disease (CHD)?**

1. Defects that *decrease pulmonary blood flow*, such as tricuspid atresia and tetralogy of Fallot
2. Defects that *increase pulmonary blood flow*, such as atrial septal defects, ventricular septal defects, atrial–ventricular canal defects, and persistent patent ductus arteriosus
3. Defects that cause *obstruction to blood flow from either the left or right ventricle*, such as coarctation of the aorta, aortic stenosis, and pulmonic stenosis
4. Defects that cause *mixed blood flow anomalies*, such as transposition of the great arteries and hypoplastic left heart syndrome

○ **What lab test in a patient with CHD is indicative of chronic hypoxemia?**

Hemoglobin or hematocrit level.

○ **What are the four questions that must be answered in a patient with CHD before proceeding with surgery?**

Functional status, anatomy of lesion including whether there is right or left ventricular outflow obstruction, direction of blood flow (left-to-right with pulmonary hypertension or right-to-left shunt with cyanosis), and associated anomalies.

○ **What is the difference between *parallel and series* blood flow?**

Series blood flow refers to normal physiologic circulation: deoxygenated blood returns to the right heart, is pumped to the lung for gas exchange, and returns to the left heart, where it is ejected via the aorta. Parallel blood flow is seen in patients with cardiac anomalies where there is no partition between the less oxygenated side (usually the right) and the more oxygenated side of the heart that receives blood from the lungs (usually the left). This causes a mixing of lesser and greater oxygenated blood in one chamber. Blood is then ejected from this one chamber into both the pulmonary and systemic circulations at the same time. One ventricle does the work of two and the balance of resistances of the pulmonary and systemic circulations is a critical determinant of blood flow. This type of physiology is seen in patients with lesions such as atrial–ventricular canal, large ventricular septal defects, and hypoplastic left heart syndrome.

○ **What are the indications for temporary epicardial or transvenous pacemaker insertion?**

Bradycardia, tachyarrhythmias, and other conduction system disturbances. The purpose of temporary transvenous or epicardial pacemaker insertion is to provide standby pacing in the event of sudden complete heart block, to increase heart rate during periods of symptomatic bradycardia, and to control sustained supraventricular or ventricular tachycardia (VT) with overdrive pacing.

○ **How does one know if capture has been achieved when a transcutaneous pacemaker is used?**

Pacer spikes are often misinterpreted as adequate capture of ventricular pacing. Ventricular pacing is established when a wide complex idioventricular ECG is generated at the same rate as one has programmed the external pacemaker to discharge. This must be accompanied by a pulse at the same rate.

○ **What are the indications for permanent transvenous or epicardial pacemaker insertion?**

Symptomatic disease of impulse formation (sinus node disease) such as sick sinus syndrome, symptomatic disease of impulse conduction such as AV node disease, hypertrophic obstructive cardiomyopathy (HOCM), and dilated cardiomyopathy (three leads – dual chamber).

○ **What are the effects of pacemaker activity on ECG morphology?**

The electrical pulse generated by the pacemaker and transmitted to the atrial and ventricular muscle can be seen as either an electrical spike on the EKG that precedes a P wave (in the case of electrical stimulation of atrial muscle) or an electrical spike that precedes a QRS wave of wide morphology (in the case of electrical stimulation of ventricular muscle). Usually patients have two or three leads placed (one for sensing and stimulation of the atrium and one or two for sensing and stimulation of the right ventricle alone or the right and left ventricle). If the patient has issues with impulse generation at the level of the sinoatrial level, then a single pacer spike will be seen prior to a P wave followed by a narrow QRS complex. If there is no issue with preliminary impulse generation but there is a problem with impulse conduction, then a P wave will be followed by a wide QRS complex that looks like an idioventricular "escape" beat.

○ **What are the usual hemodynamic effects of coordinated atrial and ventricular pacing?**

When pacing is coordinated so that atrial and ventricular pacing occurs in a manner that allows enough time for ventricular filling to occur, stroke volume, CO, and subsequently blood pressure are usually raised. This effect can be most pronounced is patients with diastolic dysfunction such as constrictive pericardial disease, chronic hypertension, late-stage hypertrophic cardiomyopathy (HCM), aortic stenosis, etc.

○ **What are the indications for placement of an implantable cardiac defibrillator (ICD)?**

Class I indications are cardiac arrest due to ventricular fibrillation (VF) or VT without reversible cause, spontaneous sustained VT with structural heart disease, arrhythmogenic right ventricular dysplasia (ARVD), and syncope with VT or VF on electrophysiology study.

Class II indications include an ejection fraction (EF) less than 35% forty days post–myocardial infarction or 3 months post–coronary artery bypass graft surgery, and EF <30% with ischemic heart disease.

○ **What is the recommended perioperative management of an ICD?**

The recommendations are similar in many ways to perioperative pacemaker management. Knowing the brand and model is important. A complete evaluation (including EKG) of the patient's dependence on the pacer portion of the ICD should always be done. The cardiology service should be aware of the patient, as they may want to interrogate the ICD preoperatively. In the operating room bipolar electrocautery is safest. If nonbipolar electrocautery is used, it is best to use the lowest possible setting with short bursts. Also, keep the path of the current as far away as possible from the surgical field.

All ICD patients should have the antitachycardic therapy disabled during the surgical procedures including prior to placement of central lines (inappropriate shock). Ability to deliver external cardioversion or defibrillation must be present [Practice Advisory for the Perioperative Management of Patients with Cardiac Implantable Electronic Devices, 2011. See reference on page 523].

○ **A 57-year-old man is scheduled for a repeat total hip replacement under general anesthesia. He had a permanent endocardial VVIR pacemaker placed 2 years ago for complete heart block, and since arriving in the operating room he has paced continuously. What is a VVIR pacemaker?**

In a pacemaker code, the first letter refers to the chamber paced (V for ventricle), the second letter refers to the chamber sensed, the third letter refers to the response to the sensed event (I for inhibition), and the fourth letter refers to the programmability (R: rate adaptive, designed to deliver a more physiologic response by changing the rate in response to exercise).

○ **In this patient, the pacer functioned normally during a recent evaluation by the cardiologist. What other preoperative evaluations are needed?**

Patients with permanent pacemakers are often elderly and have significant coexisting disease such as CAD, hypertension, or insulin-dependent diabetes or have received a heart transplant. These medical problems, medications, acid base status, and electrolytes should be evaluated preoperatively.

○ **The Surgeon is planning on using a unipolar electrosurgical cautery (ESC). What are your concerns?**

ESC, which emits radio-frequency energy, has the potential to cause transient or permanent changes in pacemaker function. The most common problem is inhibition of the pacemaker. Patients with complete heart block are more likely to be pacemaker dependent and therefore are potentially at higher risk should a malfunction occur. If ESC is to be used extensively, then consideration should be given to reprogramming the generator to an asynchronous mode preoperatively, to avoid inhibition.

○ **Can you use a magnet to convert the generator to an asynchronous mode if intraoperatively the use of the electrocautery causes the pacemaker to malfunction intermittently?**

Although most devices respond to magnet application by a device-specific single- or dual-chamber asynchronous pacing mode, routine use of magnets without knowledge of the expected pacemaker response is not advocated. Applying the magnet to a programmable generator (VVIR) in the presence of electromagnetic interference (EMI) increases the risk of reprogramming and is discouraged. Unless the planned surgery is truly emergent or poses little risk of EMI from electrocautery, the pacemaker clinic, service, or manufacturer should be contacted for advice.

The pacemaker should also be checked after surgery for program integrity, circuit damage, and myocardial damage at the electrode site.

○ **Is use of bipolar electrosurgical unit (ESU) safer than unipolar ESU in patients with a permanent pacemaker?**

Because the active and return electrodes are the two blades of the forceps in a bipolar ESU, current passes between the tips and not through the patient. Exposure of the pacemaker generator to electrical interventions is minimal. However, bipolar ESU generates considerably less power than the unipolar and is mainly used for ophthalmic and neurologic surgery.

○ **What other measures should be taken to minimize susceptibility to EMI from ESU?**

a. Locate the ESU receiving plate as remote from the generator as possible.

b. The pulse generator and leads should not be between the operative site and the receiving plate (ensure the current flows away from the pacemaker system).

c. Use the lowest current and short bursts only.

d. Pacing function should be confirmed by monitoring heart sounds or the pulse waveform.

e. Stop all diathermy if arrhythmia occurs.

○ **You are asked to assist in the management of a patient with acute CHF that is refractory to diuretic therapy (a total of 120 mg of furosemide has been administered). What important questions must you ask?**

Diuretics often require the administration of a threshold dose to be effective. The initial question you should ask is: "How was the furosemide administered?" An initial dose of 40 mg followed by a second dose of 80 mg (double the dose) would be appropriate. Often the answer will be that three doses of furosemide, 40 mg each, were administered. Furthermore, the timing and route of administration is important (IV quicker than po). Other questions include the following: "Does the patient have renal insufficiency?" and "Is the patient taking diuretics, and if so, what drug and dose?" The latter two imply a higher dose may be necessary.

○ **A 70-year-old man with systolic heart failure is refractory to appropriately administered escalating doses of furosemide. Suggest an option to treat his diuretic resistance.**

Loop diuretics are the only class of diuretics effective as single agents in moderate to severe CHF. Often, adding a second agent with a different site of action in the nephron – for example, a thiazide diuretic that prevents fluid reabsorption at a site distal to the loop of Henle – will enhance diuresis.

○ **Describe the typical findings for CO, arterial-mixed venous oxygen difference, and SVR in systolic CHF.**

CO is low, arterial-mixed venous oxygen difference is increased, and SVR is increased.

○ **Give several reasons why dobutamine is a superior inotropic drug versus dopamine for the treatment of CHF.**

Dobutamine acts as a vasodilator (SVR and PVR reduction) improving left and right ventricular systolic function, whereas dopamine, even at intermediate infusion rates, may cause peripheral vasoconstriction. Dobutamine is a direct agonist that causes less tachycardia at low doses and a greater increase in coronary blood flow, thereby increasing CO with less increase in myocardial oxygen demand.

○ **What is the effect of an increase in preload on CHF?**

The chronic response to dilated cardiomyopathy is to increase end-diastolic ventricular volume. Because of this, up to a point, the total stroke volume can be maintained in the face of decreasing systolic function. An increase in preload will therefore improve stroke volume up a point when the end-diastolic volume has caused overstretching of cardiac myofibrils. This overstretching causes inefficient interaction of actin and myosin filaments and results in decreased cardiac contractility.

○ **You place a pulmonary artery catheter in a severely malnourished alcoholic patient with peripheral edema and cardiomegaly. Findings include elevated CO, decreased arterial-mixed venous oxygen difference, and low SVR. What diagnosis should you consider?**

These are classic hemodynamic findings in beriberi heart disease (thiamine deficiency) and alcoholic cardiomyopathy in a patient with end-stage liver disease.

○ **What is the indication for venodilators (or furosemide and rotating tourniquets) in the treatment of CHF?**

To reduce preload in patients presenting with dyspnea due to high filling pressures causing pulmonary congestion [Gauthier et al., 2008. See reference on page 523].

○ **You suspect severe LV systolic dysfunction in a patient newly admitted to the ICU. A pulmonary artery catheter is inserted. However, your pressure transducer is malfunctioning and your CO machine is broken. What laboratory test will confirm your suspicion?**

Mixed venous oxygen saturation will determine whether the CO and oxygen delivery is matched to oxygen demand. The normal systemic venous oxygen saturation (SvO_2) is 75%, with a 5–10% decrease considered significant and usually preceding hemodynamic changes.

○ **A sustained VT is well controlled with lidocaine 2 mg/min in a 55-year-old man following a non-Q wave MI. He has a known history of ischemic cardiomyopathy. Day 3 of his admission, his speech becomes slurred, he is lethargic, and when he is aroused he becomes very agitated. What should you do?**

The patient has classic findings of lidocaine-induced CNS toxicity, and you should strongly consider stopping this drug. Other symptoms of lidocaine toxicity include seizures, tremors, paresthesias, nausea, and vomiting. Elderly patients and patients with heart failure or hepatic insufficiency are especially at risk due to the reduced hepatic metabolism of lidocaine.

○ **What are the acute hemodynamic effects of furosemide administration?**

Pulmonary venous pressure falls. Furosemide causes mainly venodilation and reduces preload within 15 minutes of intravenous bolus. Diuresis starts 30 minutes after administration and peaks at 1–2.5 hours.

○ **A 72-year-old woman admitted to the ICU with pulmonary edema is much improved after overnight diuresis, with a negative fluid balance of 4 L. She suddenly develops polymorphic VT requiring cardioversion. Her regular medications include furosemide 80 mg po bid. What is the likely etiology?**

Acute ischemia or infarction and electrolyte abnormalities, especially hypokalemia and hypomagnesemia, may induce torsades de pointes in CHF patients after vigorous diuresis – especially in patients on chronic diuretics.

○ **A 65-year-old man with known severe hypertension, CHF, and COPD is intubated for acute pulmonary edema and suspected pneumonia. BP is 190/110 mm Hg; oxygen saturation is 94% on 60% oxygen. You successfully lower his blood pressure to 140/80 mm Hg with intravenous SNP; however, the patient develops chest pressure and his oxygen saturation decreases to 86%. What happened?**

Three vascular effects of nitroprusside are the likely culprits, one pulmonary and two cardiac. Nonselective dilation of the pulmonary arteriolar bed can worsen ventilation–perfusion mismatch, especially in patients with COPD or pneumonia, and cause desaturation. This desaturation may make coronary oxygen delivery insufficient and cause myocardial ischemia, leading to chest pain. *Coronary steal* (reduced perfusion to coronary arteries with fixed obstruction in the setting of arteriolar dilation by nitroprusside of arteries feeding nonischemic areas) may lead to ischemia and chest pain. The decreased function of the heart may cause some degree of pulmonary congestion increase V/Q mismatch. Finally, a decrease in coronary artery perfusion pressure related to a lowered aortic diastolic pressure may be the culprit. The presenting diastolic BP of 110 mm Hg may have been necessary to perfuse the myocardium. Chest pain and arterial oxygen desaturation follow as described above.

○ **What are the hallmark signs for detecting aortic stenosis in the preoperative period?**

These signs include a systolic murmur radiating to the carotids, left ventricular hypertrophy on EKG, and calcifications (of a congenital bicuspid valve) noted on chest x-ray. The arterial pressure wave is altered with a narrowed pulse pressure (<50 mm Hg), delayed or slow rise of the systolic pressure, and a prominent anacrotic notch. Clinical presentation is often late in the course of the disease with angina, dyspnea (CHF), syncope, or sudden death.

○ **Define critical aortic stenosis.**

Critical aortic stenosis occurs when the valvular cross-sectional area is less than one fifth of normal (aortic valve index <0.5 cm^2/m^2).

○ **Why is it so critically important to avoid atrial arrhythmias in a patient with aortic stenosis?**

Narrowing of the aortic orifice from 2.5–3.5 to about 1 cm^2 leads to concentric left ventricular hypertrophy and a reduction in left ventricular compliance. Left ventricular filling during diastole depends on adequate preload as well as atrial contraction (which contributes less than 20% of filling in the normal heart, but may contribute twice this amount in aortic stenosis). Atrial fibrillation will cause loss of this valuable supply of preload volume and decrease stroke volume. As the aortic valve area diminishes below 0.5–1 cm^2, the left ventricle will begin to dilate and the patient may develop atrial fibrillation and symptoms of pulmonary congestion or syncope with exertion.

○ **Describe the pathophysiology of chronic aortic regurgitation.**

Volume overload of the left ventricle, with dilation and eccentric hypertrophy. The left ventricle generates a very large stroke volume, aided by peripheral dilation, to make up for the regurgitant backward flow through the aortic valve during diastole. The heart rate is usually elevated as this reduces the proportion of time spent in diastole. With severe, compensated AR the regurgitant flow may exceed 20 L/min, giving a total CO of 25 L/min.

○ **What is the medical management of aortic regurgitation?**

Because the left ventricle is volume overloaded and dilated, the preservation of CO is most important. Avoidance of increased impedance to forward flow by keeping the SVR low-normal is helpful to left ventricular function. Keeping the heart rate fast will reduce the regurgitant fraction. Because of the loss of part of the ejected stroke volume back into the left ventricle, the body compensates by increasing LVEDV; one must therefore endeavor to maintain adequate preload.

○ **What are the hemodynamic changes associated with MR?**

Chronic MR produces volume overloading of the left ventricle. It also causes LV hypertrophy/dilation and LA dilation, so pressures remain low in the LA and there is little effect to the pulmonary vasculature and RV until late in the progress of the disease. Acute MR results in increased left atrial pressure and decreased CO that can cause pulmonary edema, pulmonary hypertension, and RV failure. Compensatory changes lead to worsening of the MR as a result of tachycardia and increase SVR.

○ **What are the anesthetic management principles of MR?**

CO is optimized when the heart is full and reasonably fast, with the blood pressure maintained at low-normal with afterload reduction. Bradycardia should be avoided as it is associated with an increase in ventricular size leading to valvular dilation and an increase in the regurgitant fraction. Contractility of the left ventricle is difficult to determine without a PAC or TEE, so one should avoid myocardial depression acknowledging that these patients will often require inotropic support during general anesthesia.

○ **What are the consequences of hypotension in mitral stenosis?**

In patients with severe mitral stenosis, sudden decrease in SVR may not be tolerated due to reflex tachycardia that accompanies it. Therefore, SVR should be maintained with vasopressors. Phenylephrine is better than ephedrine since it is predominantly an alpha-agonist, which eliminates the concerns regarding increases in heart rate.

The development of atrial fibrillation with rapid ventricular response rates may significantly decrease CO. Treatment consists of cardioversion (25 W/s) or IV esmolol to decrease heart rate to less than 110 bpm.

○ **Describe the treatment and perioperative anesthetic management of pericardial tamponade.**

In this condition, blood or fluid collects within the pericardium preventing the ventricles from adequately filling. Treatment is pericardiocentesis in symptomatic patients. Until the tamponade is relieved, one must endeavor to keep the patient as well oxygenated as possible, maintain preload, and keep the heart rate at the high end of normal due to limited ventricular filling, but ensure that the heart rate is not so high that it may prevent adequate diastolic filling.

○ **T/F: The classic signs of traumatic cardiac tamponade include distended neck veins and muffled heart sounds.**

False. The classic signs of cardiac tamponade are usually absent. If the blood in the pericardial sac is clotted, needle pericardiocentesis will also be negative.

○   **What is pulsus paradoxus?**

Pulsus paradoxus occurs when there is a fall in systolic blood pressure of 12 mm Hg or more during inspiration. This is an exaggeration of a normal occurrence. During inspiration in a spontaneously breathing individual, there is a small decrease (hemodynamically insignificant) in stroke volume from the left ventricle. The inspiratory decrease in intrathoracic pressure leads to augmented venous return and increased right ventricular end-diastolic volume, but reduced LVEDV due to right ventricular distension and rightward shift of intraventricular septum. Pulsus paradoxus is a manifestation of an exaggerated decrease in left ventricular stroke volume. Causes include cardiac tamponade, constrictive pericardial disease, and chronic obstructive pulmonary disease (or any condition in which there are large swings in intrathoracic pressure).

○   **Describe the TEE diagnosis of pericardial tamponade versus hypovolemia.**

The TEE assessment of hypovolemia versus tamponade can be challenging.

The key element is to identify whether the patient has a moderate to large pericardial effusion. This appears as an echo lucent (black) space around the heart (circumferential and therefore seen in multiple images). However, in some situations (postcardiac surgery) the fluid collection may be localized and smaller in size.

Whether circumferential or localized, increased pericardial pressure causes diastolic collapse of one or more cardiac chambers (usually right sided initially, because RV is thinner walled than the LV). RA collapse lasting longer than one third of the R–R interval is specific for cardiac tamponade.

Typically in tamponade the heart is tachycardic, LV end-diastolic volume is low, and the LV function is normal to hyperdynamic (however, this may depend on the baseline LV function).

Additional findings of tamponade include 25% respiratory variation of mitral valve and tricuspid valve inflow (increased tricuspid valve inflow with decreased mitral valve inflow during inspiration).

The echocardiographic findings of hypovolemia can be similar in that the LV is usually tachycardic, underfilled, with normal or hyperdynamic function. However, all cardiac chambers are uniformly underfilled without compression, and, most importantly, a significant pericardial effusion is notably absent [Memtsoudis et al., 2006. See reference on page 523].

○   **A patient with HCM presents in acute heart failure and is treated with diuresis, nitrates, and inotropic agents. What would you predict would be the outcome of this therapy?**

The patient's condition becomes more critical. The correct management is volume administration, slowing the heart and increasing afterload. The key pathophysiology of HCM is a hypertrophied interventricular septum that can lead to "functional" outflow tract obstruction if the ventricle is empty or hypercontractile. An associated anomaly called systolic anterior motion (SAM; of the anterior mitral leaflet) contributes to the obstruction when the anterior leaflet bulges into the outflow tract resulting in MR. Both outflow tract obstruction and MR are exacerbated by inotropic therapy and hypovolemia.

○   **What are the forms of HCM?**

HCM is classified into three general types: symmetric hypertrophy, apical hypertrophy, and septal hypertrophy. This disease process encompasses several disease types and has gone by several names including HOCM, idiopathic hypertrophic subaortic stenosis (IHSS), and asymmetric septal hypertrophy. HOCM, in which there is obstruction of the ventricular outflow, can occur with any of the forms, but is most common in the asymmetric form of the septal hypertrophy type.

○ **What is the anesthetic management of the obstructive form of HCM?**

The general management principles are to increase preload, thereby increasing the distance between the boundaries of the left ventricle and the outflow tract. The avoidance of positive inotropic drugs such as dopamine, epinephrine, etc., and the use of negative inotropic drugs such as beta-blockers will prevent the dynamic obstruction of ventricular outflow in high stress states. Generous sedation will also reduce sympathetic discharge. Raising blood pressure, preferably with drugs that do not affect inotropy (classically phenylephrine is used), will decrease the pressure gradient between the left ventricle and aorta.

○ **What are the two most common causes of post-CPB bleeding, excluding surgical causes?**

Residual heparin and platelet dysfunction/thrombocytopenia.

○ **Name three vasodilator drugs used in cardiac surgery.**

Nitroprusside, nicardipine, and NTG.

○ **How do you treat hypertension during CPB?**

Hypertension is caused by high SVR or excessive perfusion flow and is treated with IV vasodilators such as nitroprusside. Another option is to administer isoflurane by a calibrated vaporizer in the oxygenator gas inlet line. Phentolamine can be used in pediatric patients undergoing CPB, but has a longer half-life.

○ **During CPB how does the perfusionist maintain constant venous return?**

The reservoir allows for constant venous return. With membrane oxygenators, the reservoir is the first component of the extracorporeal circuit that receives venous drainage as well as the cardiotomy drainage. Blood then passes to the arterial pump. The reservoir serves as a capacitance chamber that buffers the fluctuations between venous return and arterial outflow. This protects the patient from the risk of systemic air embolism if venous drainage is reduced and the system is effectively pumped dry. The reservoir also serves as an air trap and allows administration of blood, fluids, or drugs to the circuit.

○ **What are some of the causes of a decrease in SvO_2 during CPB?**

SvO_2 can be negatively influenced by a decrease in oxygen delivery or an increase in oxygen consumption. An inappropriate decrease in arterial flow, for whatever reason, by the CPB machine, a drop in hemoglobin, and a reduction in the ability of the machine to oxygenate the blood (malfunctioning oxygenator) can lead to a decrease in SvO_2. Also, use of methylene blue, an increase in patient temperature, awareness or "light anesthesia," as well as a preexisting condition, such as sepsis, may also decrease SvO_2.

○ **List several causes of hypotension during CPB.**

Hypotension is caused either by inadequate forward flow (low flow rate from the CPB pump) or from peripheral vasodilatation, which may be caused by a number of factors:

- Hypoxic vasodilatation, secondary to either reduced CO or the fact that the initial priming solution contains no oxygen
- The presence of NTG in the cardioplegic solution
- Hemodilution, resulting in a decreased circulating volume of catecholamines
- Release of endogenous vasoactive particles after the introduction of the patient's blood to the heart–lung machine

○   **What is the differential diagnosis of hypotension (specific to cardiac surgery) postoperatively following CPB?**

Preload: postoperative bleeding. TEE will show the left ventricular cavity is obliterated during systole as the ventricle attempts to eject all of the available volume. The ventricle is seen to pump vigorously and the midportion of the left ventricle the papillary muscles are touching (kissing papillary muscles).

Rhythm: the incidence of atrial fibrillation or flutter is 20–30%, especially on day 2 or 3 postoperative.

Left or right ventricular dysfunction and low CO: inadequate protection of the myocardium during aortic cross-clamping, pulmonary edema, acute left ventricular distension or other trauma, uncorrected valvular lesion or valvular incompetence, and reduced coronary blood flow due to graft occlusion. Pericardial tamponade must be high on the differential diagnosis list. Echocardiographic findings of right atrial collapse during systole, when the right atrial pressure is lowest, and the subsequent impact on venous return to the heart can help diagnose this cause of postoperative hypotension. Immediate guided percutaneous drainage or reopening of the mediastinum is critical.

Low serum levels of thyroid hormone.

SVR low: normothermic perfusion or longer pump times, rewarming after hypothermic CABG, sepsis, and vasodilator therapy.

○   **What is the influence of cooling during CPB on $PaCO_2$?**

As core temperature drops, carbon dioxide becomes more soluble and thus $PaCO_2$ drops (pH becomes more alkaline).

○   **What is pH stat management of CPB and deep hypothermic circulatory arrest?**

The principle behind pH stat management is the addition of carbon dioxide while the core temperature of the patient is dropped during CPB. The object is to raise the *temperature-corrected $PaCO_2$* to 40 mm Hg. In principle, this will cause cerebral vasodilatation and increase cerebral blood flow. This is clearly beneficial for pediatric patients undergoing palliative or corrective surgery for congenital cardiac lesions. But for adults, the evidence suggests this type of management may not yield the same benefits because the increased flow will also cause embolization of air and atherosclerotic debris from the aorta, which could cause postoperative cognitive dysfunction.

○   **What is the influence of cooling during CPB on PaO_2?**

As in the case of carbon dioxide, oxygen also becomes more soluble as core temperature drops. Thus, the PaO_2 drops on the *temperature-corrected* blood gas result as temperature drops. The PaO_2 drops approximately 5–6 mm Hg for every 1°C drop in core temperature below 37°C.

○   **During CPB with a temperature of 28°C and a hematocrit of 24%, the temperature-corrected $PaCO_2$ is 50 mm Hg and uncorrected $PaCO_2$ is 60 mm Hg. What is the appropriate management?**

Increase the fresh gas flow in the oxygenator. In a bubble and membrane oxygenator, CO_2 transfer is proportional to total gas flow. The higher the total gas flow, the lower the CO_2. At higher flows it may be necessary to add CO_2 to prevent hypocarbia.

○   **How do you measure the core temperature during CPB?**

The core temperature is composed of highly perfused tissues whose temperature is uniform and high, in comparison to the rest of the body. This temperature can be evaluated in the pulmonary artery, distal part of the esophagus, tympanic membrane, or nasopharynx. In a rapid changing temperature situation, like CPB, these sites remain reliable. Rectal temperature lags behind those measured in core sites and is considered an "intermediate" temperature in deliberately cooled patients. During CPB, bladder temperature is equal to rectal temperature when urine output is low but equal to pulmonary artery temperature when the urinary flow is high.

During rewarming, the adequacy of temperature increase is best evaluated by considering both "core" (nasopharynx) and "intermediate" (rectal) temperatures.

Skin surface temperatures are considerably lower than core temperature and affected by local factors (warming blanket, topical cooling device). This will lead to errors in measuring temperatures.

○ **What is the most common adverse effect of protamine administration?**

Less than 1% of patients receiving protamine develop an adverse reaction. Hypotension is the most common reaction and can be severe, especially if the medication is given too rapidly or there is underlying hypovolemia. These reactions are not always antibody mediated and can be due to complement activation.

○ **What are the proposed mechanisms for protamine reactions?**

Previous exposure to protamine can result in IgE- and IgG-mediated reactions, which cause severe hypotension and bronchospasm. Protamine is also known to cause nonimmunologic release of chemical mediators and complement activation. These anaphylactoid reactions to protamine can lead to pulmonary vasoconstriction and right ventricular failure. Protamine has also been linked to noncardiogenic pulmonary edema postbypass.

○ **Who is at high risk for a protamine reaction?**

- Diabetics taking protamine insulin preparations, for example, NPH insulin (0.6–2% incidence)
- Vasectomized men (appears to be rare)
- Fish-allergic individuals (also appears to be rare)
- Patients previously exposed to protamine for heparin reversal (increasing incidence)

○ **What are the cardiovascular effects of protamine?**

Unpredictable. The most common effect is hypotension especially if given rapidly in patients with poor LV function for heparin reversal after CPB. Causes include mediator release (histamine, thromboxane), hypocalcemia, and anaphylaxis. Systemic vasodilation and pulmonary vasoconstriction (increased PAP and PVR) are variable. Protamine has no direct action on the human heart. Maximum effect is at 1 minute, worn off by 4 minutes. Other adverse effects: bleeding, hypertension, and noncardiogenic pulmonary edema.

○ **What is the treatment for different types of protamine reactions?**

Protamine reactions are not uncommon, and can be life threatening [Porsche and Brenner, 1999. See reference on page 523].

There are several different reactions as follows:

1. When protamine is administered rapidly, it causes systemic hypotension as with other polycationic drugs (e.g., vancomycin) due to *histamine release* from mast cells.

   Always administer slowly. Rate of administration is more important than the route. Restrict its use to 1 mg/kg and 20 mg in any 60-second period.

2. Type II or *anaphylactoid reactions* (not a pure substance and can contain fish protein).

   Prior protamine reaction: Prepare a dilute solution (1 mg in 100 mL), and administer over 10 minutes. If no adverse reaction, may administer the full dose.

   Systemic hypotension within 10 minutes of protamine suggests a reaction and specific treatment depends on other hemodynamic events.

   Normal or low pulmonary pressure suggests either rapid administration or anaphylactoid reaction.

3. Type III reactions to protamine are characterized by ***pulmonary hypertension*** and vasoconstriction with possible resultant right heart failure. This side effect is mediated by protamine–heparin complex–induced release of thromboxane A2 from platelets and macrophages. Studies have shown that this reaction is attenuated by pretreatment with COX inhibitors.

Inotropes with pulmonary dilating properties, such as isoproterenol or milrinone, will support the failing heart while facilitating passage of blood across pulmonary circulation. Reinstitution of CPB may be necessary with extreme hemodynamic deterioration and will require full heparin dose (occasionally heparin alone corrects the pulmonary hypertension).

4. ***Antihemostatic*** effect – Platelet count can drop precipitously when protamine is administered after heparin. Protamine also activates thrombin receptors on platelets causing partial activation and subsequent impairment of platelet aggregation.

Alternative to protamine in patients with previous history of reactions: allow heparin effect to dissipate and administer platelet concentrates.

○   **What is a type II reaction to protamine?**

Idiosyncratic anaphylactic or anaphylactoid reaction, presumably due to prior sensitization or patients with fish allergy.

○   **If a patient experiences a possible type II reaction to protamine coming off CPB and becomes severely hypotensive, what should you do?**

Stop protamine, give 100% oxygen, discontinue anesthetic agents, aggressively address intravascular volume expansion, and selectively give a pulmonary vasodilator into the right side of the heart, and a vasoconstrictor/inotrope into the left (e.g., epinephrine). Diphenhydramine and famotidine can be used to counteract the vasodilatory effects of histamine. For refractory hypotension, reinstitute CPB.

○   **During CPB the activation of fibrinolysis results in postoperative bleeding complications. What are the treatment strategies to minimize blood loss?**

During CPB, activation of fibrinolysis results in an increased activation of plasminogen and the reduction of plasmin inhibitors. CPB also initiates elastase release that may be an indicator of postoperative inflammatory reaction and could correlate with a reduction in AT III.

The use of lysine analogs (epsilon aminocaproic acid or tranexamic acid) in cardiac surgical patients results in less chest tube drainage but significant decreases in transfusion requirements have not been consistently documented. Aprotinin inhibits thrombin activation and fibrinolysis and has a protecting effect on thrombocytes. Aprotinin, though, has been removed from the market due to increased risks of death, serious kidney damage, stroke, and cardiac toxicity.

○   **What is the incidence and risk factors for adverse neurologic outcome following CABG surgery?**

The overall incidence is reported as 6.1%. Adverse cerebral outcomes include focal injury, stupor or coma, seizures, memory deficit, and deterioration in intellectual function. Risk factors include age, proximal aortic atherosclerosis, and a history of neurologic disease. The landmark study by Newman et al. demonstrated the incidence of cognitive decline was 53% at discharge, 36% at 6 weeks, 24% at 6 months, and rising to 42% at 5 years. Possible mechanisms include progression of concomitant disease, stress of major surgery, and specific events during CABG surgery (atheroemboli, microemboli, cerebral hypoperfusion, and systemic inflammatory response) [Newman et al., 1996. See reference on page 523].

○ **What are the limitations of the ACT clotting test in monitoring high-dose heparin anticoagulation?**

The ACT is less precise than the PTT, and lacks high correlation with the PTT or with heparin antifactor Xa levels. It is influenced by a number of variables including the platelet count, platelet function, lupus anticoagulants, factor deficiencies, ambient temperature, hypothermia, and hemodilution. As the various methods are not standardized, results from different methods are not interchangeable. Aprotinin will prolong celite-based ACTs but generally not kaolin-based ACTs unless very high initial bolus doses of aprotinin are administered.

○ **How do you determine if an unexpected PTT prolongation is due to heparin contamination?**

Measure the PTT before and after heparinase treatment. Heparinase degrades unfractionated heparin, most importantly the pentasaccharide sequence which is the antithrombin-binding site required for heparin anticoagulation. The resulting small fragments lack anticoagulant activity.

○ **Which clinical situations may be associated with heparin resistance from acquired antithrombin deficiency?**

Heparin binds to plasma proteins including platelet factor 4, fibrinogen, factor VIII, and histidine-rich glycoproteins. Many of the heparin-binding proteins are acute phase reactants, so the phenomenon of heparin resistance due to altered clearance is often encountered in acutely ill patients and those with malignancy and during peripartum or postpartum periods. Drug-induced causes include aprotinin and NTG. Its association with low antithrombin levels is also a point of heated discussion in the literature and includes infective endocarditis (IE), intra-aortic balloon counterpulsation, oral contraceptives, shock, low-grade intravascular coagulation, prior heparin or streptokinase therapy, presence of clot within the circulation, neonatal respiratory distress syndrome, and increased platelets or factor VIII levels.

○ **Describe the maneuvers an anesthesiologist should perform in the event of a massive air embolism on CPB.**

Position the patient in steep Trendelenburg with bilateral compression of the carotid arteries. The surgeon and perfusionist should stop the pump and isolate the patient from the circuit, perform retrograde perfusion through an exit wound in the aorta, remove the aortic cannula, purge the arterial circuit of air, and place the aortic cannula in the SVC. The perfusate temperature should be decreased to 20°C and once all of the air is expelled from the aorta, the aortic cannula is placed in the ascending aorta and the CPB restarted at high flow rates. The coronary arteries are massaged and all four heart chambers vented. The MAP is increased to 65 mm Hg, the FiO_2 is set at 100%, and the $PaCO_2$ is maintained in the low 30s. The anesthesiologist should administer steroids and mannitol. Discontinue bypass with the systolic pressure >100 mm Hg and low filling pressures. A hyperbaric medicine consult should be considered.

○ **Describe the management of coronary air embolism.**

Coronary artery air embolism may occur as one of the sequelae of air embolism. Air embolism is usually related to surgery or trauma and is well known to occur during CPB. Arterial emboli may occur from the introduction of air via the venous circulation, even in the absence of obvious cardiac or pulmonary shunts. Coronary emboli can cause dysrhythmias, hypotension, and myocardial infarction. Diagnosis of intracardiac air may be made with echocardiography. Electrocardiographic changes may also be seen.

Management of coronary air embolism is mainly supportive with 100% oxygen and circulatory support with intravenous crystalloids, vasopressors, and intra-aortic counterpulsation as needed. Hyperbaric oxygen can accelerate the absorption of air bubbles. Hyperoxygenation increases the nitrogen gradient between air bubbles and the blood and facilitates its removal. Massive gas embolism related to CPB mandates immediate discontinuation of bypass and venting from the aortic cannulation site. Coronary air may be expressed by massage and needle venting.

○ **What are the causes of renal failure after CPB?**

CPB induces hypotension and nonpulsatile flow that promotes renal vasoconstriction and decreased RBF. Surgery and CPB cause the release of norepinephrine, as well as activation of angiotensin with a renin release that persists well after CPB. Both pump-mediated platelet activation and elaboration of thromboxane as well as tissue release of endothelin may add to renal vasoconstriction. Aortic cross-clamping may release aortic atheroemboli that circulate to the kidney.

Studies on patients undergoing mitral valve replacement have shown that when the postoperative left atrial pressure decreases by 7 mm Hg compared with the preoperative levels both sodium excretion and urine flow rate show a decrease. This coincides with decreased circulating levels of ANP. While ARF after CPB occurs in less than 2% of patients, the mortality associated with it remains between 60 and 90%.

○ **What are the physiologic effects of intra-aortic balloon pump (IABP) counterpulsation therapy?**

The tip of the IABP lies in the descending aorta just below the origin of the left subclavian artery. Inflation and deflation of the balloon are synchronized to the patient's cardiac cycle. Inflation at the onset of diastole augments diastolic pressure and increases coronary perfusion pressure as well as improves the relationship between myocardial oxygen supply and demand. Deflation occurs just prior to the onset of systole with improvement in CO, EF, and wall tension and a decrease in heart rate, PCWP, and SVR.

○ **Describe triggering and timing of inflation and deflation of the IABP as it relates to the EKG.**

The most common method of triggering the IABP is from the R wave of the patient's EKG. Inflation starts in the middle of the T wave at the beginning of diastole that is noted on the dicrotic notch on the arterial waveform and deflation is set to occur prior to the ending of the QRS complex, immediately prior to the arterial upstroke. The arterial waveform may be used if synchronization with the EKG mode is difficult, as in tachyarrhythmias or poor EKG signals.

○ **What are the contraindications to IABP?**

Contraindications include aortic aneurysm, aortic dissection, severe aortic insufficiency, severe peripheral vascular disease, and irreversible brain damage.

○ **What factors affect the function of a left ventricular assist device (LVAD)?**

LVAD is placed as a bridge to transplant, for short-term support during cardiogenic shock, or to improve quality of life in nontransplant candidates (long-term support).

LVAD output is affected by the factors that affect the device preload and afterload. These include patient's preload, patient's position, height of the device relative to the heart, and cannula size.

○ **Does a 50-year-old male with moderate MR, undergoing knee arthroplasty, require subacute bacterial endocarditis (SBE) prophylaxis?**

No. Although this patient has a valvular lesion, clean surgery through uninfected tissue does not require SBE prophylaxis.

○ **What are the cardiac conditions with an increased risk of IE and therefore require antibiotic prophylaxis?**

They include:

1. Prosthetic cardiac valve or prosthetic material used for cardiac valve repair

2. Previous IE

3. CHD including unrepaired cyanotic as well as palliative shunts and conduits, completely repaired congenital heart defect with prosthetic material or device during the first 6 months after the procedure, and repaired CHD with residual defects

4. Cardiac transplantation recipients who develop cardiac valvulopathy [Prevention of Infective Endocarditis. Guidelines From the American Heart Association, 2007. See reference on page 523].

○ **Prior to what procedures do the patients with above cardiac conditions require prophylaxis?**

All dental procedures that involve manipulation of gingival tissue or the peripheral region of teeth or perforation of the oral mucosa will require IE prophylaxis.

Patients who undergo respiratory tract procedure that involves incision or biopsy of the respiratory mucosa will also require IE prophylaxis.

In contrast to previous AHA guidelines, antibiotic prophylaxis to prevent IE is not recommended for GU or GI procedures.

○ **What are the current recommendations for SBE prophylaxis?**

First-line therapy recommended includes amoxicillin or ampicillin and if allergic to penicillin, clindamycin 600 mg or azithromycin 500 mg.

Antibiotics should be administered in a single dose 30–60 minutes before the procedure, but the dosage may be administered up to 2 hours after procedure.

The standard regimen is amoxicillin 2.0 g orally (children 50 mg/kg).

For patients who cannot take oral medications: ampicillin 2.0 g IV or IM (children 50 mg/kg IM or IV) or cefazolin or ceftriaxone 1 g IM or IV (children 50 mg/kg IM or IV).

If the patient is allergic to amoxicillin or penicillin, the guidelines call for cephalexin 2 g (children 50 mg/kg) or clindamycin 600 mg (children 20 mg/kg) or azithromycin or clarithromycin 500 mg (children 15 mg/kg) orally.

If the patient is allergic to amoxicillin or penicillin and cannot take oral medications: cefazolin or ceftriaxone 1 g IM or IV (children 50 mg/kg IM or IV) or clindamycin 600 mg IM or IV (children 20 mg/kg IM or IV).

Key Terms

Adrenergic downregulation in CHF
Adverse protamine reactions/treatment
Aortic insufficiency: hemodynamic treatment
Aortic insufficiency: medical management
Aortic valve lesions: flow volume loops
Arterial blood gas temperature correction effects
Atrial fibrillation/aortic stenosis: treatment
AV pacing: hemodynamic effects
Blood supply: AV node
Cardiac cycle: P/V loop
Cardiac pacemaker indications

Cardiac pressure–volume relationship
Cardiac surface anatomy
Cardiac tamponade: diagnosis/anesthetic management
Cardiac tamponade: pulsus paradoxus
Cardiopulmonary bypass (CPB) management
Cardiovascular physiology: left ventricle
Circulatory arrest: pH stat implications
Coronary air embolism
Coronary artery anatomy
Coronary blood flow: determinants
Coronary perfusion pressure

Coronary perfusion pressure: left versus right

CPB and temperature measurements

CPB antifibrinolytics

CPB: gas embolism management

CPB hypotension: causes

DDD pacemaker: perioperative management

Determinants: coronary blood flow

Diagnosis RV infarction

Disease states: beta1 receptor density

Dominant coronary artery: definition

ECG changes: myocardial ischemia

ECG with right coronary occlusion

Effect of preload in congestive heart failure (CHF)

Effects of junctional rhythm

Electrosurgical unit (ESU)–induced pacemaker malfunction: prevention

Enhanced ventricular function: mechanism

Factors affecting function of LVAD

Heart block: coronary occlusion

HOCM/asymmetric septal hypertrophy: anesthetic management

Hypertrophic cardiomyopathy (HOCM): hypotension treatment

Hypothermia: pH stat management

Implantable cardiac defibrillator: interventions

Intra-aortic balloon pump (IABP): physiologic effects/ hemodynamic effects/contraindications

Intraoperative myocardial ischemia: diagnosis and treatment

Ischemia: chordae tendineae rupture

Left ventricular failure diagnosis and treatment post-CPB

Left ventricular filling physiology

Left ventricular preload: measurement

Left ventricular versus right ventricular function

LV preload: best assessment techniques

Management: acute heart failure

Management of congenital heart defects

Mitral insufficiency: medical management/ pharmacological treatment

Mitral stenosis; hypotension

Myocardial compliance

Myocardial contractility: assessment

Myocardial ischemia: acute mitral regurgitation

Myocardial oxygen demand: determinants

Myocardial oxygen supply

Myocardial perfusion

Neurologic risk after CPB surgery

New York Heart Association (NYHA) functional status

Nitric oxide and increased pulmonary vascular resistance

Nitric oxide: pulmonary vasodilatation

Pacemaker: effects on cardiac output

Pacemakers: fixed versus synchronous mode

Pacemakers: nomenclature/designation

Pacer lead placement: ECG morphology

Patient with AICD: perioperative management

Perioperative ischemia: TEE diagnosis

Perioperative myocardial infarction: diagnostic tests

Post-CABG hypotension: differential diagnosis

Post-CPB creatinine increase: differential diagnosis

Pulmonary hypertension: differential diagnosis

Renal failure: CPB surgery

RV failure hemodynamics

Subacute bacterial endocarditis (SBE) prophylaxis/indications

Stroke volume: atrial fibrillation effect

SvO_2 saturation during CPB: interpretation

TEE: diagnosis: hypotension

TEE findings in mitral regurgitation

TEE: left ventricular regional wall motion

TEE: normal anatomy

TEE: tamponade versus hypovolemia

TEE views: perfusion distribution/coronary circulation

Transcutaneous pacing

Valvular insufficiency: diagnosis

Vasodilators: primary pulmonary hypertension

Ventricular pressure–volume loops

VSD: factors affecting L to R shunt

Wall motion abnormalities: TEE view

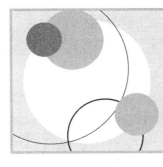

Cardiopulmonary Resuscitation

Victory belongs to the most persevering.
Napoleon

○ **Which vasoactive substances are involved in the compensatory response to acute hypovolemia?**

1. Angiotensin–renin (kidney): angiotensinogen, renin, angiotensin I, angiotensin II (lung), and aldosterone (adrenal cortex)

2. Adrenergic (adrenal medulla): norepinephrine and epinephrine

3. AVP (pituitary): ACTH and arginine vasopressin

> Blood pressure = cardiac output (contractility, sodium and water retention, capillary fluid shift)
> × systemic vascular resistance (vasoconstriction).

○ **What is the mechanism of sinus tachycardia?**

A heart rate of greater than 100 beats/min originating from the sinus node (SN) that is classified as appropriate (exercise, anxiety, panic attacks, dehydration, deconditioning, hypovolemia, hyperthyroidism, pheochromocytoma, electrolyte abnormalities, hypercarbia, hypoxia, pain, inadequate anesthesia, drug effects, fever, anemia, heart failure, pulmonary embolism) or inappropriate.

Inappropriate sinus tachycardia is a diagnosis of exclusion. The proposed underlying mechanisms include intracardiac SN abnormality (high intrinsic heart rate, depressed efferent cardiovagal reflex, and beta-adrenergic hypersensitivity) and extracardiac (length-dependent autonomic neuropathy, excessive venous pooling, beta-receptor hypersensitivity, alpha-receptor hyposensitivity, altered sympathovagal balance, and brainstem dysregulation).

○ **What is the treatment of a patient who develops chest pain suggestive of ischemia?**

- Immediate assessment: measure vital signs and oxygen saturation, obtain IV access, 12-lead ECG, brief targeted history and physical exam, obtain initial serum cardiac marker levels, check electrolytes, hematocrit and coagulation studies, and stat portable chest x-ray.
- Immediate general treatment: MONA – morphine IV, oxygen 4 L/min, nitroglycerin, and aspirin 160–325 mg.
- Twelve-lead ECG shows ST depression and new T-wave inversion: patient is at high risk for unstable or new-onset angina or nondiagnostic ECG but troponin positive; start adjunctive treatments as indicated: heparin, aspirin, glycoprotein IIb/IIIa receptor inhibitors, nitroglycerin IV, and beta-adrenergic receptor blocker.
- Cardiology consultation for monitoring or cardiac catheterization and possible revascularization.

○ **Sinus rhythm, QRS axis –64° (left-axis deviation), QRS duration 142 milliseconds, qR in lead aVL, rS in leads II, III, aVF, rsR′ in V1 and V2, and qRS in lead V5–6. What is the EKG diagnosis?**

Bifascicular block (right bundle branch block and left anterior hemiblock).

○ **What are most common causes of bifascicular block?**

Idiopathic degenerative conductive disease and ischemic heart disease.

○ **Why are epinephrine, phenylephrine, vasopressin, methoxamine, and dopamine thought to be equally efficacious in restoring blood pressure during CPR?**

All of them cause peripheral vasoconstriction through alpha-adrenergic effects that increases aortic diastolic pressure and augments cerebral and coronary perfusion. Beta stimulation has previously been thought to facilitate defibrillation by increasing the amplitude of fine fibrillation, but actually may be detrimental by increasing myocardial oxygen consumption and decreasing the endocardial/epicardial flow ratio.

○ **When is it necessary to treat an intraoperative dysrhythmia?**

When it is detrimental to cardiac output (blood pressure) and tissue perfusion, a precursor of a more life-threatening dysrhythmia, and in the presence of myocardial ischemia. Most intraoperative dysrhythmias can be explained on the basis of an autonomic imbalance and do not need treating.

○ **According to the ACLS protocol, what drugs are first choice to control the heart rate of a patient with atrial fibrillation and a rapid ventricular response?**

Diltiazem (or other calcium channel blocker), or a beta-blocker. Amiodarone is an alternative, but it may also convert the rhythm to sinus, which may be undesirable before anticoagulation. If the patient is unstable, electrical cardioversion should be considered rather than adding a second drug.

○ **What drugs can be harmful in the treatment of atrial fibrillation in a patient with Wolff–Parkinson–White (WPW)?**

Adenosine, calcium channel blockers, digoxin, and possibly beta-blockers slow conduction through the AV node, but not necessarily through the accessory pathway, which may increase the ventricular rate.

Amiodarone or procainamide are the recommended drugs in this situation.

○ **What is the treatment for acute-onset WPW syndrome?**

Synchronized direct current (DC) cardioversion in the unstable patient or beta-blockers and a primary antiarrhythmic agent (one of the following: amiodarone, flecainamide, procainamide, propafenone, sotalol) followed by cardiac consultation in the hemodynamically stable patient. WPW is characterized by short PR interval, wide QRS, and delta wave. WPW with atrial fibrillation often mimics ventricular tachycardia (VT).

○ **T/F: Atrial fibrillation or atrial flutter of greater than 48 hours duration should be treated with DC cardioversion and amiodarone.**

False. First control the rate. If atrial fibrillation is >48 hours duration, nonemergent conversion to NSR with shock or drugs may cause embolization of atrial thrombi unless the patient has been adequately anticoagulated.

○ **Successful cardioversion of atrial flutter may occur at what energy level?**

50 to 100 J.

○ **How does synchronized electrical cardioversion differ for supraventricular tachyarrhythmias compared with VT?**

SVTs – atrial fibrillation initial energy dose is 120–200 J biphasic or 200 J monophasic. Conversion of atrial flutter is initial energy dose of 50–100 J with either monophasic or biphasic. Doses may be increased in a stepwise fashion.

VT – stable VT initial energy dose is 100 J for monophasic or biphasic. Dose may be increased if no response. Unstable VT requires defibrillation doses.

○ **What factors determine the treatment of VT?**

- Hemodynamically stable versus unstable patient
- Monomorphic versus polymorphic
- Normal versus impaired left ventricular function

Hemodynamically stable monomorphic VT and polymorphic VT in patients with normal QT interval and *normal LV function*: procainamide, amiodarone, lidocaine, and sotalol; *impaired LV function*: amiodarone or lidocaine.

Ongoing polymorphic VT and unstable patients: immediate cardioversion.

Self-terminated polymorphic VT with prolonged QT interval: magnesium.

○ **What is the difference between the therapeutic effect of cardioversion and defibrillation to terminate tachycardias?**

Cardioversion (*synchronized* DC shock on the R-wave peak of the QRS complex of a stable tachycardia) terminates repetitive reentry loops, whereas defibrillation (*unsynchronized* shock in the very unstable patient in ventricular fibrillation [VF] and pulseless VT) depolarizes the entire myocardium. Delivery of a shock during cardiac repolarization (T wave) may precipitate VF.

○ **List two important factors that affect the success of defibrillation.**

1. Energy output of the defibrillator
2. Resistance to current flow during shock delivery

○ **What is the primary determinant of delivered energy?**

Transthoracic impedance. When transthoracic impedance is higher, the actual delivered energy will be lower.

○ **What factors affect transthoracic impedance?**

1. Paddle size – resistance decreases with increasing electrode size (common paddle size 8–10 cm in diameter).
2. Use of gel or paste reduces impedance.
3. Transthoracic impedance decreases with successive shocks.
4. Impedance is slightly higher during inspiration than during exhalation (air is a poor conductor).
5. Firm pressure of at least 11 kg reduces resistance by improving paddle–skin contact.

○ **What is the optimal energy for open-chest defibrillation?**

During cardiac surgery, internal paddles applied directly to the heart are used for direct defibrillation of the heart. Low energy levels, 5–25 J, are required since skin impedance is bypassed.

○ **How does epinephrine improve survival during VF?**

In VF, epinephrine's alpha1 mechanism and increase in systemic vascular resistance leads to an increased aortic diastolic pressure and therefore an increase in coronary blood flow.

○ **Explain what PATCH and 5H–5T have in common.**

Both are mnemonics for the most frequent causes of pulseless electrical activity (PEA).

5H: hypovolemia, hypoxemia, hydrogen ion (acidosis), hyperkalemia/hypokalemia, and hypothermia.

5T: tablets (drug overdose, accidents), tamponade (cardiac), tension pneumothorax, thrombosis (coronary), and thrombosis (pulmonary: PE).

○ **True/False – Atropine should be given in PEA.**

False – as per the 2010 ACLS guidelines, atropine is no longer recommended during PEA. Epinephrine and vasopressin are the two medications to be given along with CPR. Epinephrine 1 mg should be given IV or IO every 3–5 minutes. Vasopressin 40 U IV or IO may be used to substitute the first or second dose of epinephrine [Peberdy et al., post-cardiac arrest care: 2010 American Heart Association Guidelines for Cardiopulmonary Resuscitation and Emergency Cardiovascular Care. See reference on page 523].

○ **What is the osmolality of sodium bicarbonate ($NaHCO_3$)?**

One ampule (50 mL) contains 50 mEq of sodium and 50 mEq of HCO_3. $NaHCO_3$ is hypertonic, about 1,800 mOsm/L.

○ **Why were $NaHCO_3$ and calcium chloride ($CaCl_2$) removed from cardiac resuscitation protocols?**

There is concern that $NaHCO_3$ may cause paradoxical intracellular acidosis (leading to myocardial depression), hyperosmolality, and hypernatremia. Intracellular influx of calcium is intimately involved in the terminal stages of cell death, and this is a concern in the setting of resuscitation. $CaCl_2$ may also prevent reflow of blood into ischemic areas of the brain and heart, worsening outcome.

○ **What effect on CO_2 does bicarbonate administration have?**

For every 50 mEq of $NaHCO_3$ infused, 1,250 mL of CO_2 is produced. $NaHCO_3$ therapy started at a 1–2 mEq/kg bolus. Maintenance of adequate ventilation is important to prevent a concomitant respiratory acidosis. Repeated boluses can lead to hypernatremia and increased plasma osmolarity. Tris(hydroxymethyl)aminomethane (THAM) is an alternative treatment that does not result in an increased $PaCO_2$ [Miller, 2010].

Key Terms

Atrial flutter: pharmacological treatment
Defibrillation
Effect of vasopressin versus epinephrine
Myocardial ischemia, tachycardia: treatment
$NaHCO_3$ in cardiac arrest
Pressor treatment and myocardial ischemia
Pulseless electrical activity: treatment

Pulseless VT treatment
Sinus tachycardia mechanisms
Stable atrial fibrillation: treatment
Synchronized electrical cardioversion
Treatment of ventricular tachycardia (VT)
Vasoactive medications: effect on BP and HR
Ventricular fibrillation (VF): epinephrine mechanism

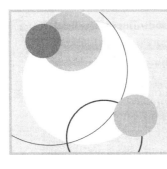

Caudal, Epidural and Spinal Anesthesia

The roots of education are bitter, but the fruit is sweet.
Aristotle

○ **What are the boundaries of the epidural space?**

The epidural space is bounded anteriorly by the posterior longitudinal ligament, laterally by the periosteum of the vertebral pedicles and the intervertebral foramina, and posteriorly by the ligamentum flavum and the anterior surface of the lamina. Superiorly the space extends to the foramen magnum, where dura is fused to the base of the skull. Caudally, it ends at the sacral hiatus.

○ **What anatomical structures are encountered during correct placement of an epidural needle, using the midline approach?**

As the epidural needle enters the midline of the back between the spinous processes, it passes through the skin and subcutaneous tissue, followed by the supraspinous ligament, the interspinous ligament, the ligamentum flavum, and, finally, the epidural space.

○ **At what level does the spinal cord proper end (conus medullaris) in an adult?**

The spinal cord descends caudally in the spinal canal and changes in conformation from a solid structure to a strand-like continuation of the nerves referred to as the cauda equina (horse's tail), usually at the level of the first or second lumbar vertebral body. The conus medullaris usually lies about the level of the L1/L2 intervertebral disc, although this is variable. In 10% of the population conus medullaris may extend lower (as low as upper body of L3).

○ **At what level does the spinal cord end in a neonate?**

Anywhere from T12 to L3, lower than the normal level in adults. During the first year of life, the spinal cord recedes to the L1 adult level.

○ **At what level does the subarachnoid space terminate in children?**

The dural and arachnoid sacs usually terminate at the level of the second sacral vertebrae in adults, but may extend to the third or fourth sacral levels in infants.

○ **What are the landmarks to performing a midline lumbar spinal block?**

The iliac crest and L4 and L5 spinal processes (and/or L3 spinous process).

○ **What would be the indication of a subarachnoid or subdural injection while test dosing an epidural with local anesthetic?**

The rapid onset of significant sensory block within 2 minutes of subarachnoid injection.

○ **What is the subdural space?**

A potential space located between the dura mater and the arachnoid.

○ **What is the largest vertebral interspace?**

The largest interlaminal interspace of the vertebral column is the L5/S1 interspace.

○ **What is the technique of the paramedian approach to subarachnoid space?**

The midline is identified and the interspace is chosen. Identify the superior aspect of the inferior spinous process. A skin wheal is raised 1 cm lateral and 1 cm caudad to this point. The spinal needle is directed 10–15° toward the midline (cephalomedial plane) and advanced. There will be only two pops felt, the ligamentum flavum and dura.

○ **What are the advantages of the paramedian approach?**

1. Calcified ligaments and osteophytes in the midline (in old patients) are avoided.
2. Opening between vertebrae through which the spinal needle passes to CSF is larger, which is advantageous in patients having difficulty with assuming flexed position (arthritis, prone position). Therefore, paramedian position does not require same level of patient cooperation and reversal of lumbar lordosis as with median approach.

○ **What is the disadvantage of the paramedian approach?**

More likely to encounter blood vessels.

The midline approach provides a relatively avascular plane because epidural venous plexus is sparse in the midline. Any obstruction to venous return involving inferior vena cava such as pregnancy causes engorgement of epidural veins.

○ **What is the Taylor approach to the subarachnoid space?**

Lumbosacral subarachnoid approach described by Taylor in 1940.

The technique is a variation of the paramedian approach carried out at the L5/S1 interspace. The lowermost prominence of the posterosuperior iliac spine is identified and the skin entered 1 cm medial and 1 cm caudad to this point. The needle is directed medially and cephalad to enter the subarachnoid space at L5/S1.

○ **Define density.**

The density of a substance is the ratio of its mass to its volume under specified conditions of pressure and temperature. The dimensions of density are weight per unit volume.

○ **Define specific gravity.**

Specific gravity is the ratio of the mass of a substance compared with a standard (mass of an equal volume of distilled water at 4°C or air or hydrogen) under prescribed conditions of temperature and pressure.

○ **Define baricity.**

Baricity is analogous to specific gravity, but the ratio is between the densities of local anesthetic solutions and cerebrospinal fluid (specific gravity 1.003–1.008 at 37°C). It is a relevant term because it indicates how the solution will "behave" after subarachnoid injection.

○ **What is meant by the terms hyperbaric, hypobaric, and isobaric?**

The density of normal human CSF at 37°C is 1.0063 to 1.008 g/mL [Levine et al., 1981. See reference on page 524]. Local anesthetic solutions with densities (at 37°C) greater than 1.008 are termed hyperbaric. Solutions with densities between 0.998 and 1.007 are considered to be isobaric. Solutions with densities less than 0.997 are termed hypobaric. Specific gravities of commonly used agents: bupivacaine 0.5% in 8.25% dextrose = 1.0278, in water = 1.0058; lidocaine 2% = 1.0066; lidocaine 5% in 7.5% dextrose = 1.0333.

○ **How does the baricity of a local anesthetic affect the level of anesthetic?**

An isobaric solution tends to remain in the immediate area of injection. It is not significantly affected by patient position. A hypobaric solution tends to move away from the dependent area in the CSF. It is useful when administered in positions such as prone jackknife. A hyperbaric solution tends to move by gravity to a lower site and is useful for a saddle block.

○ **What factors are most influential in the distribution of a spinal anesthetic?**

The most significant is the amount or dose (not volume) of local anesthetic.

Other factors include: (1) baricity of the local anesthetic, (2) position of the patient in the first 5 minutes after injection of the spinal anesthetic (hypobaric solution rises: hyperbaric solution sinks with gravity), (3) patient factors (intra-abdominal pressure), and (4) volume of CSF in the spinal canal (reduced with ascites or pregnancy).

○ **What factors are probably unrelated to the height of spinal block (least influential)?**

Factors probably unrelated include added vasoconstrictor, coughing or straining, barbotage, rate of injection (except hypobaric), needle bevel (except Whitacre needle), gender, and weight.

○ **T/F: Following a spinal block, autonomic nervous system (ANS) shows the highest dermatomal spread.**

True.

Interruption of spinal cord function begins caudally and proceeds cephalad during a spinal block.

• Level of ANS 2 or more dermatomes cephalic to level of skin analgesia
• Level of motor two to three segments caudad to level of skin analgesia

○ **Why did the Sprotte needle design initially lead to many reports of "failed spinal anesthetics?"**

The Sprotte needle has an elliptical opening, much longer than any other spinal needle. The length of this opening could allow the hole to be only partially through the dura. During injection, it would be possible for some of the anesthetic to exit into the epidural space rather than the subarachnoid space. Also, dural puncture can be more difficult with a Sprotte needle compared with a sharper Quincke needle.

○ **How can you prolong the duration of an epidural block?**

Choice of local anesthetic is the most important determinant.

Adrenergic agonists prolong the block by decreasing drug clearance and partly also due to inhibitory effect on sensory and motor neurons.

Epinephrine does not significantly prolong bupivacaine probably because the inherent duration of these drugs exceeds the duration of epinephrine's effect. However, epinephrine prolongs analgesia and improves quality of analgesia when added to more dilute solutions such as labor epidurals.

○ **T/F: When using mid-upper thoracic epidural, local anesthetic dose should be reduced relative to the lumbar dose.**

True. Unlike spinal, epidural produces a segmental block that spreads both caudally and cranially from the site of injection. Therefore, when using mid-upper thoracic epidural, local anesthetic dose should be reduced to about 30–50% relative to lumbar to prevent excessive cephalad spread.

○ **How is caudal anesthesia related to epidural anesthesia?**

Caudal anesthesia is a form of epidural anesthesia in which the injection is made at the sacral hiatus (S5) through the sacrococcygeal ligament. Because the dural sac normally ends at S2, accidental spinal injection is rare. Caudal anesthesia is primarily used in children for postoperative analgesia for hernia repair or urologic procedures.

○ **What is the sacral hiatus?**

The sacral hiatus is due to nonfusion of the fifth sacral vertebral arch immediately cephalad to the coccyx and is covered by the sacrococcygeal ligament (an extension of the ligamentum flavum).

○ **What is the sacral cornua?**

The large bony processes on each side of the sacral hiatus.

○ **At what level does the dural sac (spinal dura mater) terminate?**

The dural sac usually terminates at the level of the second sacral vertebra at the level of the posterior superior iliac spine, where the filum terminale blends with the periosteum on the coccyx.

○ **For what types of surgical procedures is caudal anesthesia used?**

Caudal blocks can be used for most of the indications recommended for lumbar block. However, there is often difficulty getting the local anesthetic to spread high enough, so the technique is usually reserved for procedures that require a blockade of the sacral nerves (cystoscopy or perineal surgery).

○ **What are the anatomical landmarks of caudal epidural block?**

Sacral hiatus can be identified by palpating the sacral cornua.

Prominent landmarks such as the triangle formed between the two posterior superior iliac spines and the apex of sacral hiatus may be used to detect the sacral hiatus easily, especially in obese patients. This is an equilateral triangle. This identification increases the success rate of caudal epidural block.

The most frequently used technique to identify the caudal epidural space is based on feeling of the "pop" on penetrating the sacral coccygeal membrane.

○ **If air or clear fluid is aspirated after needle insertion during a caudal block, should you proceed with the caudal block?**

No. Aspiration of air or fluid indicates improper needle placement. Aspiration of air may indicate entrance of the needle into the peritoneum. The "clear fluid" may be cerebrospinal fluid if the needle has advanced past the S2 level.

○ **List at least four complications associated with spinal anesthesia.**

Hypotension, bradycardia, unexpected cardiac arrest, postdural puncture headache (PDPH), high spinal (hypotension and hypoventilation), nausea and vomiting, urinary retention, and neurologic sequelae.

○ **Which dermatomes correspond to the level of innervation by sympathetic cardiac accelerator fibers?**

Dermatomal levels T1–T4.

○ **Why may significant hemodynamic changes result from an epidural blockade, but not from a subarachnoid block?**

Significant hemodynamic changes may result from spinal or epidural depending on the level of the block due to vasodilatation below the block level. Hemodynamic instability due to local anesthetic toxicity is more likely with epidural (in case of an accidental intravenous injection) because a larger total dose is utilized for epidural block.

○ **How is the function of the urinary bladder affected as a result of an epidural blockade?**

Temporary urinary bladder atony results from blockade of sacral segments S2–S4, urinary retention from reduction in the strength of the detrusor muscle of the base of the bladder (increasing the bladder capacity), and the urinary sphincters are not relaxed. Catheterization of the bladder may become necessary until resolution of the block, especially if a continuous epidural technique is to be utilized intraoperatively and/or postoperatively. Overfilling may result in a neurogenic bladder. The incidence of urinary retention is related to the type of anesthesia (any central block), the surgical procedure (pelvic and major spine surgery will decrease the voiding reflex), and its duration.

○ **A 78-year-old woman is undergoing left total knee arthroplasty. Twenty-five minutes following epidural blockade to the level of T2 the patient becomes unconscious and apneic, requiring immediate intubation and mechanical ventilation. What is the most likely cause of this complication?**

High epidural blockade will result from the introduction of large volumes of local anesthetic solutions into the epidural space. Although rare, respiratory arrest most commonly results from extensive sympathetic blockade (which may develop over 25–30 minutes), reduced cardiac output, and reduced oxygen delivery to the brain causing medullary hypoperfusion.

Epidural blockade decreases pulmonary function proportionate to the level of motor block achieved (loss of abdominal muscles impairs active expiration; loss of intercostal muscles impairs active inspiration and the ability to generate negative intrathoracic pressure, leaving the patient dependent on the diaphragm). Effects of high spinal are more marked on the parameters of exhalation than of inhalation. If all the thoracic roots are blocked, the inspiratory capacity is decreased by only 20% but the expiratory reserve volume is decreased to zero. Therefore, the ability to cough (forced expiration) is markedly decreased. In addition, high sensory blockade may blunt the respiratory response to hypercarbia. Contributory factors are more significant in patients with COPD.

○ **Epidural anesthesia is chosen for a right above-the-knee amputation in a 67-year-old male with peripheral vascular disease. Loss of resistance is obtained through a 17-gauge Tuohy needle with the patient in the lateral position. Immediately following the introduction of a 3 cm³ test dose of local anesthetic solution containing epinephrine, clear fluid is noted to flow freely from the needle hub when the syringe is removed from the hub. How can you determine that the fluid is cerebrospinal fluid?**

If the immediate, free-flowing fluid is warm to the touch, it is likely to be CSF. A solution of local anesthetic just introduced into the epidural space is likely to still be near room temperature. If the returning fluid precipitates in a container of etidocaine solution, it is CSF. Local anesthetic solutions do not precipitate in etidocaine solution. CSF will also induce a positive color change on glucose test strip, while a solution containing local anesthetic will not.

○ **What are some advantages of continuous spinal over single-dose spinal and continuous epidural anesthesia?**

Advantages include the following: (1) facilitation of the surgical schedule if the catheter is placed in the preinduction area, (2) the potential for positional hypotension is minimized since the patient may be fully anesthetized after being positioned, (3) the possibility of systemic toxic reactions is virtually eliminated due to the ability to titrate small amounts of local anesthetics, (4) titratability increases the likelihood of obtaining exactly the right level of anesthesia and decreases the likelihood of cardiovascular instability during induction, (5) employing a short-acting local anesthetic shortens the recovery period, (6) the duration of anesthesia can be prolonged indefinitely, (7) a definite end point (aspiration of CSF) assures the catheter is in the correct place and therefore enhances the likelihood of successful anesthesia, and (8) subarachnoid narcotics may be administered during a surgical procedure or continued into the recovery period to provide long-lasting postoperative analgesia.

○ **What are some disadvantages of continuous spinal anesthesia?**

Cauda equina syndrome associated with small-bore continuous spinal anesthesia.

Other disadvantages include: (1) additional time required for placement of the catheter, (2) PDPH, (3) possible catheter breakage, and (4) a potential for infection, neurologic changes, and hemorrhage.

○ **What are the causes of cauda equina syndrome after neuraxial blocks?**

Neurologic injury occurs in about 0.02–0.06% of all central neuraxial blocks. However, in most of these cases the block was not clearly proven to be the causative factor [Auroy et al., 1997. See reference on page 523].

Injury to cauda equina roots (paraplegia, lack of bowel/bladder sensation) may occur from:

1. Direct needle trauma.
2. Spinal cord ischemia.
3. Accidental injection of neurotoxic drugs or chemicals.
4. Introduction of bacteria into subarachnoid or epidural space.
5. Epidural hematoma.
6. Probable neurotoxicty of local anesthetics in high concentration. Hyperbaric 5% lidocaine has been implicated as a cause of multiple cases of cauda equina syndrome after injection through microcatheter (>24 gauge) during continuous spinal anesthesia. Nerve injury is believed to result from the pooling due to apparent maldistribution of the local anesthetics causing toxic concentrations around cauda equina nerve roots.

○ **What is a PDPH?**

This is a headache thought to be from a persistent leak of spinal fluid through the dural puncture site. Depletion of CSF, which acts as a cushion for the spinal cord and brain, is believed to allow stretching of the supporting structures (meninges) activating stretch-sensitive nociceptors. Pain may also result from distention of the blood vessels, which, because of the fixed volume of the skull, must compensate for the loss of CSF volume. The characteristic spinal headache occurs 6–12 hours after the spinal anesthetic has regressed, being worse in the upright posture.

○ **What is the classic presentation of a dural puncture headache?**

The defining feature of a dural puncture headache is a severe pounding headache that worsens as the head is elevated. The pain typically begins in the occipital area and spreads to the frontal area, and radiates to the neck and shoulders. Dizziness, nausea, vomiting, photophobia, tinnitus, deafness, and diplopia from abducens nerve palsy are possible symptoms.

○ **What are the risk factors for a dural puncture headache?**

Risk factors for dural puncture headache include parturients, younger patients (less than 50 years of age), women, use of needles with large bore, cutting needles (Quincke or diamond point) rather than conical point (Greene, Whitacre, Sprotte), and multiple punctures. Inserting a needle with the bevel perpendicular to the long axis of the trunk and glucose-containing local anesthetics can also increase the risk of spinal headache. Studies consistently have shown that 24 hours of prophylactic bed rest does not decrease the incidence or the severity of PDPH. A low incidence of PDPH is seen after continuous spinal anesthesia, and it is speculated that the presence of a spinal catheter causes an inflammatory response that promotes dural closure.

○ **What is the incidence of dural puncture headache with a 24-gauge Sprotte needle?**

The 24-gauge Sprotte needle has been reported to cause a 0.02% incidence (or less than 1%) of dural puncture headache.

○ **When is a dural puncture headache most likely to occur?**

Headache typically occurs on the first or second day after dural puncture.

○ **What complications can be associated with PDPH?**

Cranial nerve palsies, especially VI and VIII (vision and hearing disturbances due to traction on the nerves from a brain that no longer floats on a cushion of CSF). Rarely subdural hematoma and intracerebral hemorrhage occur.

○ **What is the incidence in children?**

Headache is rare under the age of 13. One study showed no headache in children under 10 years of age following lumbar puncture.

○ **Are any tests available for PDPH?**

No. PDPH is a diagnosis of exclusion. However, magnetic resonance imaging can visualize leaking cerebrospinal fluid in the lumbar spine. Abdominal pressure will transiently relieve PDPH headache but not headaches from other sources.

○ **What is the differential diagnosis?**

Subdural hematoma, pneumocephalus, meningitis, any cause of elevated intracranial pressure, nicotine withdrawal, caffeine withdrawal, postpartum headache, and migraine.

○ **Name two commonly accepted treatments for a PDPH.**

Intravenous or oral caffeine and epidural blood patch. Intravenous hydration has not been shown to be an effective treatment. Intravenous ACTH or cosyntropin (synthetic ACTH analogue) and sumatriptan (a serotonin agonist) have been reported to be efficacious. Three patients who received two to three doses of ACTH subsequently developed seizures. Although conclusion cannot be drawn about the possible contribution of ACTH, proper prospective evaluation of the value of ACTH in the treatment of PDPH is required [Hakim SM, 2010. See reference on page 523].

○ **What is the initial therapy for PDPH?**

Twenty-four-hour trial of symptomatic therapy (bed rest, hydration with oral or intravenous fluids, and analgesics) or immediate epidural blood patch, unless cranial nerve traction symptoms exist.

○ **How is caffeine thought to work?**

Evidence shows that the probable mechanism for caffeine's stimulatory effect on the CNS is its competitive inhibition of adenosine receptors, which results in vasoconstriction.

○ **What dose of caffeine is used?**

Three hundred milligrams of oral caffeine or 500 mg of intravenous caffeine sodium benzoate (which contains 250 mg of caffeine).

○ **What is the caffeine content of some common beverages?**

Freeze-dried coffee 66 mg/cup; drip coffee 142 mg/cup; tea 47 mg/cup; Coke 65 mg/12 oz can; Pepsi 43 mg/12 oz can; Mountain Dew 55 mg/12 oz can.

○ **What are the side effects of caffeine therapy?**

The most common side effects are transient flushing, palpitation, and dizziness. Very rarely seizures may occur.

○ **What other cerebral vasoconstrictors are useful?**

Sumatriptan can also be used. The usual dose is 6 mg subcutaneously.

○ **What is epidural blood patching?**

This is the technique of injecting 15–20 mL of aseptically drawn autologous blood into the epidural space near the site of the original dural puncture. Injection is performed with the volume indicated or until mild back pressure is felt. Side effects are mild back pain and fever and occasional temporary radiculopathy from nerve pressure.

○ **What are the contraindications to EBP?**

Local infection of the back, septicemia, and active neurologic disease.

○ **Can EBP be done on an HIV patient?**

Yes.

○ **How does epidural blood patch relieve headache?**

Relief of PDPH is often rapid after blood patch. It is hypothesized that injection of blood increases lumbar CSF pressure and restores intracranial pressure. A sustained (15 minutes or more) increase in lumbar CSF pressure has been noted after injection of blood. Epidural blood patch either stops the transdural leak of CSF or reestablishes the normal CSF pressure.

○ **How effective is epidural saline for treatment of a dural puncture headache?**

Bolus epidural saline is less effective than blood patch and the benefit is transient. Some have reported success with prolonged use of saline infusion of 15–20 mL/h. A high relapse rate limits use of the technique.

○ **You are called to evaluate a patient 12 hours after a spinal anesthetic for a cesarean section. She is complaining of a nonpositional headache. Is this a PDPH?**

Probably not. PDPHs are characteristically positional in nature, worse when the patient is upright and improved when the patient is recumbent. In addition, spinal headaches usually occur 1–2 days after dural puncture. Patients typically complain of pain in the frontal and occipital regions.

○ **What is meant by the term "multiorifice" catheter?**

The distal end of the catheter can be either open (single port) or closed (multiport). A closed-tip catheter has three orifices at 0.5 cm intervals, starting 0.5 cm from the tip. Each of the orifices is orientated at 120° to the axis of the catheter in order to facilitate spread.

○ **What would you do if a catheter tip is sheared off when placing an epidural catheter?**

Any attempt to withdraw a catheter through a needle with an angled bevel may produce shearing or complete transection of the plastic catheter. No direct harm usually results from this since the materials used are nonirritating and "tissue-implantable." The patient should be informed of the foreign body present, but surgical removal is usually not required.

○ **How does spinal curvature affect the level of spinal anesthesia?**

Anatomical configuration of the spinal column has a minor effect. Severe kyphosis or kyphoscoliosis, with a decreased volume of cerebrospinal fluid, can be associated with a higher than expected level of block using hypobaric techniques or rapid injection.

○ **How much 1:1,000 epinephrine must be added to 20 mL of a local anesthetic solution to obtain a 1:200,000 concentration of epinephrine?**

A 1:1,000 solution contains 1,000 μg/mL of epinephrine. A 1:200,000 solution contains epinephrine 5 μg/mL. A 20 cm^3 solution contains 100 μg or 0.1 cm^3 of epinephrine 1:1,000.

○ **What is the dermatome level of the nipple?**

T4.

○ **What is the dermatome level of the inguinal ligament?**

L1.

○ **Which dermatomes supply the inguinal region?**

Dermatomal levels T12 and L1.

○ **What is the dermatome level of the xiphoid?**

T6.

○ **What are the dermatomes that supply to the knee?**

The anterior knee is supplied by the saphenous nerve, or L1–4. The posterior knee is supplied by the posterior tibial nerve, or L4–5, S1–3.

○ **What is the dermatome that supplies the umbilicus?**

T10.

○ **What is the disadvantage of using commercially prepared solutions of local anesthetics with epinephrine added?**

Commercial preparations are more acidic (pH approximately 4.0) because epinephrine is rapidly inactivated in an alkaline solution. In such an acidic medium, very little local anesthetic is available in the unionized form for penetration of neural tissue; therefore, onset of analgesia is slower with commercial products.

○ **What recommendations should be made concerning the postoperative initiation of LMWH therapy in a patient who has had a neuraxial block technique?**

This is determined by the proposed LMWH regimen. For single-daily dosing the first dose of LMWH may be given 12 hours postoperatively, with the second dose withheld for a further 24 hours. For twice-daily dosing regimens the first dose should be given no sooner than 24 hours postoperatively. Any concomitant medications with effects on hemostasis may increase the risk of spinal hematoma [Horlocker et al., 2010. See reference on page 525].

○ **Can LMWH be administered in the presence of an indwelling epidural catheter?**

Catheters can be used for postoperative analgesia during LMWH therapy. More specifically, the timing of the catheter removal represents the highest risk of spinal hematoma. For single-daily dose regimens, the catheter should be removed a minimum of 10–12 hours after the preceding dose of LMWH and an interval of at least 2 hours before the subsequent dose of LMWH. For twice-daily dose regimens, the catheter must be removed on postoperative day 1 prior to the start of LMWH, with at least 2 hours before the first dose of LMWH.

○ **What are the guidelines for removing an epidural in a patient on IV or oral anticoagulants?**

Controversial. If on coumadin, the PT and INR should be no more than 1.5 times normal. If on IV heparin, it is our policy to discontinue the heparin 2 hours prior to removal, and if the PTT is normal, remove the epidural catheter, waiting an additional 1 hour before restarting the infusion. With low-molecular-weight heparin agents, according to the ASTRA guidelines, there may be a "window of opportunity" between 10 and 12 hours for prophylactic dose, and 24 hours after therapeutic doses (1 mg/kg) and 2 hours before the next anticipated dose (when it is safest to insert/withdraw a catheter). More studies are needed especially with newer agents such as fondaparinux (Arixtra – half-life is 17 hours and no neuraxial block is recommended for 36 hours), and a personal institutional policy is mandatory.

○ **Blood is seen in the needle during the difficult placement of an epidural catheter. What actions should be taken?**

Surgery should not be postponed by traumatic needle or catheter placement. There is an increased risk of spinal hematoma and LMWH therapy should be delayed for 24 hours.

○ **What are the common side effects with neuraxial opioids?**

Respiratory depression, urinary retention, pruritus, nausea, and vomiting. Early respiratory depression is associated with the highly soluble drugs, for example, fentanyl, whereas delayed respiratory depression (up to 24 hours) is associated with poorly soluble drugs, for example, morphine.

○ **What dose of fentanyl is commonly added to intrathecal injection?**

Fifteen to 20 μg is frequently used in combination with the shorter acting local anesthetics in the ambulatory surgery setting in order to extend the sensory block without increasing the duration of motor block.

○ **What is the primary site of action of epidural/intrathecal opioids?**

Laminae II of the substantia gelatinosa of the dorsal horn of the spinal cord.

○ **Do epidural opioids only act at the spinal cord?**

No. Depending on the physicochemical properties of the opioid, the amount reaching the spinal cord may be small and its effect may largely be due to systemic uptake and redistribution to the brain. Considerably more morphine than the more lipid-soluble fentanyl reaches the spinal cord when administered epidurally.

○ **Is fentanyl the ideal epidural opioid?**

No. Investigators have shown that a continuous intravenous infusion of fentanyl produced the same quality of analgesia and side effects as compared with a similar dose of epidural fentanyl by continuous infusion.

○ **In the recovery room, a patient has full motor and sensory recovery after spinal anesthesia. She is unable to void, and the surgeon is blaming the anesthetic. Could he be correct?**

Yes. Urinary retention has been described with longer acting local anesthetics and neuraxial narcotics. On emergence from spinal anesthesia, the bladder is the last to regain function and urinary retention is not uncommon. Neuraxial local anesthetics cause reduction in the strength of detrusor contraction (increasing bladder capacity) and contraction of the bladder sphincter. Opioids cause dyssynergia between bladder detrusor muscle and urethral sphincter.

○ **How does neuraxial anesthesia affect thermoregulation?**

Neuroaxial blocks inhibit numerous aspects of thermoregulatory control. The vasoconstriction and shivering thresholds are reduced by regional anesthesia (in the blocked segments). The result is that cold defenses are triggered at a lower temperature than normal during regional anesthesia, and substantial hypothermia often goes undetected in these patients. Sympathectomy-induced vasodilatation increases the heat loss to the cold environment.

With epidural anesthesia, shivering-like tremors occur in about 30% of patients. The decrease in core temperature triggers thermoregulatory vasoconstriction and shivering above the level of epidural anesthesia.

○ **T/F: Severe bradycardia and cardiac arrest have been reported following spinal anesthesia.**

True.

○ **How does a spinal anesthetic cause bradycardia?**

The mechanism is multifactorial:

1. Unopposed vagal tone from a high sympathectomy (T2–5).
2. Blockade of the cardioaccelerator fibers (T1–T4).
3. Decreased outflow from the intracardiac stretch receptors (slowing of the heart rate secondary to a drop in venous return). Three such intracardiac receptors have been suggested: (i) pacemaker stretch; (ii) low-pressure baroreceptors in the right atrium and vena cava; (iii) paradoxical Bezold–Jarisch reflex, mechanoreceptors in the left ventricle [Reverse Bainbridge reflex. Crystal et al., 2012. See reference on page 523].

Other considerations include ancillary drug effects (fentanyl, remifentanil), vagal maneuvers (peritoneal traction, bladder distension, vasovagal reaction), and disease processes (hypoxia, myocardial ischemia, sinus node disease).

○ **What is the management of bradycardia after spinal anesthesia?**

Maintain preload and aggressively treat moderate bradycardia with epinephrine early.

The treatment of hypotension with vasopressors such as ephedrine (a mixed alpha and beta agonist) is more appropriate than with a pure alpha agonist such as phenylephrine when bradycardia is also present.

○ **What is the Bainbridge reflex?**

The Bainbridge reflex, also called the atrial reflex, is an increase in heart rate due to an increase in central venous pressure.

○ **On placing an interscalene block, the patient develops a high spinal. Explain.**

Subarachnoid injection can occur two different ways: (1) inadvertent needle placement into the spinal canal and (2) injection through the dural sheath that at the cervical level extends out the foramina to cover the nerve root.

○ **Is ambulatory surgery a contraindication to use of a spinal anesthetic?**

Absolutely not. If appropriate local anesthetics are chosen based on the anticipated length of surgery, these patients can be discharged in a similar time course as those patients who have had a general anesthetic. In addition, regional anesthesia can result in less nausea and vomiting than general, resulting in shorter PACU stays.

○ **Does the bevel direction of an epidural needle influence the catheter direction?**

No. There is no correlation between the two.

○ **In performing a thoracic epidural in an anesthetized patient using the hanging drop technique, does it matter if the patient is under controlled or spontaneous ventilation?**

Yes. The hanging drop technique depends on the negative pressure of the epidural space to "suck" in the drop once the epidural space has been entered. This pressure is increased with controlled ventilation. The safest approach would be to place the epidural catheter in an awake patient.

○ **Four hours after your last dose of 2% lidocaine into a lumbar epidural catheter, your patient is in the recovery room with full motor and sensory blockade. She has no discomfort. What should you do?**

Inform the surgeon and order a STAT MRI of the thoracolumbar spine (upper cuts must correspond to spine segments above the catheter tip).

Two percent lidocaine (plain) has an expected duration of sensory and motor block of 60–90 minutes. The sensory block can be augmented by the addition of epidural opioids. Addition of epinephrine to 2% lidocaine will prolong the anesthetic effect. The diagnosis of epidural hematoma is extremely rare, but in the presence of leg weakness should be excluded as this represents a neurosurgical emergency.

○ **Five minutes after starting an "easy" labor epidural, the patient has complete pain relief with no motor block, but a sensory level on the left side at T1 and right side at T10. What is your diagnosis?**

Subdural catheter placement. Epidural analgesia may also produce uneven block due to uneven distribution depending on the catheter placement. In addition, analgesic strength of local anesthetic solutions that are used for labor epidural (current practice) may not produce any motor block (e.g., 0.1% ropivacaine or bupivacaine).

Subdural block presents with a very rapid onset of pain relief and an unusually variable presentation of sensory block. An inadvertent subarachnoid (spinal) injection would also present with rapid pain relief, but the patient would have motor blockade and little discrepancy in sensory levels between sides. The catheter should be removed and certainly never be used in the event of an emergency cesarean section.

○ **After using three percent 2-chloroprocaine for your epidural anesthetic, the surgeon requests epidural duramorph. What is your response?**

Duramorph has been shown to be ineffective after the use of epidural three percent 2-chloroprocaine, but it probably just shortens the duration of duramorph. Use of chloroprocaine is not a contraindication for duramorph.

In addition, one of 2-chloroprocaine's metabolites, 4-amino-2-chloroprocaine, may impair the action of bupivacaine if used concurrently.

○ **How far should an epidural catheter be advanced into the epidural space?**

Approximately 2–5 cm. If you advance the catheter greater than 6 cm, the catheter tip is likely to exit the central axis via a neural foramina. Placement at 4–5 cm has been shown to be most efficacious especially for labor epidural where the patients tend to move and turn on the bed during labor.

○ **You use 5 cm³ of normal saline in a "loss of resistance" technique to identify the epidural space. You remove the trocar and several drops of fluid run out. Is this CSF?**

Probably not. A 17-gauge needle that penetrates the dura usually runs like a faucet. To be certain, you can check the temperature (warm if it is CSF) and glucose content (positive test with a urine dipstick).

○ **How much does a spinal anesthetic affect the glomerular filtration rate?**

A spinal anesthetic to at least the T11 level will reduce the glomerular filtration rate proportionally to decreases in arterial pressure due to its effects on autoregulation.

○ **If a patient has a spinal anesthetic to the C8–T1 level, how much will this block affect her inspiratory capacity?**

It will be decreased by as much as 20%. At this level of block expiratory reserve volume will be decreased to zero; risk of aspiration should be a concern especially in OB patients with incompetent LOS.

The resting ventilation (tidal volume) is not impaired as long as the phrenic nerve (cervical 3, 4, 5 dermatomes) is intact.

○ **How does neuraxial block affect peristalsis?**

Following the sympathetic block to abdominal organs (T6–L2) after a high neuraxial block, the parasympathetic nervous system remains unopposed. This causes the intestinal sphincters to be relaxed and peristalsis to be normally active. Secretions are increased.

Nausea and vomiting is seen in up to 20% of patients after neuraxial blocks and is primarily related to hyperperistalsis (unopposed vagal activity).

○ **What spinal level is most dependent in the supine position? What is its significance?**

The T4–T6 level is most dependent in the supine position. Following placement of a hyperbaric spinal, when the patient is repositioned supine, the anesthetic will flow cephalad and may produce a T4–T6 level (depending on the dose of spinal medication). The associated sympathetic block (two levels above sensory) may affect the cardiac accelerators (T1–T4) and intercostal muscle function.

○ **Does the baricity of a spinal anesthetic impact its duration of action?**

Yes. An isobaric solution has a clinically longer duration of action than a hyperbaric or hypobaric spinal solution. The limited spread of the local anesthetic with an isobaric solution produces a higher concentration in the CSF and thus increases the time until the minimally effective concentration is reached.

○ **Hypotension frequently follows placement of a subarachnoid block. What is the etiology and treatment?**

Decreased vascular resistance and diminished cardiac output. Although hypotension is due to both venous and arterial dilatation, venodilatation effect predominates because 75% of the blood volume is in the venous system. Arterial system is able to retain significant degree of autonomic tone, and in a normovolemic patient the decrease in total peripheral resistance is about 15–18% only.

Hypotension may be ameliorated by administration of intravenous fluids and/or sympathomimetic agents (ephedrine, phenylephrine).

○ **What factors increase the incidence and severity of hypotension?**

- Hypovolemia
- Sensory level greater than T4
- Baseline systolic blood pressure less than 120 mm Hg
- Level of needle insertion at or above L2–3
- Addition of epinephrine to the local anesthetic solution
- Use of a combined spinal–general anesthesia technique

○ **A patient arrests 10 minutes after induction of spinal anesthesia. What do you do?**

The most likely cause is a high spinal, and supportive therapy is the treatment including airway control and BP support. However, unexpected cardiac arrest during spinal anesthesia has been described. Sudden severe bradycardia and asystolic arrest can develop without evidence of high spinal respiratory depression or hypoxemia and hypercarbia. Immediate resuscitation along standard ACLS guidelines is indicated. For severe bradycardia or cardiac arrest, full resuscitation doses of epinephrine should be promptly administered. Review drugs administered, actions, and therapeutic maneuvers performed prior to the arrest and correct any obvious underlying causes. The differential diagnosis includes profound sympathectomy, arrhythmia, oversedation, "high spinal," airway obstruction, and hypokalemia or hyperkalemia.

○ **What is epidural test dose?**

Currently, the most commonly used test dose is 3 mL of 1.5% lidocaine (45 mg) with 1:200,000 epinephrine (15 μg).

○ **What symptoms are seen if the test dose is positive?**

Since the function of the test dose is to allow recognition of accidental dural or intravascular placement, the amount of drug should be sufficient to produce rapid low spinal block if injected intrathecally or provide reliable indication of intravascular injection.

Usually 3 mL of 1.5% hyperbaric lidocaine intrathecal injection at lumbar level produces sensory anesthesia at S2 dermatome level within 2 minutes.

Epinephrine 15 μg injected intravascularly would rapidly produce a transient increase in heart rate of 20–30 bpm and usually a slight increase in blood pressure. The time of onset to tachycardia is within 60 seconds and the duration is about 60 seconds. Occasionally, however, epinephrine 15 μg may produce other signs such as perspiration, tachypnea, or subjective signs such as patient complaining of apprehension or unease or "funny" feeling in the chest.

○ **What are the implications of spinal anesthesia in a patient with pseudotumor cerebri?**

Spinal anesthesia poses no additional risk for this patient given the lack of a CNS lesion and mass effect in the presence of elevated ICP. This patient is actually at a lower risk for PDPH and, in fact, drainage of CSF is therapeutic to reduce headache pain associated with benign intracranial hypertension.

○ **What factors must be considered for the safe administration of epidural anesthesia?**

Observe contraindications to epidural anesthesia (patient refusal, sepsis with hemodynamic instability, uncorrected hypovolemia, and coagulopathy), an understanding of the inherent physiological effects (sympathetic blockade and respiratory changes) and need for maintaining preload, signs and symptoms of drug toxicity, proper epidural placement, and assessment of the level of the block. It has been shown that placement of the epidural at the level of the dermatome that corresponds to the incision is associated with fewer side effects, lower drug dose requirements, and better pain control.

○ **What dose adjustment is required for age when administering epidural local anesthetics?**

Older patients require a smaller dose of local anesthetic to achieve the same level of block when compared with younger patients. Less compliant epidural space and diminished adipose tissue may be primarily responsible.

Elderly patients are at risk for systemic toxicity due to the diminished clearance of drugs by the liver, especially those undergoing extensive first-pass metabolism.

○   **A patient complains of back pain after an epidural. The surgeon suspects epidural abscess. What information is important to determine the actual etiology of this patient's pain?**

Back pain can be caused by infection, hematoma, or even preexisting back pain. Assess for leg weakness and bowel or bladder dysfunction. An abscess usually appears at least 5 days postplacement, and the incidence is rare. Epidural hematoma can occur spontaneously in clinical settings outside the operating room but when associated with regional anesthesia, there is usually a preexisting coagulopathy. If the hematoma is not surgically decompressed in 6–8 hours, full neurologic recovery is compromised. Confirmation is made by MRI or CT scan.

○   **When is a caudal catheter better than an epidural catheter?**

Normally in very small children and infants, the placement of the caudal catheter is technically very easy and the space is better defined than the epidural space. In adult patients it may be a viable alternative to the lumbar approach in accessing the epidural space (multiple lumbar fractures, ankylosing spondylitis).

○   **What are the nonsurgical reasons to consider epidural analgesia?**

Patients with multiple rib fractures, pneumothorax, sternal fractures, and chronic pain syndromes (carcinoma of the lung, chronic back pain) are very good candidates for the analgesic benefits of epidural opioid/local anesthetic mixtures. Patients with angina, claudication, and severe peripheral vascular disease may benefit as well.

○   **What are some advantages of regional anesthesia?**

Outcome differences relate primarily to the epidural technique, which is most studied compared to the other neuraxial techniques. The advantages shown include decreased graft thrombosis in peripheral revascularization, decreased bleeding and DVTs in hip surgery, better postoperative pain control if the technique is continued into the postoperative period following major abdominal/thoracic/orthopedic surgery, possible reduction in phantom limb pain if used prior to amputations, and improved pulmonary function following thoracic surgery with thoracic epidural pain relief. Recently, neuraxial anesthesia is shown to reduce the surgical site infection rate when compared to general anesthesia [Sessler DI, 2010. See reference on page 524]. It bypasses many of the potential sources of minor or major morbidity associated with general anesthesia, for example, trauma to the lips, teeth, pharynx, and vocal cords; bronchospasm; aspiration; prolonged somnolence; prolonged paralysis; and potential allergy and adverse responses to other anesthetic agents. Also protracted nausea and vomiting are less common after regional anesthesia.

○   **Are there any advantages of regional versus general anesthesia for total hip replacement?**

Blood loss is decreased about 30–50%. There is less risk of transfusion and a lower incidence of DVT. There may be less acute postoperative confusion. The quality of interface between bone and methylmethacrylate may be improved.

○   **With what procedures has epidural analgesia been shown to be particularly beneficial and why?**

Procedure	Benefit
Thoracotomy	Pulmonary function
Joint replacement	Decreased DVT, earlier ambulation
Vascular procedures	Improved blood flow, decreased graft thrombosis
Pediatric cardiac	Decreased ventilator time and hospital stay
Abdominal surgery	Less ileus

○ **Is there any difference in anesthetic-related mortality in patients receiving epidural or spinal anesthesia and general anesthesia?**

Meta-analysis (141 trials, 9,589 patients, in 2000) has reported the rate of death as 2.1% in patients receiving epidural or spinal anesthesia and 3.1% in those receiving general anesthesia. This decline of 1 death per 100 patients in the regional anesthesia groups resulted from reductions in pulmonary embolism, cardiac events, stroke, transfusion requirements, infections, and respiratory depression. The type or location of surgery did not influence the result [Rodgers et al., 2000. See reference on page 524].

○ **How are dural fibers arranged? How does bevel direction of the spinal needle affect the dural hole?**

Previous investigators reported that the dural fibers were predominantly longitudinal in direction. Later electron microscopic examination has shown that the dural structure is far more complex and consists of multidirectional interlacing collagen fibers and both transverse and longitudinal elastic fibers. However, it was suggested that insertion of the needle bevel parallel to the long axis of spine causes less tension on the dural hole and therefore reduces the incidence of PDPH.

Lower headache with cone-shaped needle tips may be the result of exposing more inflammatory mediators around the opening rather than often-quoted more gentle spreading of the dura at the site of the puncture.

○ **A 36-year-old patient is to undergo lower limb surgery. He is diagnosed with ankylosing spondylitis. Is epidural or spinal anesthesia an acceptable technique?**

Yes. This is an acceptable alternative to general anesthesia and helps to avoid endotracheal intubation, which could be difficult due to stiff and deformed cervical spine with limited mobility.

However, regional anesthesia also may be difficult due to limited joint mobility and closed interspinous spaces. Ossification of ligamentum flavum is not common.

○ **What agents cause transient neurologic symptoms (TNS)?**

TNS incidence is greater (up to 40%) after lidocaine spinal anesthesia.

The incidence of TNS after spinal anesthesia with other local anesthetics: mepivacaine 30–40%, prilocaine up to 6%, tetracaine up to 12%, and bupivacaine and ropivacaine rare.

There is increased incidence associated with lithotomy position during surgery, ambulatory surgical status, arthroscopic knee surgery, and obesity.

Variables that are not shown to increase the risk of TNS include the lidocaine dose, addition of epinephrine to lidocaine, presence of dextrose, paresthesia, hypotension, and blood-tinged CSF.

○ **What are the symptoms of TNS?**

The symptoms usually include pain (VAS score 4–7) and/or dysesthesia radiating from lower back to buttock or lower extremity. The symptoms manifest within 12 hours after surgery and recover within 1 week (72 hours). Currently there are no cases with abnormal neurologic examinations or motor weakness.

Electrophyiologic studies of nerve conduction, EMG, and SSEP before and after TNS have shown no change! The pathogenesis still remains unknown [Zaric and Pace, 2009. See reference on page 524; Miller, 2010].

Key Terms

Agents causing TNS
Anesthetic effects: spinal reflexes
Ankylosing spondylitis: epidural anesthesia risks
Benefits: epidural versus general anesthesia
Cauda equina syndrome
Caudal analgesia: anatomical landmarks
Causes of failed spinal anesthesia
Diagnosis of spinal hematoma
Differential spinal block
Effect of epidural analgesia on postoperative course
Epidural anesthesia: thermoregulation
Epidural anesthetics: peristalsis effect/GI effects
Epidural: detection of CSF
Epidural test dose: effects/symptoms
High spinal effects
LMW heparin: continue versus discontinue
LMWH: neuraxial anesthesia/postoperative epidural
Mechanism of action of ephedrine
Neuraxial block: duration
PDPH: risk factors
Pseudotumor cerebri: LP effects

Regional anesthetics: LMWH
Retained epidural catheter: management
Spinal anesthesia anatomy: paramedian
Spinal anesthesia and cardiac arrest
Spinal anesthesia: complications
Spinal anesthesia: respiratory effects
Spinal anesthesia spread factors
Spinal anesthetic complications: MRI indications
Spinal anesthetics: anatomy
Spinal anesthetics: severe bradycardia
Spinal anesthetics: TNS symptoms
Spinal cord anatomy
Spinal hypotension: causes/treatment
Subarachnoid block: ECG changes
Subdural injection: symptoms
Sympathectomy: physiological effects
Thecal sac anatomy
Treatment of low SVR
Vasoconstrictors: compare mechanisms
Venous pressure: gravity effects

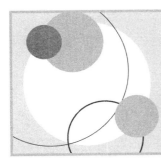

Chronic Pain Management

The worst pain a man can suffer: To have insight into much and power over nothing.
Herodotus

○ **What is chronic pain?**

Somatic, visceral, or neuropathic pain lasting more than 3 months, or that outlasts an initial injury to tissues, with symptoms greater than the underlying pathology would suggest. Some investigators use the duration of greater than 6 months.

○ **What areas in the CNS are involved in pain generation and perception?**

Afferent pathways, CNS, and efferent pathways.

Nociceptors transmit pain sensation to the dorsal horn of the spinal cord (modulation at substantia gelatinosa, laminae II) across to the contralateral spinal cord and through spinothalamic tracts to the thalamus. There are two spinothalamic tracts: neospinothalamic tract for acute pain (transmits pain sensations to midbrain, postcentral gyrus, and cortex) and paleospinothalamic tract for dull and burning pain (transmits pain sensations to the reticular formation, limbic system, and midbrain). Stimulation of the periaqueductal gray site in the midbrain results in activation of efferent pathways that inhibit pain impulses.

○ **What are C fibers?**

Small-caliber, pain-mediating fibers representing roughly 70% of the peripheral nerve system. C fibers are the slowest and smallest, mediate the sensation of warmth, and are the main component responsible for the sensation and transmission of pain, at a conduction velocity less than 2 m/s. In addition, C fibers subserve most of the autonomic peripheral functions.

○ **Describe the basic physiologic processes of pain – transduction, transmission, modulation, and perception.**

Transduction: the conversion at the periphery of the noxious surgical insult into an electrical action potential, precipitating the release of pain-producing substances such as histamines, serotonin, bradykinin, prostaglandins, etc.

Transmission: the approach of the peripheral electrical action potential to the primary sensory nerve and through the dorsal root ganglion, dorsal horn of the spinal cord, and higher central nervous system structures in an ascending, afferent pathway.

Modulation: the descending, inhibitory, or efferent neurologic pathway of the pain cycle.

Perception: the cortical response to pain.

○ **What medications may affect transduction?**

Peripheral local anesthetics and NSAIDs decrease transduction of pain.

○ **What medications effect transmission?**

Nerve blocks with local anesthetics decrease transmission.

○ **What medications enhance modulation of pain?**

Epidural/intrathecal opioids and alpha-agonists play a role in modulation as do antidepressants (tricyclic antidepressants) and antiepileptic medications.

○ **Define hyperalgesia.**

Abnormal hypersensitivity to noxious mechanical or thermal stimulation.

○ **What is the cause of hyperalgesia in neuropathic pain?**

Primary hyperalgesia is increased sensitivity in a region where noxious stimuli have already been placed, whereas secondary hyperalgesia is increased sensitivity in an area surrounding injury, on intact skin. Both are components of central sensitization, where the transmission of nociception has been changed. One component of sensitization involves C fiber input causing strengthening of synapses in the dorsal horn of the spinal cord. As a result, response to a particular stimulus is increased in intensity as well as duration. There is also decreased input from the descending inhibitory pathway.

In addition, a rearrangement of fibers within the spinal cord is thought to occur. Nociceptive neurons consist of unmyelinated C fibers or thinly myelinated A-delta fibers. A-beta fibers are large-diameter fast-conducting fibers that do not normally transmit the sensation of pain, but rather of light touch or pressure. The dorsal horn is anatomically organized in layers or laminae. Unmyelinated C fibers are located in lamina I and II and large myelinated (A-beta) fibers in laminae III–V. A-beta fibers are thought to be upregulated as well as move to lamina II in the dorsal horn. Thereby non-noxious stimuli such as touch or pressure can be perceived of as painful.

○ **What are the clinical features of lumbar radicular pain?**

Lumbar radicular pain ("sciatica") is caused by irritation of the sensory root or dorsal root ganglion of a spinal nerve. A herniated disc is a common cause, but spinal stenosis is more likely in the elderly. The pain is often described as sharp and shooting and is typically felt as a narrow band down the length of the leg in the distribution of the affected dermatome. It may be associated with sensory and/or motor dysfunction (radiculopathy) and may coexist with spinal or somatic referred pain.

○ **Are NSAIDs indicated for the treatment of acute low back pain?**

They are one of the mainstays of drug therapy. The benefit from the combined analgesic and anti-inflammatory properties of NSAIDs or acetaminophen can be seen within days of the onset of symptoms. If no medical contraindications are present, a 2- to 4-week course of acetaminophen or NSAIDs is indicated.

○ **What are Waddell signs?**

These are controversial signs that indicate a nonorganic source of pain. The presence of three of five potential Waddell signs points strongly to a nonorganic source:

• Tenderness: superficial, nondermatomal tenderness to a superficial light skin roll or pinch
• Simulation: pain in lumbar region to axial loading or to body rotation with shoulder and pelvis in line

- Distraction: inconsistent responses to a similar test (i.e., supine vs. sitting straight-leg raise)
- Regional disturbances: primarily motor or sensory loss in a nondermatomal distribution
- Overreaction: disproportionate and inappropriate responses to examination including verbal and facial expressions and unconventional movements and postures

○ **List treatment options for nonmalignant neuropathic pain.**

There are multiple causes for neuropathic pain, which can be classified into site of initial injury whether it is in the central or peripheral nervous system. There is no proven treatment to prevent or cure neuropathic pain. Treatment has traditionally been through a combination of medications and nerve blocks, implantable devices, physical therapy, transcutaneous electrical nerve stimulation (TENS), and psychological/occupational therapy. Membrane stabilizers and antidepressants such as gabapentin (Neurontin), pregabalin (Lyrica), duloxetine (Cymbalta), and amitriptyline (Elavil) are often used (especially for diabetic neuropathy or postherpetic neuralgia). Carbamazepine is indicated for trigeminal neuralgia (TN). Topical capsaicin, lamotrigine, baclofen, and opioids may also relieve pain in some patients.

○ **What is breakthrough pain and how is it managed?**

In 1990, Portenoy and Hagen proposed [See reference on page 524] a standard definition of breakthrough pain as a transient increase in the intensity of moderate or severe pain, occurring in the presence of well-established baseline pain. It is rapid in onset (within 3 minutes) and of short duration (median 30 minutes). According to the American Pain Society definition (2002) breakthrough pain is: "intermittent exacerbations of pain that can occur spontaneously or in relation to specific activity; pain that increases above the level of pain addressed by the ongoing analgesia; includes incident pain and end-of-dose failure."

Supplemental opioids (morphine, hydromorphone, oxycodone) and short-acting oral immediate-release or transmucosal opioids (fentanyl). If higher dosages of fixed-schedule opioids are maintained at all times as a prophylactic strategy, unacceptable side effects may result.

○ **During labor does a basal infusion for patient-controlled epidural analgesia (PCEA) enhance analgesia?**

The role of background infusion in the PCEA setting (in addition to on-demand dosing) seems to be still unclear in the literature. While some authors suggest that the continuous basal infusion with PCEA increases drug consumption without an analgesia benefit, other studies have demonstrated reduced need for analgesia supplementation with basal infusion.

○ **Describe the pathophysiology of phantom limb pain.**

Phantom limb pain is defined as a painful, unpleasant sensation in the distribution of a missing body part after a traumatic or surgical amputation. There is no agreement as to the mechanism, and it is likely that the cause is multifactorial and the result of disordered interactions between peripheral, spinal, and supraspinal mechanisms. The theories are divided into: peripheral causes (sensation due to a loss of previously present peripheral nerve activity, regeneration of the nerves that were injured/cut, neuroma formation with resulting painful nerve activity, alteration in ion channel activity at the site of injury), spinal causes (deafferentation), and central causes (changes in parts of the cortex and thalamus). Stress and depression may contribute to the syndrome.

○ **Phantom limb pain is frequently intractable and chronic. Are there any effective therapies available?**

Many treatment approaches have been attempted for phantom pain including medications, physical therapy, cognitive behavioral therapy, neuromodulation, and ablative procedures. Ablative surgical procedures (brain or spinal cord) have shown limited effectiveness. No single therapy has been shown to be effective for all patients. Studies examining regional or neuraxial anesthesia have failed to show consistent results to support its preemptive effects. Controlled trials using opioids, IV calcitonin, and ketamine have been shown to reduce pain in the short term. Anticonvulsants such as gabapentin, and tricyclic antidepressants such as nortriptyline, have demonstrated efficacy for neuropathic pain. NSAIDs or opioids may be indicated if the pain is thought to be secondary to somatic pain from the stump or residual limb. Baclofen or clonazepam may be useful for cramping pain or stump movement disorders. TENS and acupuncture have also been used with inconsistent long-term results. Mirror therapy is a noninvasive treatment option that is thought to restore motor cortex activity with illusory movements of the paralyzed limb.

○ Is botulinum toxin (BTX-A) effective in the treatment of myofascial pain?

Several studies have shown that BTX-A may be effective in reducing pain in myofascial disorders in a few prospective trials. However, stronger efficacy in large multicenter trials is currently lacking.

○ What is the mechanism of Botox pain relief?

Botulinum A toxin is produced by *Clostridium botulinum*. It affects the presynaptic membrane of the neuromuscular junction and prevents acetylcholine release and therefore muscle contraction. Inactivation persists until collaterals form in junction plates on new areas of muscle cell walls.

The proposed mechanism of action in pain management is due to reduction in spasticity in both dystonias and migraines. Side effects of botulinum toxin include pain, erythema, and unintended paralysis of nearby muscles.

○ Discuss the medical and surgical management of TN.

TN is a pain syndrome characterized by intermittent, sudden, often severe, lancinating pain that is typically one sided in the distribution of the trigeminal nerve. The distribution is typically in maxillary (V2) and mandibular (V3) nerve distributions (<5% is V1). Pain can occur in paroxysms and triggers include chewing, brushing teeth, cold air, or talking. There is no clinically evident neurologic deficit. Compression by an aberrant loop of artery or vein is thought to account for 80–90% of cases. The annual incidence of TN is estimated at 2–5 per 100,000. Prevalence increases with age, and there is a female predominance (1.5:1) with 90% of cases beginning after the age of 40 years. There is a slightly higher association with multiple sclerosis. The goal of treatment is to reduce significant morbidity associated with this disease. Carbamazepine (Tegretol) is the most effective medical therapy, with selected patients benefiting from Trileptal, baclofen, gabapentin, Lyrica, and clonazepam. Surgical options are reserved for those who have failed medication management. These include peripheral nerve blocks or ablation, gasserian ganglion and retrogasserian ablative procedures, craniotomy with microvascular decompression, and stereotactic radiosurgery (Gamma Knife®).

○ What is complex regional pain syndrome (CRPS), formerly known as reflex sympathetic dystrophy (RSD)?

RSD and causalgia are former terms for what is now known as CRPS types I and II, respectively. The general feature of CRPS is that it is a painful condition characterized by continuing pain, allodynia, and hyperalgesia disproportionate in time, degree, or severity to the usual course of any known trauma or lesion. The pain is regional (not in distribution of a specific dermatome), usually distal, and exhibits variable progression over time. Symptoms include severe burning pain, pathological changes in bone and skin (warm, shiny red skin turns bluish and cool), excessive sweating, tissue swelling, and extreme sensitivity to touch. Eventually disuse atrophy of the skin, muscles, and joints can result. There are two types: CRPS I (without nerve injury, replaces the term RSD) and CRPS II (with identifiable nerve injury, replaces causalgia).

○ **What are the diagnostic criteria for CRPS Type I and II [IASP, 1994 and Harden et al., 2007. See reference on page 524]?**

In 1994, a consensus group met to review the criteria for the diagnosis of CRPS/RSD and the term CRPS was used as a broad category to include patients with pain that is sympathetically mediated. CRPS is a clinical diagnosis. In order to make a diagnosis of CRPS II, there must be a definable nerve injury, whereas CRPS I develops after major or minor injuries with no obvious damage to the nerves in the involved extremity.

The following criteria must be met to make a clinical diagnosis:

1. Continuing pain, which is disproportionate to any inciting event.

2. Must report at least one symptom and one sign in three of the following four categories:

	Symptom	*Sign*
Sensory	Hyperesthesia/allodynia	Hyperalgesia to pinprick and/or allodynia to light touch
Vasomotor	Reports of temperature or skin color asymmetry or changes	Evidence of >1° temperature asymmetry and/or skin color changes or asymmetry
Sudomotor	Evidence of edema, sweating changes, asymmetry	Evidence of edema, sweating changes, asymmetry
Motor/trophic	Reports of decreased range of motion, motor dysfunction, trophic changes	Evidence of decreased ROM, motor dysfunction (weakness, tremor, dystonia), and trophic changes (hair, nail, skin)

3. There is no other diagnosis that explains the signs and symptoms.

The IASP criteria for CRPS have proven to be very sensitive. Harden et al., in 2007. [See reference on page 524] showed that when two of four sign categories were present and three of four symptom categories were present, the resultant sensitivity was 0.85 and the specificity was 0.69 for a clinical diagnosis of CRPS.

○ **What is the progression of CRPS?**

Traditionally, RSD has been described as *three consecutive phases of disease* (*acute, dystrophic, and atrophic*) with the early symptoms like those of a disturbance of sympathetic function. In the *acute stage*, during the first 1–3 months, there is burning pain disproportionate to the degree of injury and extreme sensitivity to touch, with skin color and temperature changes. The *dystrophic stage* at 3–6 months involves constant pain and swelling, increased muscle tone, stiffness, and wasting, and early bone loss. During the *atrophic phase* of skin, muscle, and bone, the skin becomes cool and shiny, with muscle stiffness, weakness, spasm, and tremor, and symptoms may spread to another limb. Depression and anxiety may be present.

Recently, however, the idea of stages of CRPS has been discounted and features of different stages can be found at different times.

○ **What are the complications of regional pain syndrome 1 (RSD)?**

The signs and symptoms of sympathetic nervous system involvement are discussed above. In addition, signs of motor system dysfunction include difficult in starting movement, increased muscle tone, muscle spasm, tremor, and weakness. Additional problems are infections, migraine headache, excessive sweating, fatigue, dermatitis, eczema, depression, and anxiety. Skin, muscle, and bone atrophies with reduced function of the limb are frequent.

○ **T/F: The goal of treatment of CRPS is pain control through drug therapy and immobilization of the affected limb.**

False. Medications are targeted to alleviating symptoms as the goals are pain control and mobilization of the affected limb with physical therapy. Treatment employs multimodal pharmacologic therapy using, for example, a combination of NSAID anticonvulsants, antidepressants, and opioids. Sympathetic nerve blocks can be helpful for diagnosis and treatment, allowing for analgesia and ability to effectively perform physical therapy. Intrathecal baclofen for refractory dystonia has been utilized as well as TENS. There is also increasing evidence in favor of spinal cord stimulators for patients with suboptimal benefit from conventional therapy.

○ **What are the indications for sympathetic blockade?**

Diagnosis and treatment of sympathetically mediated acute or chronic pain. The most common indications include CRPS types I and II, visceral pain, acute herpetic neuralgia, postherpetic pain, and peripheral vascular disease. Sympathetic blockade to a region is indicated by increased temperature and blood flow to the skin, while somatic sensation should be unaltered.

○ **Where is the stellate ganglion?**

It is formed by the fusion of the lower cervical and first thoracic ganglions (cardiothoracic ganglion), present in 80% of individuals. It lies on the anterior surface of the seventh cervical transverse process.

○ **What features indicate a successful stellate ganglion block?**

The development of a unilateral Horner syndrome: partial ptosis, meiosis, apparent enophthalmos, lack of sweating, and nasal congestion. Sympathetic blockade in the upper extremity should also be evident.

○ **What are the complications of stellate ganglion block?**

CNS toxicity (intra-arterial injection of local anesthetic into the vertebral artery) resulting in seizures, vasovagal reactions, phrenic nerve block, brachial plexus blockade, spinal or epidural injection, and recurrent laryngeal nerve palsy with hoarseness. Pneumothorax is possible if the needle is inserted in a caudad direction. Horner syndrome (unilateral meiosis, ptosis, and enophthalmos) is an expected side effect that can occur. Intercostal neuralgia has been described manifesting as severe chest wall pain. Bilateral stellate ganglion blocks are contraindicated.

○ **What is the difference between unilateral right and left stellate ganglion blockade on left ventricular function?**

With TEE assessment, blood pressure and heart rate are not significantly changed.

Following right stellate ganglion blockade there are no significant differences in systolic and diastolic functions. Left stellate ganglion block results in denervation of the left ventricle without a change in systolic function, but relaxation is prolonged. Left ventricular end-diastolic volume (LVEDV) and left ventricular end-systolic volume (LVESV) are significantly increased. In patients without cardiovascular disease (ASA I), these effects are not clinically significant as the heart responds with a small stroke volume increase to offset the simultaneous decrease in afterload.

○ **Describe options for pain management related to pancreatic disease.**

Medical management (opioids, antidepressants, anticonvulsants, antiarrythmics), *radiographically guided injections* (celiac plexus block, peripheral nerve block, neuraxial blocks), *behavioral* (psychotherapy, relaxation, biofeedback), *acupuncture, neuromodulation* (spinal cord stimulation [SCS], TENS), and *intrathecal drug delivery systems.*

○ **What is the anatomy of the celiac plexus block?**

The celiac plexus surrounds the celiac artery at the level of L1 vertebrae, anterior to the aorta. Blockade involves preganglionic fibers from the greater and lesser splanchnic nerve, postganglionic sympathetic fibers, preganglionic parasympathetic fibers, afferent visceral nociceptive fibers, and branches of the right vagus. This results in denervation of the stomach, liver, gallbladder, pancreas, kidneys, gut to the transverse colon, diaphragm, spleen, and abdominal aorta [Polati et al., 2008. See reference on page 524].

○ **Does the celiac plexus supply the pelvic organs?**

No. The hypogastric plexus supplies the pelvic organs.

○ **List the complications of celiac plexus block.**

Common side effects due to sympathetic denervation includes hypotension (mostly postural, and in up to one third of patients) and transient diarrhea due to hyperperistalsis (in up to 40% of patients). Other complications are rapid absorption of the drug leading to systemic toxicity (more common from injection into vena cava than accidental intra-aortic injection). Other less common complications are pneumothorax, retroperitoneal hemorrhage, subarachnoid injection, or injury to pancreas or kidney.

○ **What is postthoracotomy pain syndrome?**

Chronic pain persisting at least 2 months after thoracotomy resulting from surgical trauma or fibrosis.

The pain is thought to be a combination of myofascial and neuropathic components, usually in the distribution of the affected intercostal nerve. Management of the pain includes the use of tricyclic antidepressants and anticonvulsants. Repetitive local anesthetic intercostal blocks, epidural analgesia, or trigger point injections of a neuroma may be useful. Neuromodulation has also been used with SCS, or also with targeted subcutaneous therapy.

○ **What are the proposed mechanisms of TENS therapy?**

It is proposed that TENS therapy may work by the gate control theory (closing the gate and disallowing pain transmission). Also, it is speculated that a mechanism of action occurs through the stimulation and release of endogenous opioids. TENS works best in patients with myofascial syndromes, peripheral nerve injuries, phantom limb pain, and stump pain. It is unsatisfactory in patients with chronic pain that has no peripheral nociceptive cause (central pain state) and in patients with a physiologic and/or psychological dependence on drugs.

○ **What are the diagnostic criteria for *fibromyalgia syndrome* (FMS)?**

According to the American College of Rheumatology (1990) criteria for the classification of fibromyalgia:

1. History of widespread pain in all four quadrants of a patient's body for a minimum of 3 months. Pain is considered widespread when all of the following are present: pain in both sides of the body, pain above and below the waist, and axial skeletal pain (cervical spine, anterior chest, thoracic spine, or low back pain). Low back pain is considered lower segment pain.

2. Pain in 11 of 18 tender point sites on digital palpitation that cluster around the neck, shoulder, chest, hip, knee, and elbow regions.

However, it is important to note that the above criteria do not include the symptoms of fatigue, sleep disturbance, and cognitive dysfunction that are important components of the disease.

○   **What is the difference between FMS and myofascial pain syndrome (MPS)?**

MPS is a painful musculoskeletal condition characterized by the development of trigger points in muscle (painful palpable taut band) and "referred pain." It presents as local pain with fatigue and morning stiffness is uncommon. The prognosis is good, and often resolves with treatment, consisting of physical therapy, trigger point injections, muscle relaxants (such as tizanidine), relaxation techniques, and acupuncture. FMS is chronic pain syndrome characterized by diffuse pain, fatigue, morning stiffness, and tender points (with the absence of taut bands), with a poor prognosis.

○   **What are some of the therapies for the treatment of MPS?**

Trigger point therapy (myofascial release therapy, myotherapy, medical massage therapy)

Spray and stretch technique (vapocoolant spray on the trigger point and then PT-directed stretch therapy)

Trigger point injections (local anesthetic injected directly into the trigger points)

Dry needling (the use of a needle to disrupt the trigger point with no injection)

Chiropractic manipulation

Craniosacral therapy

Exercise

Improvement of nutrition

Changing sleeping habits

TCA in low doses

Elimination of stress, biofeedback, and counseling for depression

For MPS there is no role for injected steroids.

○   **Is fentanyl useful in the treatment of chronic pain?**

Fentanyl is an ideal agent for delivery via the transdermal therapeutic system due to its low molecular weight, high potency, and lipid solubility. These systems release the drug into the skin at a constant rate ranging from 25 to 100 uq/h. Compared with oral opioids, the advantages of transdermal fentanyl include a lower incidence and impact of adverse effects (constipation, nausea and vomiting, and daytime drowsiness), a higher degree of patient satisfaction, improved quality of life, improved convenience and compliance resulting from administration every 72 hours, and decreased use of rescue medication. Therapeutic blood levels are attained 12–16 hours after patch application and decrease slowly with a half-life of 16–22 hours following removal.

○   **What types of neurolytic blocks are used for treatment of pain related to head and neck cancer?**

Neurolytic blocks can be conducted for divisions of the trigeminal nerve and the trigeminal nerve as well as the occipital nerve. Neurolytic blocks for pain in the trigeminal (V) distribution are being used less frequently and have been replaced by surgical techniques such as posterior fossa microvascular decompression or radio frequency. This is due to the high incidence of side effects such as anesthesia dolorosa (pain in an area of anesthesia). Glycerol rhizolysis and balloon decompression are also utilized in the gasserian ganglion for neurolysis. Controlled lesioning is thought to be the primary advantage of radio-frequency neurolysis over glycerol rhizolysis or balloon decompression. Nasal endoscopically guided neurolytic sphenopalatine ganglion block with 6% phenol after a prognostic block with local anesthetic solution has also been described.

○ **What is postherpetic neuralgia?**

Herpes zoster results from reactivation of the varicella-zoster virus from the dorsal root ganglia that remains dormant after the primary "chickenpox" infection. It presents with a classic dermatomal rash and burning pain that precedes the rash and may persist well after the resolution of the rash. The pain associated with herpes zoster can be grouped into three phases. Acute herpetic neuralgia accompanies the rash and lasts for 30 days following the onset of the rash. Subacute herpetic neuralgia is defined as pain persisting from 30 to 120 days after rash onset. Postherpetic neuralgia is the pain that persists for at least 120 days after rash onset. Tricyclic antidepressants, anticonvulsants, capsaicin, lidocaine patches, and nerve blocks have been used in selected patients. The pain may be very debilitating and require narcotics for adequate pain control.

○ **How do you avert the progression of acute herpes zoster to postherpetic neuralgia?**

Few approaches have been proved beneficial and postherpetic neuralgia remains a painful source of frustration for both patients and physicians. Antiviral drugs (oral acyclovir started within 72 hours after the onset of the rash), oral corticosteroids (reduces pain of herpes zoster and the incidence of postherpetic neuralgia), nerve blocks, and combination therapy have been described.

○ **Describe the use of autonomic nerve block for chronic nonmalignant pain originating in the pelvis.**

It has been claimed that some chronic perineal pain syndromes respond to bilateral lumbar sympathetic block and superior hypogastric block has been used for chronic nonmalignant pelvic pain syndromes.

○ **Describe the efficacy of neurolytic blocks in the treatment of chronic pelvic pain associated with cancer.**

The pain of rectal tenesmus due to pelvic carcinoma may be helped with celiac plexus block. Neurolytic superior hypogastric plexus blocks have been used for chronic pelvic pain and block of the ganglion impar at the inferior end of the sacrum has been used for perineal pain in cancer.

○ **Describe diagnostic and neurolytic lumbar sympathetic block.**

The lumbar sympathetic chain consists of four or five paired ganglia that lie along the anterolateral surface of the lumbar vertebral bodies, containing preganglionic and postganglionic fibers to the pelvis and lower extremities. It is most frequently located at L2 or L3 level at the medial margin of the psoas muscle in the retroperitoneal connective tissue. Blocks for the lower limb are performed in the prone or lateral position, usually targeting the anterior anterosuperior portion of L3 or anteroinferior edge of the vertebral body of L2. A volume of 5–20 mL is injected incrementally.

Neurolytic injections are made with 2–3 mL of aqueous phenol (3–6%) or alcohol (50–100%). Phenol is used more often due to a decreased incidence of neuritis after the procedure. Radio-frequency techniques can also be utilized, allowing for more controlled lesions compared with radio frequency. However, chemical neurolysis can create a larger lesion, depending on volume used.

○ **What is clonidine and how is it used to provide analgesia?**

Clonidine is a direct centrally acting alpha-2 adrenergic receptor agonist. Alpha-2-Agonists are used primarily as anesthetic adjuvants for the treatment of acute and chronic pains (intractable pain, RSD, and neuropathic pain). Oral clonidine can augment spinally mediated opioid analgesia, whereas epidural or intrathecal clonidine can provide effective analgesia alone. Intrathecal clonidine does not provide surgical anesthesia. Clonidine decreases postoperative oxygen consumption and adrenergic stress response and only mildly potentiates opiate-induced respiratory depression. It does not cause urinary retention.

○ **What is the mechanism of action of epidural clonidine?**

Clonidine produces analgesia by binding to the alpha-2 adrenergic receptors in the dorsal horn of the spinal cord to inhibit the release of substance P. Neuraxial clonidine also increases acetylcholine levels in the cerebrospinal fluid.

Analgesia is produced when acetylcholine binds to the spinal cord receptors (muscarinic and nicotinic) and stimulates the nitric oxide synthesis.

○ **What are the common side effects of epidural clonidine?**

Significant hypotension, bradycardia, and sedation are dose-dependent side effects of IV and epidural clonidine. A meta-analysis reported no evidence of respiratory depression by pulse oximetry.

○ **Describe the nerve fibers that transmit pain.**

Somatic pain versus visceral pain.

The nociceptive pain information is transmitted by small-diameter, unmyelinated C fibers (visceral pain which is usually dull and aching) and lightly myelinated A-delta fibers (somatic pain, which is sharp). These fibers end at the substantia gelatinosa of the dorsal horn (lamina II), the gate of the spinal cord. C fibers have a diameter of 0.4–1.2 mm and a conduction velocity of 0.5–2 m/s. A fibers have a diameter of 2–5 mm and a conduction velocity of 12–30 m/s.

○ **What is the mechanism of SCS (Spinal Cord Stimulation)?**

There are multiple theories that explain the mechanism of action of SCS [Oakley and Prager, 2002. See reference on page 524]:

1. Antidromic activation of A-beta afferents. This gate control theory explains the segmental mechanism.

    In chronic pain states large myelinated A-beta fibers, after a "reorganization process," also terminate at this gate of the spinal cord producing touching or vibration effect, and turning off or closing the gate to reception of small-fiber information.

2. Blocking of transmission in the spinothalamic tract.

    This segmental theory explains the effect of SCS blocking the transmission of electrochemical information anywhere in the spinothalamic tract.

3. *Supraspinal pain inhibition* by stimulating the dorsal column nucleus.

4. *Activation of central inhibitory mechanism influencing sympathetic efferent neurons.*

5. *Activation of putative neurotransmitters or neuromodulators.*

SCS produces neurochemical changes at the dorsal horn and produces pain relief lasting minutes, hours, or even days.

○ **What are the indications for SCS?**

SCS treats the symptoms and does not affect the underlying problem.

Failed back surgery syndrome, peripheral vascular disease and associated ischemic pain, and CRPS are probably the most important entities that respond well to SCS treatment. Other conditions such as phantom pain and postherpetic neuralgia may also respond.

○ **What is WHO analgesic ladder?**

WHO has developed a three-step "ladder" for cancer pain relief.

If pain occurs, there should be prompt oral administration of drugs in the following order: nonopioids (aspirin and paracetamol); then, as necessary, mild opioids (codeine); then strong opioids such as morphine, until the patient is free of pain. Adjuvants should be given to relieve anxiety when necessary. Appropriate nerve blocks should be performed for further pain relief. The drugs should be prescribed "by the clock," that is, every 3–6 hours, not "on demand."

This three-step approach is inexpensive and 80–90% effective.

○ **What is the mechanism of action of COX-2 inhibitors?**

The cyclooxygenase enzymes 1 and 2 are responsible for conversion of arachidonic acid to various mediators of inflammation including prostaglandins. COX-2 enzyme is believed to be produced more in response to injury and its concentration is believed to be more in areas of inflammation. Selective inhibitors of COX-2 have preference for this enzyme, hence producing selective inhibition of prostaglandin synthesis in specific areas. This reduces some of the side effects of traditional NSAIDs, especially gastric irritation.

○ **What are the symptoms of multiple myeloma?**

This is malignancy of the plasma cells in the bone marrow. Common symptoms include bone pain, usually in the back and ribs, broken bones (spine), weakness and tiredness, frequent infection and fever, and weight loss.

Key Terms

Acute low back pain treatment
Back pain: differential diagnosis
Botox: pain relief mechanism
Breakthrough pain management
Cancer pain: management
Celiac plexus block: distribution
Celiac plexus block: physiology/indications/
 complications/side effects
C-fiber stimulation
Chronic pain terminology
Chronic pain treatment: fentanyl
CRPS: diagnostic nerve block
CRPS I: diagnosis
CRPS I: early symptoms
CRPS II: diagnosis/treatment
Epidural clonidine: complications
Epidural clonidine: mechanism of action
Fibromyalgia: diagnostic criteria
Head and neck blocks: diagnosis
Herpes: acute
Indication: superior hypogastric plexus block
Lumbar sympathetic block: effects

Lumbar sympathetic neurolytic block
Management: lumbosacral radiculopathy
Mechanism of COX-2 inhibitors
Multiple myeloma: symptoms
Myofacial pain syndrome: diagnosis/treatment
Neurolytic blocks: head and neck carcinoma
Neuropathic pain: treatment/treatment with epidural
Phantom pain: mechanism/treatment
Postherpetic neuralgia: prevention/treatment/location
Radiculopathy: steroid epidural
Somatic pain pathways
Somatic pain versus visceral pain
Spinal cord stimulation: indications/mechanism
Spinal stenosis: diagnosis
Stellate ganglion block: signs/effects/complications
Sympathetic block: indications
Sympathetic nerve block: diagnosis pelvic pain
Transdermal fentanyl: indications
Trigeminal neuralgia: treatment
Trigger point injection indications
Upper extremity sympathetic block
WHO analgesic ladder

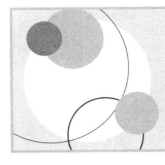

Clinical Pharmacology

*Imagination was given to man to compensate him for what he isn't; and a sense of humor
to console him for what he is.*
Unknown

○ **Compare the terms drug potency and efficacy.**

Potency is described as the dose required to achieve a maximal response, and is represented by the *dose axis* on the dose response curve.

Efficacy is the maximal effect of a drug and is represented by the *plateau* in the dose response curve.

○ **Describe the pharmacology of nicardipine.**

It is a calcium ion influx inhibitor (slow channel-blocking agent) mainly used in small boluses or infusion to treat hypertensive emergencies. It has high cerebrovascular selectivity, hence its usefulness in neurovascular emergencies.

Nicardipine is selective for vascular smooth muscle compared with myocardium and therefore acts primarily as a vasodilator. Hypotensive effects are accompanied by reflex tachycardia. It is available in both PO and IV formulations. Peak onset for IV injection is within 1–2 minutes. Almost 95% protein bound. Elimination: renal 60% (less than 1% unchanged); biliary/fecal 35%.

○ **Describe sodium nitroprusside (SNP) metabolism.**

SNP is a direct-acting nonselective peripheral vasodilator acting on both arterial and venous smooth muscles. Its immediate short-lived action is caused by release of nitric oxide (NO). Metabolism begins with transfer of an electron from iron of oxyhemoglobin to SNP → methemoglobin and unstable SNP → unstable SNP breaks down to release five cyanide ions → one cyanide ion combines with methemoglobin → cyanomethemoglobin.

Remaining cyanide ions are converted by rhodanase enzyme from liver and kidneys to thiocyanate, which is excreted. The thiosulfate ions are used as sulfur donors for this reaction. (Cyanide ions also bind cytochrome oxidase, which interferes with oxygen use, resulting in toxicity.)

○ **What are the problems with the use of SNP in renal impairment?**

Thiocyanate is a renally excreted metabolite of SNP, with a half-life of 4–7 days, which is further prolonged in renal failure. Hypoxia, nausea, tinnitus, muscle spasm, and psychosis can occur when levels exceed 10 mg/100 mL. Hypothyroidism can result as thiocyanate inhibits iodide ion uptake by the thyroid gland. Oxyhemoglobin can oxidize thiocyanate to sulfate and cyanide, but it is too slow to be of clinical importance.

○ **What are the signs of nitroprusside toxicity?**

Nitroprusside toxicity is a result of the breakdown of the molecule to release five free cyanide ions. The cyanide enters the electron transport chain, where it binds to and inactivates cytochrome oxidase. Clinically, this manifests in symptoms such as tachycardia, hypertension, altered mental status, and arrhythmias, and signs such as metabolic acidosis, increased venous oxygen content, and tachyphylaxis to the nitroprusside.

○ **What are the toxic effects of nitroglycerine?**

Severe hypotension, tachycardia, blurred vision, convulsions, coma, and methemoglobinemia.

○ **What are the pharmacodynamics of vasodilator drugs?**

Vasodilators work to relax smooth muscle in the arterial tree, the venous system, or both (balanced vasodilators). Drugs that work on the arteries reduce afterload, and are primarily used to treat hypertension and heart failure; they are typically not used to treat angina, due to the reflex tachycardia they produce. Drugs that act primarily on the venous side reduce preload, and are useful for treating angina and edema.

○ **What are the effects of vasodilators on renal blood flow?**

Vasodilators may lead to an initial increase in RBF due to relaxation of the renal arteries. However, autoregulation of renal blood flow typically returns the RBF back to its baseline flow rate shortly after the initiation of the vasodilator therapy. Persistent increase in RBF is more reliably achieved by the use of dopamine receptor (D1) agonists.

○ **What are the cardiorespiratory effects of dexmedetomidine?**

Hypotension is the most significant side effect, seen in almost one third of patients receiving dexmedetomidine. Tachycardia is also seen, but may be a reflex secondary to the drop in blood pressure. Respiratory effects are not typical, but higher doses can lead to respiratory depression.

○ **What is the mechanism of vancomycin-induced hypotension and how can it be minimized?**

Red man syndrome: chills or fever, fainting, tachycardia, hives, hypotension, cardiac arrest, itching, nausea or vomiting, and rash or redness of the face, base of neck, upper body, back, and arms from histamine release due to rapid infusion. Parenteral vancomycin should be administered as an infusion over at least 60 minutes.

○ **Describe the therapeutic action and mechanism of magnesium sulfate.**

Second most common intracellular cation after potassium; normal plasma level 0.7–1.1 mmol/L and anticonvulsant level 2–3.5 mmol/L; exists in three forms: ionized, protein bound, and ion bound:

- Magnesium supplement
- Antiarrhythmic and direct cardioprotectant: ventricular tachycardia: monomorphic or torsade de pointes
- Anticonvulsant (obstetrics: preeclampsia)
- Cofactor in enzymatic reactions involving energy metabolism and nucleic acid synthesis
- Also: hormone receptor binding, gating of calcium channels, transmembrane ion flux and regulation of adenylate cyclase, neuronal activity, control of vasomotor tone (coronary and systemic vasodilation), decreases cardiac excitability, depression of neurotransmitter release and muscle contraction, physiological calcium antagonist, and inhibition of platelet aggregation.
- Toxic effects: hypotension, cardiac conduction defects/cardiac arrest (antidote: calcium chloride), and CNS depression.

○ **Describe the main therapeutic uses of adenosine.**

The heart: inhibitory effect on the AV node resulting in cardiac arrest that makes it the drug of choice for AV nodal reentrant tachycardia (SVT). Important in myocardial preconditioning and may be helpful in heart failure. Adenosine induces collateral circulation, reduces noradrenaline/endothelin release and renin/angiotensin/aldosterone axis activation, and protects against reperfusion.

The brain: Parkinson disease, neuropathic pain, drug addiction, schizophrenia, and Alzheimer disease.

The lungs: marker of airway inflammation with provocative inhalational testing.

The immune system: immunosuppression in chronic illness and inhibits tumor growth.

The blood: inhibits platelet aggregation.

○ **What is the duration of action of adenosine?**

Less than 10 seconds. Metabolism is very rapid by circulating enzymes in erythrocytes and vascular endothelial cells. Adenosine is deaminated to inactive inosine (further degraded to hypoxanthine and uric acid) and by phosphorylation to adenosine monophosphate (AMP).

○ **What are the hemodynamic effects of amiodarone?**

Amiodarone, a potent drug used to treat ventricular tachycardia and SVT, causes both a negative inotropic effect on the heart and peripheral vasodilation. In patients without preexisting cardiac disease, these effects tend to cancel each other out, and cardiac output is maintained. However, amiodarone has been shown to reduce cardiac index and increase RV pressures in patients with preexisting LV dysfunction (EF <35%).

○ **Describe the side effects of amiodarone.**

The side effects are common particularly at daily doses higher than 400 mg. They include:

Pulmonary alveolitis

Prolongation of QT interval that may lead to torsade

Corneal microdeposits, photosensitivity, and cyanotic discoloration

Displacement of digoxin from protein binding sites and increase in its plasma concentration

Hypothyroidism or hyperthyroidism

○ **A patient is receiving amiodarone for suppression of ventricular ectopy. What are your concerns for administering anesthesia for femoral–popliteal bypass surgery?**

Amiodarone causes a peripheral neuropathy and has been associated with intractable hypotension and bradyarrhythmias unresponsive to catecholamines under general anesthesia. Despite recommendations to discontinue 2 weeks prior to elective surgery, patients often require continuation for intractable arrhythmias.

○ **What is the pharmacology of milrinone?**

Milrinone is a phosphodiesterase inhibitor currently approved for IV administration to treat decompensated congestive heart failure. It inhibits type III phosphodiesterase, thereby increasing intracellular cAMP.

○ **What are the cardiovascular effects of milrinone?**

Milrinone administration results in a positive inotropic effect on the heart, vasodilatation in the periphery, and a decreased pulmonary vascular resistance. The hemodynamic consequences of this action produce biventricular afterload reduction, with an increase in cardiac output and a reduction in total peripheral resistance.

○ **Describe cardiac arrhythmias caused by digitalis toxicity.**

The therapeutic dose of digoxin is 0.5–2.0 ng/mL. Digoxin toxicity can lead to cardiac arrhythmias especially in the presence of hypokalemia. The cardiac arrhythmias can be atrial or ventricular. The initial feature may be prolongation of the PR interval. The most common arrhythmia is atrial tachycardia with AV block. Ventricular fibrillation is the most frequent cause of death from digoxin toxicity.

○ **What electrolyte abnormality is a risk factor for precipitating digitalis toxicity?**

Hypokalemia (K^+ <4 mEq/L). Other factors that predispose to digitalis toxicity include hypercalcemia, hypoxia, drugs (propranolol, amiodarone, verapamil, quinidine), hypothyroidism, advanced age, and renal insufficiency. Since magnesium is a cofactor of the Na^+/K^+-ATPase pump, alterations of its concentration will affect the pump's actions (not really increased toxicity).

○ **What does the arterial blood gas (ABG) reveal in cases of salicylate toxicity?**

Aspirin initially stimulates the respiratory center, resulting in hyperventilation and a resultant respiratory alkalosis. Later, it interferes with the Krebs cycle, resulting in increased lactate production and the development of a wide anion gap metabolic acidosis. Thus, patients tend to present with a mixed respiratory alkalosis/metabolic acidosis with a wide anion gap. If toxicity results in hypoventilation, a pure acidosis may be seen.

○ **What is the therapy for salicylate toxicity?**

Activated charcoal is the primary therapy, as early administration can reduce aspirin absorption by up to 80%. Fluid replacement is mandatory, and should be accompanied by alkalinization of the urine. Alkalinizing the urine from a pH of 5 to 8 increases renal clearance from 1.3 to 100 mL/min. Alkalinization is easily accomplished by administering a sodium bicarbonate bolus of 1–2 mEq/kg, followed by a slower infusion rate. Hypokalemia must also be corrected.

○ **What are the signs and symptoms of acetaminophen toxicity?**

Acetaminophen toxicity is divided into four phases, depending on the time of the ingestion. During Phase 1, occurring 0–24 hours after ingestion, the patient either is asymptomatic or complains of generalized symptoms such as nausea, vomiting, anorexia, and malaise. A subclinical rise in liver transaminase enzyme levels occurs approximately 12 hours after initial ingestion. During Phase 2, which occurs 18–72 hours after ingestion, the patient continues to display GI symptoms and will begin to complain of right upper quadrant pain. Labs will reveal a further increase in transaminase levels. Phase 3, at 72–96 hours, is the period of centrilobular hepatic necrosis. The patient will have worsening RUQ abdominal pain, jaundice, coagulopathy, renal failure, and hepatic encephalopathy, and may ultimately succumb. Phase 4, from 96 hours to 3 weeks, is marked by a gradual resolution of symptoms and organ failure for patients who survive Phase 3.

○ **Describe the perioperative implications of angiotensin-converting enzyme (ACE) inhibitors and potassium homeostasis.**

ACE inhibitors interfere with the stimulus to release aldosterone. This can lead to hyperkalemia especially in the presence of renal function impairment and concomitant use of K-sparing diuretics.

There is also a risk of hemodynamic instability and hypotension occurring during anesthesia, especially with surgery involving major body fluid shifts. This is mainly due to decreased sympathetic nervous system vasoconstrictive responses. This exaggerated hypotension has been responsive to crystalloids and sympathomimetics such as ephedrine or phenylephrine. If resistant, a vasopressin agonist such as terlipressin may be effective. Anesthetic drugs should be titrated down to limit the magnitude of hypotension due to ACE inhibitors.

○ **What is the role of ACE inhibitors in MI survival?**

ACE inhibitors have been shown to reduce mortality by about 20% when used on a long-term basis in high-risk postinfarction patients. Full-dose ACE therapy administered within the first postinfarct day results in greater improvement in LV function than lower-dose or delayed ACE therapy [Pfeffer et al., 1997. See reference on page 524].

ACE inhibitors should be used in all patients with a STEMI without contraindications. They are also recommended in patients with NSTEMI who have diabetes, heart failure, hypertension, or an ejection fraction less than 40%. In such patients, an ACE inhibitor should be administered within 24 hours of admission and continued indefinitely. Contraindications to ACE inhibitor use include hypotension and declining renal function [2007 focused update for the management of STEMI. See reference on page 524].

○ **What are the physiological effects of amiloride?**

Amiloride is a potassium-conserving (antikaliuretic) drug that possesses weak natriuretic, diuretic, and antihypertensive activity. It is typically administered in conjunction with a loop or thiazide diuretic to reduce the excretion of potassium and magnesium in the urine.

○ **What is the mechanism of action of acetazolamide?**

Acetazolamide inhibits carbonic anhydrase, which accelerates the reversible conversion of carbon dioxide and water to bicarbonate and hydrogen ions. Prevention of the renal reabsorption of bicarbonate leads to alkalinization of the urine and increased sodium, and water loss. Acetazolamide decreases the production of aqueous humor in the eye, and is used to treat glaucoma.

○ **How does acetazolamide work in ophthalmology?**

It inhibits carbonic anhydrase, an enzyme important in aqueous humor synthesis in the ciliary processes. As such, it decreases the production of aqueous humor and lowers the intraocular pressure.

○ **What effect does acetazolamide have on acid base status?**

It causes a mild hyperchloremic metabolic acidosis. Acetazolamide causes alkalinization of urine by significantly interfering with hydrogen ion secretion in the proximal tubule and impairing bicarbonate reabsorption. In exchange for this filtered bicarbonate, more chloride is absorbed in the kidney. Because of this, acetazolamide results in diuresis of alkaline urine, causing hyperchloremic metabolic acidosis.

○ **How does furosemide acts as a diuretic?**

Furosemide prevents concentration of urine by inhibiting the absorption of sodium and chloride in the thick ascending limb of the loop of Henle. It also inhibits magnesium and calcium reabsorption, which are dependent on sodium and chloride concentrations.

○ **What are some prolonged metabolic effects of furosemide?**

Increased blood glucose and impaired glucose tolerance has been reported with furosemide administration. Increased reabsorption of uric acid in the proximal tubules is associated with elevated serum concentrations.

Adverse effects are largely related to fluid or electrolyte imbalance. Hyponatremia, hypochloremic metabolic alkalosis, hypokalemia, hypomagnesemia, as well as volume depletion. It may cause prerenal azotemia, particularly in the elderly. Although furosemide also causes increased excretion of Ca^{2+} ions, they are reabsorbed later in the distal convoluted tubule; hypocalcemia is therefore not seen with furosemide use.

○   **How do diuretics affect potassium homeostasis?**

Diuretics increase sodium delivery to the distal tubules, resulting in a lumen-negative gradient that promotes potassium secretion. Volume depletion causes a secondary hyperaldosteronism, which stimulates distal tubular sodium reabosrption in exchange for potassium and hydrogen ions. All diuretics, except carbonic anhydrase inhibitors, cause chloride depletion, which independently promotes potassium loss.

○   **What is the mechanism of action of hydrochlorothiazide (HCTZ)?**

HCTZ inhibits sodium reabsorption at the distal convoluted tubule (as opposed to loop diuretics, which work on the ascending tubule). This results in natriuresis and water loss, as well as loss of potassium. HCTZ also promotes calcium reabsorption at the same site.

○   **What are the effects of HCTZ on the blood chemistry panel?**

HCTZ primarily results in hypokalemia. Also causes metabolic alkalosis (increased hydrogen secretion) and hyponatremia (impairment of renal diluting capacity). Since calcium and magnesium are competing ions, increased calcium absorption may result in hypomagnesemia. Glucose tolerance is also reduced, so HCTZ is sometimes associated with hyperglycemia (believed to be related to hypokalemia and impaired insulin secretion). Hyperuricemia occurs due to increased net reabsorption of uric acid in the proximal tubule. Finally, HCTZ results in increased levels of LDL cholesterol, total cholesterol, and triglycerides.

○   **What is the pharmacology of fenoldapam?**

Fenoldapam binds to the dopamine D1 receptor, resulting in arterial vasodilation and a lowering of blood pressure and afterload. It is especially active in the renal and mesenteric vascular beds, where it increases renal perfusion, due to the large concentration of D1 receptors in these areas. It may be useful preoperatively in the prevention of contrast media–induced acute renal failure.

○   **Describe bleomycin toxicity.**

Most serious toxic effect is dose-related pulmonary interstitial fibrosis that is estimated to involve 4% of all patients treated. The other side effects are mucocutaneous reactions, alopecia, and hyperpigmentation. Some patients with lymphoma may develop an acute reaction characterized by hyperthermia, hypotension, and hypoventilation.

○   **A patient is to have a hysterectomy for endometrial carcinoma. What are the implications of prior chemotherapy?**

Doxorubicin (Adriamycin) used in the treatment of endometrial carcinoma causes myelosuppression and has well-recognized cardiac side effects. The risk of irreversible cardiomyopathy increases with a cumulative dose greater than 550 mg/m^2, prior radiotherapy, and concurrent cyclophosphamide treatment. Cisplatin causes acute renal failure, peripheral neuropathies, and severe nausea.

○   **Describe the toxicity related to doxorubicin.**

Cardiotoxicity usually manifests in the form of congestive heart failure. It usually appears within 1–6 months after initiation of therapy. Cardiomyopathy has been reported to be associated with persistent voltage reduction in the QRS wave, systolic interval prolongation, and reduction of ejection fraction. It may develop suddenly and may not be detected by routine ECG. It may be irreversible and fatal but responds to treatment if detected early.

○ **A 27-year-old man with past history of receiving chemotherapy for a hematologic malignancy presents with worsening dyspnea on exertion for several months. Exam reveals jugular venous distension and rales throughout both lung fields. X-ray of the chest demonstrates cardiomegaly. Echocardiogram shows four-chamber dilation with severely reduced LV function. What chemotherapeutic agent might the patient have received?**

Doxorubicin, which can present with cardiomyopathy even years after its initial administration.

○ **Is preoperative cardiac testing recommended for patients who have received doxorubicin (Adriamycin)?**

Female gender, age at treatment (younger is worse), cumulative dose, thorax radiation, and more time since treatment are risk factors for myocardial dysfunction after doxorubicin. These factors, and the type of surgery, must be taken into account when deciding whether to perform cardiac testing before anesthesia.

○ **What are the principal toxicities of cyclophosphamide?**

Plasma cholinesterase inhibition and hemorrhagic cystitis.

○ **Discuss the extrapyramidal effects of antiemetics used in anesthesiology practice.**

The antiemetics associated with the extrapyramidal side effects are phenothiazines such as chlorpromazine. Promotility agent metoclopramide is also known to cause the same. The mechanism of action for antiemesis of both groups of drugs is by dopamine antagonism in the dopaminergic receptors in the CNS, especially the chemoreceptor trigger zone (CTZ). This is also the reason for the side effects. The extrapyramidal side effects include tardive dyskinesia (abnormal involuntary movements that may affect the tongue, facial and neck muscles, extremities, and sometimes muscles involved in breathing and swallowing) caused by chronic phenothiazine administration. The other effects are acute dystonias, opisthotonus, oculogyric crisis, and muscle cramping and rigidity. Very rarely laryngospasm has been seen causing sudden respiratory distress. Akathisia, a feeling of unease and restlessness in the lower extremities, is also seen.

○ **What is the treatment of extrapyramidal drug effects?**

Most of the acute extrapyramidal reactions respond very well to diphenhydramine 25–50 mg IV. If severe life-threatening effects occur, then complete life support measures are required.

○ **How would you manage an overdose of carbamazepine?**

Carbamazepine toxicity is marked by ataxia, drowsiness, slurred speech, seizures, and nonspecific GI symptoms. Physical exam may reveal bullous skin formations, mydriasis, tachycardia, hypotension, respiratory depression, and CNS depression progressing ultimately to coma. A CBC will show pancytopenia. Therapy involves the repeated use of activated charcoal (1 g/kg) and is mostly supportive: IV fluids, airway management, and benzodiazepines for seizure control.

○ **Describe phenytoin and its drug interactions.**

Phenytoin is a hydantoin derivative that is used to treat partial and generalized seizures. It is also used to treat ventricular dysrhythmias and trigeminal neuralgia.

The drug is 90–93% protein bound in the plasma and is a potent enzyme inducer. The oxidative metabolism of many lipid-soluble drugs, including carbamazepine, valproic acid, ethosuximide, anticoagulants, and corticosteroids, may be increased.

Chronic therapy with phenytoin leads to resistance to neuromuscular-blocking drugs. The resistance appears to result from a pharmacodynamic mechanism. Upregulation of receptors has also been suggested.

Phenytoin increases defluorination of isoflurane but enzyme induction has not produced serum F concentrations of clinical significance.

Sinus node activity may be depressed in patients treated with phenytoin. As some volatile anesthetics also depress the sinoatrial node, coadministration of phenytoin during general anesthesia should be carried out with caution.

○ **Describe the pharmacology of mannitol.**

Mannitol ($C_6H_{14}O_6$) is an alcohol and a sugar (polyol) available as a sterile, nonpyrogenic solution for intravenous injection only. It is a vasodilator and obligatory osmotic diuretic available in concentrations of 5–20%. The 5% concentration has 5 g/100 mL, 274 mosm/L and is pH adjusted to 6.3 (4.5–7). Dose: 0.25–1.5 g/kg IV slow over 10 minutes. $T_{1/2}$ elimination is about 30–60 minutes. It is used mainly to reduce intracranial pressure and to treat patients with oliguric renal failure. Nonosmotic actions include decrease in blood viscosity, decrease in SVR, mild positive inotropic effect on the heart, and free radical scavenger. Side effects include variable effects on blood pressure, acute heart failure in patients with impaired renal function, rebound phenomena with unexpected rise in ICP, hypovolemia, electrolyte disturbances, and plasma hyperosmolarity.

○ **What are the toxic effects of metformin?**

Lactic acidosis is the most serious side effect. This is caused by binding to mitochondrial membranes and reducing intracellular concentration of ATP, hence anaerobic glucose metabolism and accumulation of lactate. Other side effects include anorexia, nausea, and diarrhea.

○ **Should metformin be discontinued prior to elective surgery?**

Most clinicians discontinue metformin the day before surgery and restart it when the patient's renal function is stable. Older textbooks state that metformin needs to be discontinued several days before surgery, as metformin may cause metabolic acidosis in patients with hypovolemia or renal insufficiency.

A recent Cochrane meta-analysis of 37,000 patient-years showed no increase in lactic acidosis with metformin use [Salpeter et al., 2006. See reference on page 524]. However, many of the these studies excluded patients with chronic renal insufficiency, liver function abnormalities, congestive heart failure, peripheral vascular disease, pulmonary disease, or age greater than 65. Therefore, these conditions continue to be relative contraindications to proceeding to surgery without discontinuation of metformin therapy.

○ **What is the concern if a patient taking metformin receives contrast dye?**

Metformin is eliminated via renal metabolism. Since contrast media may temporarily decrease renal function, the blood concentration of metformin may rise to levels high enough to cause significant lactic acidosis. Patients who are scheduled to receive contrast media should therefore temporarily discontinue the use of metformin prior to the study.

○ **What are the perioperative implications of herbal medicine preparations?**

Although herbal supplements have pharmaceutical properties and may interact with anesthetic drugs, >50% of patients neglect to mention them during their preoperative interview [Jacqueline et al., 2001. See reference on page 524]. The misconception that herbal drugs are not as potent as pharmaceutical drugs may lead to unexpected complications during anesthesia. The ASA recommends that herbal supplements should be discontinued 2–3 weeks prior to surgery. The following herbs are known to have significant side effects:

- *Echinacea*, used for its supposed immunostimulation properties, may antagonize the immunosuppressive actions of corticosteroids and cyclosporine. It also inhibits the hepatic cytochrome P-450 system.
- *Ephedra*, used to promote weight loss and increase energy, may result in hypertension and cardiac arrhythmias. Prolonged use depletes peripheral catecholamine stores and may cause profound hypotension and bradycardia that is resistant to ephedrine.
- *Valerian*, used as a sedative, potentiates the effects of sedatives that act at the GABA receptor (e.g., midazolam).
- *St. John's wort*, used to manage depression, increases the metabolism of drugs that rely on the cytochrome P-450 system.

○ **What are the perioperative effects of garlic?**

Garlic has the potential to modify the risk of developing atherosclerosis by reducing blood pressure and thrombus formation and lowering serum lipid and cholesterol levels. However, garlic inhibits platelet aggregation in a dose-dependent fashion and may augment the effects of warfarin, heparin, NSAIDs, and aspirin, resulting in abnormal bleeding.

○ **What other herbal supplement may possess anticoagulation effects?**

Ginseng, which is used as an aphrodisiac, has been reported to significantly increase INR. In addition, it has been suggested that ginseng exerts an irreversible antiplatelet activity similar to aspirin.

Key Terms

ACE inhibitors: anesthetic hypotension
ACE inhibitors: MI survival
Acetaminophen toxicity
Acetazolamide: mechanism of action
Amiloride: Physiological effects/electrolyte effects
Amiodarone: hemodynamic effect/side effects
Arrhythmias: digitalis toxicity
Arterial blood gases (ABG): salicylate toxicity
Aspirin toxicity: treatment
Carbamazepine toxicity
Chemotherapeutic agents: toxicity
Cyanide toxicity
Cyclophosphamide: anesthetic implications
Dexmedetomidine: cardiorespiratory effects
Digitalis toxicity: perioperative causes/treatment
Doxorubicin: complications/toxicity/anesthetic implications
Drug efficacy versus potency
Extrapyramidal drug effects: treatment
Fenoldopam: pharmacology
Fenoldopam: renal effects

Furosemide: effects
Furosemide: prolonged metabolic effect
Herbal medications: anticoagulation effects
Herbal medicine: perioperative implications
Herbals: garlic
Hydrochlorothiazide: blood chemistry effect
Hydrochlorothiazide: mechanism of action
Hyperkalemia with ACE inhibitors
Mannitol: metabolic side effects
Metformin: contrast dye interaction
Milrinone: cardiovascular effects
Milrinone: pharmacology
Nicardipine: pharmacology
Nitroprusside toxicity: blood chemistry/signs
Pharmacology of mannitol
Phenytoin: drug interactions
Toxicity of nitroglycerine
Vasoactive drug: mechanism
Vasodilators: pharmacodynamics
Vasodilators: renal blood flow

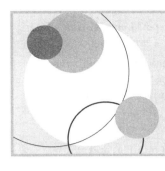

Critical Care Medicine

Any idiot can face a crisis – it's day to day living that wears you out.
Anton Chekhov

○ **Name the statistically significant independent risk factors for stress ulceration in critically ill patients.**

Coagulopathy (platelets <50,000, INR >1.5, or aPTT >2 × normal) and prolonged (>48 hours) mechanical ventilation. These are absolute indications for gastrointestinal (GI) prophylaxis. All other risk factors are relative, although patients with multiple risk factors (e.g., second- or third-degree burns over 20% of body surface area [BSA], renal failure, severe head injury) may also be considered at high risk. Note that there is a clear association between GI prophylaxis and *Clostridium difficile* infection, and a possible association between GI prophylaxis and pneumonia; thus, these pharmacologic agents should be used judiciously.

○ **Describe the cardiovascular changes associated with sepsis?**

Clinical presentation of sepsis: hypotension with adequate fluid resuscitation and impaired end-organ perfusion. Hallmarks include a high cardiac output and high mixed or central venous oxygen saturation (SvO_2 or $ScvO_2$). Cardiovascular changes include low systemic vascular resistance (SVR), high pulmonary vascular resistance (PVR), leaky capillaries, and a potential decrease in myocardial contractility with a reduction in oxygen extraction.

○ **What are the two most commonly cited underlying pathophysiologic mechanisms of sepsis at the cellular/subcellular level?**

Microcirculatory derangements (leading to shunting of oxygenated blood) and inability of mitochondria to utilize oxygen provided to them, both of which can lead to an elevated $ScvO_2$ or SvO_2.

○ **Name some of the stress response mediators thought to be implicated in septic shock?**

TNF-α (gram-negative infections), IL-1 and IL-6 (gram-negative infections), and IL-8 (gram-positive infections).

○ **Which interventions have been shown, by prospective, randomized controlled trials, to improve outcomes in sepsis?**

Goal-directed therapy initiated within 6 hours (Goals: mean arterial pressure >65 mm Hg, central venous pressure ≥8 mm Hg, urine output 0.5 mL/kg/h, ±central venous oxygen saturation [$ScvO_2$] ≥70%), early (<24 hours) enteral nutrition, and administration of activated protein C (if APACHE score 25 or two or more organs failing). Note that empiric, broad-spectrum coverage is based on large, retrospective data showing that inappropriate initial coverage is highly correlated with poor outcomes. Based on these data a prospective study would not be ethical. Adrenocortical axis testing (cortisol stimulation with ACTH) with steroid replacement in nonresponders and strict glucose control are controversial [Jones et al., 2001. See reference on page 524].

151

○ **In the patient with septic shock following adequate fluid resuscitation and persistent hypotension, which vasopressor should be used?**

Goal: attempt to normalize SVR and in doing so reestablish normal delivery of oxygen to tissues. Norepinephrine and/or dopamine are the first-line drugs, with vasopressin second line according to the Surviving Sepsis Guidelines (2008). If patients have a diminished cardiac output, then dobutamine should be considered to augment contractility.

○ **A patient presents in septic shock, CVP <8 mm Hg, mean arterial pressure <60 mm Hg, and SvO_2 = 70%. Would you fluid resuscitate this patient or start pressors?**

Pressors are drugs that make the blood pressure go up. There are five components of blood pressure: preload, contractility, afterload, rate, and rhythm. Resuscitation should start with oxygenation SpO_2 >95%, pH >7.3 and <7.5, and crystalloid or colloid infusion to CVP 8–12 mm Hg. Drug causing profound alpha constriction should be avoided if systolic pressure >90 mm Hg as renal blood flow increases to that point, and then decreases. If the SvO_2 is <70%, transfuse with packed RBC to an Hct >30% and then start inotropes to maintain the SvO_2 >70%.

○ **What strategies can be employed to lower the incidence of ventilator-associated pneumonia (VAP)?**

Avoid intubation altogether (use continuous positive airway pressure [CPAP] instead, when possible); use an endotracheal tube equipped with a supraglottic suctioning device (recommended by the CDC, 2008); most authors recommend maintaining the head of the bed at 45°, especially when feeding; unresolved issues include selective gut decontamination, using antiseptic impregnated endotracheal tubes, intensive glycemic control, and avoidance of H_2 antagonist or proton pump inhibitors for patients who are not at high risk for developing GI bleeding.

○ **What is the frequency of sinusitis during mechanical ventilation?**

Sinusitis is most common in patients with nasotracheal intubation (2–27%), facial trauma, and nasal tube feeding.

○ **What are the characteristic features of adult respiratory distress syndrome (ARDS)?**

Acute ARDS is characterized by rapid onset of respiratory failure with arterial hypoxemia resistant to supplemental O_2. Diffuse infiltrates appear on the chest x-ray, and may appear before symptoms develop. Pulmonary capillary wedge pressure is usually normal (<18 mm Hg).

○ **What is the management of ARDS?**

Mechanical ventilation may be required and FiO_2 adjusted to obtain PaO_2 between 60 and 80 mm Hg. Application of PEEP may help to maintain FiO_2 <0.5 to avoid oxygen toxicity from prolonged use.

Underlying cause of ARDS should be sought, and sepsis is associated with the highest risk of progression to ARDS.

○ **What are the effects of PEEP?**

Pulmonary effects: improved oxygenation through redistribution of extravascular water and increased FRC through distention and recruitment of alveoli, and decreased shunt.

Cardiovascular effects: diminished cardiac output due to decreased venous return to right heart, right ventricular dysfunction, and alterations in left ventricular distensibility.

○ **What is optimal PEEP in ARDS?**

PEEP level that provides maximum oxygen delivery and lowest dead space ventilation. Clinically this is the PEEP level that will result in adequate perfusion and a PaO_2 of 60 mm Hg or greater, with an adequate hemoglobin (Hb) level at an FiO_2 of less than 50%.

○ **Mention two circumstances where PEEP is indicated in adult patients.**

1. If the PaO_2 remains below 60 mm Hg with an FiO_2 of 60%
2. If the shunt estimation is greater than 25%

○ **What are the major causes of ARDS?**

Sepsis, multisystem organ failure, shock, aspiration, trauma, infection, embolism, inhalation of toxic gases, drug overdose, poisons, and numerous miscellaneous causes.

○ **Name five different modes of mechanical ventilation.**

1. *Controlled mechanical ventilation (CMV)*: fixed tidal volume (TV) and a fixed rate.
2. *Assist–control ventilation (ACV)*: Assist/control is essentially the same as CMV except that the patient may, if desired, trigger the set-volume machine breaths at a more rapid rate. In other words, the machine senses the patient's inspiratory effort and delivers a set TV when inspiratory effort is made. If no inspiratory effort is made, the ventilator functions as in control mode. Common problem associated with ACV is respiratory alkalosis in patients breathing at high respiratory rates.

   ACV or CMV could be volume controlled (VCV) or pressure controlled (PCV).
3. *Intermittent mandatory ventilation (IMV)*: A fixed TV and rate are delivered. In addition to this mandatory ventilation, the patient is able to take spontaneous breaths. The TV and rate of the spontaneous breaths is determined by the patient's respiratory efforts. In SIMV mode, the machine creates timing windows around the scheduled mandatory breaths in order to synchronize each machine's breath with the patient's inspiratory effort, which might vary the machine cycle times slightly. If no inspiratory effort is detected within the time window, the machine delivers a mandatory breath at the scheduled time.
4. *Pressure support ventilation*: Maintains a predetermined positive pressure throughout inspiration. This helps overcome increased resistance from the mechanical components of the breathing system (ETT, tubing, etc.). It is often combined with IMV. In this mode provider sets the trigger sensitivity and the inspiratory pressure. The patient determines the respiratory rate, and the TV varies according to the inspiratory gas flow, lung mechanics, and patient's own respiratory effort.
5. *Inverse ratio ventilation*: This is ventilation in which the inspiratory time is greater than the expiratory time, the opposite of normal breathing.

○ **How is TV determined on a ventilator?**

By the ventilator mode: in volume preset modes the TV is selected; in pressure preset modes the set pressure limit determines the end of each inspiration and TV.

○ **Is the use of PCV necessary in ARDS?**

Damage to lung parenchyma can occur from overdistension due to volutrauma or barotrauma. TVs of 6 mL/kg and plateau pressures <30 cm H_2O are ideal and can be achieved through volume- or pressure-limited mechanical ventilation. Note that VCV was used in the ARDSNet trial [The acute respiratory distress syndrome Net work, 2000. See reference on page 524] demonstrating improved survival with 6 mL/kg versus 12 mL/kg TVs.

○   **Compare the pressure waveforms of volume- and pressure-controlled ventilatory modes.**

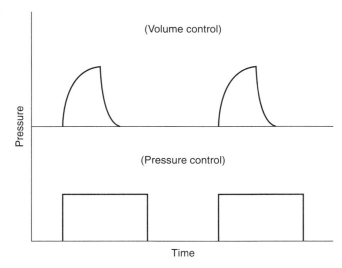

It has been shown that especially in obese patients PCV could provide sufficient minute ventilation and improve oxygenation while using lower plateau pressure than VCV.

○   **What is the proposed mechanism for improved oxygenation with prone position mechanical ventilation in ARDS?**

Prone position may be a rational approach for a patient whose hypoxemia appears life-threatening [Briccard, 2003. See reference on page 524].

Several mechanisms proposed for improved oxygenation:

1.   Increased end-expiratory lung volumes (FRC).

2.   Better V/Q matching – reduction in ventilation/perfusion heterogeneity with improvement in ventilation and reduction in shunt.

3.   Recruitment of collapsed alveolar units.

4.   Mobilization of secretions.

○   **What are the distinguishing features of pressure support ventilation?**

Augments every breath during spontaneous breathing. Practically, a breath is initiated by the patient's respiratory effort and supported with rapid flow until a preset pressure is reached. Inspiration then ceases and the exhalation valve is opened allowing expiration. Advantages over IMV include increased TV and decreased work of breathing. Methods of setting pressure include: (a) maximum inspiratory pressure (pressure = [maximum inspiratory pressure]/3) and (b) proximal airway pressure (pressure = [peak pressure] – [plateau pressure]).

○   **What triggers the ventilator to deliver a breath in pressure support ventilation?**

Patient inspiratory effort. The ventilator delivers the gas flow required to maintain a selected positive pressure during inspiration.

○ **What are the symptoms of carbon monoxide (CO) poisoning?**

Symptoms of CO toxicity as a function of the blood carboxyhemoglobin (COHb) level:

Blood COHb Level (%)	Symptoms
<15–20	Headache, dizziness, and occasional confusion
20–40	Nausea, vomiting, disorientation, and visual impairment
40–60	Agitation, combativeness, hallucination, coma, and shock
>60	Death

Tachypnea is absent, because the ***carotid bodies are sensitive to the arterial O_2 tension and not to the O_2 content***.

The classical cherry red color of the blood is also absent in most patients because it occurs only at COHb concentrations above 40%, and it may also be obscured by coexistent hypoxia and cyanosis.

○ **What are the major effects of CO on oxygen delivery?**

1. Decreased oxygen delivery as Hb has a 200-fold higher affinity for CO than for O_2. Example: at a PCO of 0.16 mm Hg, 75% Hb is combined with CO as COHb, that is, small amount of CO can tie up a large proportion of Hb in blood.

2. Left shift of the Hb–O_2 dissociation curve that results in a decreased ability to unload O_2 at the cellular level.

Thus, it reduces:

1. Oxyhemoglobin concentration.

2. Blood oxygen content.

3. Oxygen-carrying capacity.

And impairs the release of oxygen to tissues.

Initially, it was thought that these were the primary mechanisms for injury in CO poisoning. More recently, it has been suggested that CO binding to myoglobin, cytochrome aa3 (cytochrome c oxidase), and mitochondrial cytochrome oxidase, and brain lipid peroxidation, may also contribute to CO toxicity (Miller, 2009).

○ **What is the treatment of CO poisoning in pregnancy?**

In pregnant patients, the fetal COHb may be higher than the maternal level.

Treatment with hyperbaric O_2 at 2–3 atm for 1 hour may be needed to reduce fetal and maternal COHb levels rapidly.

However, even a high inspired O_2 (FiO_2) not only improves oxygenation but also promotes elimination of CO.

FiO_2 of 1.0 decreases blood half-life of COHb from 4 hours seen in room air to <1 hour.

○ **What is the effect of carboxyhemoglobin (COHb) on ABG analysis and pulse oximeter reading?**

HbCO affects the O_2 saturation (true measured SaO_2 value) and O_2 content, but not PaO_2. The pH may be normal (initially). Hypoxemia can be missed if the O_2 saturation is calculated in the laboratory based on the PaO_2 and standard O_2 dissociation curve. Pulse oximeters are not reliable. The oxygen saturation is read as *too high* as it does not differentiate Hb bound to CO from Hb bound to oxygen; the machine reports oxygen saturation as the sum of both values. Blood co-oximeters use four wavelengths of light to separate out oxyhemoglobin from reduced Hb, metHb, and HbCO, whereas pulse oximeters utilize only two wavelengths of light that do not detect Hbs that cannot bind oxygen.

○ **What laboratory tests will detect CO toxicity in burn patients?**

As compared with the pulse oximeter, the arterial blood gas will show lower oxygen saturation, an anion gap metabolic acidosis, and increased carboxyhemoglobin levels (normal <5%). Co-oximetry is needed to detect CO. Nonsmokers should have carboxyhemoglobin levels of 1–3% and smokers 4–9%. Patients are generally asymptomatic if carboxyhemoglobin levels are less than 10%, with overt signs developing at ~15%.

○ **Describe the acute physiologic changes seen in burn patients.**

Massive intravascular fluid loss with fluid replacement calculated using the Parkland formula, which is 4 mL/kg for each percent of BSA burned, half in the first 8 hours *after the burn* (not from admission to your ICU) and the other half over the next 16 hours.

Increased risk of infection compared with normal ICU patients.

A systemic inflammatory response, which can manifest with fever >39°C, hyperglycemia, disorientation, and ileus. A hypermetabolic state starts 24–36 hours after injury, which may double the patient's normal energy expenditure. Proliferation of extrajunctional acetylcholine receptors, risk of hyperkalemia with succinylcholine and an increased need for nondepolarizing muscle relaxants, limited IV access, exaggerated heat loss, and hemodynamic instability are challenges for the anesthesiologist.

○ **How long should you wait before starting total parenteral nutrition (TPN) in the critically ill patient?**

At least 8 days, according to the Early Parenteral Nutrition Completing Enteral Nutrition in Adult Critically Ill Patients Study [EPaNIC, 2011; Casaer et al., 2011. See reference on page 524], a prospective, randomized controlled, parallel-group, multicenter investigator-initiated trial in 4,640 patients that showed waiting 8 days to start TPN (as opposed to 48 hours) shortened ICU stay and lowered infection rates. This study compares early (European guideline) with late (American/Canadian guideline) initiation of parenteral nutrition when enteral nutrition fails to reach a caloric target.

○ **T/F: A recognized complication of TPN is hypophosphatemia.**

True. Hypophosphatemia (defined as phosphate <2.5 mg/dL) is reported in 17–28% of critically ill patients. It can result from increased renal excretion of phosphate, decreased absorption by the GI tract, or, most commonly, an increase in intracellular movement of phosphate. Glucose loading, as occurs with administration of TPN, results in intracellular glucose movement. As TPN is instituted, glucose transport and oxidative phosphorylation acutely increase, resulting in increased demand for intracellular phosphate to support the formation of ATP. Hypophosphatemia can lead to impaired myocardial contractility and cardiovascular collapse, as well as respiratory failure, rhabdomyolysis, seizures, delirium, and death.

○ **Why do some patients on TPN have an increased minute ventilation?**

The respiratory quotient (RQ) of a nutritional substance is defined as RQ = (CO_2 eliminated)/(O_2 consumed). The RQ of glucose is 1.0, whereas the RQ of proteins is 0.8–0.9, and the RQ of fats is ~0.7. Overfeeding patients or providing too much carbohydrate causes an increase in carbon dioxide production. The patient compensates by increasing his or her respiratory rate in order to breathe off the excess CO_2.

○ **What are the potential complications of TPN?**

Catheter sepsis can occur as a primary or secondary infection. Metabolic complications arise from too much or too little energy source and electrolyte abnormalities. These include hyperglycemia, nonketotic hyperosmolar coma, hypoglycemia, prerenal azotemia, hypercarbia, hypertriglyceridemia, fatty acid deficiency, metabolic acidosis, hypophosphatemia, hypomagnesium/hypermagnesium, hypokalemia/hyperkalemia, hypocalcemia/hypercalcemia, and alteration in liver function tests.

○ **How should a patient on TPN scheduled for surgery be managed perioperatively?**

The patient should be changed from TPN to 10% dextrose at the same rate to maintain glucose homeostasis. This prevents rebound hypoglycemia.

Serial accuchecks for serum glucose should be performed every hour to avoid hypoglycemia/hyperglycemia.

○ **During prolonged surgery, what laboratory tests should be monitored when a patient is receiving TPN?**

Plasma glucose, potassium, and pH.

○ **Discuss the anesthetic management of a patient with DNR order.**

When a patient with a DNR order undergoes anesthesia or conscious sedation, the DNR order needs to be reconsidered. An informed patient's (or patient's health care proxy) decision to suspend a DNR order (meaning proceed with full code during surgery) for a procedure should be respected.

After the patient has recovered from anesthesia and leaves the recovery room, one should ensure that reinstitution of the DNR order occurs.

Electronic medical records can help alert physicians about a patient's DNR order before surgery and require them to reconsider this order at specified times, such as at a preoperative anesthesia visit, on transfer from the postoperative recovery room, and every few days thereafter while in the intensive care unit.

○ **What are the predisposing factors and clinical manifestations of critical illness myoneuropathy?**

Critical illness myopathy (CIM)/polyneuropathy (CIP), either singly or in combination, is usually manifested as severe weakness with respiratory failure or difficulty with weaning from the ventilator in critically ill patients in the ICU with sepsis or multiorgan failure. Flaccid weakness of the extremities, often severe, and loss of tendon reflexes are associated findings. The exact etiology of CIP and CIM remains to be determined. Physical therapy is the only effective rehabilitation therapy available.

Multiorgan failure and sepsis predispose to the neuropathy. Other serious illnesses such as pneumonia, severe asthma, liver/lung transplantation, and use of certain drugs predispose to myopathy. These drugs include high-dose corticosteroids and nondepolarizing neuromuscular blocking agents. Prevention of CIP and CIM involves early and effective treatment of sepsis, tight glycemic control, and cautious use of muscle relaxants and corticosteroids on the ICU [Latronico et al., 2005. See reference on page 524].

○ **What are the clinical features and treatment of *Clostridium tetani* infection?**

Tetanus is caused by *C. tetani* infection at a laceration or break in the skin. It can also occur as a complication of burns, puerperal infections, umbilical stumps (tetanus neonatorum), and surgical site infection. Tetanus is caused by tetanospasmin (exotoxin). It is manifested mostly by neuromuscular dysfunction. It starts with tonic spasms of the skeletal muscles and is followed by paroxysmal contractions. The muscle stiffness initially involves the jaw (lockjaw) and neck and later becomes generalized.

Treatment goals include interrupting the production of toxin, neutralizing the unbound toxin, controlling muscle spasms (sedation, muscle relaxants, and ventilator support), managing dysautonomia, and appropriate supportive management.

Specific therapy includes IM tetanus immunoglobulin to neutralize circulating toxin before it binds to neuronal cell membranes.

The disease can be prevented by immunization with tetanus toxoid and appropriate wound care.

Key Terms

Acute septic shock
ARDS: diagnosis
ARDS: optimal tidal volume
ARDS: prone position mechanism
Brain death: diagnosis criteria
Burns: carbon monoxide poisoning
Carbon monoxide poisoning: clinical features/
    management/mechanism/treatment
Carboxyhemoglobin effect on ABG
Clostridium tetani infection
Critical illness myoneuropathy
DNR and anesthesia
Hyperalimentation: perioperative management/anesthetic
    implications
Hyperbaric O_2 therapy/indication
Hypoxemia: ventilator management
Low tidal volume ventilation: protective effect
Lung-protective ventilation: pressure goal
Measurement of carbon monoxide in burn victims
Mechanism of carbon monoxide toxicity

Mode of ventilation: ventilatory pattern
PEEP effect on PAOP
PEEP: LV effect
Pressure-limited ventilation in ARDS
Pressure support ventilation: triggering
Pressure versus volume ventilation: ICU
Septic shock: hypotension treatment
Septic shock: stress response mediators
Septic shock: vasopressin therapy
Total parenteral nutrition (TPN) discontinuation:
    complications
TPN: metabolic effects
TPN: phosphorous deficiency
TPN: respiratory quotient
Ventilator-associated pneumonia management
Ventilator: low tidal volume
Ventilator management: PEEP indications
Ventilators and pulmonary compliance
Ventilatory management: acute respiratory disease
Ventilatory modes: pressure waveform

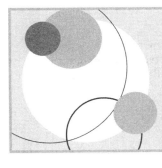

Electrical and Fire Safety in the Operating Room

If you can't explain it simply, you don't understand it well enough.
Albert Einstein

○ **What is the potential, in volts, between the ground wire in the OR and the "hot" wire?**

Electricity from a main power source is delivered to the OR through an isolation transformer. No wires are grounded; hence, there is no potential created that would allow flow of current. If a wire does become grounded, then a potential of 117 V is created, and current will flow to ground depending on the resistance to completing a circuit.

○ **What is an isolation transformer?**

An isolation transformer is required to provide ungrounded power. This device uses electromagnetic induction, and converts the grounded power on the primary side to an ungrounded power system on the secondary side of the transformer.

○ **What is the purpose of using an isolation transformer in the electrical supply to the operating room?**

The isolation transformer converts the grounded electrical power from the utility company into ungrounded power in the OR. This decreases the risk of shock because there is no electrical potential between the wire and ground, only between the two wires. Thus, to receive a shock from an ungrounded power supply, a person must contact two wires. To receive a shock from a grounded system, however, a person must merely be in contact with ground and also touch the "hot" wire.

○ **Most operating rooms have ungrounded electrical power supply. Why?**

Ungrounded power provides an extra measure of safety from gross electric shock (macroshock).

○ **In an operating room with ungrounded power, what is the function of the equipment ground wire?**

All equipment plugged in to the isolated power system has an equipment ground wire that is attached to the case of the instrument.

Equipment ground wire serves three functions:

1. Low-resistance path for fault current and thereby reduces the risk of macroshock
2. Dissipates leakage currents that are potentially harmful to the electrically susceptible patients
3. Provides information to line isolation monitor (LIM) on the status of the ungrounded power system

○ **What is the significance of the LIM sounding its alarm?**

The LIM measures the potential for current flow from the isolated operating room power supply to ground. It determines the amount of current that could flow if a second short circuit should develop and sounds the alarm if this current exceeds 2 or 5 mA (third-generation LIM set to alarm at 5 mA), depending on the particular monitor used.

○ **What determines the difference between microshock and macroshock?**

Macroshock is 60-Hz current in excess of 1 mA (threshold of perception), which is applied to tissue at locations remote from the heart, whereas microshock refers to the application of small currents (100 μA, which will induce ventricular fibrillation) directly to the heart.

○ **Why is the LIM more useful for preventing macroshock than microshock?**

Macroshock is the current delivered to the body surface and current up to 5 mA is accepted as harmless. The LIM alarms when there is potential for current flow of 2 or 5 mA. Microshock (current delivered directly to the heart) can cause ventricular fibrillation with current as low as 0.1 mA, well below the alarm point of an LIM.

○ **Which patients are susceptible to microshock hazards?**

Any patient having a low-resistance pathway to the heart is at risk for microshock (pacing wire, saline-filled central venous catheter, or pulmonary artery catheter).

Currents as low as 100 μA can cause ventricular fibrillation. The source for such tiny currents can be the "leakage current" associated with any AC-powered device. Recommended maximum allowable 60-Hz leakage current is 10 μA.

○ **How can you protect patients from microshock hazard?**

Protection from microshock is achieved by:

1. Intact equipment ground wire – prevent microshock by providing a low-impedance path in which the majority of leakage current can flow.

2. Electrically isolate all direct patient connections from the power supply in the patient monitor by an isolation transformer in the main unit.

Other things an anesthesiologist can do to reduce the incidence of microshock include:

- Never simultaneously touch an electrical device and a saline-filled central line or external pacing wire.
- Whenever handling a central line, insulate oneself by wearing gloves.
- Never let any external current source (e.g., nerve stimulator) come in contact with the intracardiac catheter or wires.

○ **How does a ground fault circuit interrupter (GFCI) prevent macroshock?**

GFCI prevents individuals from receiving macroshock in a grounded power system. It interrupts the power when it detects a difference (5 mA) in the current flowing in hot and neutral wires due to short circuit.

○ **Compare and contrast LIM with GFCI.**

Both monitor macroshock hazard due to faulty equipment leakage current (short circuits).

LIM continuously monitors leakage current (5 mA) in an ungrounded system, and alarms, but the equipment can still be used. GFCI, which is used in a grounded power system, interrupts the power without warning if leakage current of more than 5 mA is detected; defective equipment could no longer be used.

○   **What is the difference between monopolar and bipolar electrosurgery?**

Electrosurgery is the standard method of "power" coagulating or cutting body tissue using radio-frequency electrical current. In both techniques, electrical current passes from an active electrode to heat or burn tissue, and then through body tissue to a return inactive electrode. In the monopolar technique, the return electrode is a grounding pad placed on the patient's buttock or thigh, as far away from the heart as possible. The bipolar technique uses two closely spaced electrodes, often the two jaws of a surgical instrument (e.g., forceps) with no return plate.

○   **Is it possible to cause ventricular fibrillation with electrocautery?**

No.

Ventricular fibrillation is prevented by the use of alternating current of ultrahigh frequency (0.5–3 million Hz, radio-frequency range) compared with line power (50–60 Hz). These high-frequency currents can pass directly across the precordium without exciting contractile cells or causing ventricular fibrillation due to low tissue penetration.

○   **What causes unintentional burns at the site of the ESU return plate or alternate return pathway?**

A properly applied ESU return plate does not cause burns because the surface area of the return plate over which the current diffuses is large (low current density) and the resistance to flow is low resulting in insignificant heating. If the ESU return plate is improperly applied or the cord connecting the return plate to the ESU is damaged, ESU will seek alternate return pathways. Anything attached to the patient, such as ECG leads or temperature probe, can provide this alternate pathway. The current density at these alternate sites will be considerably higher than that of the ESU return plate because its surface area is much smaller, potentially resulting in serious burns.

○   **Is there a fire hazard when chlorhexidine with alcohol is used for skin preparation prior to surgery utilizing ESU?**

Yes.

One must wait 3 minutes for dry time after using chlorhexidine (CHG) as a prep. Do not drape the patient until this 3-minute dry time has occurred. Time it! CHG has alcohol (usually 70%) as an ingredient, making it extremely flammable.

Key Terms

Line isolation monitor (LIM) function
Protection from microshock

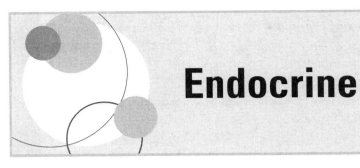

Endocrine

Estimated amount of glucose used by an adult human brain each day, expressed in M & Ms: 250
Harper's Index, October 1989

○ **What is the hormonal stress response to surgery?**

1. Autonomic response: catecholamines, insulin, and glucagon.
2. Hypothalamic–pituitary: cortisol, thyroxine, arginine vasopressin, growth hormone, ACTH, angiotensin, aldosterone, and renin–angiotensin.
3. Local tissue, vascular endothelial response: cytokines and other mediators.

○ **What happens to serum concentrations of antidiuretic hormone (ADH) and aldosterone after surgery?**

ADH, aldosterone, renin, and angiotensin increase resulting in sodium and water retention and a secondary expansion of the extracellular space.

○ **Where is aldosterone produced and what is its stimulus for secretion?**

Aldosterone is a mineralocorticoid secreted from the zona glomerulosa of the adrenal gland. Its secretion is stimulated by pituitary ACTH, angiotensin II (renin–angiotensin system), and increased serum potassium concentration. Hypovolemia, hypotension, congestive heart failure, and surgery also increase aldosterone levels.

○ **Where does aldosterone exert its primary effect and what is this effect?**

Aldosterone secretion enhances sodium reabsorption in the distal nephron of the kidney in exchange for potassium and hydrogen ions. The net effect is fluid retention and expansion of the extracellular fluid space, with a reduction in serum potassium concentration and metabolic alkalosis.

○ **What is the mechanism of hyperkalemia with the use of ACE inhibitors?**

Since aldosterone is responsible for the excretion of potassium, hyperkalemia is a potential complication of the use of angiotensin-converting enzyme inhibitors, angiotensin receptor blockers, aldosterone receptor antagonists, and direct renin inhibitors. Changes in potassium tend to be small (0.1–0.3 mmol) and may not be clinically significant.

○ **What are the hormones that regulate electrolyte homeostasis?**

Sodium homeostasis is regulated by the effects of ADH, aldosterone, and the natriuretic peptides (ANP, brain natriuretic peptide [BNP], and C-type natriuretic peptides).

Potassium is affected by aldosterone, epinephrine, and insulin.

Calcium levels are regulated by parathyroid hormone (PTH) and vitamin D. The latter two hormones also have minor effects on the regulation of magnesium levels.

○ **What are the effects of alpha- and beta-adrenergic stimulation on insulin and glucagon secretion?**

Beta islet cells (insulin secreting) have both alpha- and beta-adrenergic receptors. The stimulation of the alpha-receptors inhibits insulin secretion while stimulation of the beta-receptors increases insulin release. The alpha islet cells (glucagon secreting) only have beta-receptors that lead to an increase in glucagon release when stimulated.

○ **What enzymes and organs are involved in the production of angiotensin II from its precursors?**

Renin (from kidneys) converts angiotensinogen (from liver) to angiotensin I. Angiotensin I is then rapidly converted, primarily in the lungs, by angiotensin-converting enzyme to angiotensin II. Kidney, liver, and lungs are involved.

○ **Which has a more potent effect during stress, angiotensin I or II, and what are these effects?**

Angiotensin II, a potent direct vasoconstrictor, potentiates the actions of norepinephrine and increases the secretion of aldosterone, while directly increasing sodium reabsorption in the proximal renal tubules.

○ **Describe the endocrine function of the pituitary gland.**

Pituitary gland consists of anterior and posterior pituitary.

Anterior pituitary secretes six hormones under the control of hypothalamus. The posterior pituitary hormones that are synthesized in the hypothalamus are transported for storage in the gland. These are vasopressin (ADH) and oxytocin.

○ **What are the presenting symptoms of a pituitary adenoma?**

Overproduction of anterior pituitary hormones is most often due to hypersecretion of ACTH (Cushing syndrome). Hypersecretion of other tropic hormones rarely occurs.

The anterior pituitary gland is the only endocrine gland where adenoma leads to destruction by compressing the gland against the bony confines of sella turcica. The features of panhypopituitarism are highly variable since it depends on the rate of growth/destruction and age of the patient.

Acromegaly occurs due to excessive secretion of growth hormone in adults by an adenoma in the anterior pituitary. Presenting symptoms include headache, papilledema (increased intracranial pressure), visual disturbances, as well as symptoms due to excessive growth hormone.

○ **What are the signs/symptoms of hypothyroidism?**

The signs and symptoms of hypothyroidism are nonspecific and difficult to diagnose. These include fatigue, decreased mental acuity, depression, somnolence, cold intolerance, constipation, dry skin, brittle hair, menorrhagia, and weight gain. Physical exam reveals hypothermia, periorbital edema, decreased or absent deep tendon reflexes, sinus bradycardia, and hoarseness. Myxedema coma is characterized by hypoventilation, hypothermia, hypotension, congestive heart failure, hyponatremia, hypoglycemia, obtundation, and adrenal insufficiency. This condition is frequently fatal and often seen in patients with severe long-standing unrecognized hypothyroidism who are subjected to cold exposure, surgery, trauma, infection, or antidepressants.

○ **What happens to the cardiac output in hypothyroidism?**

Cardiac output is decreased due to a reduction in heart rate and stroke volume. In addition, decreased blood volume, baroreceptor reflex dysfunction, and pericardial effusion make the patient susceptible to the cardiodepressant effects of anesthetic agents.

○ **What laboratory findings (excluding abnormal thyroid function tests) are characteristic in hypothyroidism?**

Hyponatremia, hypoglycemia, hypercholesterolemia, and a normochromic normocytic anemia. Chest x-ray may show an enlarged heart secondary to pericardial effusion and the EKG characteristically shows sinus bradycardia, low voltage, and a prolonged QT interval.

○ **What are the CNS manifestations of myxedema?**

Depression, memory loss, ataxia, frank psychosis, and ultimately coma.

○ **How would you treat refractory hypotension in myxedema coma?**

IV thyroid supplement (T3 or T4) and steroid replacement (hydrocortisone 100 mg IV q 8 hours) should be given until the hypothalamic–pituitary–adrenal axis can be evaluated.

○ **What are the clinical signs and symptoms of hyperthyroidism?**

Goiter, tachycardia, anxiety, insomnia, and tremor are seen in over 90% of patients. Heat intolerance, fatigue, weight loss, ocular signs (proptosis), skeletal muscle weakness, alopecia, pretibial myxedema, congestive heart failure, and atrial fibrillation are reported as well.

○ **What are the ocular signs in hyperthyroidism?**

Exophthalmos from an infiltrative process involving the retrobulbar fat and eyelids, lid sag, lid retraction, and periorbital swelling. The extraocular muscles, cornea, and optic nerve are also involved.

○ **What are the associated laboratory findings in hyperthyroidism?**

Hypercalcemia, hypokalemia, hyperglycemia, hypocholesterolemia, mild anemia, thrombocytopenia, lymphocytosis, granulocytopenia, hyperbilirubinemia, and increased alkaline phosphatase.

○ **How does thyroid storm manifest?**

Thyroid storm is an acute exacerbation of hyperthyroidism usually caused by a stress such as surgery or infection. The patients present with hyperthermia, extreme tachycardia with a high cardiac output, peripheral vasodilation, and possibly profound hypotension and altered mental state with severe agitation. Congestive heart failure, dehydration, hyperglycemia, shock, and death also may occur.

Typically, it occurs 6–18 hours postoperatively.

○　**How is thyroid storm different from thyrotoxicosis?**

Thyroid storm is a severe and life-threatening exacerbation of thyrotoxicosis usually precipitated by a nonthyroidal illness such as an infection, surgery, withdrawal of iodine therapy, diabetic ketoacidosis, vigorous palpation of the thyroid gland, and radioactive iodine therapy.

○　**What is the differential diagnosis of thyroid storm?**

Differential diagnosis includes other hypermetabolic states: sepsis, pheochromocytoma, cocaine/amphetamine overdose, a neuroleptic malignant syndrome in those receiving antipsychotic medications, and malignant hyperthermia (MH).

○　**Are thyroid function tests necessary prior to the initiation of treatment for thyroid storm?**

No. This is a medical emergency that requires immediate and aggressive management. Presumptive diagnosis is made on the basis of history and clinical findings.

○　**What is the initial treatment of thyroid storm?**

First, treat life-threatening changes in vital signs. Then, make the diagnosis, correct precipitating causes, and treat high circulating levels of thyroid hormone and resulting effects with β-blockers (maintain heart rate <90 beats/min), IV fluids for volume replacement, cooling and acetaminophen (antipyretic), and antithyroid drugs: propylthiouracil via nasogastric tube (PTU 600–1,000 mg, followed by 200–400 mg q 8 hourly), followed 1 hour later by an iodide preparation.

Hydrocortisone (100–200 mg q 8 hourly) has been reported to increase survival. The duration of storm averages 3 days. Supportive therapy may be needed for fever, tachycardia, hypotension, volume depletion, hyperglycemia, and altered consciousness.

○　**How does one differentiate between MH and thyroid storm?**

Sustained tachycardia, hyperthermia, and increased oxygen consumption are shared by both. An acute significant elevation in end-tidal CO_2, arterial CO_2, metabolic acidosis, and muscle rigidity are features of MH.

○　**A thyroidectomy patient in the PACU is having respiratory distress. What is your differential diagnosis?**

Vocal cord dysfunction from recurrent laryngeal nerve damage, cervical hematoma with airway compression, tracheomalacia, and pneumothorax.

○　**What is the main determinant of hypocalcemia after total thyroidectomy?**

Hypoparathyroidism, is usually transient.

According to the study by Wingert et al., involving 221 patients undergoing thyroidectomy Eighty-three percent of all patients experienced hypocalcemia postoperatively, with 13 percent requiring some treatment for symptoms [Wingert et al., 1986. See reference on page 525].

○　**Describe the symptoms of hypocalcemia following thyroidectomy.**

Usually appearing within 72 hours postoperatively; numbness and tingling around the mouth, hands, and feet; muscle cramps and spasms; headaches; anxiety; depression.

○ **What is the mechanism of hyponatremia in hypothyroidism?**

Although previously thought to be secondary to syndrome of inappropriate ADH secretion (SIADH), it is currently thought to be a function of impaired water excretion related to decreased delivery of sodium and volume to the distal renal tubules as a result of decreased renal blood flow.

○ **Describe the pulse pressure in thyrotoxicosis.**

Widened, reflecting increased flow and vasodilation.

○ **A patient with symptomatic hyperthyroidism is scheduled for elective surgery the next day. What should you do for this patient?**

Cancel the case and refer the patient to an endocrinologist for preoperative assessment and preparation.

Treatment includes antithyroid drugs (propylthiouracil, iodine), radioactive iodine, and surgical subtotal thyroidectomy. If one must proceed, anesthetic risks include acute exacerbation of hyperthyroidism caused by surgical stress (thyroid storm) resulting in tachycardia, hyperthermia, hemodynamic instability, and arrhythmia. Induction with volatile agents is slowed due to the increased cardiac output and the rate of drug metabolism is increased, with no change in MAC. Emergent cases should be treated intraoperatively with invasive monitoring, beta-adrenergic blockade, resuscitation with IV fluids, and temperature control. Refractory hypotension from relative cortisol deficiency may respond to corticosteroids. The first dose of PTU can be administered down the nasogastric tube. Thyroid storm usually occurs 6–18 hours after surgery, so the patient should be monitored in a surgical critical care setting postoperatively.

○ **What is the percentage of cortisol that is not protein bound?**

Five to 10%.

○ **What causes Addison's disease?**

This occurs when adrenal glands do not produce enough cortisol (and aldosterone in some cases).

The disease is characterized by weight loss, muscle weakness, fatigue, low blood pressure, and pigmentation of the skin.

○ **Primary adrenal insufficiency (Addison's disease) refers to disruption of which component of the hypothalamic–pituitary–adrenal axis?**

Adrenal gland.

○ **Secretion of which adrenal hormone is not impaired by secondary adrenal insufficiency?**

Aldosterone.

Secondary adrenal insufficiency is caused by inadequate ACTH secretion by the anterior pituitary. The adrenal cortex produces cortisol and aldosterone. Aldosterone secretion is regulated by the renin–angiotensin system (angiotensin II).

○ **What is the characteristic hemodynamic pattern of adrenal insufficiency?**

Refractory hypotension due to decreased systemic vascular resistance and, to a lesser degree, decreased cardiac contractility, hypovolemia, and electrolyte disturbances (hypercalcemia, hypoglycemia, hyponatremia, hyperkalemia, metabolic acidosis).

○   **Which sedating agent used for prolonged periods has been shown to increase mortality in critically ill patients by inducing primary adrenal insufficiency?**

Etomidate.

In induction doses, etomidate is a selective inhibitor of adrenal 11β-hydroxylase, the enzyme which converts deoxycortisol to cortisol. Mortality rates may be increased when etomidate is used as a long-term continuous infusion for sedation in mechanically ventilated critically ill patients.

○   **What is the treatment for adrenal insufficiency perioperatively?**

Preoperative replacement of missing cortisol, usually given as 100 mg of hydrocortisone phosphate every 24 hours, and aldosterone (fludrocortisone). Preparation also includes treatment of hypovolemia, hyperkalemia, and hyponatremia.

Intraoperative crisis (Addisonian crisis): presents with hypotension, syncope, lethargy, confusion, convulsions, hypoglycemia, nausea/vomiting, metabolic acidosis, hyponatremia, and hyperkalemia.

Treatment consists of intravenous glucocorticoids and volume resuscitation with crystalloid solutions (saline solution with glucose).

○   **Is there any evidence to support the use of corticosteroids in septic shock?**

No. Only animal studies have shown improved survival with steroid treatment in sepsis. Guidelines for the use of steroids in septic shock recommend use of low-dose steroids for septic shock unresponsive to fluids and vasopressors (2008). CORTICUS [the Hydrocortisone Therapy of Septic Shock Study. See reference on page 525] demonstrated a lack of benefit in the administration of steroids to patients in septic shock, regardless of response to corticotropin stimulation testing. Based on this, the 2008 Surviving Sepsis Guidelines no longer recommend the use of the corticotropin test in patients with septic shock.

○   **In which disease states have randomized prospective trials shown improved outcome with the use of corticosteroids?**

Bacterial meningitis, acute spinal injury, typhoid fever, pneumocystis carinii pneumonia, and, possibly, treatment of the fibroproliferative phase of acute respiratory distress syndrome.

○   **How much cortisol is produced per day in patients undergoing minor and major surgery?**

The adrenal cortex normally produces 20–30 mg of cortisol per day. The amount increases in response to minor stress (50 mg) and major stress (75–100 mg). Production rates of cortisol seldom exceed 200–300 mg per day. Current dosing recommendations for supplemental corticosteroids in patients with suspected adrenal insufficiency are:

Minor stress	25 mg hydrocortisone
Moderate stress	50–75 mg per day or 25 mg intraoperatively, followed by IV infusion 100 mg over 24 hours
Major stress	100–150 mg per day or 200–300 mg/70 kg in divided doses per day

○   **What type of malignancies are commonly associated with hypercalcemia?**

Breast cancer is the most common cause. Others include lung cancer, squamous cell carcinomas of the head, neck, and esophagus, gynecologic tumors, renal cell carcinoma, and multiple myeloma. The secretion of humoral mediators by solid tumors (PTH-like substances, cytokines, or prostaglandins) may produce hypercalcemia through increased bone osteoclastic activity, even without bony metastases.

○ **Hypercalcemic crisis is a life-threatening emergency. Describe management options.**

The most common causes of hypercalcemia are primary hyperparathyroidism and malignancy. Aggressive intravenous rehydration (normal saline [0.9% NaCl] at 300–400 mL/h, with normal renal and cardiac function) to obtain euvolemic status, reduce bone resorption, and increase urinary excretion of calcium is the mainstay of therapy. For hypercalcemia greater than or equal to 4 mmol/L, calcitonin and pamidronate or zoledronic acid IV. For hypercalcemia unresponsive to other measures, mithramycin IV. The clinical manifestations primarily affect the neuromuscular, gastrointestinal, renal, skeletal, and cardiovascular systems.

○ **Describe the clinical symptoms of hyperparathyroidism.**

Symptoms are due to hypercalcemia that primarily affects the nervous system: weakness and fatigue, depression, bone pain, osteoporosis, myalgias, decreased appetite, nausea and vomiting, constipation, kidney stones, polyuria, polydipsia, and cognitive impairment.

○ **What are the two types of diabetes insipidus (DI)?**

Central (insufficient ADH secreted by the anterior pituitary) and nephrogenic DI (renal tubules do not respond to ADH).

Urine is dilute despite high serum osmolarity. Central DI may result from head injury, or diseases or surgery to the pituitary. Nephrogenic DI can result from electrolyte abnormalities, illnesses such as sickle cell anemia, myeloma, renal insufficiency, uropathy, or drugs such as lithium. While both types of DI are treated with fluid resuscitation (usually with normal saline), only central DI is treated with DDAVP every 12–24 hours, along with adequate fluid to match losses. The next dose of desmopressin is administered when the specific gravity of urine has fallen to less than 1.008–1.005, with an increase in urine output.

○ **What findings are diagnostic of DI?**

Large volumes (usually greater than 3 L per day) of dilute urine (osmolality <300 mosm/L; specific gravity <1.010) and hypernatremia.

○ **A diagnosis of DI may be confirmed by what test?**

Failure of urine osmolality to increase more than 30 mosm/L in the first hours of complete fluid restriction is diagnostic with confirmation by increased plasma ADH levels. Aqueous vasopressin will test the responsiveness of renal tubules.

○ **How is DI treated?**

Aqueous pitressin 5–10 U q 4–6 hours intravenously or DDAVP 10–20 U q 12–24 hours intranasally. Chronic therapy with chlorpropamide (stimulates ADH release) and thiazide diuretics have been used successfully.

○ **Characterize urine sodium level and plasma osmolality in SIADH.**

SIADH features elevated urinary sodium (>20 mEq/L) with hypotonic plasma (<270–280 mosm/L) and low serum sodium (<130 mEq/L).

○ **How is the SIADH diagnosed?**

ADH (also known as vasopressin) is stored in the posterior pituitary and regulates plasma osmolarity. SIADH occurs when ADH continues to be secreted at an abnormally high threshold despite low osmolality. The diagnosis is made on the basis of hyponatremia <135 mEq/L and plasma osmolality $P_{Osm} <270$ mosm/kg in the presence of high urine osmolality (urine sodium >20 mEq). The patients exhibit a characteristic response to water restriction.

○ **How is the release of ADH (AVP or arginine vasopressin) regulated?**

ADH, or vasopressin, is typically secreted when the serum osmolality exceeds the set point of hypothalamic osmoreceptors, typically between 280 and 290 mosm/L. Psychiatric stress can also stimulate its secretion. Hypovolemia, detected by left atrial and pulmonary vein stretch receptors, and hypotension signaled from aortic and carotid baroreceptors are more potent and overriding triggers and a large amount of AVP $(10–100 \times$ normal) is released. Surgical stress is also a profound stimulus and typically lasts 2–3 days after the surgical procedure.

Anesthetics have little effect on AVP secretion, but surgery is a major stimulus.

○ **What are frequent causes of SIADH?**

1. Malignancies producing ADH-like compounds.
2. Pulmonary disease (bronchogenic carcinoma, tuberculosis, pneumonia, and asthma).
3. CNS disorders (meningitis, tremor, tumors, subarachnoid hemorrhage, and acute intracranial hypertension).
4. Drugs (chlorpropamide, oxytocin, vincristine, cytoxan, nicotine, narcotics, clofibrate, vinblastine, cyclophosphamide).
5. Pain in the postoperative period.
6. Hypothyroidism.
7. Adrenal insufficiency.

In contrast, patients in septic shock have inappropriately low ADH levels although the pathologic mechanism is unknown.

○ **How is hyponatremia treated?**

Water restriction is the first treatment of hyponatremia, with sodium-containing fluids used if sodium is <120 mEq/L. Correction of sodium >0.5 mEq/h may cause central pontine myelinolysis.

○ **What is the anatomy and physiology of carcinoid syndrome?**

Carcinoid syndrome occurs in about 20% of patients with carcinoid. The two most common symptoms are flushing and diarrhea.

While carcinoid tumors secrete bradykinin, histamine, prostaglandins, and kallikrein, the secretion of serotonin and/or 5-hydroxytryptophan is mainly responsible for the syndrome. The most common location of these tumors is the appendix, ileum, and rectum; however, they can be found in bronchus, stomach, pancreas, duodenum, and colon. Symptoms are related to the location of the tumor, with tumors in the small bowel and proximal colon more likely to produce the characteristic flushing, bronchoconstriction, gut hypermotility, and hyperglycemia. The liver generally clears the mediators of this symptom complex, unless there are liver metastases.

○ **What are the cardiac manifestations of carcinoid syndrome?**

These manifestations are due to fibrosis of the endocardium, primarily on the right side. Pulmonic stenosis is usually predominant. Tricuspid valve is often fixed open resulting in regurgitation.

Carcinoid triad is cardiac involvement with flushing and diarrhea.

○ **How are the symptoms of carcinoid syndrome treated?**

Octreotide (a somatostatin analog) blocks release of serotonin and mediators, as well as prevents the peripheral effects of mediators. A carcinoid crisis with severe hypotension and bronchoconstriction may require fluids and vasopressors, as well as intravenous octreotide (100 μg bolus and 100 μg/h).

○ **What is a pheochromocytoma?**

A pheochromoctyoma is a catecholamine-secreting tumor usually found in the adrenal medulla (90%) or paravertebral chromaffin tissue. It may secrete epinephrine, norepinephrine, or other catecholamines. Ten percent are bilateral, and some may be familial or associated with a multiple endocrine neoplasia (MEN) syndrome or neurofibromatosis. Symptoms of hypertension, palpitations, headache, sweating, flushing, anxiety, tremor, and weight loss reflect excess catecholamines. Plasma metanephrine testing has the highest sensitivity (96%) for detecting a pheochromocytoma, but it has a lower specificity (85%). In comparison, a 24-hour urinary collection for catecholamines and metanephrines has a sensitivity of 87.5% and a specificity of 99.7% [Sawka et al., 2003. See reference on page 524].

○ **Why are β-blockers not used alone for preoperative preparation of patients with pheochromocytoma?**

If β-receptors are blocked in these patients before the administration of phenoxybenzamine (α-receptor antagonist), norepinephrine and epinephrine will produce unopposed alpha stimulation, resulting in a further increase in peripheral vascular resistance and worsening hypertension.

○ **How is pheochromocytoma managed intraoperatively?**

Intraoperative management depends on optimal preoperative preparation including α-adrenergic receptor blockade (phenoxybenzamine or prazosin for 10–14 days), reexpansion of fluid volume, and β-adrenergic receptor blockade for patients with persistent arrhythmias or tachycardia. Patient readiness is suggested with adequate blood pressure control to 165/90 mm Hg, orthostatic hypotension, resolution of ST-T changes on EKG, and no more than one PVC every 5 minutes. All anesthetic agents have been used with success (isoflurane, sevoflurane, fentanyl, sufentanil, remifentanil, and regional anesthesia). Invasive monitoring is essential, anticipating hypertension (treated with IV nitroprusside, phentolamine, or magnesium) and transient arrhythmias (esmolol) on induction. After the tumor is isolated and the venous supply is secured, resuscitation with volume and direct-acting vasopressors (phenylephrine, dopamine, vasopressin, or catecholamine infusions) may be required. Rarely, patients may remain hypertensive perioperatively. Dilutional anemia, hypotension, and hypoglycemia should be anticipated following surgery.

○ **Following resection of a pheochromocytoma, the patient becomes hypoglycemic in the PACU. What is the cause?**

The high serum catecholamine levels in this disorder cause increased glycogenolysis, and gluconeogenesis and decreased insulin secretion. With removal of the tumor, rapid decrease in catecholamine levels can result in marked hypoglycemia.

○ **Why does epinephrine cause hyperglycemia?**

Epinephrine causes glycogenolysis in the liver and inhibits insulin release from the pancreas.

○ **What are preoperative considerations in diabetes mellitus (DM)?**

The type of DM, current treatment regimen, and complications from DM are the most important items to assess preoperatively; in addition, these patients may have related complications, such as atherosclerotic heart and peripheral vascular disease. The patient with type 1 DM with an absolute deficiency of insulin will be prone to ketoacidosis if insulin is omitted, whereas the patient with type 2 DM will have insulin resistance and may in fact have high levels of endogenous insulin; this second patient may be on oral agents, insulin, or both, and may be susceptible to nonketotic hyperosmolar coma. Classic complications from DM include the *triopathy* of nephropathy, neuropathy, and retinopathy.

The treatment regimen and degree of blood glucose control, as well as the prior considerations mentioned, will determine recommendations for medication management; preoperative instructions should include being NPO for surgery and treatment of potential hypoglycemia.

○ **What is the most common type of neuropathy that develops in DM?**

Symmetrical peripheral polyneuropathies.

Sensory changes of the lower extremities (numbness, tingling, burning).

Carpal tunnel syndrome.

Segmental demyelination of nerves (cranial, median, ulnar).

Autonomic neuropathy is also common and is associated with a 50% mortality rate over a 5-year period.

○ **What are some clinical manifestations of diabetic autonomic neuropathy?**

Orthostatic hypotension, cardiac arrhythmias, loss of heart rate response to valsalva maneuver or respirations (loss of beat-to-beat variability in heart rate), resting tachycardia, gastroparesis, bladder dysfunction, impotence, hypoglycemia, painless myocardial ischemia, unexpected cardiac arrest, and impaired pupillary reflexes.

○ **What features of the history and physical examination would suggest diabetic autonomic neuropathy?**

A clue about autonomic neuropathy may be a resting tachycardia, because parasympathetic neuropathy occurs before sympathetic neuropathy. Other cardiac effects of autonomic neuropathy include postural hypotension and silent ischemia. Gastroparesis may present as vomiting undigested food before breakfast, as well as having a "full stomach" despite strict observance of NPO guidelines. Other GI/GU manifestations include diarrhea, neurogenic bladder, and impotence. These autonomic symptoms appear in parallel with the peripheral nervous system symptoms of pain and/or a characteristic stocking–glove pattern of numbness.

Dysesthesias (impairment of sensation and unpleasant sensation produced by normal stimuli) of the lower limbs are a common complaint of patients and are indicative of peripheral neuropathy.

○ **Describe the complications of hyperglycemia in the perioperative setting.**

Diabetic ketoacidosis, osmotic diuresis, hypovolemia, cerebral edema, hyperviscosity and thrombogenesis, worsened wound healing, increased risk of infection, and length of hospitalization.

○   **What is considered ideal perioperative glucose control?**

Hemoglobin A1C goal for nonpregnant adults with DM of <7%. Tight control of perioperative glucose ≤110 mg/dL reduces morbidity (septicemia and wound healing) with the increased risk of hypoglycemia [Preiser et al., 2009. See reference on page 524; The NICR-SUGAR study, 2009. See reference on page 525].

○   **What effect does glucagon have on blood glucose?**

Glucagon causes the liver to convert stored glycogen into glucose, which raises blood glucose levels.

In other words, glucagon has opposing effects to that of insulin, causing release of glucose from glycogen, release of fatty acids from stored triglycerides, and stimulation of gluconeogenesis.

Key Terms

Addison's disease: blood chemistry
Addison's disease: perioperative treatment
Antidiuretic hormone (ADH) regulation
Carcinoid crisis: prevention
Carcinoid crisis: treatment
Carcinoid-induced bronchospasm: treatment
Carcinoid syndrome/symptoms
Cardiac lesions in carcinoid
Diabetes insipidus: diagnosis and treatment
Diabetes insipidus: diagnostic test
Diabetes perioperative complications
Diabetic neuropathy signs dysesthesia: diabetic neuropathy
DM control: glycosylated Hb
Electrolyte homeostasis: hormones
Endocrine function of the pituitary gland
Glucagon effects
Hormonal regulation of osmolality
Hyperaldosteronism: drug treatment
Hypercalcemia: acute treatment
Hyperglycemia: complications
Hyperglycemia: preoperative treatment
Hyperparathyroidism: signs
Hyperthyroid: metabolic/circulatory effects

Hyperthyroidism: signs
Hypoglycemia: glucagon
Hypothyroidism: anesthetic concerns
Lab diagnosis of hypothyroidism
Malignant hyperthermia (MH) versus thyroid storm
Management of complications of carcinoid
Parathyroid hormone effects: calcium and phosphate
Pheochromocytoma and intraoperative hypotension
Pheochromocytoma: diagnostic markers/preoperative preparation
Pheochromocytoma: hypertension treatment
Pheochromocytoma: initial treatment
Pheochromocytoma: preoperative medications
Pituitary adenoma deficiencies
Postthyroidectomy: hypocalcemia
Primary hyperaldosteronism
Steroid prophylaxis: indications
Surgical stress response hormones
Syndrome of inappropriate antidiuretic hormone (SIADH): laboratory values
Thyroidectomy: complications/hypocalcemia
Thyrotoxicosis: treatment
Vasodilators: pheochromocytoma
Vasopressin treatment in diabetes insipidus (DI)

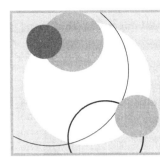

ENT Surgery

It is the tragedy of the world that no one knows what he doesn't know — and
the less a man knows, the more sure he is he knows everything.
Joyce Cary

○ **What special anesthetic considerations are necessary for patient safety during laser surgery?**

Unintentional injury during a laser procedure may include direct laser exposure in nontarget areas and indirect injury due to ignition of the drapes or endotracheal tube (ETT) resulting in burns. Preventive measures include wearing appropriate protective eyewear (for patient and staff), moistening combustible materials, maintaining deep anesthesia or using muscle relaxants to prevent unintentional movement, limiting FiO_2, considering nasotracheal intubation, and/or using a laser-safe tube. All personnel must complete a laser safety module and be prepared to extinguish a flame.

○ **What potential complications occur during laser surgery?**

Bleeding, pneumothorax, and airway fire.

○ **What are the requirements in order to have an airway fire?**

Ignition source, oxidizing agents, and combustible material.

○ **What measures can be taken to reduce the risk of laser-generated airway fires?**

The goal is to limit laser beam contact with flammable materials and high concentrations of gases that support combustion.

Three strategies used are:

1. Reduction of the flammability of the ETT

2. Reduction of the available O_2 content

3. Removal of the flammable material from the airway (anesthesia without ETT)

It must be emphasized that **no** cuffed ETT is completely laser-proof. In order to reduce the hazard of fire, use of proper gas mixtures is important during laser airway surgery.

The measures that can be taken are:

• Use of a specially designed metal and wrapped or laser-proof ETT.
• Inflation of the ETT cuff with saline or water. The fluid acts as a heat sink and allows more energy to be absorbed before perforation and if penetrated the escaping liquid helps extinguish any fire (may use methylene blue as a signal for cuff rupture).

- Moistening exposed flammable surfaces. Place saline-soaked pledgets in the airway to limit risk of ignition.
- Avoid nitrous oxide that supports combustion.
- Reduction in inspired oxygen concentration to the lowest tolerated by the patient less than 30% (helium or air).
- Choice of ventilation techniques not requiring an ETT such as jet ventilation.
- Apneic technique – anesthetized and immobilized (using muscle relaxants), patient's lungs are ventilated by mask between laser applications. However, there is a greater potential for debris to enter the trachea.
- Nasotracheal intubation.
- Reduction of heat by limiting laser exposure (short, frequent bursts).

○ **How does "jet" ventilation work?**

A small (16-gauge) cannula in the airway delivers a high-pressure jet of gas (usually oxygen). Additional air is entrained via the Venturi effect. A cone-shaped wedge of gas actually reaches alveoli, although total volume delivered per jet ventilation puff is less than anatomic dead space. Exhalation is passive.

○ **What is the appropriate management of an airway fire?**

The ETT fire is the most serious fire in the patient.

Immediately stop ventilation, disconnect the oxygen source, remove the ETT, flood the surgical field with saline, ventilate the patient by mask with 100% oxygen, reintubate, examine the extent of damage and remove debris by laryngoscopy/bronchoscopy, ventilate with humidified oxygen and continue monitoring in critical care setting for 24 hours, use short-term steroids, and continue ventilatory support and antibiotics as needed. Obtain CXR and monitor for pulmonary dysfunction.

○ **What risk do lasers pose to patients and health care providers?**

Damage to eyes and skin from reflection of laser light by surgical instruments, electrical shock, fire and explosion, and contamination of the atmosphere (smoke and diseased particulate matter).

○ **Name the types of lasers available for clinical use.**

Carbon dioxide, argon, krypton, neodymium-doped yttrium aluminium garnet (Nd:YAG), and neodymium-doped: yttrium–aluminum–garnet: potassium-titanyl-phosphate (Nd:YAG–KTP).

○ **Which types of lasers are used during airway surgery, and how do techniques differ for proximal and distal airway surgery?**

A YAG solid state laser (emits near-infrared invisible light at 1,064 nm) is typically used for debulking, coagulating, and removing obstructing tumors in the airway. CO_2 laser has limited penetration.

Proximal airway laser surgery requires a rigid bronchoscope with intravenous anesthesia and jet ventilation; a flexible bronchoscope passed through a large (>8.0) ETT may be used for distal airway surgery.

○ **What is the disadvantage of using polyvinyl chloride (PVC), red rubber, or silicone ETTs during laser surgery?**

Each of these tubes can be ignited by the carbon dioxide laser in an environment of 100% oxygen. PVC tubes are the least flammable.

○ **What are the characteristics of laser-safe ET tubes?**

Two types: common one is a PVC tube with a double cuff, to ensure protection of the airway in the event of a cuff rupture. Special flexible metal tubes are also available, which prevent reflected laser beam scattering – these have a larger diameter. Use of laser-resistant metal ETTs requires extra care to prevent mucosal abrasions. These tubes are bulkier and more rigid than conventional tubes.

○ **What effect can CO_2 laser have on the eyes?**

The nature of the ocular damage depends on the wavelength of the laser light. Exposure to a 10,600 nm wavelength produced by the CO_2 laser can cause corneal opacification because energy is largely absorbed on the surface of the eye (limited penetration of the *CO_2 laser*. The *Nd:YAG laser* has tissue penetration of 2–6 mm, and may cause retinal injury and scarring.

○ **What is the advantage of helium when using a small-bore tube?**

Helium improves laminar flow and decreases airway resistance; therefore, it improves overall air flow through the narrow lumen of a small-bore tube.

○ **How does helium work to alleviate subglottic stenosis?**

A mixture of helium and oxygen (heliox) is less dense than air or oxygen; as a result, it provides more laminar flow in the obstructed airway, and is believed to reduce work of breathing, respiratory distress, and postextubation stridor.

○ **Name three anesthetic techniques for microlaryngoscopy.**

1. Ninety-five percent of operations can be done with a small 5.0 mm I.D. ETT placed near the posterior commissure. Only 5% of microsurgical laryngeal procedures involve the lower third of the vocal cords.
2. Jet ventilation through the laryngoscope. This technique is contraindicated in children.
3. Apneic oxygenation technique with intermittent ventilation.

○ **How do you assess adequacy of ventilation when using jet ventilation?**

Low-frequency jet ventilation for microlaryngoscopy requires an oxygen supply at 30–50 psi, an inspiratory time of 1.5 seconds, and passive free egress of gas over an expiratory time of 6 seconds. This will result in a ventilation rate of 6 or 7 breaths/min. Movement of the chest wall is assessed to determine adequacy of tidal volume. Arterial blood gas measurements are used to determine CO_2. Pulse oximetry is used to monitor oxygenation.

High-frequency jet ventilation delivers a *small tidal volume breath* from an O_2 source of 5–50 psi through a small-bore cannula with an interposed cycling mechanism allowing high frequencies of 10–15 Hz. Arterial blood gas measurements are used to determine CO_2.

○ **List common problems associated with middle ear surgery.**

Nitrous oxide–induced changes in middle ear pressure, bleeding, facial nerve injury, cervical spine injury secondary to improper head positioning, nausea, vomiting, and vertigo.

○ **What are the consequences of N_2O administration in middle ear surgery?**

Inhaling a high concentration of nitrous oxide can result in increasing pressure in a noncompliant cavity such as the middle ear. Normally the pressure in the middle ear is passively vented via the Eustachian tube but surgical trauma, edema, or underlying disease may obstruct the Eustachian tube and prevent decompression.

○ **Is nitrous oxide contraindicated in middle ear surgery?**

Middle ear pressure rises with N_2O administration and with its removal negative pressure may develop as the N_2O is rapidly reabsorbed if the middle ear does not communicate with the atmosphere. Rupture of the tympanic membrane, nausea, vomiting, and development of serious otitis have been documented. It is generally recommended that the N_2O be discontinued 10–30 minutes before closure of the middle ear.

○ **What are the anesthetic implications in the management of bleeding during middle ear surgery?**

Successful surgery in the middle ear requires a bloodless operative field. Infiltration of the surrounding tissues with epinephrine-containing solutions provides some hemostasis, but often intraoperative hypotension must be induced. Care should be taken to choose appropriate patients for this technique, as hypotension may induce ischemia of perfusable organs and tissues. A recent article has advocated the use of propofol versus isoflurane for this technique because propofol helps to maintain middle ear blood flow autoregulation. Elevation of the head of the OR table to reduce CVP and improve venous drainage of the head and neck may be helpful, but can predispose the patient to venous air embolism.

○ **Is a recent upper respiratory infection (URI) a contraindication to myringotomy and tube insertion?**

Typically this procedure is accomplished using mask inhalation anesthesia. The children often have accompanying URIs and it is the drainage of middle ear fluid that eradicates this problem. No significant difference in postoperative morbidity has been observed in children asymptomatic and those with uncomplicated URIs who undergo myringotomy and tube placement and do not require endotracheal intubation.

○ **What is the most feared complication of infection in the retropharyngeal space?**

Descending necrotizing mediastinitis, with mortality rates approaching 50%.

○ **What facial space(s) is involved in Ludwig's angina?**

The submandibular space, with secondary involvement of the submental space.

○ **What is Ludwig's angina?**

It is a cellulitis of the floor of the mouth caused by bacterial infection of the sublingual and/or submandibular tissues. It can rapidly lead to stridor and eventually asphyxia and death due to acute airway obstruction. Antibiotic therapy is usually ineffective due to mixed bacterial flora and poor penetration into the space.

○ **How is the airway secured in a patient with Ludwig's angina?**

Awake intubation or cricothyroidotomy under local anesthesia is preferred. The patient should not be anesthetized prior to securing the airway.

○ **What is the most common origin of infection in patients with Ludwig's angina?**

Dental abscesses.

○ **What are the most common local findings in patients with Ludwig's angina?**

Swelling of the floor of the mouth and tongue, fever, and suprahyoid firmness without fluctuation.

○ **What is the most common cause of death in Ludwig's angina?**

Airway compromise is always synonymous with the term Ludwig's angina, and it is the leading cause of death [Saifeldeen and Evans, 2004. See reference on page 525].

○ **What are the most important organisms in Ludwig's angina?**

Aerobic streptococcus, staphylococcus, bacteroides, and peptostreptococcus.

○ **What are the most common presenting signs of anterolateral pharyngeal space infections?**

Trismus, fever, chills, swelling at the angle of the mandible, and medial bulging of the pharyngeal wall.

○ **What are the most common findings on lateral neck x-rays in patients with retropharyngeal abscess?**

Prevertebral soft tissue widening, air-fluid levels, loss of cervical lordosis, and cervical osteomyelitis.

○ **What are the risks of general anesthesia in a patient with peritonsillar abscess?**

Difficulty in intubation should be expected due to distorted anatomy, edema, and trismus. Accidental rupture of the abscess with spillage of pus into an unprotected airway is a risk. If possible, the abscess should be drained by needle aspiration under local anesthesia prior to induction of general anesthesia.

○ **Are nondepolarizing muscle relaxants contraindicated in surgery where facial nerve preservation is a concern?**

To identify the facial nerve at least 10–20% of the muscle twitch response must be preserved. Realistically, the use of nondepolarizing muscle relaxants may be implicated as contributory if the patient demonstrates facial nerve dysfunction postoperatively. Despite monitoring, the surgical risk of facial nerve paralysis is 0.6–3.0% [Dulguerov et al., 1999. See reference on page 525].

○ **What is the risk of hemorrhage and mortality after elective tonsillar and adenoid surgery?**

Postoperative hemorrhage occurs at a rate of 2–4% in various studies. Mortality has been reported at 1:10,000 in the 1960s; with more recent studies, mortality has been estimated to be 1:15,000, unadjusted for age [Windfuhr et al., 2009. See reference on page 525].

○ **What are some signs of ongoing bleeding after T&A in the PACU?**

Frequent swallowing, tachycardia, and hypotension (or occasionally hypertension). Aspiration of large amounts of blood can produce intrapulmonary shunting and hypoxemia. The child may be hypovolemic, anemic, agitated, and/or in shock.

○ **When is bleeding after adenotonsillectomy likely to occur?**

Three fourths of bleeds after adenotonsillectomy occur within the first 6 hours after surgery. The remaining 25% occur in the remaining 24 hours. Occasionally bleeding occurs as late as 5–10 days after surgery and is usually associated with infection.

○ **How should a child with post-tonsillectomy bleed be induced?**

Awake intubation is not practically feasible in an anxious frightened child. Options include either rapid sequence induction or mask induction with cricoid pressure. Regardless of the method chosen, two suction catheters, duplicate laryngoscopes, and ETTs are prepared and a physician experienced in emergent cricothyroidotomy should be present. If hemorrhage is brisk, laryngoscopy and intubation may be performed with the head turned to the lateral position.

○ **A 5-year-old presents 10 hours after tonsillectomy vomiting frank blood. He is tachypneic, hypotensive, and anxious. Can he undergo mask induction before an IV is established?**

No. An IV or IVs should be started and intravascular volume replaced prior to induction and a rapid sequence planned. If no IV can be started, and emergent induction is required to control bleeding, IM ketamine would be a better choice, with the most rapid control of the airway possible to prevent aspiration. Transfusion of blood should be dictated by following serial hematocrits. The end point of fluid replacement should be return of blood pressure and heart rate toward normal.

○ **Beyond fluid replacement how should the child be prepared for surgery?**

The child should be typed and cross-matched as indicated by hematocrit. Coagulation studies should be obtained. The child should be treated as a full stomach.

○ **A patient develops worsening hoarseness after tonsillectomy. How should you respond?**

Hoarseness is a common problem following extubation. Usually hoarseness resolves within 5–7 days. Hoarseness that worsens or persists for >7 days requires evaluation by an otolaryngologist to rule out vocal cord injury.

○ **What complications should one be aware of in surgery for head and neck cancer?**

Open neck veins allow entrainment of air into the venous system. This potentially devastating complication can be reduced, if not eliminated, by placing the patient in a slightly head-down position. Tumors involving the major vessels in the neck can require sacrifice of one or both internal jugular veins resulting in decreased cerebral perfusion pressure and cerebral edema. Cardiac arrhythmia is also a concern. Occasionally a carotid artery may need to be ligated if infiltrated with tumor.

○ **A patient develops ventricular ectopy during right radical neck dissection. Does this operation raise specific concerns of arrhythmia?**

Prolonged Q-T interval resulting in a lower threshold for ventricular arrhythmia is commonly associated with right but not left radical neck dissection. This presumably results from trauma to the right stellate ganglion and cervical autonomic nervous system during dissection. Torsade de pointes is a possible arrhythmia.

○ **What are the consequences of bilateral denervation of the carotid bodies in bilateral neck dissection?**

Bilateral carotid body denervation is associated with increased resting $PaCO_2$ and the loss of the normal respiratory and blood pressure responses to acute hypoxia. Hypertension is also common and should be aggressively treated. Serious respiratory depression may occur after opioid administration.

○ **What are the limits of epinephrine injection when given for hemostasis?**

Classically, epinephrine administration during anesthesia is limited to 2.5 mcg/kg with halothane, 10 mcg/kg with enflurane, and 5 mcg/kg with isoflurane and sevoflurane. Children seem to be able to tolerate higher doses than adults. Volatile anesthetics sensitize the myocardium to the atrial and ventricular arrhythmogenic effects of epinephrine.

○ **A surgeon is applying a 4% topical cocaine solution to the nasal mucosa in preparation for surgery. What is the recommended maximum dose of cocaine?**

The maximum recommended dose of intranasal cocaine is 3 mg/kg.

○ **What are the risks of intranasal cocaine?**

Cocaine may cause agitation, hypertension, and tachycardia.

Increased risk of ventricular fibrillation or other severe ventricular arrhythmias and cardiac arrest especially in patients with preexisting heart disease.

Inhalational anesthetics such as halothane (chloroform, cyclopropane, and trichloroethylene), more than isoflurane, sensitize the myocardium to the effects of sympathomimetics.

○ **In what patients and with what medications should the use of cocaine for topicalization be avoided?**

In hypertensives and patients taking adrenergic-modifying drugs such as guanethidine, reserpine, tricyclic antidepressants, and monoamine oxidase inhibitors. A combination of these drugs may produce a hypersympathetic response. Ketamine, because of its sympathomimetic effects, may also exaggerate hypertension.

○ **Why should cocaine-induced cardiovascular instability be treated with labetalol and not propranolol?**

Labetalol offers the distinct advantage of both an alpha-adrenergic and a beta-adrenergic receptor blockade, whereas a lethal hypertensive exacerbation has been attributed to the unopposed alpha stimulation following propranolol.

○ **What is the difference between a unilateral and a bilateral mandibular fracture?**

A unilateral mandibular fracture is stable; a bilateral fracture is unstable. With a bilateral mandibular fracture the posterior fragment may be distracted posteroinferiorly by the muscles of the floor of the mouth leading to obstruction of the pharynx by the base of the tongue.

○ **How does a Le Fort I fracture complicate anesthetic management?**

A Le Fort I fracture is a horizontal fracture through the maxilla that results only in a mobile palate and it presents little problem to the anesthesiologist. Patients may be intubated either orally or nasally providing intranasal damage has been ruled out.

○ **What are the anesthetic concerns with a Le Fort II fracture?**

A Le Fort II fracture involves the nose and, therefore, nasal intubation is relatively contraindicated. Because the force necessary to create this fracture is substantial, one must be suspicious of an occult fracture at the base of the skull.

○ **What are the causes of recurrent laryngeal nerve (RLN) injury?**

Stretching of the nerve (retraction or positioning injury), direct surgical trauma, ischemia, or misadventure during endotracheal intubation.

○   **How is the diagnosis of RLN injury made?**

The patient may complain of hoarseness or a weak voice. Direct or indirect laryngoscopy reveals the ipsilateral vocal cord in a paramedian position due to the unopposed action of the cricothyroid muscle on the same side, resulting in an incompetent glottis. The RLN innervates all the intrinsic muscles of the larynx except for the cricothyroid and inferior pharyngeal constrictors. Bilateral injury results in closure of the glottis following extubation, creating a true asphyxial emergency.

Key Terms

Airway burn: management

Airway laser: gases

Anesthesia for laser surgery

Apneic oxygenation: blood gases

Foreign body aspiration: physical exam

Helium advantage: small-bore tube

Heliox: airway resistance

Intraoperative middle ear bleeding management

Jet stylet: advantages

Jet ventilation and ABGs

Laser: endotracheal tube (ETT) fire prevention

Laser-safe ETT tubes

Laser surgery and airway fire

Lasers: management of airway fires

Nd:YAG laser characteristics

Recurrent laryngeal nerve injury

Subglottic stenosis: helium

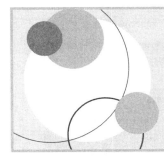

Genitourinary and Renal Surgery

The illiterate of the 21st century will not be those who cannot read and write,
but those who cannot learn, unlearn and relearn.
Alvin Tofler

○ **What are the significant risk factors of perioperative renal failure?**

Acute kidney injury (AKI) occurs in about 1% of patients undergoing general surgery procedures. An AKI risk prediction model developed has found significant independent risk factors to be:

- Age ≥56 years
- Male sex
- Active congestive heart failure
- Hypertension
- Emergency surgery
- Intraperitoneal surgery
- Renal insufficiency – mild or moderate
- Diabetes mellitus – oral or insulin therapy

The risk index is classified according to the number of risk factors: Class I–V representing 0–6+ risk factors present. Compared with Class I, the hazard ratio for Class II–V AKI risk was 3.1, 8.5, 15.4, and 46.2, respectively.

Predictors of AKI for patients undergoing cardiac surgery are related to poor cardiac performance and advanced atherosclerotic disease.

○ **What are the strategies for perioperative preservation of renal function?**

Very few evidence-based strategies exist for perioperative preservation of renal function. The goal of fluid and hemodynamic management should be to avoid renal hypoperfusion due to hypotension and volume depletion. Although colloids are more effective in maintaining plasma volume, there is no clear evidence that they provide better renal protection. Goal-directed therapy, aimed at providing an adequate cardiac output (CO) and oxygen delivery, has been shown to lower the risk of postoperative renal impairment.

Tight blood glucose control appears to be beneficial in both cardiac and noncardiac surgical patients and critically ill patients. For patients undergoing aortic surgery, the level of aortic clamping highly impacts the degree of impairment of renal perfusion. Post-infrarenal clamping has an incidence of AKI of 5% versus 13% for post-suprarenal clamping.

Promising pharmacologic agents for renal protection include: (1) fenoldopam, a selective DA-1 agonist that increases medullary and cortical blood flow and decreases oxygen demand; (2) atrial natriuretic peptide, which produces vasodilation of the preglomerular artery, inhibition of the renin–angiotensin axis, and prostaglandin release.

○ **When is renal insufficiency diagnosed?**

Renal insufficiency occurs with a GFR 25–40% of normal. Elevated BUN and creatinine are seen. Nocturia, due to decreased concentrating ability, may be the only symptom.

○ **What are the causes and management of perioperative oliguria?**

Decreased urine output may be a normal part of the stress response to surgery. Norepinephrine, released in response to pain, trauma, and shock, leads to activation of the renin–angiotensin–aldosterone system and causes ADH release. Intense stress, however, can cause afferent arteriole constriction and, if not relieved, can lead to acute renal failure.

Perioperative renal dysfunction may be subdivided into prerenal, intrinsic renal, and postrenal causes.

Prerenal causes are the most common because of hypovolemia (e.g., due to acute hemorrhage), and should respond to fluid boluses. There is a linear relationship between mean arterial pressure (MAP) >50 and urine output.

Perioperative oliguria (<0.5 mL/kg/h) is almost always prerenal in origin and only rarely due to acute renal failure. If fluid and hemodynamics are optimized and oliguria persists, diuretics should be considered.

Other causes of renal hypoperfusion are related to cardiac dysfunction or other conditions such as hepatorenal syndrome, which should be managed accordingly. In congestive heart failure and fluid overload, diuretics should be given. During sepsis, systemic vasodilation produces severe hypotension and requires aggressive fluid resuscitation along with inotropic–vasopressor agents. Certain drugs interfere with the mechanism of renal perfusion, such as nonsteroidal anti-inflammatory agents.

Intrinsic reasons for postoperative renal failure include ischemia, toxins (such as myoglobin, aminoglycosides, and radiocontrast), and renal parenchymal diseases (often preexisting).

Intrinsic renal failure is treated conservatively by maintenance of adequate renal perfusion pressure and stimulation of diuresis with furosemide, mannitol, or low-dose dopamine infusion. More aggressive treatment includes dialysis. The attempts to pharmacologically prevent intrinsic renal failure have not been met with success. However, the negative effects of specific toxin exposures can be diminished. For example, the use of homocysteine and aggressive hydration along with nonionic contrast dyes provides some benefit in high-risk situations. Calcium channel blockers have been found to ameliorate the effects of cyclosporine, cisplatin, and contrast dye as long as hypotension is avoided. Minimizing acute tubular necrosis (ATN) in the setting of hemolysis or rhabdomyolysis can be attempted with aggressive fluid management and urine alkalinization. A low urine pH (<5.6) leads to myoglobin precipitation as ferrihematin in the proximal tubule, and hypovolemia causes a low tubular flow and sludging. If oliguric ATN cannot be avoided by these measures, however, there has been much interest generated recently in using ANP to promote dialysis-free survival.

Postrenal causes involve obstruction of the urine collecting system anywhere from the renal pelvis to the distal urethra. Voiding dysfunction can result from disruption of sacral parasympathetic motor innervation of the bladder from residual spinal or epidural block or neuraxial opioids. Once these causes and a malfunctioning Foley catheter have been ruled out, renal ultrasound or other imaging should be considered.

○ **What are the initial clinical effects of ATN on renal function?**

Initial effects are loss of urinary concentrating ability and inability to conserve sodium. ATN occurs following the breakdown of the energy requiring Na–K-ATPase pump in the thick ascending loop of Henle (LOH). Abnormal tubular integrity and necrosis of tubular cells results in obstruction of tubular flow by cellular debris and backleak of ultrafiltrate.

○ **What are the diagnostic criteria for ATN?**

The diagnosis of ATN is based on a consideration of the clinical history as well as physical and laboratory findings. A 50% decrease in glomerular filtration rate or an increase in creatinine (Cr) 0.5 mg/dL is a commonly used criterion for diagnosis.

Patients may be oliguric or nonoliguric, the latter case having a better prognosis. With tubular dysfunction, urine sodium is elevated (>40 mEq/L) as well as fractional excretion of sodium (FENa = [urine sodium/plasma sodium]/[urine Cr/plasma Cr] × 100) above 2%. The inability to concentrate the urine results in urine osmolality below 450 mosm/kg (usually below 350 mosm/kg). A normal BUN/Cr ratio of 10–15:1 suggests ATN, as opposed to prerenal failure which is >20:1. Examination of urine sediment reveals muddy brown granular casts, amorphous debris, epithelial cell casts, and free renal tubular epithelial cells.

○ **Describe the methods of lab assessment of renal function.**

- Serum BUN and Cr
  - Elevation only a late sign of decreased GFR
  - BUN levels affected by urea load (intake), production, and tubular reabsorption
  - Cr levels affected by muscle mass, increase in catabolic states
  - Prerenal azotemia ratio ≥20:1
  - ATN ratio = 10–15:1
- Urine sodium excretion
  - Prerenal azotemia <20 mEq/L
  - ATN >40 mEq/L
- Urine osmolality (mosm/kg)
  - Prerenal azotemia >400
  - ATN <500
- FENa (%)
  - Prerenal azotemia <1
  - ATN >2
- Urine sediment
  - Prerenal azotemia – normal, occasional hyaline and finely granular casts
  - ATN – epithelial cells, granular and muddy brown casts
- Free water clearance – less sensitive than Cr clearance (CrCl)
- CrCl – requires 24-hour urine collection
  - $CrCl = \dfrac{urine\ cr \times urine\ volume}{Plasma\ cr}.$

○ **Which renal function test is the most reliable predictor of imminent acute renal failure?**

At present, out of the above-mentioned tests, measured CrCl remains the most reliable predictor of renal dysfunction (indicator of imminent acute renal failure) in critically ill surgical patients. CrCl is a direct reflection of GFR. A 2-hour CrCl facilitates sequential monitoring of renal function during rapidly changing patient status, and it is shown to correlate well with 24-hour CrCl.

○ **What is the FENa?**

FENa is defined by (urinary Na/plasma Na) divided by (urinary Cr/plasma Cr) × 100%. A prerenal picture is suggested by a ratio <1% and intrinsic renal disease by a ratio >3%. Diuretic therapy can overcome the kidneys' ability to retain sodium; thus, a high urine Na does not necessarily reflect loss of tubular function. However, low urine Na in the setting of diuretics indicates an intense prerenal state.

○   **How does urine specific gravity and osmolality help determine renal tubular function?**

A high specific gravity (>1.030) or an osmolality (>1,050 mosm/kg) means that there is unimpaired tubular function. Low urine specific gravity (1.010) or osmolality (290 mosm/kg) that is the same as plasma is suggestive of renal disease. A dilute urine (50–100 mosm/kg) may still indicate renal disease as the urine dilution mechanism fails after the concentrating ability.

○   **What are the hormonal causes of oliguria?**

Normal urine output does not rule out renal failure, just as oliguria may be due to a number of factors independent of GFR. Urine output depends on tubular excretion of solute and water, which is determined hormonally by levels of circulating renin, ADH, aldosterone, and catecholamines. Surgical stress is a profound stimulus for the release of ADH, typically persisting for 2–3 days after the surgical procedure. It also leads to the elaboration of high levels of angiotensin II, which causes increased NaCl resorption at the proximal tubule, elaboration of aldosterone and contraction of the glomeruli mesangial cells with a physiologic decrease in GFR.

○   **When does hyperkalemia manifest in patients with renal insufficiency?**

Hyperkalemia occurs in severe renal insufficiency secondary to decreased clearance. Normal potassium levels may be maintained as long as GFR exceeds 8 mL/h since excretion is reliant on tubular excretion.

○   **How is magnesium excreted?**

Because circulating Mg is partially protein-bound, only 70–80% is filtered across the glomerulus. In general, only 3% of the filtered magnesium escapes reabsorption and is excreted, although this can increase or decrease depending on magnesium status. Mg is unique in that most of it (50–60%) is reabsorbed in the thick ascending LOH or distal convoluted tubule rather than in the proximal convoluted tubule (20–30%). It is also unique that alterations of Mg excretion are dependent on changes in loop transport. Most of Mg transport is passive, diffusing with NaCl down an electrical gradient. Mg wasting can therefore be induced with a loop diuretic.

○   **What electrolyte abnormalities are associated with renal failure?**

Electrolyte changes associated with uremia are hyponatremia, hyperkalemia, hypercalcemia or hypocalcemia, hyperphosphatemia, hypermagnesemia and anion gap metabolic acidosis.

○   **What are some of the laboratory abnormalities that may accompany acute renal failure?**

The major problem arising from acute renal failure is the inability to maintain the dynamic balance between dietary intake of essential substances and production of waste products. This results in:

- A decrease in serum sodium and calcium
- A daily rise in serum potassium of 0.3–3 mEq/L except when there is concomitant potassium loss from diarrhea or vomiting
- Metabolic acidosis
- A progressive rise in serum urea, creatinine, uric acid, magnesium, sulfate, phosphate, some amino and organic acids and polypeptides
- A decrease in serum proteins, particularly albumin
- Elevation of total lipids, cholesterol, phosphorus and neutral fats
- Hyperglycemia, which may or may not be insulin resistant

○ **What are some of the metabolic and systemic effects that may accompany acute renal failure?**

The kidney functions both as an endocrine and an excretory organ. Thus, disorders of renin–angiotensin and aldosterone secretion occur, contributing to the hypertension that develops in patients with severe renal disease. Heart failure and abnormalities in liver function and blood coagulation may also occur. Infection is common and difficult to treat because the altered excretion of antibiotics leads to rapid development of toxic levels of these drugs.

○ **What are some of the laboratory or electrolyte effects that accompany chronic renal failure?**

Metabolic acidosis, hyperkalemia, hypocalcemia, hypermagnesemia and hyperphosphatemia are seen. Reduced erythropoietin production results in chronic anemia. Coagulopathies occur due to platelet dysfunction. Accumulation of compounds such as guanidine succinic acid and hydroxyphenolic acid is thought to produce platelet dysfunction by interfering with the platelet's ability to expose a phospholipid surface, termed PF3 activity. Both are dialyzable and dialysis frequently improves the hemostatic defect.

○ **What are some of the systemic effects that accompany chronic renal failure?**

There is altered hydration status with unpredictable intravascular fluid volume. Systemic hypertension, congestive heart failure and attenuated sympathetic nervous system (SNS) activity are often seen. Chronic anemia due to decreased erythropoietin production and depression of the bone marrow by uremic toxins results in increased CO and shifts the oxyhemoglobin dissociation curve to the right. In addition, there is increased susceptibility to infection, as there is decreased activity of phagocytes. Most chronic renal failure patients succumb to sepsis. Pathophysiology of uremic pruritus is poorly understood.

○ **What percentage of the filtered sodium is reabsorbed by the renal tubules?**

Of the 25,000 mEq sodium filtered each day, 65% is reabsorbed in the proximal tubule, 25% is actively reabsorbed in the ascending LOH and 9% by the distal tubule under aldosterone regulation. Only 1% of the filtered sodium is excreted in the urine.

○ **How does urinary sodium measurement reflect renal tubular function in the oliguric patient?**

Prerenal oliguria due to reduced renal perfusion is associated with a urinary sodium concentration <20 mEq/L. A urine sodium >40 mEq/L is indicative of intrinsic renal disease.

○ **Describe the countercurrent exchange mechanism and its function in the kidney.**

Countercurrent exchange mechanism is where the incoming and outgoing fluids run parallel and close to each other retaining a high concentration of a dissolved substance at one point in the system.

Juxtamedullary nephrons have LOH that course deep into the medulla. These loops participate in the countercurrent exchange mechanism with the counterflow arrangement of the vasa recta, and make possible formation of highly concentrated urine.

○ **What are juxtamedullary nephrons?**

Each kidney consists of cortex and medulla.

The cortex of the kidney is made up primarily of glomeruli and proximal and distal convoluted tubules.

The medulla is subdivided into an inner and an outer layer and includes the LOH and collecting ducts. Nephrons are grouped by location of their glomeruli into cortical and juxtamedullary types.

○   **Describe the renal blood flow (RBF) physiology.**

RBF = 25% of the CO or 1 L/min.

GFR = 10% of RBF (or 15% of renal plasma flow [RPF]).

The kidneys are the most highly perfused major organ of the body, only 0.4% of body weight, but receive 25% of the CO. Eighty to 90% of RBF goes to cortical nephrons (short LOH), and only 10–15% to juxtamedullary nephrons (larger glomeruli and long LOH). The glomerular capillary network is the filtering apparatus. At the distal end, efferent arterioles dip into the corticomedullary junction to form the vasa recta that surround the collecting tubules. The vasa recta, which play an important role in generating the countercurrent mechanism, receive <1% of the RBF.

The medulla receives only 6% of the RBF and medullary hypoxia is present under normal conditions due to high rate of O_2 consumption. Normal O_2 extraction in the outer medulla is the highest in the body, and is about 79%, which is more than the heart (65%). Medullary thick ascending LOH is especially vulnerable to hypoxic as well as nephrotoxic injury.

In the outer cortex, adenosine induces vasoconstriction by stimulation of adenosine A1 receptors. In the deep juxtamedullary zone, nitric oxide and endogenous prostaglandins promote vasodilation. The net effect is diversion of blood flow to the hypoxic medulla as much as possible. The NSAIDs (prostaglandin synthesis inhibitors) can inhibit this process and cause medullary hypoxia.

However, the low medullary blood flow and countercurrent O_2 escape due to parallel arrangement of entering and exiting capillaries is essential to create and maintain urea gradient to concentrate urine.

○   **Are NSAIDs bad for kidney function?**

Unless there is a massive overdose, usually NSAID causes problems only in patients with coexisting renal problems (advanced age, hypovolemia, CHF, sepsis, major surgery).

Ketorolac causes ischemic acute renal failure in critically ill and elderly, even with a single dose.

○   **How does cyclosporin affect renal function?**

It causes renal injury partly through induction of sympathetic hyperactivity, and renal vasoconstriction.

○   **How does the kidney preserve stable blood flow over the physiologic range of MAP?**

Autoregulation preserves stable blood flow to the kidney over a range of arterial blood pressures. The RBF is regulated by vascular smooth muscle tone. For example, anesthesia may decrease RBF by dropping CO or MAP. However, autoregulation works to preserve RBF by decreasing renal vascular resistance as MAP decreases. This occurs in normal and denervated kidneys over a range of 60–160 mm Hg. Outside the autoregulatory limits, RBF becomes pressure dependent. Glomerular filtration generally ceases when mean systemic arterial pressure is less than 40–50 mm Hg.

○   **Autoregulation of the kidney is based on what mechanisms?**

The mechanisms are based on the myogenic response (MR) and tubuloglomerular feedback (TGF). MR refers to the ability of smooth muscle to contract in response to a stretching force. Tubuloglomerular mechanism is involved in constriction of the afferent arteriole in response to increases in sodium chloride concentration in the early distal tubule, which itself is a function of tubular flow rate. A third mechanism is believed to exist, which is independent of TGF and slower than MR.

○ **How is RBF determined?**

It is most commonly measured by para-aminohippurate (PAH) clearance, which at low concentrations is assumed to be cleared by filtration and secretion in one pass through the kidney. Therefore, RPF = clearance of PAH = ([PAH]urine/[PAH]plasma) × urine flow.

Knowing the hematocrit allows RBF calculation by: RBF = RPF/(1 − Hct).

○ **Can RBF be accurately determined in a hypovolemic patient?**

No. There are several instances where PAH clearance does not accurately reflect GFR. Hypovolemia is one such instance, as the kidney will sequester PAH. Other inaccuracies are engendered by too high a plasma concentration of PAH, proximal tubule deterioration, and oliguria.

○ **How is GFR calculated?**

In the absence of the polysaccharide inulin that is filtered but neither secreted nor absorbed, CrCl will reflect GFR and is calculated as:

$$CrCl = \frac{[creatinine]urine}{[creatinine]plasma} \times \text{urine flow rate}$$

An alternate formula that can provide an estimate when only a single plasma creatinine value is known is as follows:

$$\text{Male CrCl} = \frac{(140 - age) \times \text{lean body weight}}{72 \times [creatinine]plasma}$$

The product of this equation needs to be multiplied by 0.85 to accurately estimate female GFR.

○ **What is the filtration fraction?**

It is the amount of RPF that is actually filtered by the glomerulus.

It can be simply stated as: FF = GFR/RPF.

○ **Why is a normal serum creatinine still consistent with impaired renal function, especially in the elderly?**

Serum creatinine concentrations are dependent on dietary protein intake and muscle tissue turnover. Elderly people have less muscle mass and thus lower serum creatinines. Creatinine is freely filtered at the glomerulus with minimal secretion in the distal tubule and no reabsorption. Because of the wide ranges of normal for serum creatinine, a 50% increase may still be within the normal range yet represent a significant reduction in glomerular filtration rate that will not be recognized unless a baseline value is known or a formal CrCl study is performed.

○ **What degree of nephron loss and fall in CrCl is associated with uremia?**

The loss of 95% of functioning nephrons. The full manifestations of the uremia syndrome are seen only after the GFR decreases below 25 mL/min. Patients with clearances below 10 mL/min are dependent on dialysis for survival until successfully transplanted.

○ **What level of spinal or epidural blockade is required to suppress the vasoconstrictor response to sympathetic stimulation that results in a reduction in RBF and GFR?**

Neuraxial blockade from the level of T6 and below is required, as sympathetic renal constrictor fibers are derived from T6 to L1 spinal cord segments through the celiac plexus. Sympathetic stimulation occurs secondary to surgical stress, general anesthesia, hypoxia, hypotension, pain, severe bleeding, and strenuous exercise. Aortic cross-clamping below the renal arteries will increase renal vascular resistance despite adequate thoracic epidural blockade.

Resistant hypertension represents a significant challenge in everyday clinical practice. Catheter-based renal sympathetic denervation (RSD) represents an innovative new technique to effectively reduce blood pressure in these patients [Papademetriou et al., 2011. See reference on page 525].

○ **What are the effects of airway pressure and PEEP on renal function?**

PEEP can decrease CO and thus RBF, GFR, and urine output. Renin and aldosterone levels rise but not antidiuretic hormone. These effects are seen at 15 cm H_2O PEEP.

○ **Can hyperventilation cause intraoperative oliguria?**

Hyperventilation increases air trapping and raises intrathoracic pressures. This decreases preload to the heart, decreases left ventricular compliance, and increases right ventricular afterload due to high pulmonary vascular resistance. The decrease in CO likely leads to a baroreceptor-mediated increase in sympathetic outflow, renin production, and subsequent renal vasoconstriction. It is speculated that various hormones also play a role in renal dysfunction: ANP, ADH, aldosterone, prostaglandin, epinephrine, and norepinephrine.

It has been postulated that increased renal vein and inferior vena caval pressure are a cause of decreased venous drainage; however, this is not believed to be clinically significant. Intrarenal redistribution of blood flow from the cortex to the juxtamedullary nephrons has been demonstrated in animal studies but other studies have shown conflicting results.

Finally, activation of inflammatory mediators as a result of ventilator-associated lung injury has recently been speculated to play a role in multiple organ dysfunction.

○ **Can rhabdomyolysis affect renal function?**

Myoglobinuria occurs in the setting of the skeletal muscle breakdown during rhabdomyolysis. Above the renal threshold of 0.5–1.5 mg/dL, myoglobin begins to appear in the urine. At 100 mg/dL, the urine becomes reddish brown.

Myoglobin is nephrotoxic and decreases GFR, resulting in oliguria. The pathogenesis appears to be related to intrarenal vasoconstriction. Myoglobin is absorbed by the renal tubules, where it inhibits nitric oxide, leading to medullary vasoconstriction and ischemia. Nephrotoxicity is compounded by hypovolemia and acidemia. Acidemia is thought to enhance precipitation of pigment in the tubules, with tubular obstruction playing a role in acute renal failure.

○ **What factors predispose to renal failure from myoglobinuria secondary to rhabdomyolysis?**

A low urine pH (<5.6) leads to myoglobin precipitation as ferrihematin in the proximal tubule. Hypovolemia, which causes a low tubular flow, is another risk factor. Both of these contribute to renal failure by promoting tubular obstruction.

○ **What are the problems with renal function and sevoflurane?**

The metabolism of some inhaled anesthetics including sevoflurane produces inorganic fluorides, which can cause high-output renal failure. Fluoride causes injury to the collecting tubules leading to nephrogenic diabetes insipidus. The patients with inorganic fluoride levels of less than 50 μmol/L do not develop renal injury. Clinical studies indicate that with sevoflurane the serum fluoride levels often peak above that level even during surgery of average duration. However, with sevoflurane the serum fluoride levels fall rapidly due to sevoflurane's low blood gas solubility and rapid elimination, and renal toxicity is therefore not expected to occur.

Two factors explain the absence of renal injury with sevoflurane:

1. The duration of systemic increase in fluoride concentration and not the peak concentration determines renal injury.

2. The liver is the primary organ of sevoflurane metabolism. There is minimal renal defluorination of sevoflurane compared with methoxyflurane. It is thought that high intrarenal fluoride from methoxyflurane causes renal toxicity.

Sevoflurane interacts with carbon dioxide absorbent (strong bases) and forms degradation product compound A (an olefin compound), which is shown to be a dose-dependent nephrotoxin in animals. However, the levels found during administration of sevoflurane are far below the toxic level, even with low FGF (1 L/min). Therefore, even under low flow anesthesia sevoflurane does not seem to result in adverse effects in humans.

○ **What are the effects of renal failure on the elimination of vecuronium, atracurium, cisatracurium, and mivacurium?**

The duration of neuromuscular blockade in renal failure is prolonged with vecuronium due to increased elimination half-life and lower plasma clearance. These effects are a consequence of 30% elimination by the kidneys in healthy patients. Atracurium and cisatracurium undergo pH-dependent Hoffman elimination and are not dependent on renal excretion for termination of action. The duration of mivacurium can be prolonged to 10–15 minutes in renal failure, which has been attributed to low plasma pseudocholinesterase levels in uremic patients or in patients presenting after hemodialysis.

○ **What are some physiologic effects of preoperative hemodialysis?**

Hemodialysis can produce significant intravascular fluid volume shifts, resulting in hypovolemia and intraoperative hypotension. A too rapid shift in fluid and electrolytes causes a disequilibrium syndrome featuring weakness, nausea, vomiting, and occasionally convulsions and coma. Because of heparinization, patients are at risk of bleeding. Patients are also at risk of infection.

○ **A chronic renal failure patient requiring regular hemodialysis develops weakness and mild respiratory distress in the postanesthetic care unit. The patient has received vecuronium that has been reversed with neostigmine and atropine in full and appropriate doses. What is the most likely explanation?**

The excretion of cholinesterase inhibitors (neostigmine, pyridostigmine, and edrophonium) is delayed in patients with impaired renal function. This offsets the increased elimination half-life of vecuronium and makes recurarization an unlikely explanation. One should consider an interaction between antibiotics, diuretics and electrolyte disturbances with the muscle relaxant. In addition, mild hypothermia may be a contributory factor in the prolongation of action of any NMB due to slowed metabolic clearance.

○ **What effect does renal failure have on the reversal agents for muscle relaxants?**

Fifty percent of neostigmine and 70% of pyridostigmine and edrophonium are excreted in the urine. Renal failure may prolong the duration of action of these drugs up to 100%.

○   **Is succinylcholine a safe choice in the renal failure patient?**

If the patient has been dialyzed within 8–12 hours and the potassium concentration is normal, then succinylcholine is an appropriate choice. In most cases, renal failure patients are no more susceptible to an exaggerated hyperkalemic response induced by succinylcholine than those with normal renal function (unless they have uremic neuropathy). If the patient is hyperkalemic (the upper limit of normal to proceed with surgery is controversial but stated as 5.5 mEq/L), use of nondepolarizing muscle relaxants minimally dependent on the kidney for elimination would be appropriate (cisatracurium, vecuronium, mivacurium). The concern is that the 0.5–1.0 mEq/L increase temporarily seen after succinylcholine use might push an asymptomatic hyperkalemia into the range where cardiac conduction is affected.

○   **What is the mechanism of renal dysfunction following abdominal aortic aneurysm surgery?**

Contributing factors leading to ATN include intravascular volume depletion, embolization of atherosclerotic debris to the kidneys, and iatrogenic surgical trauma to the renal arteries. Aortic cross-clamping reduces RBF whether above the renal arteries (80–90%) or below (40%). Renal vasoconstriction and intrarenal redistribution of blood flow may account for the deterioration in renal function, but the pathophysiology is unclear. Mannitol, loop diuretics, and renal vasodilators may be used for renal protection, although studies demonstrate little or no benefit.

○   **What are the compensatory mechanisms for systemic hypotension?**

Several interrelated compensatory mechanisms exist:

Autonomic nervous system: Arterial baroreceptors in the carotid sinus and aortic arch survey MAP. They act via the vasomotor center in the brainstem to activate the SNS, releasing epinephrine and norepinephrine, producing increased heart rate and contractility as well as venous and arterial vasoconstriction. Venous baroreceptors located in the right atrium and great veins respond to reduced venous pressure with decreases in heart rate.

Capillary shift mechanisms: Fluid shifts from the interstitium into the central circulation to restore blood volume in response to hypotension. Movement of fluid depends on the balance between capillary hydrostatic pressure, interstitial hydrostatic pressure and colloid osmotic pressure of the plasma (Starling's equation).

Hormonal and renal influence on fluid balance: ADH or vasopressin, released from the posterior pituitary gland, produces vasoconstriction and increased reabsorption of water in the distal collecting ducts of the kidney. While primarily released in response to changes in plasma osmolality, other triggers are decreased central blood volume (via low-pressure atrial receptors) and hypotension (via the carotid baroreceptors).

The renin–angiotensin–aldosterone system: Renin is released in response to hyponatremia, decreased renal perfusion pressure, and ANS stimulation via beta receptors on juxtaglomerular cells. This acts on plasma angiotensinogen to form angiotensin I, which is then converted to angiotensin II by angiotensin-converting enzyme (ACE). Angiotensin II is a powerful direct arterial vasoconstrictor. It also acts on the adrenal cortex to release aldosterone and on the adrenal medulla to release epinephrine. It augments norepinephrine release via presynaptic receptors, thus enhancing SNS tone.

Via the renin–angiotensin–aldosterone system, the kidneys act to increase blood volume by retaining sodium and water reabsorption in the collecting ducts and distal convoluted tubules.

○   **What effect does renin–angiotensin have on blood pressure?**

Renin cleaves angiotensinogen (liver) into the angiotensin I. ACE in the lung and kidney cleaves angiotensin I into the potent vasoconstrictor angiotensin II. It takes about 20 minutes for the renin–angiotensin system to fully exert its effect.

Angiotensin II increases systemic blood pressure at the site of the arteriole. It has 10 times the vasoconstrictor potency at the renal efferent arteriole as it does systemically. Thus, moderate levels of angiotensin II can maintain

GFR even in the face of moderately decreased RBF. Angiotensin II further enhances systemic blood pressure by stimulating NaCl reabsorption by the proximal tubule, ADH secretion by the posterior pituitary, and aldosterone production by the adrenal cortex. Profound hypotension, however, leads to renal decompensation. The kidney ceases its high-energy-consuming transport of sodium in the ischemic renal medulla and switches strategies to decrease GFR. High levels of angiotensin II work toward this end by causing constriction of the glomerular mesangial cells, decreasing ultrafiltration. Angiotensin II also exerts negative feedback control by inhibiting further renin release, stimulating intrarenal prostaglandins, and stimulating ANP release.

○ **How do the different vasodilators used for induced hypotension differ in their effects on RBF?**

The selective DA_1-dopaminergic agonist fenoldopam is capable of providing deliberate hypotension, without any significant decrease in RBF. Nitroglycerin decreases RBF less than sodium nitroprusside, which is associated with renin–angiotensin and sympathetic stimulation. Trimethaphan abolishes autoregulation and causes the greatest decrease in RBF.

○ **What are the complications of lithotripsy?**

The complications of lithotripsy vary depending on the technique. Any of the techniques can cause renal parenchymal damage and bleeding with subsequent postoperative urine outflow obstruction. Bacteremia and septicemia can also ensue.

Laser lithotripsy raises specific concerns for ureter mucosal damage or perforation with the rather sharp wire over which the laser is transmitted. Eye damage can occur from stray laser energy.

Percutaneous lithotripsy can result in perforation of bowel or great vessels. Patients are subject to all the risks of a prone patient, including loss of airway, blindness, neuropathy, and positioning-induced ischemia to the nose, breasts, or genitalia. As the surgical site is near the diaphragm, pneumothorax is a possibility.

ESWL can induce cardiac dysrhythmia (10–14%), fatal pulmonary hemorrhage, hypotension, bony fracture, and flank ecchymosis or hematoma. It can trigger congestive heart failure. Epidural space localisation using a 'loss of resistance to saline' technique is recommended, in order to avoid the possible risk of damage to the spinal cord and emerging nerves (due to the presence of an air-water interface) [Abbott et al., 1985. See reference on page 525]. It can cause orthopedic implant or pacemaker destruction and inappropriate AICD firing. It could even cause fetal demise or AAA rupture in the poorly selected patient.

○ **What level of regional anesthesia is required for extracorporeal shock wave lithotripsy (SWL)?**

A T6 sensory level assures adequate anesthesia, as renal innervation is derived from T6 to L4.

○ **What concerns are there following a regional technique for extracorporeal SWL?**

The patient may initially become severely hypotensive due to vasodilation from the regional technique, compounded transiently by the warm water of the bath. On the other hand, hydrostatic pressure from the water bath on the legs and abdomen causes a redistribution of venous blood centrally, as well as a hydrostatically mediated increase in SVR. As a result, arterial blood pressure is likely to stabilize. The sudden increase in central venous volume, however, can precipitate congestive heart failure in patients with marginal cardiac reserve. When the patient leaves the bath, the compressive effects of the bath are lost and the blood pressure again falls. If an epidural technique with loss of resistance to air is used and a large volume of air injected, this air can provide an interface for energy absorption that can result in epidural tissue damage. Foam tape used to secure epidural catheters should be clear of the blast path as this tape can absorb up to 80% of the shock wave energy and result in a failed lithotripsy.

○   **What is the importance of the EKG during extracorporeal SWL?**

There is a risk of cardiac dysrhythmias due to the discharge of shock waves independent of the cardiac cycle. To minimize this problem the EKG is coupled to the lithotripsy so that the shock waves are triggered by the R wave of the EKG. Therefore, it is important that a good reliable EKG signal is obtained preferably with waterproof EKG electrodes. Shock wave–induced cardiac arrhythmias occur in 10–14% of patients undergoing lithotripsy despite the fact that shock waves are synchronized with the patient's ECG and are delivered in the refractory period of the cardiac cycle. These arrhythmias are believed to be due to mechanical stresses on the conduction system exerted by the shock waves and can manifest as PACs, PVCs, atrial fibrillation, or SVT. EKG artifact during ESWL is also common.

○   **What are the absolute contraindications to extracorporeal SWL?**

Pregnancy, untreated bleeding disorders, and abdominal pacemakers are the only absolute contraindications to extracorporeal SWL. Orthopedic instrumentation and abdominal aortic aneurysms are acceptable as long as they are not in the blast path.

○   **What is TURP syndrome?**

Transurethral prostatic resection syndrome. Acute hyponatremia and cerebral edema resulting from excessive absorption of irrigating fluid cause restlessness, agitation, confusion, seizures, and coma. Fluid overload may result in hypertension and bradycardia. Hypotension, widened QRS and ventricular ectopy, pulmonary edema, congestive heart failure, and cardiac arrest may result. Hemolysis, septicemia, glycine toxicity with visual disturbances, and air embolus can be associated.

○   **A patient is undergoing a TURP under spinal anesthesia and becomes disorientated and hypertensive, 1 hour into the case. What is your next step?**

Ensure adequate oxygenation, ventilation, and patency of the airway. Inform the surgeon of the change in the patient's mental status. Treatment consists of administering diuretics and fluid restriction, cautery of open venous sinuses, and rapid completion of the surgical resection. Retarding further fluid absorption by lowering the height of the irrigant is prudent. Nitroglycerine can be employed as a temporary measure to treat excessive preload. Check serum sodium levels and treat accordingly.

○   **Can you use normal saline for irrigation during TURP?**

Electrolyte solutions cannot be used because they disperse the electrocautery current.

Water has excellent visibility, but hypotonicity lyses red blood cells. Significant absorption leads to water intoxication.

○   **What determines the absorption of irrigating solution in transurethral resection of the prostrate?**

The following principles govern the amount of irrigating solution: (1) the height of the container of irrigating solution above the surgical table determines the hydrostatic pressure driving fluid into prostatic veins and sinuses (it is recommended to have a height <30 cm above OR table, 15 cm above for the final stage of resection); (2) the duration of surgical time for resection is proportional to the quantity of fluid that is absorbed. On an average 10–30 mL of fluid is absorbed per minute of resection time, with as much as 6–8 L absorbed in some cases lasting up to 2 hours. Whether patients suffer complications as a result of absorption of irrigating fluid depends on the amount and type of fluid absorbed.

○ **What are the current concerns of irrigating fluids for TURP?**

The problem associated with the absorption of large volumes of irrigating solution, *overhydration, still remains.*

Incidence of *severe CNS problems associated with extreme hyponatremia, such as convulsions and coma, has been reduced.*

Replacement of distilled water with *nearly isosmotic solutions (sorbitol, glycine) has eliminated hemolysis and its sequelae* as a complication of TURP.

○ **What happens if the serum sodium falls below 100 mEq/L?**

Loss of consciousness, seizures, arrhythmias, hypotension, pulmonary edema, and cardiovascular collapse can occur.

○ **What is the cause of transient blindness after transurethral resection of the prostate?**

Systemic absorption of glycine.

Glycine is a nonessential amino acid that has a distribution similar to γ-aminobutyric acid, one of the inhibitory neurotransmitters. It has been suggested that glycine also is a major inhibitory transmitter acting in the spinal cord, brainstem, and retina. In addition, absorption of glycine may result in CNS toxicity as a result of its oxidative biotransformation to ammonia. Blood ammonia levels as high as 500 μM have been detected. Deterioration of CNS function is said to occur when ammonia levels exceed 150 μM. In a prospective study examining glycine metabolism, blood ammonia levels were increased postoperatively in 12 of 26 patients in whom 1.5% glycine levels were also measured. Of interest, glycine and ammonia levels did not correlate; in fact, the opposite relationship was prevalent. Furthermore, high ammonia levels were not necessarily associated with CNS symptoms of toxicity.

○ **What is the management of TURP syndrome?**

Prompt management is required.

- Ensure adequate oxygenation and ventilation. Provide circulatory support as needed.
- Consider invasive monitors if cardiovascular instability present.
- Terminate surgery as soon as possible.
- Laboratory studies: electrolytes, creatinine, glucose, and arterial blood gases.
- Obtain a 12-lead electrocardiogram.
- Mild hyponatremia ($Na^+ > 120$ mEq/L): fluid restriction and loop diuretic. Severe hyponatremia ($Na^+ < 120$ mEq/L): 3% sodium chloride IV at <100 mL/h. Discontinue when serum $Na^+ > 120$ mEq/L. Rate of rise of sodium should not be >12 mEq/L over 24 hours.

○ **What are some of the bleeding complications associated with a TURP?**

A hypertrophied prostate is highly vascular and operative bleeding could be significant (2–5 mL/min of resection time, 20–50 mL/g of prostate). Abnormal bleeding after TURP occurs in less than 1% of cases. The coagulopathy is deemed by some to be due to systemic fibrinolysis caused by prostatic release of plasminogen activator, which converts plasminogen into plasmin. Others believe that the bleeding diathesis is secondary to DIC triggered by the systemic absorption of resected prostate tissue, which is thromboplastin rich. If primary fibrinolysis is suspected, an intravenous bolus and infusion of aminocaproic acid may be an effective antidote.

○ **What level of spinal anesthesia is desirable for a TURP?**

An anesthetic level to T10 is necessary. A spinal anesthetic provides adequate anesthesia for the patient and good relaxation of the pelvic floor and the perineum for the surgeon. The signs and symptoms of water intoxication and fluid overload can be recognized early in an awake patient. An anesthetic level above T10, however, may delay the recognition of a bladder perforation.

○ **What symptoms may be associated with bladder perforation during TURP?**

Bladder perforation during TURP is a relatively common complication approximately 0.7% incidence [Hahn et al., 1993. See reference on page 525] and may result in the urologist noting a diminished return of irrigating fluid. Most bladder perforations are extraperitoneal and occur during difficult resections with the cutting loop, knife electrode, or resectoscope tip, although others can occur from bladder overdistension with irrigation fluid. An extraperitoneal perforation typically results in pain in the periumbilical, inguinal, or suprapubic region. An intraperitoneal perforation may cause back pain or referred pain to the upper abdomen, the precordium, or the shoulder. Other signs and symptoms may include pallor, sweating, abdominal rigidity, nausea and vomiting. The differential diagnosis for such symptomatology is broad and can range from myocardial ischemia or infarction to abdominal aneurysmal leak or rupture to tension pneumothorax. Epidural hematoma might be suspected with severe back pain and a working spinal block. Less critical considerations could range from acute appendicitis or cholecystitis to gastritis or peptic ulcers.

○ **What are the contraindications to robotic prostatectomy?**

Relative contraindications to robotic prostatectomy include:

- Previous radiation
- Morbid obesity
- Previous androgen deprivation (hormone) therapy
- Large-volume prostate
- Previous endoscopic or open prostate surgery
- Previous abdominal surgery
- Previous history of intra-abdominal infection or ruptured viscera
- Previous hernia repair

○ **Describe laser resection of the prostate and its advantage over TURP.**

This new clinical approach to treating benign prostatic hypertrophy (BPH) is termed "holmium laser resection of the prostate."

Potassium-titanyl-phostate (KTP) laser is another advancement.

Advantages:

1. Decreased amount of irrigation solution required, decreased bladder pressures, and improved hemostasis result in less absorption of irrigant solution.

2. It is irrelevant whether irrigant can conduct electricity, so normal saline may be used. This avoids osmotic complications of absorbing large amounts of glycine, mannitol, and sorbitol.

3. Case may be done under GA or IV sedation (no TURP syndrome).

○ **What are the particular complications of laparoscopy associated with urogenital surgery?**

While unintentional extraperitoneal insufflation can always occur in laparoscopic cases, genitourinary surgery often intentionally demands such extravasation of gases. This carries additional risk of CO_2 subcutaneous emphysema. The large retroperitoneal area has facile communication with the thorax and can extend via the subcutaneous tissue to the head and neck. Postoperative pharyngeal swelling from submucosal CO_2 can lead to airway compromise. The large surface area exposed can lead to marked acidosis. Postoperative oliguria may be caused by increased perirenal pressure from the insufflated gas.

Key Terms

Acute renal failure: tests
Acute renal impairment
Acute tubular necrosis: diagnosis
Anesthesia for shock wave lithotripsy (SWL)
Arrhythmias during extracorporeal SWL
Contrast CT: renal function preservation
ESRD: preoperative laboratory abnormalities
Evaluation of postoperative oliguria
Hemodialysis: effects
Hormone response to hypovolemia
Hypotension: compensatory mechanisms
Intraoperative oliguria: hyperventilation
Intraoperative oliguria: management
Lithotripsy: complication
Mechanism of action of angiotensin
Oliguria: hormone etiology
Perioperative/postoperative oliguria: cause/treatment/
   endocrine causes

Postoperative ATN: differential diagnosis
Preoperative renal failure: predictors
Prerenal oliguria: laboratory evaluation/diagnosis/
   treatment
Renal blood flow physiology
Renal failure: electrolytes
Renal function: hormonal regulation of osmolality
Renal function: perioperative preservation
Renal insufficiency: diagnosis
Renal insufficiency: hyperkalemia
Renal perfusion
Renin–angiotensin cardiovascular physiology
Rhabdomyolysis: oliguria
Robotic prostatectomy: contraindications
TURP syndrome: treatment

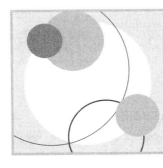

Geriatric Patients

I intend to live forever, or die trying.
Groucho Marx

○ **T/F: The American Society of Anesthesiologists (ASA) physical status classification takes into consideration the age of the patient.**

False. The ASA classification is a preoperative physical status classification of patients taking into consideration severity of systemic disease, functional limitations, and the need to proceed as elective or emergency surgery.

○ **The response of an elderly patient to premedication is unpredictable. Why?**

Doses of narcotics and benzodiazepines should be reduced 20–40% in elderly patients. Contributing factors include an increase in CNS sensitivity, decrease in volume of distribution, and decrease in liver blood flow producing high initial plasma levels and prolonged drug effects. Narcotic administration may produce apnea and episodic respiration, predisposing to airway obstruction.

○ **What happens to the elimination half-life ($t_{1/2}$) of benzodiazepines in the elderly?**

The $t_{1/2}$ of midazolam is almost doubled when compared with younger adults. The $t_{1/2}$ of diazepam increases with age. A rule of thumb is that the $t_{1/2}$ of diazepam in hours equals the patient's age in years.

○ **Even though anesthetic agents such as propofol, methohexital, ketamine, and etomidate are eliminated by hepatic metabolism, the clinical effects of these drugs are not significantly prolonged in the elderly. Why?**

For induction doses, the termination of the clinical effects of these drugs occurs when they are redistributed from the vessel-rich organs to vessel-poor groups. Once redistribution sites are saturated with larger doses or prolonged infusions, metabolism does affect clinical length of action.

○ **T/F: The induction dose of barbiturates should be reduced in elderly patients because their CNS is more sensitive to the hypnotic action of these drugs.**

False. The induction dose of barbiturates should be reduced, but for pharmacokinetic and not pharmacodynamic reasons. A smaller initial volume of distribution and altered distribution of cardiac output result in a slower intercompartmental transfer and redistribution of the drug from the central compartment. This results in apparent drug sensitivity due to a transiently higher initial plasma concentration of the injected drug.

○   **T/F: Propofol causes less hypotension in the elderly when compared with younger adults.**

False. Hypotension is more marked in the elderly. Termination of clinical drug effect depends on the rate constant for intercompartmental drug transfer, similar to thiopental. The induction dose should be reduced by 20–40% in elderly patients, and administered slowly. Remember: "Start low and go slow."

○   **Compare and contrast the cardiovascular effects of thiopental and propofol in the elderly.**

Thiopental IV produces peripheral vasodilation with a moderate reduction in blood pressure. In the elderly patient with a diminished baroreceptor reflex and increased vascular wall stiffness, thiopental can cause a significant hypotension. As a result of an increased volume of distribution at steady state, the elimination half-life of thiopental is twice as long in the elderly (13–25 hours) as compared with the young patient. In addition, the thiopental dosage requirement decreases 25–75% in the geriatric patient and it may take longer to induce unconsciousness.

In the elderly patient the induction dose of propofol is half that of the younger patient. Propofol clearance is reduced in the elderly patient, resulting in reduced dose requirements for maintenance. The cardiovascular depression seen with propofol is greater than that seen with thiopental. These effects can be minimized if propofol is injected slowly.

○   **How is the speed of anesthetic induction affected by aging?**

Intravenous induction is prolonged in the presence of reduced cardiac output that increases arm–brain circulation time. In contrast, inhalational induction may be faster than in young adults, because a decrease in cardiac output results in decreased anesthetic uptake, faster increase in alveolar anesthetic partial pressures, and a greater percentage of cardiac output going to the brain.

○   **Do anesthetic requirements increase or decrease with aging?**

The minimum alveolar concentration (MAC: minimum alveolar concentration of an inhaled anesthetic) decreases 4–5% each decade after the age of 40 years. ED_{50} (median effective dose of an intravenous drug) is also reduced. The physiologic basis for these changes is multifactorial.

○   **What are the physiologic reasons for a decrease in MAC with age?**

The reasons include an increase in body fat, decrease in cardiac output, decreased rate of drug clearance, reductions in metabolism, and a generalized atrophy of the organ systems, especially the CNS.

○   **T/F: The dose of succinylcholine should be reduced in the elderly.**

Some elderly men demonstrate an increased sensitivity to succinylcholine due to reduced plasma cholinesterase enzyme activity and therefore require a dose reduction. In most elderly patients the impact is clinically insignificant.

○   **How are the pharmacokinetic profiles of nondepolarizing muscle relaxants altered in the elderly?**

Decreased volume of distribution (reduced skeletal muscle mass) and reduced clearance.

Nondepolarizing muscle relaxants are required in about the same quantity in elderly and younger patients to provide the same degree of paralysis, but their duration of action is prolonged if they require hepatic or renal elimination and/or biotransformation. Antagonism of neuromuscular blockade with neostigmine is not altered, but the incidence of arrhythmias is higher in the elderly with cardiovascular disease.

○ **How does the pharmacokinetics of rocuronium differ between young and elderly patients?**

Elderly patients have a similar speed of IV onset, but a prolonged duration of action attributed to decreased hepatic clearance. The pharmacodynamic effects of rocuronium do not differ between these two age groups [Zeeh and Platt, 2002. See reference on page 525].

○ **Are elderly patients more sensitive to the effects of opioids?**

Yes. Pharmacodynamic changes are primarily responsible for the increased potency of opioids in the elderly. In addition, reduced central volume of distribution and clearance produce a high peak plasma concentration after a bolus dose and prolonged drug effect. Dose requirements should be reduced 30–50%.

○ **What is the most important physiologic effect of aging on the heart of a healthy patient?**

Aging makes patients volume-dependent yet volume-intolerant due to an increase in cardiac chamber stiffness (decrease in ventricular compliance) such that hemodynamic function is optimal only within a narrow range of end-diastolic pressure and volume.

Additional functional changes include decreased arterial compliance, reduction of maximal cardiac output due to reduction of maximal heart rate, and prolongation of time required for both myocardial contraction and relaxation.

○ **How is the myocardium affected by aging?**

Reduced elasticity in the peripheral vasculature causes increased afterload and leads to left ventricular hypertrophy, dilation of the aorta, and elevated systolic blood pressure. This thickening and stiffening of the heart results in loss of contractility and adversely affects diastolic relaxation. The role of atrial contraction in ventricular filling becomes increasingly important, with the onset of atrial fibrillation adversely affecting cardiac output. Disturbances in cardiac rhythm are associated with fibrosis of the sinoatrial node, atrophy of conduction pathways, and loss of normal pacemaker cells. Common findings include sick sinus syndrome, left anterior hemiblock, bundle branch blocks, and supraventricular and ventricular ectopic beats.

Changes in autonomic function leave the elderly in a state of *physiologic beta-blockade*. Patients have reduced chronotropic and inotropic response to beta-adrenergic agonists, lower maximal heart rates in response to stress, and diminished heart rate response to hypotension.

○ **How is cardiac output affected by aging?**

Elderly patients who exercise regularly and maintain their skeletal muscle mass show little or no change in cardiac output at rest and during moderate exercise. Maximal cardiac output does decrease 1% per year after age 30 years due to a progressive decrease in maximum heart rate.

Aging produces ventricular hypertrophy and diastolic dysfunction; therefore, cardiac output is more dependent on the atrial contribution to ventricular filling. The elderly increase cardiac output by increasing stroke volume (Frank–Starling mechanism) rather than increasing heart rate or by stimulation of β-adrenergic agonists.

○ **How does aging affect heart rate and blood pressure?**

Maximal heart rate and α_1-adrenergic responsiveness is decreased. Systolic blood pressure is increased and diastolic blood pressure is unchanged or reduced producing a widening of the arterial pulse pressure.

○ **Are systemic and pulmonary vascular resistance affected by advancing age?**

SVR and PVR are elevated due to decreased elasticity and arterial compliance.

○ **Is β-adrenergic receptor sensitivity increased or decreased in the elderly?**

β-Adrenergic responsiveness is reduced to both agonists and antagonists, the so-called endogenous "β-blockade of aging." The receptor density is unchanged.

○ **What is the cause of a slow heart rate response to hypotension in the elderly?**

This reflects the slower autonomic reflex responses.

○ **What EKG findings should lead to further investigation in an elderly patient prior to elective surgery?**

Left anterior bundle branch block, atrioventricular conduction delays, and atrial flutter or fibrillation suggest underlying cardiac disease and require further investigation. Disturbances in cardiac rhythm associated with aging and not necessarily indicative of pathology include sick sinus syndrome, right bundle branch block (RBBB), and premature ventricular and supraventricular beats.

○ **What percentage of myocardial infarctions in the elderly are "silent?"**

Almost 50% [Woon and Lim, 2003. See reference on page 525]. Elderly patients with EKG findings that support the diagnosis of ischemic heart disease and those with decreased exercise tolerance for unclear reasons or with unreliable histories should be referred for further cardiac evaluation.

○ **Is the presence of peripheral vascular disease a predictor of coronary artery disease in the elderly?**

Yes. The incidence of cardiovascular disease is 50–65% in the elderly, and may be found in patients who are completely symptom-free. Another significant predictor is the presence of cerebrovascular disease.

○ **How do elderly patients increase their cardiac output in response to exercise?**

By increasing stroke volume (Frank–Starling mechanism) rather than increasing heart rate or stimulation of β-adrenergic agonists.

○ **A 69-year-old, otherwise healthy patient with no significant past medical history is scheduled for repair of an inguinal hernia. He has good exercise tolerance, but a routine 12-lead EKG shows a RBBB. What further cardiac evaluation is indicated?**

None. An isolated RBBB in an elderly patient, who is otherwise asymptomatic, does not appear to be associated with an increased incidence of cardiac disease. Further evaluation would be justified if there were Q waves or evidence of prior myocardial infarction, left anterior hemiblock, atrioventricular conduction delays, and atrial flutter or fibrillation.

○ **A 74-year-old patient with a history of non-insulin-dependent diabetes mellitus is scheduled for peripheral vascular surgery. He has a normal resting EKG. Does he need further cardiac evaluation?**

The 2007 ACC/AHA guidelines [See reference on page 525] stipulate that relatively few patients will benefit from advanced preoperative testing. This patient has no active cardiac conditions (unstable coronary syndrome, decompensated heart failure, significant arrhythmias, or severe valvular disease). He has one clinical risk factor: diabetes mellitus. The clinical risk factors are history of ischemic heart disease, history of compensated or prior heart failure, history of cerebrovascular disease, diabetes mellitus, and renal insufficiency.

According to the guidelines, if a patient with one or two clinical risk factors is to undergo one of the high-risk surgeries (aortic and other major vascular surgery or peripheral vascular surgery), it is reasonable to proceed with planned surgery with heart rate control or consider noninvasive testing if it changes the management.

○ **What techniques can be utilized to reduce perioperative MI in the geriatric patient?**

Preoperative beta-blockade that is continued into the intraoperative and postoperative periods has been shown to decrease perioperative MI [2009 ACCF/AHA Focused Update on Perioperative Beta Blockade. See reference on page 525]. Thorough evaluation of cardiac function is required looking for evidence of ischemic heart disease. Continue all cardiac medications throughout the perioperative period. The goal of anesthesia is to maintain the balance between myocardial O_2 supply and demand throughout the perioperative period. The most sensitive ECG lead for detecting ischemia is V_5. Transesophageal echocardiography will detect regional wall motion abnormalities and is the most sensitive monitor for myocardial ischemia.

○ **What are the predominant changes in the respiratory system in the elderly patient?**

Decreased lung volumes and reduced gas exchange, with a decrease in resting PaO_2.

The PaO_2 is decreased and the alveolar–arterial oxygen gradient is increased primarily due to mismatching of ventilation and perfusion and reduced alveolar surface area. There is a reduction in the efficiency of gas exchange.

Breakdown of alveolar septae reduces total alveolar surface area, increasing both anatomic and alveolar dead space. This disrupts the normal matching of ventilation and perfusion, increasing both physiologic shunting and dead space.

○ **What is the effect of aging on FRC and CC?**

Both FRC and CC increase with age, but CC increases to a greater extent until they overlap at 44 years of age (supine) and 66 years of age (standing). When CC >FRC, airway closure occurs during normal tidal breathing leading to air trapping and uneven inhaled gas distribution.

○ **What changes are seen in the pulmonary function tests (PFTs)?**

Changes in PFTs include increased residual volume, FRC, CC, and dead space. VC is progressively reduced as residual volume increases, with TLC remaining relatively unchanged (10% reduction by age 80) unless physical stature is reduced.

Chest wall mechanics is altered due to fibrosis and calcification of the rib cage and declining respiratory muscle strength. Diminished elastin and an increase in connective tissue reduce elastic recoil of the lungs. There is an increase in lung compliance; however, total pulmonary compliance changes are minimal.

○ **What is the effect of age on ventilatory response to imposed hypoxia and hypercarbia?**

In the elderly the ventilatory responses to hypoxia and hypercapnia are markedly reduced in the awake state. These patients are at increased risk for apnea, episodic respiration, and airway obstruction in the recovery room. In addition, there is a general loss of muscle mass in the airways resulting in a reduced responsiveness of protective airway reflexes with increased risk of aspiration.

○ **How would you calculate the expected PaO_2 and A–a gradient for a given age?**

PaO_2 (mm Hg) = 110 − (age × 0.4); A–a gradient = (age/4) + 4; $PaCO_2$ changes very little with age because CO_2 is 20 times more diffusible than O_2.

○ **How does the oxyhemoglobin curve change with advancing age?**

The curve shifts slightly to the left as age increases, resulting in a lower PaO_2 at a given SpO_2. The p50, which is normally 27 mm Hg, may drop to the low 20s by age 80.

○ **Why is aspiration pneumonitis a common complication in the elderly during debilitating illness and in the postoperative period?**

Decreased airway reflexes, swallowing disorders, delayed gastric emptying, residual drug effects, and postoperative delirium (metabolic or subclinical neurologic disease) increase the patient's risk of aspiration.

○ **What changes occur in the kidneys with aging?**

The kidneys become smaller with age. Glomerulosclerosis results in a progressive reduction of renal mass, with as much as 30% lost by the age of 70 years. Consequently, there is a reduction in both renal blood flow (RBF) and glomerular filtration rate (GFR). RBF decreases 10% per decade in the adult years with relative sparing of the renal medulla. GFR decreases at the rate of approximately 1 mL/min per 1.73 m^2 per year or 1–1.5% per year. Creatinine clearance decreases by 1% per year after age 40 and can be estimated using the following equation: creatinine clearance = (140 − age) × weight (kg)/72 × serum creatinine. Serum creatinine levels remain within normal limits despite the reduction in GFR because of reduced muscle mass and less creatinine production.

Elderly patients have a reduced ability to concentrate the urine (less responsive to ADH) and to excrete acid load, with impaired ability to conserve sodium.

○ **In spite of the age-related decline in renal function, the serum creatinine of the elderly remains within normal limits. Why?**

A decrease in skeletal muscle mass leads to decreased production of creatinine that parallels the decline in creatinine clearance.

○ **What is the cause of mild elevations in the serum potassium levels in the elderly?**

Renovascular changes that occur in the juxtaglomerular apparatus cause decline in the production of renin and aldosterone. Functional hypoaldosteronism leads to decreased renal excretion of potassium. This is offset by a loss of lean body mass and reduction in exchangeable potassium.

○ **What are the major complications seen with NSAID use in the elderly population? How can they be avoided?**

Elderly patients are prone to developing NSAID-induced nephrotoxicity or gastropathy. Resolution typically occurs with reduction in the NSAID dose, or possibly complete elimination of the drug. Fortunately, alternative medications (nonacetylated salicylates, acetaminophen, COX-2 inhibitors) offer comparable analgesia without the above-mentioned side effects.

○ **How is cerebral autoregulation of blood flow affected in a healthy elderly patient?**

It is unaffected in the healthy elderly patient.

○ **Summarize the effect of aging on baroreceptor function.**

Advancing age is associated with impairment of baroreflex responsiveness and increased risk of orthostatic hypotension. Baroreceptors are stretch receptors located in the aortic arch and carotid sinus. The decrease in arterial compliance associated with aging can reduce the ability to transduce changes in pressure at the baroreceptors, diminishing the magnitude of the reflex.

○ **Is cerebral autoregulation and the cerebrovascular response to hyperventilation altered in the elderly?**

Both autoregulation of cerebrovascular resistance in response to changes in arterial blood pressure and cerebral vasoconstrictor response to hyperventilation remain largely intact in elderly patients who are free of cerebrovascular disease.

Cerebrovascular autoregulation may however be somewhat impaired, especially in the elderly patient with systolic hypertension. Impaired autoregulation and baroreceptor dysfunction may lead to episodic cerebral hypoperfusion during sleep and in the postprandial period. There may be an association between episodic hypotension, impaired autoregulation, and silent strokes in the elderly.

○ **How are the pharmacokinetics of spinal anesthesia affected by age?**

Anticipate a higher level of spinal anesthesia, with faster onset of action and prolonged duration due to decreased blood flow to the subarachnoid space resulting in slower absorption of anesthetic solutions, increased cephalad spread due to a smaller volume and higher specific gravity of the cerebrospinal fluid, and exaggerated lumbar lordosis or thoracic kyphosis. The incidence of postdural puncture headache is lower.

○ **Are geriatric patients prone to develop exaggerated reductions in blood pressure with spinal anesthesia compared with younger patients?**

Yes. This is due to lower residual inherent vascular tone and lack of adequate compensatory reflexes with reduced adrenergic responsiveness. Age also influences the level of spinal anesthesia, with greater cephalad spread per injected dose, especially when larger volumes of anesthetic solution are used.

○ **Is spinal anesthesia better for the elderly patient's postoperative mental function?**

There may be a benefit if the patient does not receive any sedation.

○ **Are the elderly more prone to hypothermia?**

Yes, primarily due to impaired temperature regulation.

Factors that increase their susceptibility include less insulation due to smaller amounts of subcutaneous tissue, decreased reflex cutaneous vasoconstriction, and decreased heat production (decline in basal metabolic rate by 1% per year after age 30 years).

○ **What are the possible detrimental effects of hypothermia in the elderly?**

Delayed emergence; prolongation of neuromuscular blockade (reduced metabolism), and the effects of inhaled anesthetic agents (decreased MAC); postoperative shivering and tachycardia (increased oxygen consumption, increased myocardial oxygen demand, ischemia, myocardial depression, or ventricular arrhythmia); cold diuresis (hypovolemia); hypoxemia (V/Q mismatch); and impaired coagulation (platelet dysfunction or reduced clotting factor activity). Elderly patients are at risk for hypothermia due to impaired autonomic vascular control.

○ **T/F: Advancing age has a clinically significant adverse effect on liver metabolism.**

False. The liver becomes smaller with age, but has a wide margin of functional reserve. Enzymatic function is preserved, so drug metabolism will be minimally affected given the loss of liver mass and parallel decrease in liver blood flow. There is a slight decrease in the clearance of drugs extensively dependent on first-pass drug extraction.

○   **Does an elderly patient need a larger or a smaller volume of local anesthetic solution injected into the epidural space to achieve the same level of block compared with younger patients? Why?**

Smaller local anesthetic dose.

Segmental dose requirements for epidural anesthetics are reduced with the injection of large volumes resulting in a markedly exaggerated cephalad spread of the solution. Injection of small volumes of local anesthetic solutions produces no significant change. Less compliant epidural space together with diminished adipose tissue may be primarily responsible for age-related changes in epidural dose requirements. Initially, this was thought to be related to decrease in the size of intervertebral foramina and less leakage of epidural medication with increasing age. However, studies have failed to demonstrate a correlation between leakage of radiocontrast material through the intervertebral foramina and age.

○   **How does body composition change with aging?**

Body mass index and the proportion of body fat are increased, skeletal muscle mass is decreased approximately 10%, and there is a reduction in intracellular water, with maintenance of intravascular volume in healthy individuals.

○   **How is energy production changed by the structural changes described above?**

Energy expenditure gradually decreases 1–2% from the ages of 20 to 80 years. Increased levels of norepinephrine reflect increased basal sympathetic activity in the aged; however, sympathetically mediated metabolic responses are blunted. This is seen with the decreased responsiveness of maximal heart rate and β-adrenergic activity. It has been postulated that the elderly's blunted thermogenic response may be a manifestation of this phenomenon and results in increased fat stores. Loss of skeletal muscle results in a decrease in maximal and resting oxygen consumption and diminished production of body heat. Combined with less insulating subcutaneous tissue and diminished reflex cutaneous vasoconstriction to prevent heat loss, body temperature may be difficult to control in older patients.

○   **T/F: You can tell you are growing older when …**

You get winded playing checkers.

Your children begin to look middle-aged.

You look forward to a dull evening.

You know all the answers, but nobody's asking the questions.

You join the health club – and don't go.

You sit in a rocking chair and can't get it going.

Your knees buckle, and your belt won't.

You burn the midnight oil at 9:00 PM.

Dialing long distance wears you out.

Your back goes out more often than you do.

The little gray-haired lady you help across the street is your wife.

You have too much room in the house and not enough in the medicine cabinet.

You sink your teeth into a steak, and they stay there.

Everything hurts, and what doesn't hurt doesn't work.

All of the above.

Key Terms

Age related: p50

Anemia and myocardial ischemia in older patients

Cardiac function in elderly patients

Elderly spirometric volumes

Geriatric anesthesia: pulmonary changes

Geriatric: autonomic function

Geriatrics: muscle relaxants

Geriatrics: NSAID use

Left ventricular function: geriatric

Minimum alveolar concentration (MAC) reduction in elderly: pathophysiology

Normal arterial oxygenation: age

Pharmacology of induction agents in the elderly

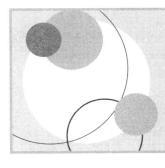

GI Disorders and Obesity

The difficult is that which can be done immediately; the impossible is that which takes a little longer.
George Santayana

○ **Define obesity and morbid obesity.**

Obesity is body weight 20% greater than ideal weight. Morbid obesity is body weight more than two times ideal weight or greater than 100 lb over ideal weight.

○ **Define body mass index (BMI). Is BMI gender specific?**

BMI is independent of gender and defined as the ratio of an individual's weight in kilograms to his or her height in square meters. It is a method of calculating ideal body weight (IBW).

IBW = BMI of 22–28.

$$BMI = \frac{weight\ (kg)}{height\ (m^2)}$$

○ **Define obesity and morbid obesity in terms of BMI.**

The World Health Organization (WHO) defines overweight = 25−29.9 and obesity as >30 (obesity class 1 = 30−34.9; obesity class 2 = 35−39.9; obesity class 3 ⩾40).

Morbid obesity ⩾40 kg/m^2.

○ **Define lean body weight (LBW) and IBW.**

IBW (kg) = height (cm) − x, where x = 100 for adult males and 105 for adult females.

In nonobese patients with a normal muscular build (excluding those with a tremendous increase in muscle mass), total body weight (TBW) should approximate IBW.

LBW is TBW minus adipose tissue. It should approximate 80% of TBW in males and 75% of TBW in females. In morbidly obese patients, LBW can be estimated by increasing IBW by 20−30% [Miller, 2010].

○ **Is an obese patient at greater perioperative anesthetic risk? Why?**

Yes, mostly due to cardiopulmonary morbidity.

1. Associated comorbidities: adult-onset diabetes mellitus, sleep apnea, pulmonary HTN, deep venous thrombosis (DVT), pulmonary embolism, hypothyroidism, Cushing disease, electrolyte abnormalities, fatty liver, cholelithiasis, obesity surgery, or drug therapies.

2. Systemic physiologic changes: pulmonary (hypoxemia, impaired ventilatory response to CO_2), cardiac (hypertension, increased CO and blood volume, CAD, pulmonary hypertension, RVH, LVH, CHF, arrhythmia), GI (aspiration risk, cholelithiasis, fatty liver, or cirrhosis), and unpredictable drug metabolism.

3. Technical challenges: difficult airway and ventilatory management, arterial and venous access, blood pressure monitoring, invasive monitoring, and positioning.

○ **What changes in pulmonary volumes and function tests are associated with morbid obesity?**

The pulmonary function tests of obese patients show a restrictive pattern. Lung volumes are decreased including functional residual capacity (FRC), vital capacity, and total lung capacity. The decrease in FRC is mainly due to a decrease in expiratory reserve volume. Tidal volume and residual volume remain unchanged. Closing capacity, the volume at which small airways begin to close, remains unchanged; however, the reductions in FRC can lead to lung volumes below closing capacity and subsequent increased V/Q mismatching and right-to-left shunting. A decrease in lung compliance can be seen as a result of increased pulmonary blood flow due to the overall increase in blood volume. Polycythemia secondary to chronic hypoxia also contributes to decreased pulmonary compliance [Barash et al., 2009]. FEV_1 and maximum midexpiratory flow rate are normal or slightly decreased.

○ **Are oxygen consumption, carbon dioxide production, and basal metabolic rates changed in obesity?**

Total oxygen consumption and carbon dioxide production are increased because metabolic rate is proportional to body weight.

○ **What are the physiologic causes of hypoxemia seen in obese patients?**

As mentioned above, decreases in lung volumes below closing capacity lead to airway closure, atelectasis, V/Q mismatch, and right-to-left shunting. Furthermore, oxygen consumption is increased. Obese patients are prone to hypoventilation and obstructive sleep apnea (OSA). Baseline PaO_2 values in obese patients breathing room air are therefore generally less than similarly aged nonobese patients [Barash et al., 2009].

○ **In obese patients, to what degree is the FRC decreased? How is this affected by anesthesia and patient positioning?**

FRC declines exponentially as BMI increases. This is further exacerbated by the supine and Trendelenburg position. In the anesthetized obese patient, FRC is decreased by 50% compared with 20% for the nonobese patient.

○ **What deleterious physiologic effects may result from supine positioning in the obese patient?**

Acute restrictive lung disease resulting in hypoxemia and hypercarbia; decreased FRC and shorter time to desaturation following apnea and high peak inspiratory airway pressures causing hypoventilation or barotrauma; endobronchial intubation; and reduced preload to the heart (compression of the vena cava or high peak pressures) decreasing cardiac output and worsening ventilation–perfusion mismatch.

○ **Why is the morbidly obese patient at risk for hypoxemia following induction of anesthesia?**

Morbid obesity is accompanied by hypoxemia due to V–Q mismatching. Changes in lung volumes result in closure of small airways and tidal volumes resting below closing volumes during normal breathing. FRC is greatly decreased, which is further exacerbated by anesthesia and the supine position. Total oxygen consumption is increased due to the large tissue mass. Consequently, following induction of anesthesia, with smaller oxygen stores and greater demands, the onset of hypoxemia can be rapid even in the setting of adequate preoxygenation. In addition, mechanical ventilation may be difficult due to decreased chest wall compliance and cephalad excursion of the diaphragm.

○ **What are the airway considerations for intubation of an obese patient?**

Obesity is a classical predictor of a difficult airway. Airway evaluation should include atlanto-occipital and temporomandibular range of motion, thyromental distance, and visualization of the oral airway. Increased neck fat may limit cervical extension and a shortened distance between the mandible and sternal fat pads may impede laryngoscopy. Maintaining a tight mask fit and manual ventilation may be difficult. The extra tissue within the oropharyngeal cavity may make laryngoscopy and intubation difficult.

○ **Would you perform general anesthesia without endotracheal intubation in an obese patient?**

Intubation is generally required for oxygenation, positive pressure ventilation, and protection of the airway from aspiration.

○ **What alternative to an awake sedated fiber optic intubation would be useful?**

The "awake look" with direct laryngoscopy is a useful practice. Topically anesthetize the mouth, pharynx, and supraglottic area with a local anesthetic solution and then gently introduce a standard laryngoscope and attempt to visualize the epiglottis and possibly arytenoids. If it is possible to see these structures, it is likely that intubation of the trachea following preoxygenation and rapid sequence induction with cricoid pressure can be performed. However, muscle relaxation may lead to loss of pharyngeal tissue support, and lack of visualization can still be a problem even if the "awake look" is reasonable.

○ **If an obese patient is to be intubated, following induction of general anesthesia, what considerations are important?**

Cricoid pressure (Sellick maneuver) should be applied in all cases. Adequate preoxygenation and denitrogenation of the patient using 3 minutes of spontaneous breathing with 100% oxygen should be performed. The availability of a second pair of experienced hands to facilitate two-man ventilation or adjust patient positioning is recommended. Availability of difficult airway devices is prudent.

○ **T/F: OSA in obese adult patients is a risk factor for both difficult mask ventilation and intubation.**

True. High closing pressure of the pharyngeal airway in OSA patients may contribute to difficult mask ventilation. Both obesity (a high Mallampati score, limited mandibular protrusion, and large neck circumference) and craniofacial abnormalities possibly contribute to difficult tracheal intubation.

○ **How is the diagnosis of sleep apnea syndrome confirmed?**

The cardinal symptoms of OSA include the "3 *S*'s": *s*noring, *s*leepiness, and *s*ignificant – other report of apnea episodes during sleep. The STOP-Bang Scoring Model may be used to identify individuals at high or low risk of OSA. The diagnosis of sleep apnea is based on the evaluation of clinical symptoms and of the results of a formal sleep study (polysomnography). A commonly adopted definition of an apnea (for an adult) includes a minimum 10-second interval between breaths, with either a neurological arousal (a 3-second or greater shift in EEG frequency, measured at C3, C4, O1, or O2) or a blood oxygen desaturation of 3–4% or greater, or both arousal and desaturation.

Although OSA occurs in both obese and nonobese people, obesity is considered the greatest risk factor [Miller, 2010].

○ **What causes sleep apnea?**

There are three forms of sleep apnea: central (CSA), OSA, and complex or mixed sleep apnea constituting 0.4%, 84%, and 15% of cases, respectively. In CSA, breathing is interrupted by a lack of respiratory effort; in OSA, breathing is interrupted by a physical block to airflow despite respiratory effort, and snoring is common.

○ **What is the Pickwickian syndrome?**

Pickwickian syndrome is also referred to as obesity-hypoventilation syndrome (OHS). It arises secondary to CNS-mediated apneic events believed to result from chronic OSA. Symptoms include obesity, decreased ventilatory response to CO_2 and O_2, sleep apnea, hypoxemia, hypercarbia, pulmonary hypertension, polycythemia, and biventricular failure; it is evident in 5 – 10% of morbidly obese patients. A BMI over 30 and evidence of arterial hypercapnia ($PaCO_2$ >45) in an awake patient support the diagnosis [Barash et al., 2009]. The term originates from Charles Dickens' portrayal of Joe, the fat, somnolent, red-faced boy in the *Posthumous Papers of the Pickwick Club*, written in 1837. (Good cocktail info, but won't be on the boards.)

○ **What is the relationship between Pickwickian syndrome and body weight?**

Body weight is typically more than 130 kg and, in most cases, a very rapid increase in weight has occurred.

○ **Describe the classic triad of the OHS.**

Obesity, alveolar hypoventilation, and hypersomnolence.

○ **What is the pathophysiology of cor pulmonale in the Pickwickian syndrome?**

Right ventricular hypertrophy and failure results from chronic hypoxemia, hypercarbia, polycythemia, and pulmonary hypertension.

○ **Why is the supine position potentially fatal in the morbidly obese patient?**

There have been reports of sudden cardiac arrest with positional change in morbidly obese surgical patients [Tsueda et al., 1979. See reference on page 525]. The mechanism of cardiovascular collapse was believed to be 3-fold: (a) further decrease in lung volume and vital capacity secondary to high intra-abdominal pressure in the supine position while there was an increase in the ventilation requirement; (b) inability to increase ventilation due to respiratory center dysfunction; (c) inability of the already failing hypoxic myocardium to handle the shift of blood to the central circulation on assuming the supine position.

○ **How can respiratory mechanics be improved postoperatively in obese patients?**

Aside from supplemental oxygen, it has been shown that positioning obese patients in a semirecumbent position (30° head of bed elevation) postoperatively significantly increases the arterial oxygen tension above that seen in the supine position.

○ **What is the effect of morbid obesity on preload, afterload, and cardiac output?**

Cardiac output, blood volume (and therefore preload), and stroke volume increase in proportion to weight gain. Cardiac output increases 100 mL/(min kg) of additional adipose tissue perfused. Systemic hypertension (increased afterload) occurs due to increases in CO and blood volume and the vascular changes inherent in the obese/diabetic patient.

○ **What is the incidence of hypertension and coronary artery disease in the obese patient?**

Systemic hypertension is 10 times more prevalent in morbidly obese patients, moderate in 50% and severe in 5 – 10% of these patients. The incidence of coronary artery disease is doubled compared with the nonobese population [Brown et al., 2000. See reference on page 525].

○ **Which hemodynamic monitors would you choose for the obese patient?**

Noninvasive blood pressure monitoring may be difficult due to a discrepancy between cuff and upper arm size. A small cuff falsely elevates blood pressure readings and a large cuff gives falsely low readings. Intra-arterial pressure measurements may be more accurate and permit arterial blood gas analysis for monitoring ventilatory status. Volume status and myocardial function may be followed with CVP or PAP monitoring or TEE if medical comorbidities warrant their use. A five-lead EKG should be used for detection of ischemia.

○ **What are the indications for use of a pulmonary artery catheter or TEE in an obese patient?**

Evidence of significant cardiovascular disease (LV compromise, pulmonary hypertension, and cor pulmonale), pulmonary dysfunction, or hypoxia is an indication for invasive monitoring if the surgery is complex or will involve significant volume shifts.

○ **Is a preoperative fasting period of 8 hours for solids and milk prior to elective surgery sufficient for an obese patient?**

According to Barash, obese patients who do not suffer from diabetes or symptomatic GERD and are not premedicated should follow the same fasting guidelines as nonobese patients. They should be allowed clear liquids up to 2 hours prior to elective surgery.

However, obese patients are at risk of regurgitation and aspiration due to increased incidence of hiatal hernia, gastroesophageal reflux, gastroparesis, diabetes mellitus, and the potential for difficult airway management.

○ **Describe hepatobiliary disease in the obese patient.**

Fatty infiltration of the liver is typical. This can progress to nonalcoholic fatty liver disease (NAFLD). This fatty infiltration is more related to duration, not degree of obesity [Barash et al., 2009]. Hepatomegaly, inflammation, focal necrosis, and cirrhotic changes may be present. Liver enzymes are generally elevated, most commonly alanine aminotransferase (ALT). Cholelithiasis is commonly associated with obesity.

○ **How does obesity affect the risk of DVT?**

Morbid obesity is an independent risk factor for the development of DVT, pulmonary embolism, and subsequent sudden death. Four risk factors have been associated with an increased risk of postoperative DVT: BMI ≥ 60, venous stasis, truncal obesity, and OHS/OSA. DVT prophylaxis with subcutaneous heparin or low-dose unfractionated heparin in the perioperative period has been shown to decrease the incidence of DVT. If possible, prophylaxis should begin prior to surgery. If contraindicated, an IVC filter should be considered prior to surgery [Barash et al., 2009].

○ **Are obese patients insulated and therefore at less risk of hypothermia?**

No. Cutaneous radiant heat loss depends on exposed body surface area and accounts for 90% of heat loss. Hypothyroidism and hypothalamic lesions may increase the risk of hypothermia.

○ **How is the volume of distribution of drugs affected by obesity?**

According to pharmacokinetic principles, a loading dose is dependent on volume of distribution, V_D, and a maintenance dose should be calculated based on clearance. Obese patients have reduced total body water, increased total body fat and lean body mass, increased cardiac output, blood volume, and splanchnic blood flow.

Highly lipophilic drugs have an increased volume of distribution, with the exception of fentanyl.

○   **How do you calculate the IV dosage of muscle relaxants in the obese patient?**

Nondepolarizing muscle relaxants are ionized compounds that have a volume of distribution equal to that of the extracellular fluid. Since they are hydrophilic, they are poorly distributed to adipose tissue. In obesity, the volume of distribution, elimination half-lives, and clearance for muscle relaxants are not significantly different from those of nonobese individuals. Thus, when dosing nondepolarizing muscle relaxants, the patient's IBW should be used for dose calculations.

The rapid onset and short duration of action makes succinylcholine the neuromuscular blocking agent of choice in morbidly obese patients. Two factors that determine the duration of action of succinylcholine, namely, the pseudocholinesterase level and the amount of extracellular fluid, are increased in the morbidly obese patients. Therefore, a larger dose of succinylcholine based on TBW is recommended to achieve optimal intubating conditions.

○   **How do you calculate sedatives and opioids dosing in obese individuals?**

Morbidly obese patients show exaggerated respiratory depression with opioids and are more susceptible to obstruction of the upper airway and hypoxemia when administered in the perioperative period [Ingrande and Lemmens, 2010. See reference on page 525]. Almost half of the adverse respiratory events secondary to opioids were reported in obese or morbidly obese patients. If opioids are required in this patient population, the dosing should be calculated according to LBW, titrated as needed, and the need for continuous monitoring in a high dependency unit seriously considered.

Thiopental and propofol are commonly used intravenous induction agents. Administration of these agents based on TBW may result in overdose and profound hemodynamic changes in obese patients. When morbidly obese subjects were given propofol based on LBW, they required similar doses and had similar time to hypnosis as lean control subjects given propofol based on TBW.

○   **What are other pharmacokinetic characteristics affected by obesity?**

Hyperlipidemia and increased alpha-1-acid glycoprotein concentrations may affect protein binding, leading to a decreased concentration of free drug. Plasma albumin concentration is unaffected. Drugs undergoing phase 1 metabolism are usually unaffected by obesity, whereas drugs undergoing phase II metabolism are enhanced.

Despite potential alterations in liver function tests and fatty infiltration, hepatic clearance is usually not affected. On the other hand, an increase in renal blood flow, glomerular filtration, and tubular secretion can lead to enhanced renal excretion. Drugs highly dependent on renal excretion may necessitate an increased dose [Barash et al., 2009; Miller, 2010].

○   **How does obesity alter the pharmacokinetic profile of benzodiazepines and barbiturates?**

Benzodiazepines and barbiturates are highly lipophilic and therefore have an increased volume of distribution, more selective distribution to fat stores, and decreased elimination half-life, resulting in lower serum drug concentrations and decreased clearance.

○   **What precautions should be taken with the administration of premedication in morbidly obese patients?**

Preoperative sedation and narcotics should not be given until the patient is in a safely monitored environment. This is particularly true if the patient has a history of OSA, hypoxia, hypercapnia, pulmonary hypertension, or an anticipated difficult airway. Due to the patient's increased risk of aspiration, H_2-receptor antagonists, metoclopramide, and nonparticulate antacid prophylaxis may be prudent.

○ **Is the intramuscular route adequate for the obese patient?**

All drugs should be administered intravenously. Attempts to give intramuscular injections may result in a subcutaneous injection, which leads to unpredictable absorption and drug response.

○ **Do obese patients metabolize inhaled anesthetics differently from nonobese patients?**

Yes. The rate of biotransformation of methoxyflurane, enflurane, and halothane is increased resulting in increased serum levels of fluoride ions, which may be potentially nephrotoxic. This is not seen with isoflurane and desflurane or sevoflurane.

○ **What are the inhalational anesthetic agents of choice in an obese patient?**

Isoflurane, sevoflurane, and desflurane. The potential for inhalational anesthetic agents to cause end-organ injury is primarily dependent on the extent of their liver metabolism. All potentially decrease hepatic blood flow but are relatively safe if the mean arterial blood pressure and cardiac output are maintained. Isoflurane has the least detrimental effect on liver blood flow. A simultaneous decrease in the liver's metabolic demand tends to balance the oxygen supply–uptake ratio. Furthermore, these agents tend to be less fat soluble so residual anesthetic effects are minimized. Desflurane has the lowest fat solubility of the potent agents.

○ **Is nitrous oxide a good choice in obese patients?**

Nitrous oxide is a logical choice for maintaining anesthesia unless high inspired oxygen concentrations are required to prevent hypoxia. N_2O is fat insoluble, rapid in onset and offset. However, N_2O increases pulmonary vascular resistance and may exacerbate RV dysfunction in patients with pulmonary hypertension. In obese patients with COPD, positive pressure ventilation can result in overdistended and possible rupture of alveolar blebs. N_2O should also be avoided in these patients.

○ **Is regional anesthesia safe for the morbidly obese patient?**

Yes. Technical difficulties include layers of adipose tissue obscuring landmarks and necessitating the use of longer needles and positioning difficulties. For peripheral nerve blocks, calculation of local anesthetic solution requirements should take into consideration estimated lean body mass. The potential for a difficult airway or aspiration risk is not circumvented. Cardiovascular and respiratory effects of high spinal may be detrimental to the patient. The patient must be able to tolerate the required surgical positioning. Laparoscopic surgery requires securing the airway due to further increasing elevated gastric pressure and the increased CO_2 load for which the patient may not be able to compensate.

○ **Does obesity affect block height during spinal anesthesia?**

Controversial. Many factors affect block height during spinal anesthesia. The obese patient has decreased subarachnoid compliance, particularly when the patient is in the supine position. Using a hyperbaric spinal technique when the patient is given an injection while sitting and then placed supine may cause cephalad movement of the drug and an unpredictable increase in the height of the block. A reduction of drug dose 20–30% may be prudent. Other authors suggest weight is not related to block height during spinal anesthesia [Miller, 2010].

○ **What are the advantages of combined epidural–general anesthesia in the obese patient?**

Earlier ambulation, reduced risk of DVT, increase in postoperative pulmonary function, and possibly a shorter hospital stay.

○ **What are the postoperative complications associated with morbid obesity?**

Obese patients are at an increased risk of atelectasis from general anesthesia, which can be further enhanced by pain. In the face of preexisting OSA/OHS, they may require BiPAP or CPAP postoperatively. Obese patients are more prone to respiratory depression due to an enhanced sensitivity to opioids. A multimodal approach to postoperative analgesia is recommended, including regional anesthesia and nonopioid analgesics. These patients, as mentioned above, are at an increased risk for DVT. There is an increased risk of surgical site infections [Miller, 2010; Barash et al., 2009].

• • • GI DISORDERS • • •

○ **What are the most common causes of small bowel obstruction?**

Adhesions account for approximately 60% of all small bowel obstructions followed by tumors (20%), hernias (10%), and Crohn's disease (5%). Other causes include intra-abdominal abscess from a ruptured appendix or diverticulum and intussusception [Foster et al., 2006. See reference on page 525].

○ **What is the primary anesthetic goal during induction for a patient with small bowel obstruction?**

Prevent regurgitation and subsequent aspiration of intestinal contents into the trachea and lungs.

○ **Why are patients with small bowel obstruction at high risk for aspiration?**

Risk factors for aspiration include elderly, emergency surgery involving the upper abdomen, and obstruction to gastric and intestinal emptying resulting in large volumes (>0.4 mL/kg) of acidic (pH <2.5) and nonacidic fluids containing bile, particulate, and fecal material.

The small bowel is a secretory organ. Normally up to 9 L of fluid can be secreted each day. When an obstruction occurs, fluid and air accumulate above the obstruction. In early obstruction, up to 1.5 L of fluid can be sequestered in the gut. By the time a high-grade obstruction is established, up to 6 L of fluid may be present [Nellgård, 1996. See reference on page 525].

○ **What measures can be taken to prevent aspiration?**

Preoperatively, the stomach should be emptied. This is usually achieved using a nasogastric tube for suctioning. Intubation of the trachea should be achieved either with the patient awake or with rapid sequence induction using cricoid pressure (Sellick maneuver).

○ **What is the pathophysiology of ischemia–reperfusion injury?**

Tissue hypoxia and acidosis are generally regarded as the major factors that mediate the pathological alterations associated with ischemia. But it is the intrinsic ability of tissues to initiate and sustain an inflammatory response that may explain the vascular dysfunction and tissue injury produced by ischemia–reperfusion. Ischemia–reperfusion injury is initiated when the ischemic tissue is reperfused and production of reactive metabolites of oxygen and nitrogen causes accumulation of activated neutrophils. With neutrophil–endothelial adhesion, tissue damage results due to secretion of additional reactive oxygen species as well as proteolytic enzymes, in particular elastase. If the area of ischemic tissue is large, neutrophils also sequester in the lung, liver, splanchnic circulation, and cardiovascular system resulting in the development of systemic inflammatory response syndrome (SIRS) and multiple organ dysfunction syndrome (MODS).

○ **What implications might this have for the gastrointestinal tract?**

The cellular damage caused by splanchnic ischemia is less than that associated with ischemia and reperfusion injury. An example may be perinatal asphyxia and ischemia–reperfusion causing necrotizing enterocolitis or delayed primary function of a transplanted liver following reperfusion in the recipient.

○ **What is gastric tonometry?**

Gastric tonometry is a monitoring technique measuring carbon dioxide partial pressure in the gastrointestinal mucosa (stomach or intestine) as an indicator of tissue perfusion.

○ **What is the clinical significance of gastric tonometry?**

Early detection of splanchnic hypoperfusion and restoration of adequate splanchnic tissue perfusion may reduce the incidence of multiorgan failure. The difference between the arterial PCO_2 and the tonometry $PgCO_2$ is a reflection of stomach perfusion. In normally perfused mucosa, gastric mucosal $PgCO_2$ is close to $PaCO_2$. During hypoperfusion the calculated difference increases. If $PgCO_2$ minus $PaCO_2$ is greater than 20, perfusion is inadequate and fluids and/or inotropes should be considered.

○ **What are the medical complications of jejunoileal bypass?**

Hypokalemia, hypocalcemia, hypomagnesemia, anemia, renal stones, gout, and liver abnormalities.

○ **A patient with bile duct obstruction due to stones and cholangitis is scheduled for cholecystectomy. Are there any laboratory findings that would distinguish this cholestatic liver injury from that of viral hepatitis?**

Conjugated hyperbilirubinemia and a liver biopsy showing centrilobular cholestasis and neutrophils within edematous portal stroma.

○ **What electrolyte abnormalities are associated with chronic diarrhea?**

Patients will exhibit a non-anion gap metabolic acidosis secondary to bicarbonate loss. They will also develop hyponatremia, hypokalemia, and hypophosphatemia [Barash et al., 2009; Miller, 2010].

○ **T/F: Dehydration and electrolyte disturbances in patients with chronic diarrhea suggest a secretory process, such as endocrine tumors or laxative abuse.**

True. Secretory diarrhea is caused by abnormal secretion or inhibition of absorption by the intestinal epithelium. Other mechanisms for diarrhea include osmotic, inflammatory, and conditions associated with deranged motility.

○ **What acid base disturbance is seen in severe pyloric stenosis?**

Hyponatremic, hypokalemic, and hypochloremic metabolic alkalosis.

○ **A patient admitted after 1 week of persistent vomiting from gastric outlet obstruction is expected to have what acid base disturbance?**

Persistent vomiting results in:

• Loss of hydrogen ions from the stomach
• Loss of sodium and chloride ions from the extracellular fluid
• Excretion of potassium by kidneys in exchange for hydrogen ions in an effort to maintain normal arterial pH

Loss of gastric secretions results in ECF depletion and avid sodium reabsorption by the kidney. Ionic neutrality is maintained by hydrogen secretion and reabsorption of bicarbonate in the face of insufficient chloride availability. Result is dehydration with hypokalemic, hypochloremic metabolic alkalosis.

Key Terms

ABG: morbid obesity and vomiting
Chronic diarrhea: electrolyte imbalance
Diagnosis of obstructive sleep apnea
Hypoxemia in morbid obesity: causes
Morbid obesity: DVT
Morbid obesity: PFTs

Morbid obesity: postoperative complications
Morbid obesity: rapid desaturation/causes
Obesity: pharmacokinetic considerations
Obesity: pulmonary effects/function
Pickwickian syndrome: ABGs
Vomiting: electrolyte imbalance

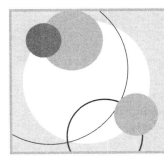

Hemostasis

It's not the size of the dog in the fight – it's the size of the fight in the dog.
Mark Twain

○ **List the vitamin K–dependent coagulation factors.**

Factors II, VII, IX, and X. Vitamin K activates each factor with the addition of a carboxyl group, which then enables them to bind via calcium to the phospholipid surface.

○ **Which of the vitamin K–dependent coagulation factors has the shortest half-life?**

Factor VII, with a half-life of 6 hours.

○ **Where are the coagulation factors produced?**

All are manufactured in the liver except factor VIII that is synthesized by vascular endothelium.

○ **How should the coagulation deficiency be treated in a patient with biliary disease secondary to gallstone obstruction?**

Biliary obstruction leads to deficiency of coagulation factors.

Activation of some factors (factors II, VII, IX, and X) depends on the presence of vitamin K. Absorption of vitamin K depends on the excretion of bile into the gastrointestinal tract. Usually, if the coagulation disorders are moderate, parenteral vitamin K corrects the problem. If this treatment is not fully effective, suspect that the disease is not purely cholestatic, and that hepatic parenchymal disease exists because long-lasting biliary obstruction leads to liver injury.

Should such patients need urgent surgery, fresh frozen plasma will be required to correct the coagulopathy.

○ **Describe how heparin functions as an anticoagulant.**

Heparin alone has no intrinsic anticoagulant activity. It acts as a catalyst to accelerate the interaction between antithrombin III (AT-III) and the activated forms of factors XIII, XII, XI, X, and II.

○ **How does AT-III work?**

AT-III is a circulatory serine protease inhibitor that irreversibly binds and inactivates thrombin and factor X. It also inhibits factors VIIa, IXa, Xa, and XIa. Thrombin is necessary for clot formation and platelet activation.

○ **When should heparin-induced thrombocytopenia (HIT) be suspected?**

HIT should be suspected in association with thrombocytopenia (platelets <100,000/μL), tachyphylaxis to heparin, and thrombotic complications appearing 7–10 days after the initiation of heparin therapy in those never exposed to heparin previously.

In vitro platelet aggregation to heparin disappears in 4–8 weeks, but may persist up to 12 months. Administration of heparin to sensitized patients will decrease the platelet count dramatically and/or produce thromboemboli. Elective cardiac or vascular surgery should be delayed until resolution of platelet aggregation studies. For urgent cardiac surgery, other strategies avoiding heparin exposure are necessary.

○ **What is the treatment of HIT?**

HIT may occur with standard heparin therapy (or low-molecular-weight heparin), after IV or SC, and the occurrence is not dose dependent.

There are two syndromes:

1. Mild: 30–40% patients; platelet count drops to 100,000 and is seen 3–5 days after initiation of therapy.
2. More severe: 0.5–6% patients; platelet count drops below 50,000 and often seen with resistance to the heparin effect. One of the serious complications is venous and arterial occlusion, even if platelet counts are low (HIT syndrome).

When HIT is diagnosed, heparin should be discontinued and fast-acting non-heparin anticoagulant should be initiated promptly (lepirudin, bivalirudin). Warfarin also should be avoided because it is slow acting, causes early reduction in proteins C and S, and promotes thrombosis. Give the anticoagulants for 1 month or more (3–6 months) if thrombosis present [Warkentin et al., 2004. See reference on page 525].

○ **What are the molecular events in heparin-associated thrombocytopenia?**

It is believed to be caused by a heparin-dependent IgG platelet antibody interaction with platelets that initiates platelet activation and aggregation (complement-mediated, heparin-dependent IgG platelet antibody).

○ **What is the nature of thrombosis in heparin-induced thrombocytopenia (HIT)?**

Arterial or venous and is a characteristic "white clot" (platelets and fibrin). Major thrombotic complications occur in 20% of HIT patients (coronary, cerebral, splanchnic, and peripheral artery).

○ **When does the syndrome of heparin-associated thrombocytopenia usually occur in patients who were never previously exposed to heparin?**

Seven to 10 days after heparin administration.

○ **Is the heparin used in catheter flush solutions, or bonded to vascular catheters, sufficient to cause this syndrome?**

Yes.

○ **How does a patient with AT-III deficiency usually present?**

Homozygotes usually die in infancy; 85% of heterozygotes have suffered a thrombotic event by age 50.

The diagnosis should be suspected in a patient with thromboembolic disease or a resistance to anticoagulation with heparin administration.

○ **Can this AT-III disorder be acquired as well as congenital?**

Yes.

○ **What are some of the causes of acquired AT-III deficiency?**

Liver disease, malignancy, nephrotic syndrome, DIC, malnutrition, or increased protein catabolism.

○ **What is the treatment for AT-III deficiency?**

Depends on the patient's risk of recurrent thromboembolic disease. Patients with a history of arterial or venous clot may require anticoagulation (warfarin, heparin, or low-molecular-weight heparin).

Fresh frozen plasma can be used as a source of AT-III when heparin is necessary.

AT-III concentrate is also available.

○ **What is the advantage of enoxaparin (LMWH) and how do you monitor its effects?**

Enoxaparin is derived from chemical depolymerization of standard heparin and has one third the size of heparin molecule. The antiactivated factor X to antiactivated factor II activity is about 4:1 to 2:1.

It has a superior bioavailability at low doses, and more predictable. HIT is relatively uncommon.

It has a longer elimination half-life and one per day dosing is adequate.

Anti-Xa activity is the only way to monitor LMWH. However this is not usually done due to long waiting time for the results to be back.

○ **How does sodium warfarin (coumadin) work as an anticoagulant?**

Coumadin is a vitamin K antagonist that blocks the carboxylation of the vitamin K–dependent factors by competing with vitamin K for binding sites on the hepatocyte where the carboxylation occurs.

○ **What other factors does coumadin inhibit?**

Proteins C, S, and Z.

○ **How can you reverse warfarin anticoagulation?**

The half-life of warfarin is approximately 36–42 hours. Reversal of warfarin anticoagulation is achieved by administering either vitamin K or FFP 5–8 mL/kg.

International normalized ratio (INR) will normalize in 4 days once warfarin is discontinued.

When vitamin K is given, normalization of INR occurs in 24 hours with oral therapy and 6–12 hours with IV administration.

Prothrombin complex concentrates (PCCs) from pooled plasma (solvent detergent treated) when given IV over 5–10 minutes correct INR within 60 minutes. IV PCC dose is 10–40 IU/kg [Koutrouvelis et al., 2010. See reference on page 525]. (However, this is not yet approved by the FDA.)

○ **What is the fastest way to reverse coumadin?**

PCC administration.

○ **What is PCC?**

Prothrombin complex concentrate.

It is a lypolized combination of concentrates of prothrombin, proconvertin, Stuart factor, and antihemophilic factor B (factors II, VII, IX, X) derived from pooled plasma.

The FDA has approved its use in hemophilia B (factor IX deficiency). It is used to hasten INR correction instead of FFP in Europe.

Comparison with other methods of reversing INR:

With vitamin K INR normalizes in 24 hours with oral administration and 6–12 hours with IV administration.

PCC needs to be reconstituted (takes only minutes). IV PCC administered over 5–10 minutes corrects INR within 60 minutes. Dose 10–40 IU/kg over 5–15 minutes.

FFP takes >60 minutes to obtain from the blood bank (ABO blood typing, thawing, transport).

However, the effect of vitamin K lasts beyond the short half-lives of FFP and PCCs.

Cost: FVIIc > PCC ($1,000) > FFP ($600).

○ **Is recombinant factor VIIa (rFVIIa) useful in coagulopathy? How does it work?**

rFVIIa initiates thrombin generation via two pathways:

1. Active complex with tissue factor (TF) via extrinsic pathway

2. Acts directly on factor IX/X on membrane of activated platelets

At pharmacological doses this results in a "thrombin burst."

The clot that forms is morphologically different: greater fibrin cross-linking and more resistant to fibrinolysis.

However, rFVIIa should have enough cofactors to enable it to work. Therefore, within 30 minutes of administration, transfuse with:

• Six units of platelets
• Four FFP
• Two pooled packs of cryoprecipitate

○ **A patient undergoing a vascular procedure receives high-dose heparin. Shortly thereafter, the surgeon reports clot formation. Laboratory work shows normal PTT. What is the likely diagnosis and how is it treated?**

AT-III deficiency. The treatment is with FFP transfusion or AT-III concentrate to increase AT-III levels.

○ **What drug is used to reverse the anticoagulant effects of heparin?**

Protamine. Protamine (a positively charged protein) binds and neutralizes heparin (a negatively charged polysaccharide), with the complex then cleared by the reticuloendothelial system.

One milligram protamine for each 100 U of heparin given, repeating the activated clotting time (ACT) measurement 3–5 minutes after reversal. The protamine dose may be calculated based on the heparin dose–response curve.

○ **What happens to clotting if too much protamine is given to antagonize heparin?**

Excess protamine has anticoagulant activity (1/100 that of heparin).

○ **How is the effectiveness of coumadin therapy evaluated?**

Monitoring INR or prothrombin time (PT). The recommended therapeutic range for standard oral anticoagulant therapy is an INR = 2–3, and with high-dose therapy INR = 2.5–3.5.

○ **What are the new oral anticoagulants, which received approval by the FDA recently?**

1. Dabigatran: This is a thrombin inhibitor. Dabigatran received the FDA approval to be used for the prevention of stroke in patients with AF in October 2010 [Gogarten et al., 2010. See reference on page 525].

2. Rivaroxaban and apixaban: These are potent direct factor Xa inhibitors. These are approved by the FDA for the prevention of venous thromboembolism after hip and knee arthroplasty in July 2011. Rivaroxaban is also effective for the treatment of symptomatic venous thromboembolism and for preventing strokes in patients with nonvalvular AF. It is also being evaluated for secondary prevention after acute coronary syndromes.

Both groups of drugs are administered orally at fixed doses and no monitoring is necessary. The drawback is these drugs lack an effective antidote or reversal agent. rFVII and PCC do not seem to reverse rivaroxaban-induced bleeding.

○ **What is INR?**

INR is a means of converting the PT ratio to a value obtained using a standardized PT method. The INR is calculated as $(PT_{patient}/PT_{normal})^{ISI}$, where ISI is the international sensitivity index assigned to the test system. This testing system was devised to improve the consistency of dosing coumadin.

○ **What does aPTT and PTT measure and what are the normal values?**

aPTT is the activated partial thromboplastin time. Maximal activation of the contact factors XII and XI is achieved with the addition of diatomaceous earth, kaolin, or crushed glass to the test tube before the addition of partial thromboplastin. Normal aPTT is 25–35 seconds.

PTT is the partial thromboplastin time and is used to assess all the coagulation factors in the intrinsic and common pathways, except factor XIII. Normal values are 40–100 seconds, with >120 seconds abnormal.

○ **What does PT measure and what are the normal values?**

PT is prothrombin time. It is a measure of the coagulation reactions of the extrinsic and common pathways, and the patient's response to oral anticoagulant therapy. Normal values are 10–12 seconds.

○ **A patient develops postoperative bleeding. What common causes should you consider?**

Surgically correctable bleeding, clotting factor problem, platelet deficiency, DIC, hypothermia, or residual heparin effect.

○ **Describe the most commonly used tests to evaluate primary hemostasis.**

Platelet count and bleeding time.

Normal platelet count is between 150,000 and 450,000/mm³. Patients with platelet counts greater than 100,000/mm³ and normal function have normal primary hemostasis. The IV bleeding time performed in a standardized fashion is 4–9 minutes and is abnormal if greater than 15 minutes. Unfortunately, there is a lack of correlation between bleeding time and intraoperative bleeding and the test is now considered obsolete.

○   **What is the ACT and when is it used?**

ACT is activated clotting time, which is used primarily to monitor heparin therapy during cardiopulmonary bypass (CPB). An activator (celite or kaolin) is added to a blood sample, causing contact activation of the intrinsic pathway, and the time to clot formation is measured. Baseline values are usually 100–120 seconds, and an ACT of 480 seconds or longer is considered acceptable anticoagulant activity of heparin for instituting CPB.

○   **What are the uses and limitations of measuring ACT?**

ACT is used to monitor heparin effect during CPB, interventional cardiology, and hemodialysis. Limitations include:

- New technology (instruments and reagents) gives varying results for IV heparin dosing when trying to achieve a standard target ACT for CPB (480 seconds using Hemochron 801).
- Choice of activator (celite or kaolin); if aprotinin is administered concomitantly, the celite ACT becomes significantly higher than the kaolin ACT due to decreased thrombin generation; insufficient anticoagulation using C-ACT may result.
- ACT may lack correlation with heparin levels because of its lack of specificity for heparin and variability during hypothermia and hemodilution on CPB. Changes in the ACT can reflect changes in heparin–AT-III, changes in thrombin, or both.

○   **Describe when a thromboelastogram (TEG) may be helpful.**

TEG is a viscoelastic measure of coagulation function and is preferable to conventional coagulation assays (aPTT, PT). It assesses coagulation by measuring viscosity and elasticity of the clot as it forms. TEG provides a rapid interpretation of coagulation function (which would otherwise require analysis of a combined number of tests) particularly useful in patients receiving massive transfusions or at risk of bleeding from multiple causes (platelet dysfunction, factor deficiencies, fibrinolysis), that is, liver transplantation or cardiac surgical patients. Majority of PT/aPTT still performed in the lab and has a time delay. TEG performed as a point-of-care hemostasis monitoring when trained personnel available. The accuracy of TEG may be greater than that of routine coagulation tests in predicting clinical bleeding.

○   **Describe the typical TEG pattern and variables measured. What is the treatment for abnormal TEG values?**

Reaction times (r) are related to the PTT and normally range from 6 to 8 minutes.

Reaction time >15 minutes can be treated with FFP.

MA — related to platelet function and is normally 50–70 mm.

MA <40 mm is treated with platelet concentrate.

Clot formation rate (alpha) is related to fibrinogen function and is normally >50°.

Clot formation rate <45° can be treated with cryoprecipitate.

MA +30 measures clot retraction, which is abnormal in fibrinolysis.

TEG provides information about:

1. Clotting cascade
2. Platelet function
3. Clot lysis

○   **What is the most common inherited bleeding disorder?**

von Willebrand disease (vWD).

What are the two key functions of von Willebrand factor (factor VIII:vWF)?

vWF is necessary for platelet adhesion to collagen in the subendothelial layer of injured blood vessels and formation of the hemostatic plug through regulation and release of factor VIII antigen.

What is the molecular abnormality in vWD?

Defective vWF, or low levels of a normal vWF resulting in an inability of platelets to bind to collagen.

Factor VIII is bound to vWF while inactive in circulation; it degrades rapidly when not bound to vWF. Factor VIII is released from vWF by the action of thrombin. A deficiency of vWF can result in decreased factor VIII levels. In vWD bleeding time is prolonged and factor VIII level may be decreased causing bleeding similar to hemophilia.

What are the different types of vWD?

vWD is the most common inherited bleeding disorder (1:800–1,000); 2–3% incidence.

Type 1 and 3 vWD — quantitative defects in the protein (type 1, partial; type 3, severe).

(Normal vWf level 5–10 mg/L.)

Type 1: accounts for 70% of all cases.

Type 2: qualitative abnormality (20% of all vWD).

Unique subtype, type 2B (20% of the patients in type 2 vWD belong to the type 2B): in this type there is an increased affinity of vWF for platelet glycoprotein 1b. This leads to spontaneous binding and clearance of both.

What is the treatment for vWD?

Depends on the type (1, 2, or 3), severity of the disorder, and type of surgery. The aim of treatment is to correct the dual defect of hemostasis: the abnormal intrinsic coagulation pathway caused by low factor VIII levels and the prolonged bleeding time resulting from abnormal platelet adhesion. Desmopressin (DDAVP) is the treatment of choice for type 1 vWD because it corrects the FVIII/vWF levels and the prolonged bleeding time in the majority of cases. In type 3 and in severe forms of types 1 and 2 vWD, DDAVP is not effective and plasma virally inactivated concentrates containing FVIII and vWF are the mainstay of treatment [Federici and Mannucci, 2007. See reference on page 525].

A patient with type I vWD is to have a breast reduction. What should be the first line of therapy?

DDAVP 0.3 μg/kg, 30 minutes before surgery, to increase vWF levels. Desmopressin usually increases plasma vWF and factor VIII concentrations 2- to 5-fold. Cryoprecipitate or factor VIII concentrates are administered to nonresponders.

What is DDAVP?

DDAVP (desmopressin acetate) is an analogue of vasopressin without vasopressor activity. Infusion of DDAVP increases the release of vWF and factor VIII from the endothelium; intravenous peak effect in 15–30 minutes, with an increase in vWF seen over 3 hours and an increase in factor VIII over 4–24 hours.

What are the hemostatic uses for DDAVP?

It is useful in treating the coagulopathy associated with vWD and hemophilia A. DDAVP has also shown utility in treating uremia-induced platelet dysfunction.

○ **What are the laboratory findings in patients with vWD?**

A prolonged bleeding time, normal platelet count, decreased factor VIII activity, and decreased plasma factor VIII:vWF. A history of easy bruising or excessive bleeding during surgery or following ingestion of aspirin or nonsteroidal anti-inflammatory drugs may be the only clue to this disease.

○ **How does vWD manifest itself?**

Most patients have a history of bleeding excessively with surgery, tooth extractions, trauma, or following ingestion of aspirin or NSAIDs. Nosebleeds or menorrhagia are the most frequent clinical problems.

Typical laboratory findings: prolonged PTT and bleeding time, with qualitative platelet dysfunction.

○ **What is the molecular abnormality in hemophilia A?**

X-linked recessive disorder due to defective factor VIII:C molecules.

○ **What are the clinical manifestations of hemophilia A?**

Bleeding into joints and muscles, epistaxis, hematuria, and bleeding after minor trauma.

○ **What is the laboratory abnormality associated with hemophilia A?**

Prolongation of aPTT.

○ **What is the minimum level of factor VIII required for hemostasis?**

Thirty percent.

○ **What is the molecular abnormality in hemophilia B?**

X-linked hereditary deficiency of factor IX (Christmas factor).

○ **Is hemophilia B clinically distinguishable from hemophilia A?**

No.

○ **How do you correct hemophilia B?**

Factor IX deficiency is corrected with FFP to at least 30% of normal or with the administration of recombinant or monoclonal purified factor IX.

○ **A patient develops postoperative bleeding. What common causes should you consider?**

Surgically correctable bleeding, clotting factor problem, platelet deficiency, DIC, hypothermia, or residual heparin effect.

○ **A patient with hemophilia A is to have surgery. What is the half-life of factor VIII and how do you decide the dose of factor VIII needed preoperatively?**

Factor VIII has a half-life of 6–10 hours. The dose of factor VIII needed can be calculated on the assumption that each unit of factor VIII infused per kilogram of body weight raises plasma VIII levels by 2%. The minimal factor VIII concentration necessary for hemostasis during major surgery is 30–40% of normal, but many recommend increasing factor VIII levels to more than 50% prior to surgery. FFP contains 1 U factor VIII activity/mL, cryoprecipitate 5–10 U/mL, and factor VIII concentrates 40 U/mL. Twice-a-day transfusions are recommended following surgery. DDAVP may be a good adjuvant. In the patient with no factor VIII activity, 20 U/kg should be the initial dose, followed by 1.5 U/(kg h). Additional factor VIII is given on the basis of factor levels for 6–10 days postoperatively.

○ **Does ketorolac have a significant effect on platelet function?**

Yes. Ketorolac is a cyclooxygenase inhibitor that decreases prostaglandin synthesis (thromboxane B2) resulting in a reversible impairment in platelet aggregation. Bleeding time is prolonged. Platelet dysfunction following ketorolac 0.4 mg/kg IV may persist beyond 24 hours.

○ **Describe the mechanism of action of antiplatelet drugs.**

Drugs may interfere platelet membrane function, prostaglandine synthesis, phophodiesterase activity or platelet receptor activity. See examples below.

Interference with platelet membrane function: Amitryptiline, imipramine, cocaine, lidocaine, procaine, isoproterenol, diphenhydramine, nafcillin, and ticarcillin.

Cyclooxygenase inhibitors: Aspirin (irreversible inhibitor), indomethacin, phenylbutazone, ibuprofen, naproxen, furosemide, and verapamil.

Inhibition of phosphodiesterase: Cyclic AMP is an inhibitor of platelet aggregation; caffeine, dipyridamole, aminophyllin, and theophyllin.

Adenosine receptor antagonists: Ticlopidine and clopidogrel. Used for stroke prophylaxis. The effect is probably irreversible.

Glycoprotein IIb/IIIa receptor antagonists: These antagonize the sites to which fibrinogen and vWF bind. Used for acute coronary syndrome and include abciximab, tirofiban, and eptifibatide. The effect is reversible.

○ **What are the key laboratory values suggestive of acute DIC?**

There is no one pathognomonic test for DIC; prolonged PT and PTT in 75% and 50–60% of patients, respectively, reduced platelet count, and fibrinogen with elevation of fibrin degradation products.

○ **What are the major causes of DIC?**

Septicemia, amniotic fluid embolism, trauma, hemolytic transfusion reactions, massive transfusion, liver disease, viremias, burns, and leukemia.

○ **What is the main fibrinolytic enzyme?**

Plasmin.

○ **What are the major endogenous activators of plasminogen?**

Tissue plasminogen activator (TPA) released from endothelium and factor XIIa and kallikrein formed in the contact phase.

○ **What exogenous substances activate plasminogen?**

Streptokinase, urokinase, and TPA.

○   **How do you reverse fibrinolytic agents?**

Fibrinolytics (streptokinase, urokinase, alteplase, reteplase, and tenecteplase) are used for the acute treatment of DVT and myocardial infarction to break up thrombi by activating the conversion of plasminogen to plasmin, which degrades fibrin.

Management of toxicity:

- Discontinue the drug.
- Consider treating hemorrhage with fresh blood, PRBC, cryoprecipitate, fresh frozen plasma, platelets, desmopressin, and antifibrinolytics (tranexamic acid or aminocaproic acid) if hemorrhage is unresponsive to conventional therapy.
- Avoid dextrans for volume expansion due to platelet inhibiting effect.

○   **How does ε-aminocaproic acid (EACA) work?**

EACA (Amicar) is a synthetic monoamine carboxylic acid that interferes with the conversion of plasminogen to plasmin, thus attenuating primary fibrinolysis.

○   **What is aprotinin and how does it work?**

Aprotinin is a serine protease inhibitor that has been used to diminish perioperative blood loss and transfusion requirements. The exact mechanism is unclear but may be due to inhibition of plasmin-mediated fibrinolysis. There is also evidence that aprotinin maintains platelet adhesiveness by preventing plasmin-mediated degradation of platelet glycoproteins.

○   **Which commonly used herbs may increase bleeding?**

Feverfew, garlic, ginger, *Ginkgo biloba*, ginseng, and vitamin E.

Key Terms

Antiplatelet drugs: mechanism of action
Antithrombin III deficiency: treatment
Antithrombotic drugs: duration
Antithrombotic drugs: preoperative management
Aspirin: platelet effects
Cholestasis: coagulopathy treatment
Desmopressin for von Willebrand
Elevated INR: factor treatment
Enoxaparin: assessment of effects

Factor VII: hemostatic in liver disease
Heparin: anticoagulation
Heparin-induced thrombocytopenia: treatment
Heparin: resistance
Platelet inhibitor drug: tirofiban mechanism
Refractory hemophilia
Reversal of fibrinolytics
TEG: decreased MA: diagnosis and treatment
Warfarin: urgent perioperative reversal

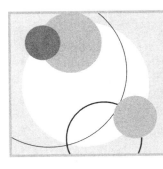

Hypothermia

The most effective means of cooling a man is to give him an anesthetic.
Pickering (1958)

○ **Why is the maintenance of body temperature of biological importance?**

Homeothermic organisms have a relatively constant body temperature ensuring optimum enzymatic function. These protein catalysts integrate the body's complex biochemical reactions. Their action is temperature dependent.

○ **What is core temperature?**

Central compartment (core) blood temperature corresponding to the vessel-rich group organs. The body is divided into three temperature compartments: central, peripheral, and the skin.

○ **What is "normal" body temperature?**

$37 \pm 0.2°C$, in humans.

○ **Are certain groups of patients more susceptible to becoming hypothermic?**

Heat loss during anesthesia is greatest at extremes of age. Geriatric patients have reduced autonomic vascular control, and neonates have a large surface area-to-mass ratio.

The high-risk surgical procedures are those involving exposure of large skin and serosal and mucosal surfaces during lengthy procedures under general anesthesia (with no humidification of gases) in a "cold" operating room, with the patient receiving cold IV solutions. Disruption of the hypothalamic thermoregulatory center will cause the patient to become poikilothermic.

○ **What mechanisms are used to reduce hyperthermia?**

Vasodilation and sweating.

○ **Where is the best noninvasive site for measuring core temperature?**

External auditory meatus. The thermoregulatory center is in the hypothalamus. The closer a temperature monitoring site is to this area, the more reflective measurements will be of the "core" temperature. Since the tympanic membrane is in close proximity to the internal carotid artery and brain stem, it is considered the "gold standard." It has also been suggested that a nasopharyngeal probe placed close to the ethmoid plate similarly reflects brain temperature.

○ **What are the most common sites for measuring core temperature?**

Sites for accurate monitoring of core temperature include the lower one third of the esophagus, tympanic membrane, and pulmonary artery catheter. Repeated measurements of tympanic membrane temperature are not practical for a variety of reasons, such as danger of eardrum perforation. Central core temperature is higher than skin temperature by 3–4°C. Transitional zones (peripheral compartment) include axillary temperature (1°C less), bladder, and mouth. Rectal temperatures are unreliable. Skin temperature (outer shell) is influenced by changes in the external environment.

○ **Is forehead temperature a good reflection of core temperature?**

No. Forehead temperature is typically 2°C cooler than the core.

○ **Define hypothermia.**

A core temperature of less than 36°C.

○ **What is the typical pattern of unintentional hypothermia during general anesthesia?**

Typically, a precipitous drop in core temperature during the first hour (phase I redistribution), followed by a gradual decline during the next 3–4 hours (phase II heat loss), eventually reaching a steady state (phase III equilibrium).

Anesthetic-induced vasodilatation causes the initial core-to-peripheral redistribution of body heat.

○ **What are the mechanisms of intraoperative heat loss?**

• Heat of vaporization (respiratory tract moisture and heat loss)
• Conduction (heat loss from warm body surfaces in contact with colder surfaces)
• Convection (cold air mass moving across exposed areas of a patient)
• Radiation (heat from the patient into the atmosphere)

Among these radiation and convection contribute most (70%) to perioperative heat loss.

Heat transfer by **radiation** is proportional to the fourth power of the absolute temperature difference between the surfaces, and radiation is the major type of heat loss in most surgical patients.

○ **Can laminar flow in the operative room increase heat loss from patient's body?**

Yes. When the layer of still air adjacent to the skin is disturbed, insulative properties decrease and heat loss increases. This increase is termed **convection** and is proportional to the square root of air speed. The operative rooms are equipped to provide laminar flow, and because of the increase in air speed, convective loss increases. Although surgical draping provides considerable thermal insulation, convective loss is usually the second most important mechanism by which heat is transferred from patient to the environment.

○ **How important is operating room temperature in regards to heat loss of surgical patients?**

Operating room temperature determines the rate at which metabolic heat is lost by radiation and convection from the skin and by evaporation from the opened surgical wounds. Therefore, operating room temperature is the most critical factor influencing heat loss.

However, room temperature higher than 23°C (infants >26°C) is required to maintain normothermia in most surgical patients and is uncomfortably warm for operating room personnel.

○ **What are the different causes of intraoperative hypothermia under anesthesia?**

- Altered normal thermoregulatory mechanisms
- Peripheral vasodilation with increased heat loss
- Reduced heat production from muscle
- Reduced basal metabolic rate
- No shivering
- Decrease in the threshold for peripheral vasoconstriction
- Altered sympathetic response to hypothermia
- Cold environment (room temperature, skin preparation solutions, irrigation, cold IV fluids)
- Exposure of pleural, pericardial, and peritoneal surfaces
- Prolonged surgery (rate of heat loss is greatest in the first hour, with as much as 1°C reduction in core temperature within the first 15 minutes of induction)

○ **Is the use of passive insulation with blankets alone enough to prevent hypothermia during surgery?**

The easiest method of decreasing cutaneous heat loss is to apply passive insulation to the skin such as cotton blankets, plastic sheeting, and space blankets. A single layer of each reduces about 30% heat loss. Warming the blanket provides little benefit, and the insulation is provided by the layer of still air trapped beneath the covering. The loss from the head can be substantial in infants. However, the amount of skin covered is more important than which surfaces are insulated.

However, the passive insulation alone is insufficient during large operations to maintain normothermia. The most common perioperative active warming system is forced air and is effective even during the largest operations.

When cutaneous heat losses are eliminated, metabolic heat production will increase mean body temperature approximately 1°C/h.

○ **How effective is the circulating-water mattress in preventing intraoperative hypothermia?**

Circulating-water mattresses are nearly ineffective because little heat is lost from the back of the patient to the 5-cm foam insulation covering the operating room table. Circulating water is more effective when placed over the patient than under him or her.

○ **Can warming fluids aid in the prevention of hypothermia?**

Yes. One unit of refrigerated blood or 1 L of room-temperature crystalloid decreases the body temperature by about 0.25°C. However, fluid warmers minimize heat losses, especially when large amounts of cold intravenous fluid or blood are administered. If a massive transfusion is anticipated, then a rapid infusion system that can deliver blood at 37°C at rates of 250–500 mL/min should be used.

○ **Describe different methods available for intraoperative rewarming.**

Warming the blood (cardiopulmonary bypass, countercurrent heat exchanger using an endovascular heat exchange catheter, fluid warmers), surface skin rewarming methods (circulating-water warming garment, forced air warming, heating blanket, Mylar Foil wrapping), lavage body cavities, and airways (humidifier and heat–moisture exchanger).

○ **Can hypothermia be beneficial?**

Yes. Mild hypothermia reduces metabolic oxygen requirements (9% for every degree in temperature drop) that may limit warm ischemia and cerebral and myocardial injury. Preservation of vital organs for transplantation is inherent on rendering the organ metabolically inert by reducing the core temperature to 4°C through cold preservation techniques. For organ-specific protection, lowering the body temperature to 33°C for 12 or 24 hours in comatose survivors of cardiac arrest has been shown to improve neurologic outcome.

○   **What are the complications of mild hypothermia?**

- Increased perioperative blood loss and need for blood transfusion
- Decreased antibody and cell-mediated immunity
- Decreased availability of oxygen in peripheral tissues
- Increased risk of wound infection with increased hospital stay
- Activated sympathoneural (norepinephrine) and adrenomedullary (epinephrine) responses
- Increased incidence of postoperative adverse myocardial events
- Hypertension and tachycardia in the elderly
- Shivering — postoperative
- Marked patient thermal discomfort
- Prolonged recovery room stays

○   **When does hypothermia become detrimental?**

At 34°C problems with hemostasis begin to increase in a linear fashion due to platelet dysfunction and fibrinolysis. Delayed reversal of muscle relaxation and increased risk of myocardial ischemia occur. At 32°C arrhythmias, cold diuresis, and delayed awakening are seen.

○   **What is the effect of general anesthesia on basal metabolic rate?**

A reduction of approximately 15%. Greater if muscle relaxants are used (up to 50%) and some degree of hypothermia occurs.

○   **What happens to temperature regulation during anesthesia?**

While under anesthesia, behavioral responses to temperature changes are abolished. General anesthetics disrupt normal thermoregulatory control. Warm-response thresholds are slightly elevated and cold-response thresholds (vasoconstriction and shivering) are significantly lowered. Sweating is therefore relatively well preserved in response to hyperthermia.

Under neuraxial anesthesia, central thermoregulatory control is slightly diminished. The degree of impairment is proportional to the number of spinal segments blocked. The cold-response threshold that triggers vasoconstriction and shivering is decreased by 0.6°C above the level of the block. The gain and maximal intensity of the shivering response are also decreased by about half.

○   **What are the effects of hypothermia on the central nervous system?**

Mild hypothermia (32–35°C).

- Decrease in cerebral blood flow, increase in cerebral vascular resistance, and normal arteriovenous oxygen difference.
- Decrease in cerebral metabolic oxygen and glucose consumption 7–10% per °C decrease in temperature.
- MAC of volatile agents is reduced by approximately 5–7% per °C decrease in temperature.
- Delayed emergence, sedation, and confusion <33°C.
- Narcosis at <30°C.
- Increase in latency in motor and SSEP.
- Slowing of the EEG, isoelectric at 20°C.

○ **What changes does hypothermia produce in the cardiovascular system?**

- Preload: increase in CVP.
- Afterload: increase in systemic vascular resistance due to vasoconstriction, with vasodilation below 20°C.
- Heart rate and rhythm: bradycardia and arrhythmias (nodal, PVC, AV block, and ventricular fibrillation or asystole).
- Contractility: decreases; reduced cardiac output.
- Effect on coronary blood flow is variable; coronary artery resistance decreases.
- Pulmonary vascular resistance is increased.
- Increased myocardial oxygen demand with shivering (300%).
- EKG: sinus bradycardia, prolonged PR and QT intervals, and widened QRS complexes.

If the sympathetic adrenergic response is functional, the initial response is sympathetic stimulation with an increase in heart rate, blood pressure, and cardiac output.

○ **Is respiratory function compromised by hypothermia?**

Yes. Hypothermia has been cited as one of the primary reasons for reintubation in the recovery room following general anesthesia.

Pulmonary effects of hypothermia include:

- Increase in pulmonary vascular resistance.
- Decrease in hypoxic pulmonary vasoconstriction.
- Increased V/Q mismatch and hypoxemia.
- Depression of the hypoxic ventilatory drive and no change in the CO_2 ventilatory response.
- Bronchodilation (increase in anatomic dead space).
- Increase in carbon dioxide and oxygen solubility; a rule of thumb is that the body temperature (°C) should equal the $PaCO_2$ in mm Hg.
- The pH rises 0.015 U per °C decrease in temperature.

○ **What are the hematologic consequences of hypothermia?**

- Thrombocytopenia secondary to platelet aggregation and sequestration in the portal circulation
- Increased fibrinolysis and DIC with tissue damage
- Reduced clotting factor activity
- Sequestration of leukocytes
- Increase in blood viscosity due to increase in hematocrit and plasma protein (2–3% with each °C decrease in temperature)
- Increase in hematocrit and rouleaux formation
- Shift of the oxygen–hemoglobin dissociation curve to the left
- Decrease in plasma volume (cold diuresis and impaired sodium resorption)

○ **How is renal function affected by hypothermia?**

Renal blood flow and GFR are decreased. Cold-induced diuresis and impaired tubular transport of sodium, chloride, and water may lead to hypovolemia. Reabsorption of potassium is decreased. The ability to concentrate or dilute urine is impaired.

○ **How does hypothermia affect the metabolism of anesthetic drugs?**

Hypothermia impairs both hepatic metabolism and renal clearance of drugs due to a reduction in blood flow. Half-life is prolonged for vecuronium (liver) and pancuronium (kidney). Metabolism of drugs dependent on Hoffman elimination or esterases is delayed (cisatracurium and atracurium). Protein binding increases as body temperature decreases.

○ **T/F: Inhalational induction of anesthesia is facilitated by the decrease in MAC seen in hypothermic patients.**

False. The MAC of inhalational agents is decreased 5–7% per °C decrease in core temperature, but decreased cardiac output and increased blood solubility offset this effect resulting in no change in the speed of inhalational induction.

○ **Which modalities are available in order to treat shivering?**

Ideally, passive or active rewarming will prevent perioperative hypothermia. The most effective drug therapy is IV meperidine 12.5–25 mg.

○ **How do you respond to the surgeon who demands that the operating room temperature be reduced because of the increased risk of wound infection?**

Recent evidence shows that the risk of wound infection is increased in hypothermic patients, [Kurtz et al., 1996. See reference on page 526] possibly due to impaired neutrophil function and vasoconstriction with hypoperfusion of peripheral tissues and tissue hypoxia. The ideal temperature for vascular surgery is 70°F.

○ **What are the consequences of postoperative rewarming?**

If a patient is hypothermic in the immediate postoperative period, and then rewarmed, the physiologic consequences include vasodilation, shivering, and increased basal metabolic rate (increased O_2 consumption and CO_2 production). Vasodilation may unmask underlying hypovolemia resulting in hypotension and tachycardia.

○ **Why is shivering undesirable in the postoperative period?**

Shivering will increase oxygen consumption (up to 2- or 3-fold). Increased oxygen demands may be detrimental in patients with intrapulmonary shunts, fixed cardiac output, and limited respiratory reserve. In addition, peripheral vascular resistance and CVP are increased, all of which may be especially detrimental in patients with microsurgery for replantation and rotational flaps. In an awake patient, shivering may cause significant discomfort, increase wound pain, and increase intracranial and intraocular pressures.

○ **What are the causes of intraoperative hyperthermia?**

- Prevention of convective heat loss by covering the patient
- Prolonged closed or semiclosed systems that increase heat and moisture from the carbon dioxide–soda lime reaction
- Malfunction or overuse of a humidifier, heat–moisture exchanger, or fluid warmer
- High ambient temperature
- Sepsis
- Malignant hyperthermia and thyroid storm
- Thermal instability (osteogenesis imperfecta)
- Drugs

○ **Discuss the physiology of deliberate hypothermia.**

Deliberate hypothermia is used as a neuroprotective strategy to decrease cerebral metabolic requirements in patients at risk for cerebral hypoperfusion and postoperative neurocognitive dysfunction [2010 American Heart Association Guidelines for Cardiopulmonary Resuscitation and Emergency Cardiovascular Care. See reference on page 526]. The temperature required to achieve electrocortical silence ranges from 12.5°C to 27.2°C (median 18°C).

○ **Where is the thermoregulatory center found in poikilothermic animals?**

The hypothalamus and thalamus. Hypothalamic and thalamic pathways can result in cortical excitation that is involved in behavioral changes. Efferent vasomotor, piloerector, sweating, and shivering efferents are generated in the hypothalamus. *CNS thermosensors* are found in the preoptic nucleus and anterior hypothalamus. The posterior hypothalamus is the location of the *set point for thermoregulation.*

Key Terms

Causes: hyperthermia

Hypothermia: cold OR mechanism

Hypothermia patients: most effective warming

Hypothermia: systemic effects

Intraoperative warming methods

Laminar flow and heat loss

Mechanism of intraoperative hypothermia

Mild hypothermia: adverse effects

Neutral thermal environment: advantages

Postoperative shivering: prevention

Temperature regulation during anesthesia

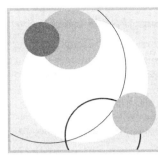

Inhalation Agents

Flaming enthusiasm, backed up by horse sense and persistence, is the quality that most frequently makes for success.
Dale Carnegie

○ **Define vapor pressure of a volatile liquid.**

When a volatile liquid resides in a closed container, the molecules of the substance will equilibrate between the liquid and gas phases. At equilibrium, the pressure exerted by molecular collisions of the gas against the container walls is the vapor pressure.

○ **Is vapor pressure dependent on the volume of liquid in the container?**

No. As long as any liquid remains in the container, the vapor pressure is independent of the volume of that liquid. Vapor pressure is dependent on temperature and the physical characteristics of the liquid.

○ **What happens to the vapor pressure and solubility of an inhalation agent as its temperature increases?**

The vapor pressure increases and the solubility decreases.

○ **T/F: Vapor pressure is dependent on the atmospheric pressure.**

False. Vapor pressure is dependent on the temperature and the physical properties of the inhalation agent, and independent of the atmospheric pressure.

○ **List the inhalation agents in order of increasing solubility.**

Desflurane (0.42), N_2O (0.47), sevoflurane (0.61), isoflurane (1.4), enflurane (1.91), halothane (2.3), and methoxyflurane (15) (blood/gas partition coefficients at 37°C).

○ **T/F: The blood/gas partition coefficient is a measure of the anesthetic potency of the inhalation agent.**

False. The oil:gas partition coefficient parallels the minimum alveolar concentration (MAC) of the inhalation agent, which is a measure of its potency. MAC = 150 divided by oil:gas partition coefficient. The blood/gas partition coefficient is a measure of the relative solubility of the agent in blood, and determines the speed of onset of action of the agent. The lower the blood/gas partition coefficient, the lower is the blood solubility, and faster the onset of action.

○ **T/F: Changes in alveolar ventilation affect the rate of rise of alveolar partial pressure (P_A) of a soluble agent more than an insoluble agent.**

True. The rate of rise of P_A of a poorly soluble agent is rapid, and independent of alveolar ventilation because of its limited uptake. The uptake of a soluble agent is large, and increasing alveolar ventilation provides more agent to the lungs to offset the loss due to uptake.

○ **T/F: Changes in cardiac output affect the rate of rise of P_A of an insoluble agent more than a soluble agent.**

False. Cardiac output and alveolar ventilation influence the rate of rise of P_A of soluble agents more than insoluble agents. Increasing the cardiac output will increase the uptake of a soluble agent, slowing the rate of rise of the P_A, whereas the rate of rise of P_A of an insoluble agent is rapid regardless of changes in cardiac output.

○ **What are the B/G partition coefficients, the vapor pressures (at 20°C), and lipid solubilities of the inhaled anesthetics?**

	B/G	VP (mm Hg)	Oil/gas (O/G)
Halothane	2.5	244	224
Enflurane	1.8	172	96.5
Isoflurane	1.4	240	90.8
Desflurane	0.45	664	18.7
Sevoflurane	0.65	162	47.2
Nitrous oxide	0.47	39,000	1.4

○ **What is the importance of F_A/F_I?**

F_A is the alveolar gas concentration and F_I is the inspired gas concentration of inhaled anesthetic agent. Following the ratio of fractional concentration of alveolar anesthetic to inspired anesthetic over time (F_A/F_I) is a simple way to assess anesthetic uptake.

○ **What determines the F_A/F_I?**

The F_A/F_I ratio is ultimately determined by the balance between the delivery of anesthetic by ventilation and its removal by uptake. Factors determining F_I include fresh gas flow rate, volume of the breathing system, and circuit absorption. Factors determining F_A include uptake, ventilation, and the concentration and second gas effects.

○ **What are the uptake factors that affect F_A/F_I?**

There are three factors: blood:gas solubility of anesthetic (λ), cardiac output (Q), and alveolar to venous partial pressure difference ($P_A - P_V$).

○ **T/F: Uptake is a sum of those three factors.**

False. Uptake is the product of the three factors. This means that if any factor approaches zero, uptake must approach zero, and ventilation is free to rapidly drive the alveolar concentration upwards.

$$\text{Uptake} = (\lambda) \times (Q) \times (P_A - P_V).$$

○   **What happens to F_A/F_I if cardiac output approaches zero (cardiac arrest)?**

Uptake would be minimal and F_A/F_I would quickly equal 1.

○   **What factors determine the input of anesthetic into alveoli (F_A)?**

These factors include: (a) concentration of inspired anesthetic (F_I), (b) alveolar ventilation, and (c) characteristics of the anesthetic delivery system. In addition, the patient's functional residual capacity (FRC) influences the F_A that is achieved.

○   **Name three ways to increase the inspired concentration (F_I) and speed of inhalational induction.**

  a. Start with higher vaporizer setting.

  b. Increase fresh gas flow.

  c. Rebreathing bag can be collapsed prior to starting the FGF (capacity in the circuit is less).

○   **What is anesthetic overpressure?**

Overpressure is compensation for the uptake of anesthetic (especially the highly soluble ones) by delivering a higher concentration than we hope to achieve in the alveoli. For example, on induction of anesthesia, one may use 4–5% of halothane to produce an alveolar concentration of 1%.

○   **The blood/gas partition of desflurane is less than the blood/gas partition of nitrous oxide, yet the rise in the F_A/F_I ratio of nitrous oxide is more rapid than desflurane. How is this possible?**

The concentration effect increases the rate of rise of the F_A/F_I ratio for nitrous oxide, because nitrous oxide is conventionally delivered at 10 times the concentration of desflurane. Also, the lipid solubility, as measured by the oil/gas partition coefficient partition, is higher for desflurane than it is for nitrous oxide (18.7 vs. 1.4). The rate of rise of the alveolar concentration is slower for desflurane than for nitrous oxide because desflurane has a larger volume of distribution.

○   **Why is the concentration effect greater with nitrous oxide than with the volatile anesthetic?**

Because nitrous oxide can be used in much higher concentrations.

○   **List two effects of using nitrous oxide and oxygen for induction of anesthesia with sevoflurane versus 100% oxygen and sevoflurane.**

  1. *Concentration effect:* Nitrous oxide uptake increases alveolar sevoflurane concentration – uptake of N_2O (first gas) reduces the total gas volume and therefore increases the concentration of sevoflurane (second gas) given concomitantly.

  2. *Second gas effect:* Tracheal inflow of sevoflurane is greater than it would be without nitrous oxide – the uptake of N_2O (the primary gas) increases the inspiratory volume, which in effect increases ventilation, and increases the alveolar concentration of sevoflurane (all inspired gases), regardless of the inspired concentration.

○   **What are the anesthetic implications of the use of intraocular sulfur hexafluoride (SF_6)?**

SF_6 is injected into the posterior chamber of the eye to facilitate retinal reattachment. In patients with an intact globe, SF_6 can absorb nitrous oxide resulting in bubble enlargement and an increase in intraocular pressure. If used, N_2O should be replaced with 100% oxygen 15 minutes before the injection procedure. In addition, N_2O should be avoided in any subsequent general anesthetic administered within 10 days.

○ **Why should N_2O be avoided when SF_6 is injected into the eye during repair of a retinal tear?**

Because N_2O use can diffuse into and cause the injected intravitreal bubble to expand in size triggering a rapid and substantial increase in IOP (14–30 mm Hg). This may compromise retinal blood flow, causing retinal ischemia. Nitrous oxide is 117 times more soluble than SF_6.

○ **What is the effect of age on the uptake of inhaled anesthetics?**

Decreased cardiac index and decreased alveolar ventilation to FRC ratio would be expected to reduce the uptake of inhaled anesthetics with advancing age.

○ **What factors determine the speed of induction of inhalational anesthesia in the child versus the adult?**

The rate of rise of the alveolar concentration is more rapid in infants and neonates than adults. The factors speeding induction are alveolar ventilation, solubility, tissue water, and cardiac index. The alveolar ventilation to FRC ratio is 5:1 in the infant and 1.5:1 in the adult. The solubility of agent in blood is 18% less in neonates and the elderly compared with young adults. The agents are 50% less soluble in infant tissues owing to the greater water content of infants. The greater cardiac index of infants speeds the rate of equilibration of the inspired to alveolar gradient.

○ **What physical characteristic of inhaled anesthetics predicts potency?**

Lipid solubility (i.e., oil/gas partition coefficient) predicts MAC. The greater the lipid solubility, the lower the MAC.

○ **What is the best estimate of anesthetic potency for inhaled agents?**

MAC.

○ **What is MAC?**

The minimum alveolar concentration of an inhaled anesthetic required to abolish movement in 50% of patients, in response to a noxious stimulus. It is a reflection of the partial pressure of the agent in the brain.

○ **What is the stimulus used for determination of MAC in humans?**

Surgical incision.

○ **Using variations on the MAC concept, can you estimate the potency of anesthetic agents using other clinical end points?**

MAC awake (Stoelting), MAC skin incision, MAC intubation (Yakaitis), and MAC-bar (Roizen).

MAC awake = the alveolar concentration of anesthetic at which a patient opens his or her eyes to command (0.15–0.5 MAC).

MAC intubation = MAC of anesthetic that would inhibit movement and coughing during endotracheal intubation.

MAC-bar = alveolar concentration of anesthetic that prevents adrenergic responses (bar) to skin incision. MAC-bar = 1.5 × MAC.

MAC_{95} is the alveolar concentration at which 95% of patients will not respond to a skin incision. MAC_{95} = 1.3 × MAC.

○ **What is the relationship between alveolar concentration (end-tidal concentration) and partial pressure of anesthetic in the CNS?**

After a short period of equilibration (8–10 minutes), alveolar concentration directly represents the partial pressure of anesthetic in the CNS (the site of anesthetic action).

First, arterial blood (Pa) equilibrates with the alveolar partial pressure (P_A). Next, the brain equilibrates with the arterial blood, at which point the P_A mirrors brain partial pressure (Pbr).

○ **Does equilibration between two phases mean equal concentrations?**

No. Equilibration means the same partial pressure exists in both phases (not concentration). It is the partial pressure gradient that propels the inhaled anesthetic across various barriers (alveoli, capillaries, cell membranes) until an equilibration is reached.

○ **T/F: When the blood:gas partition coefficient of an anesthetic is 2.0, 1 mL of blood contains two times more anesthetic molecules than 1 mL of alveolar gas, at equilibrium.**

True.

○ **Two anesthetic agents are in equilibrium with blood. With agent A, there are 1,050 volumes in the alveoli and 651 volumes in blood. With agent B, there are 355 volumes in the alveoli and 415 volumes in the blood. From this information can you predict that induction with agent A is faster than with agent B?**

Yes. Since the two anesthetic agents have reached the equilibrium, it is possible to calculate the blood–gas coefficient of these agents.

For the agent A, blood:gas coefficient = 651/1,050 = 0.62.

For the agent B, blood:gas coefficient = 415/355 = 1.16.

Agent A has lower blood–gas solubility than agent B and therefore, we can predict that the induction (and recovery) with agent A will be faster than with agent B.

○ **Two volatile agents are identical except that the blood:gas partition coefficient of anesthetic A is 0.75 and that of anesthetic B is 1.5. Can you conclude that at equilibrium, the partial pressure of anesthetic B in the blood will be twice that of anesthetic A?**

Yes. At equilibrium, there will be twice the volume of anesthetic in blood with agent B compared with agent A.

○ **What happens to MAC when body temperature decreases?**

The MAC of volatile anesthetics decreases 5–7% per °C decrease in core body temperature. The speed of inhalational induction is not changed due to a decrease in cardiac output and increased blood solubility.

○ **What is the effect of age on MAC?**

MAC is usually specified for the 30-year-old. It peaks at 6 months of age at 1.6 MAC, falls to 0.8 MAC at 60 years, and is 0.6 MAC at age 80 (gradually decreases 4–5% per decade after age 40 years).

○ **How do electrolyte abnormalities affect MAC?**

Hypernatremia increases MAC, while hyponatremia decreases MAC.

Hyperkalemia or hypokalemia has no effect on MAC.

○ **List some notable factors that do not alter MAC.**

Duration of anesthesia, gender, type of surgical stimulation, hypocarbia or hypercarbia, metabolic acid–base status, hypertension, isovolemic anemia, and magnesium levels.

○ **What is the effect of a right-to-left shunt on the speed of inhalational induction?**

Slows the rate of induction, in proportion to the size of the shunt. These effects are most marked for insoluble gases, and small or moderate with gases of intermediate solubility.

○ **What is the effect of a left-to-right shunt on the rate of inhalational induction?**

Little or no effect, with normal cerebral perfusion and a normal forward flow.

○ **What are desflurane's essential pharmacologic characteristics?**

Desflurane has a low blood–gas partition coefficient (0.42), is associated with a modest decrease in blood pressure (BP) and increase in heart rate (HR), produces some muscle relaxation, and has a MAC of 6%.

○ **How do the pharmacokinetics of desflurane differ from isoflurane?**

Desflurane has a significantly lower blood–gas coefficient (0.42 vs. isoflurane 1.4) making induction and emergence very rapid (lower blood–tissue coefficient means less drug deposited in peripheral tissues and less hangover after prolonged cases).

○ **Is the blood–gas partition coefficient of sevoflurane high or low?**

Sevoflurane has a low blood–gas partition coefficient (0.69).

○ **What factors govern rate of recovery after a sevoflurane anesthetic?**

Rate of decrease in alveolar concentration is inversely related to lipid solubility (O/G = 50), duration of administration, and B/G partition coefficient (0.63).

○ **Why is it that despite the low blood:gas solubility of sevoflurane, the washout compared with other volatile inhaled anesthetics is essentially the same?**

Although the blood:gas partition coefficient is considerably lower for sevoflurane compared with halothane, the solubility in other tissues, for example, muscle, is very similar. Thus, when the inspired concentration of the inhaled drug is abruptly reduced to zero at the conclusion of an anesthetic, muscle will continue to release the drug back to the blood (for delivery to the lungs for exhalation) at an essentially similar rate for both drugs and therefore prolongs the washout of sevoflurane in spite of its low blood:gas solubility.

○ **What is the effect of inhalational agents on cerebral blood flow (CBF) and cerebral metabolic rate?**

Inhalational agents increase CBF and decrease $CMRO_2$, thus uncoupling the $CBF:CMRO_2$ relationship. The mechanism of increased CBF is cerebral vasodilation, and the order of vasodilator potency is halothane $>>$ enflurane $>$ isoflurane $=$ desflurane $=$ sevoflurane $>$ N_2O.

○ **What is critical CBF?**

As defined by Michenfelder, critical CBF is "that flow below which the majority of subjects develop ipsilateral EEG changes indicative of ischemia within 3 minutes following carotid occlusion." It varies depending on the volatile agent used. The critical CBF for halothane is 18–20 mL/100 g per minute, which is the highest of the volatile agents, whereas for isoflurane the critical CBF is 10–12 mL/100 g per minute, which is the lowest of the volatile agents.

○ **What effects do the inhaled anesthetics have on cerebral autoregulation?**

These potent agents are cerebral vasodilators and at higher MAC levels, all will uncouple the relationship between CBF and CMR such that CBF may equal the awake CBF, despite a reduction in CMR. The relative order of dilation is halothane >> enflurane > isoflurane = sevoflurane = desflurane.

○ **Describe the effects of the inhalation agents on CSF production and reabsorption.**

Halothane: decreases production and decreases reabsorption.

Isoflurane does not appear to alter CSF production, but may increase, decrease, or leave unchanged the resistance to resorption depending on the dose.

Sevoflurane at 1 MAC depresses CSF production up to 40%.

Desflurane at 1 MAC leaves CSF production unchanged or increased.

Overall effect of CSF production and absorption on ICP is however far less important than effect through CBF change.

○ **T/F: Desflurane causes greater increases in intracranial pressure than equipotent doses of isoflurane.**

True, especially in patients with altered intracranial elastance (i.e., space-occupying lesions). Desflurane increases the rate of CSF formation with no significant effect on the rate of CSF reabsorption. Induction of hypocapnia does not consistently prevent the increase in ICP. Isoflurane remains the anesthetic of choice for patients with, or at risk for, cerebral ischemia.

○ **What are effects of nitrous oxide on cerebral circulation?**

Nitrous oxide alone increases: CBF, ICP parallel to increased CBF, and CMR. When nitrous is added to an established inhalation anesthetic, the CBF is modestly increased.

○ **Which potent inhaled agent is associated with seizure activity at higher concentrations?**

Enflurane. Seizures can be produced at 1.5–2 MAC of enflurane, especially when combined with hypocarbia.

○ **What is the effect of inhalational agents on evoked potentials?**

Dose-related decrease in amplitude and increase in latency of somatosensory evoked potentials (SSEP), visual evoked potentials (VEP), and brainstem auditory evoked potentials (BAEP). Decrease in amplitude is more marked than increase in latency. Evoked potentials of cortical origin (VEP and SSEP) are more readily affected by inhalation agents than those of brainstem or subcortical origin. The most sensitive are VEP, followed by SSEP, and the least sensitive are BAEP.

○ **What is an acceptable MAC level for monitoring SSEP?**

0.5–1 MAC isoflurane or sevoflurane.

○ **Which inhalation agents cause the most myocardial depression? List them in order of most to least effect.**

Enflurane = halothane > isoflurane = desflurane = sevoflurane >> N_2O.

Experiments in papillary muscle and isolated heart preparation have consistently demonstrated that N_2O produces a direct negative inotropic effect. This may be offset by concomitant increase in sympathetic nervous system. Negative inotropic action is more pronounced in the presence of preexisting LV dysfunction.

○ **What is the effect of inhalation agents on the HR?**

Halothane causes no change or a decrease in HR due to impairment of the baroreceptor reflex. Isoflurane, desflurane, and enflurane increase HR. The increase in HR with desflurane is more pronounced at deeper levels of anesthesia. Sevoflurane produces little to no change.

○ **What are the circulatory effects of the volatile anesthetics?**

Reduce contractility: enflurane > halothane > isoflurane = desflurane = sevoflurane.

Reduce SVR: isoflurane = desflurane > sevoflurane > enflurane and halothane.

Reduce BP: enflurane > halothane > isoflurane = desflurane > sevoflurane.

Cardiac output is reduced: halothane = enflurane, minimal change with isoflurane, desflurane, or sevoflurane.

HR is increased: enflurane > isoflurane = desflurane >> sevoflurane, and unchanged by halothane.

○ **What effect does desflurane have on the sympathetic nervous system?**

Rapid changes in inspired desflurane, whether at induction or during the anesthetic, result in sympathetic nervous system discharge producing tachycardia (more pronounced at deeper levels of anesthesia) and hypertension. Desflurane is a potent vasodilator, with a reduction in systemic vascular resistance causing hypotension.

○ **A patient is anesthetized with N_2O/O_2 and desflurane. His BP is 140/85 mm Hg and his HR is 95 bpm. The anesthesiologist thinks that the patient is "light," and increases the inspired desflurane concentration from 3% to 10%. The BP increases to 200/110, and the HR to 130. Why?**

A sudden increase in inspired desflurane concentration causes sympathetic nervous system stimulation and increase in circulating levels of catecholamines, causing tachycardia and hypertension. This can be prevented by a more gradual increase in desflurane concentration, or by prior administration of fentanyl or a beta-adrenergic blocker (e.g., esmolol or labetalol).

○ **How may the use of halothane lead to the occurrence of arrhythmias?**

All volatile agents sensitize the myocardium to epinephrine. Isoflurane, sevoflurane, and desflurane all require 3- to 6-fold greater doses of epinephrine to cause dysrhythmia when compared with halothane.

Epinephrine 1 μg/kg during halothane anesthesia is unlikely to produce PVCs. The ED_{50} for subcutaneous epinephrine causing PVCs is 2.1 μg/kg for halothane, 3.7 μg/kg when lidocaine is added to halothane anesthesia, 6.7 μg/kg with enflurane, and 10.9 μg/kg with isoflurane. Children appear to tolerate epinephrine better than do adults. Unlike isoflurane, enflurane, and desflurane, which increase HR, halothane may cause no change or decrease HR.

○ **What pharmacokinetic property of nitrous oxide makes both induction and emergence with this agent rapid?**

Low blood–gas solubility (blood/gas partition coefficient 0.47).

○ **List some disadvantages of nitrous oxide [Myles et al., 2007. See reference on page 526].**

1. It can diffuse readily into air-containing spaces in the body expanding them.
2. Potentially could contribute to postoperative nausea and vomiting.
3. It has a low potency when used alone (MAC 105).
4. Prolonged exposure may result in bone marrow depression (megaloblastic anemia) and neurological deficiencies (peripheral neuropathies and pernicious anemia).
5. May exacerbate pulmonary hypertension.
6. Diffusion hypoxia.

○ **What is diffusion hypoxia and how do you prevent it?**

Hypoxemia seen on recovery from general anesthesia due to the outpouring of large volumes of (very soluble) nitrous oxide into the alveoli, thereby displacing alveolar oxygen and diluting alveolar and arterial carbon dioxide and decreasing respiratory drive. Prevented by high inspired fractions of oxygen and adequate ventilation during the postoperative washout period.

○ **What are the effects of nitrous oxide on DNA synthesis?**

Nitrous oxide oxidizes cobalt in vitamin B_{12} by a physicochemical reaction with nitrous oxide. Vitamin B_{12} is a cofactor for the enzyme methionine synthase (MS). However, the cobalt atom has to be in the reduced from for it to function as a cofactor. Recovery of activity takes 3–4 days because of oxidation, which is irreversible. New enzyme must be synthesized to regain activity. MS is the key enzyme of one-carbon transfer reactions needed to synthesize thymidylate. It is a critical enzyme for DNA replication and cell growth because it is the only de novo source of thymine nucleotide precursors for DNA synthesis.

The neurological disease, subacute combined degeneration of the spinal cord, develops only after several months of daily exposure to nitrous oxide.

○ **What changes in red cell production result from chronic exposure to high concentrations of nitrous oxide?**

The inactivation of MS by N_2O results in a clinical picture of pernicious anemia, with megaloblastic hematopoiesis. Twelve hours of 50% nitrous is sufficient to produce mild megaloblastic changes. The half-life for (irreversible) *inactivation of methionine synthetase is shown to be 46 minutes* when 70% N_2O is administered to patients.

○ **Is isoflurane a suitable agent for use in patients with aortic regurgitation? Why?**

Yes. The regurgitant fraction is reduced by decreasing systemic vascular resistance and increasing HR.

○ **What systemic effects are expected if beta-blockers are administered concomitantly with isoflurane?**

Beta-blockers will abolish the increase in HR associated with isoflurane and increase its negative inotropic. The result is a stable to decreased HR, a decrease in cardiac output, and a more significantly reduced BP.

○ **What are the effects of general anesthetics on the control of respiration?**

The potent inhalational anesthetics reduced the respiratory drive decreasing the hypoxic drive and hypercarbic drive in a dose-related fashion such that the hypoxic drive is abolished at 1.1 MAC and the apneic threshold for hypercarbia is progressively increased.

○ **What is the effect of isoflurane on ventilation?**

Isoflurane depresses the normal response to both hypoxia and hypercarbia and is associated with a decrease in tidal volume and stable respiratory rate. Increases in $PaCO_2$ as a function of inhaled agent are:

Enflurane > desflurane = isoflurane > sevoflurane = halothane.

○ **What is the CO_2 response curve?**

The CO_2 response curve is a graph with the $PaCO_2$ (end-expiratory PCO_2) plotted on the x-axis and the minute ventilation (alveolar ventilation of pulmonary minute volume, L/min) on the y-axis. This curve describes the ventilatory response to carbon dioxide. The relationship between the $PaCO_2$ and MV is nearly linear, such that in the range of 20–80 mm Hg for every 1 mm Hg increase in $PaCO_2$, the MV increases by 2 L/min. Very high arterial $PaCO_2$ tensions depress the ventilatory response.

○ **How do the inhalation agents affect the CO_2 response curve?**

As the inhalational agent is increased, the curve is shifted to the right with a decrease in the slope, indicating a decreased minute volume response to increasing hypercarbia.

○ **T/F: Subanesthetic concentrations of inhalation agents do not affect the ventilatory response to CO_2, but do affect the ventilatory response to hypoxemia.**

True. The ventilatory response to hypoxemia is decreased at 0.1 MAC, and abolished at 1 MAC.

○ **What is the apneic threshold?**

The maximum $PaCO_2$ that does not initiate spontaneous respiration. This is 5 mm Hg below the resting $PaCO_2$, and corresponds to the x-intercept on the CO_2 response curve at which ventilation is zero.

○ **What is the relevance of the apneic threshold to the anesthetic management of the patient?**

It limits the amount of assisted ventilation that can occur. If the patient is allowed to breathe spontaneously under anesthesia, the $PaCO_2$ will increase (e.g., to 50 mm Hg). In an effort to decrease the $PaCO_2$, the anesthesiologist may decide to assist the patient's respirations. But when the $PaCO_2$ drops to 45 mm Hg, the patient will become apneic (he or she will have reached the apneic threshold which is 5 mm Hg below the resting value). Respirations will then have to be controlled rather than assisted.

○ **What effects do inhalational agents and nitrous oxide have on hypoxic pulmonary vasoconstriction (HPV)?**

Inhalational agents including nitrous oxide can inhibit HPV in high doses; for modern volatile agents ED_{50} is about 2 MAC.

○ **What is the effect of inhalation agents on uterine tone?**

Dose-dependent uterine relaxation, with halothane, enflurane, and isoflurane equally depressant at equipotent doses. The effect is modest at 0.5 MAC, but substantial at 1 MAC. N_2O has little or no effect on the uterus. At lower concentrations (less than 1 MAC), the uterine response to oxytocin is preserved. Furthermore, inhalational agents in low concentrations do not increase the blood loss from C-section.

○ **A female patient with hypothyroidism is scheduled for surgery. How does decreased thyroid function affect MAC in females?**

Thyroid gland dysfunction and gender of the patient have no effect on MAC.

○ **T/F: Isoflurane and halothane in equipotent doses produce the same degree of potentiation of nondepolarizing muscle relaxants.**

False. All inhalational anesthetics potentiate nondepolarizing blockade; isoflurane, enflurane, sevoflurane, desflurane > halothane > N_2O/O_2/narcotic. The degree of augmentation depends on the inhalational agent and the choice of muscle relaxant, that is, pancuronium > vecuronium and atracurium.

○ **Name the inhalation agents in order of production of inorganic fluoride ions from most to least.**

Methoxyflurane > sevoflurane > enflurane > isoflurane, desflurane, and halothane (negligible release of fluoride on metabolism). The plasma level associated with nephrogenic diabetes insipidus using methoxyflurane is 50 μmol/L. Despite higher fluoride concentrations associated with sevoflurane, nephrogenic DI has not been reported in humans.

○ **Which receptors are thought to mediate the CNS effect of the potent inhaled anesthetic agents?**

GABA receptors.

○ **For inhaled anesthetics, what percentage of elimination is dependent on metabolism?**

Halothane: 25–45%.

Isoflurane: 0.2%.

Desflurane: 0.02%.

Sevoflurane: 1–5%.

○ **What are the metabolic products of biotransformation of inhaled anesthetics?**

Halothane is 25–45% metabolized in the liver and transformed via the P-450 system to trifluoroacetic acid (TFA), chloride, and bromide. Reductive metabolism of halothane in the relative absence of oxygen produces bromide, fluoride, 1,1-diflouro-2-chloroethylene (CDE), 1,1,1-trifluoro-2-chloroethane (CTE), and 1,1-difluoro-2-bromo-2-chloroethylene (DBE).

Isoflurane is 0.2% metabolized by P-450 to fluoride and TFA.

Desflurane is minimally metabolized but TFA has been recovered from the urine.

Sevoflurane is 1–5% metabolized by P-450 and produces hexafluoroisopropanol and increases serum fluoride concentration.

Nitrous oxide is not metabolized by human tissue but can be reductively metabolized by gut bacteria to molecular nitrogen and free radicals.

○   **What factors increase the risk for "halothane hepatitis?"**

Multiple exposures, female gender, obesity, middle age, and familial factors.

○   **Describe the proposed mechanisms of halothane-induced hepatotoxicity.**

Hypoxia and hypoperfusion

Reductive metabolism

Altered calcium homeostasis

Immune-mediated (trifluoroacetylation of hepatocyte membranes leading to the production of IgG antibodies: anti-TFA antibody)

○   **According to the most recent evidence, what is the most likely cause of halothane hepatitis?**

Recent evidence suggests an idiosyncratic reaction that is immunologically mediated. Liver microsomal proteins, which have been modified by TFA, apparently act as triggering antigens (membrane–hapten complex) and promote the formation of antibodies, which bind to hepatocytes and result in hepatic necrosis. TFA is a product of halothane metabolism by the liver.

○   **What is the hepatitis risk from inhaled anesthetic agents?**

Halothane – 1:35,000. Enflurane has been associated with immune-mediated hepatitis (incidence of 1:800,000). There have been only a few case reports (six) of isoflurane hepatitis. There has been a case report of fatal hepatitis occurring after exposure to desflurane, in a patient who had a halothane anesthetic several years prior. There have been no case reports of fatal hepatitis occurring after exposure to sevoflurane (no TFA proteins) [Nijoku et al., 1997. See reference on page 526].

○   **What effect does nitrous oxide has on air trapped in a compliant body cavity?**

Nitrous oxide will move down the concentration gradient and expand trapped air. The space will increase in volume or pressure until equilibrium is achieved.

The blood–gas partition coefficient of N_2O (0.47) is much greater (34 times) than that of N_2 (0.015) and thus the movement of nitrous into the space is much more rapid than the movement of trapped nitrogen out. The theoretical limit of expansion for an oxygen/nitrous mixture is the reciprocal of the inspired oxygen fraction, that is, if the mix were 50/50, the oxygen fraction = 1/2 and the reciprocal = 2, and thus the volume could double; if the mix were 75% nitrous/25% O_2, the oxygen fraction = 1/4 and the reciprocal = 4, and thus the volume could quadruple.

The magnitude of increase in the space is influenced by the:

1. Partial pressure of N_2O
2. Blood flow to the air-filled cavity (expansion of bowel occurs at a much slower rate compared with pneumothorax)
3. Duration of N_2O administration

○   **A trauma patient presents to the operating room with an undiagnosed pneumothorax and is being ventilated with a mixture of N_2O (75%) and O_2 (25%). What will happen to the size of the pneumothorax?**

The size of the pneumothorax will double in 10 minutes and equilibrate to quadruple the original size by about 30 minutes.

○ **Describe the properties of xenon as an ideal inhaled anesthetic.**

1. The inert noble gas xenon has many characteristics of an ideal inhaled anesthetic agent, that is, blood:gas = 0.14.

2. MAC in humans 0.7 atm or 71%; its use as a sole anesthetic is possible.

3. Provides analgesia (similar to methoxyflurane) due to inhibition of NMDA receptors, but no emergence delirium.

4. Nonexplosive, nonpungent, and odorless.

5. Does not produce significant myocardial depression.

6. Produces no direct systemic organ toxicity and there is evidence that it has cardioprotective and neuroprotective effects, including attenuation of cognitive dysfunction after cardiopulmonary bypass in an animal model.

7. Has no toxic metabolites.

8. Shown to be unusual in that it increases tidal ventilation and decreases respiratory rate, opposite to that of other inhaled anesthetics.

Xenon does not deplete atmospheric ozone or contribute to global warming and greenhouse effect.

However:

1. Xenon cannot be synthesized and is present in atmospheric air at 0.086 ppm so it has to be removed from air by fractional distillation of liquid air, which is costly. Presently, the cost of xenon in the United States is about $10/L (100 × N_2O).

2. The scarcity requires recycling (very low FGF, closed system)!

3. Xenon has a greater density (5.87 g/L) than air (1 g/L) or nitrous oxide (1.53 g/L) and can increase pulmonary resistance and work of breathing.

4. It is similar to nitrous oxide in that it causes air space expansion.

○ **What are the pharmacodynamic and pharmacokinetic effects of inhaled nitric oxide (NO)?**

NO is an endothelium-derived directly acting vasodilator that is administered as an inhaled gas. It decreases pulmonary artery pressure in patients with reactive pulmonary vasoconstriction. This may improve PaO_2 in patients with preexisting pulmonary hypertension and ARDS (without improving mortality). Because NO is active only at the site of administration (which is the pulmonary circulation), right ventricular afterload is reduced without causing systemic hypotension. Its effects are evanescent.

It is administered as a gas at concentrations of 5–100 ppm. Termination of action is by binding with hemoglobin with an affinity 200,000 times that of oxygen.

○ **What physiologic effects are associated with NO?**

Selective pulmonary vasodilation (mediated by an increase in cyclic GMP), maintains coronary perfusion pressure, improves oxygenation, inhibits platelet adhesion and aggregation, modifies sickle RBC and reduces elevated P_{50} toward normal, reduces O_2 toxicity and increases survival during hyperoxia, decreases leukocyte activation, and blunts inflammatory response to reperfusion.

○ **Discontinuation of NO therapy requires what considerations?**

Patients may have a rebound effect with a decrease in oxygenation and an increase in pulmonary vascular resistance, in some cases to values worse than prior to institution of NO. Recommendations for withdrawal of NO include low dose requirements (<5 ppm), FiO_2 40%, PEEP <5, and stable hemodynamics, followed by an increase in FiO_2 to 60–70%, with vasopressor support, if necessary.

Key Terms

Anesthetic uptake: R to L shunt
Anesthetic uptake: solubility coefficient
Anesthetic uptake: ventilation
Blood/gas partition coefficient
Bowel distension
Desflurane, sympathetic response
Diffusion hypoxia after nitrous oxide
Factors affecting recovery from sevoflurane
HPV: factors increasing
Inhalation agents: respiratory effects
Inhalation agents: uptake and delivery
Inhalational anesthetics: ventilator effects
Inhaled anesthetic: metabolism
Inhaled anesthetic: vapor pressure
Inhaled anesthetics: pharmacokinetics
Isoflurane and beta-blockers: cardiac effects
Isoflurane and ventilation
Isoflurane: $CMRO_2$ effect
Isoflurane: effect on cerebral physiology
MAC: age-related changes
MAC and partial pressure

MAC-bar
Megaloblastic hematopoiesis: N_2O
Myocardial contractility: anesthetic effects
Nitric oxide (NO): consequences of discontinuation
NO hemodynamic effects
NO: mechanism of action
N_2O and intraocular gas
N_2O: CBF and $CMRO_2$
N_2O: cerebral effects
N_2O + volume change in gas spaces/bowel distension/
    intestinal obstruction
Recovery from isoflurane
Sevoflurane uptake: infants versus adults
Surgical stimulation: effect on MAC
Uptake and distribution of gases/infant versus adults
Uptake of inhaled anesthetics: V/Q mismatch
Vapor pressure + anesthetic concentration
Volatile agents: CBF and metabolism
Volatile anesthetics: physical properties
Xenon, N_2O, MH

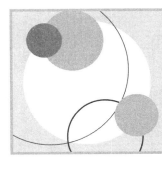

Local Anesthetics

Thanks to modern medicine we are no longer forced to endure prolonged pain, disease, discomfort and wealth.
Robert Orben

○ **What is the mechanism of action of local anesthetics?**

Local anesthetics reversibly bind the intracellular portion of voltage-gated sodium channels at the neural membrane and prevent subsequent channel activation.

Local anesthetics may also block to some degree calcium and potassium channels as well as *N*-methyl-D-aspartate (NMDA) receptors.

Local anesthetics slow the rate of depolarization (slow impulse conduction), decrease the magnitude of action potential, raise the threshold for excitation progressively, and prolong the refractory period.

Local anesthetics do not alter the resting membrane potential.

○ **Do other agents bind and block sodium channels?**

General anesthetics, substance P inhibitors, alpha-2-agonists, tricyclic antidepressants, and nerve toxins also bind and inhibit sodium channels. The latter two classes of drugs have been tested as possible replacements for local anesthetics.

○ **Which regional block site is associated with the highest peak serum level of local anesthetic?**

The absorbance of local anesthetics is highest from the intercostal space. This is followed in descending order by the caudal epidural space, the remainder of the epidural space, the brachial plexus, the lower extremity peripheral nerves, and subcutaneous tissue.

The rate of absorption: intravenous > tracheal > intercostal > caudal > paracervical > epidural > brachial plexus > sciatic > subcutaneous.

The rate of systemic vascular absorption of local anesthetics is proportionate to the vascularity of the site of injection.

○ **What are the main ester-type local anesthetics and how are they metabolized?**

The main ester local anesthetics, procaine, tetracaine, chloroprocaine, and cocaine, undergo hydrolysis by plasma pseudocholinesterases.

○ **What are the main amide-type local anesthetics and how are they metabolized?**

The main amide-type local anesthetics are bupivacaine, lidocaine, etidocaine, mepivacaine, and ropivacaine. Amide local anesthetics contain an "i" in the drug name followed by "caine." Amides are metabolized in the liver by microsomal enzymes (hydroxylation, *N*-dealkylation, and hydrolysis). Metabolism is reduced by drugs that reduce hepatic enzyme activity (i.e., propranolol, cimetidine). Drugs such as barbiturates that induce microsomal enzymes in the liver may slightly increase metabolism.

○ **Which class of local anesthetics is more rapidly metabolized – esters or amides?**

In general, the esters are more rapidly metabolized.

○ **What is the amide local anesthetic with the shortest half-life?**

Prilocaine. It has a short half-life because it is also metabolized in the lung and kidney.

○ **Cimetidine administration will likely increase plasma levels of which class of local anesthetics?**

Cimetidine decreases hepatic clearance of amide anesthetics. Ester metabolism is independent of hepatic blood flow and cytochrome P450 action.

○ **A patient states she had a severe allergic reaction to an unknown anesthetic. What class of local anesthetic is most likely responsible?**

The overall incidence of true allergic reactions to local anesthetics is very low, the majority being esters. The common metabolite of esters, *para*-aminobenzoic acid, is frequently present in the chemical environment and prior exposure may lead to sensitization. Alternatively, intravascular injections in the dentist's office associated with epinephrine-induced side effects (tachycardia and arrhythmias) and tinnitus may be reported as an "allergic reaction."

○ **What compound is responsible for the majority of allergic reactions to the amide class of local anesthetics?**

Methylparaben, the preservative in multidose vials. Preservative-free amides should be used in patients who are allergic to ester local anesthetics.

○ **A patient allergic to PABA should not be given which type of anesthetic?**

Allergic reactions to *para*-aminobenzoic acid have been associated with cross-reactivity to ester anesthetics. The preservative methylparaben may also cross-react with PABA. In general, any patient allergic to PABA should be given an amide local anesthetic from a single-dose vial.

○ **If a patient is allergic to Novocaine™, can he or she receive lidocaine?**

Yes. Novocaine™ is the trade name for procaine, an ester local anesthetic, and lidocaine is an amide. Cross-sensitivity between esters and amides is very rare.

○ **What is the value of skin testing in determining the safety of a local anesthetic?**

Skin testing has limited value and can actually cause anaphylactic reactions, so it is not entirely safe. Even a normal skin test does not rule out a potential allergic reaction to a local anesthetic.

○ **Which patients are at increased risk for systemic toxicity with lidocaine administration?**

Reduced drug metabolism due to impaired liver function or decreased liver blood flow (e.g., in cirrhosis or CHF) as well as severe hypoproteinemia (less protein binding means more free drug in plasma) places patients at increased risk for toxicity with lidocaine.

○ **What are the premonitory symptoms associated with toxic blood levels of a local anesthetic?**

The patient may complain of ringing in the ears, difficulty hearing, a metallic taste in the mouth, numbness around the lips, and a general feeling of restlessness or impending doom.

○ **While performing an axillary block, 15 mL of 0.25% bupivacaine was accidentally injected intravascularly. What signs and symptoms should you look for?**

Systemic administration may produce both central nervous system and cardiac toxicity. Initially there may be CNS excitation (light-headedness, perioral numbness, dizziness, blurred vision) followed rapidly by disorientation, drowsiness, generalized convulsions, and respiratory depression/arrest. Arrhythmias and cardiovascular collapse may occur when the heart sees a high plasma concentration through either very large IV administration or a high concentration returning to the heart as a bolus (as in an injection of 0.75% bupivacaine traversing the route from the epidural veins to azygos veins and then directly to the heart).

○ **While performing an intercostal block, the patient suddenly seizes. Describe appropriate management.**

CNS toxicity can occur from intravascular injections.

Recommendations for treatment of LA systemic toxicity (LAST):

Airway management is the first step. Hyperventilation is helpful to decrease local anesthetic levels in the brain and to increase the PaO_2 of the patient during the seizure.

Seizure suppression: benzodiazepines or small doses of barbiturates should be administered to terminate the seizure.

BCLS/ACLS:

Use small initial doses of epinephrine (10–100 µg boluses).

Vasopressin is not recommended.

Avoid Ca channel blockers, beta-blockers, and local anesthetics.

Consider lipid emulsion therapy at first signs of LAST:

1.5 mL/kg bolus of 20% lipid emulsion.

Infusion at 0.25 mL/kg per minute for at least 10 minutes after return of circulatory stability.

Consider giving a second bolus and increasing infusion to 0.50 mL/kg if circulatory stability is not attained.

Upper limit of lipid emulsion recommended is 10 mL/kg over the first 30 minutes.

Consider cardiopulmonary bypass if lipid emulsion treatment fails [Jeng et al., 2010. See reference on page 526].

○ **What is the antiarrhythmic drug of choice in treating bupivacaine cardiotoxicity?**

Amiodarone now seems to be the drug of choice for treatment of bupivacaine-induced ventricular arrhythmias.

○ **T/F: More potent, more lipid-soluble local anesthetic agents have greater cardiac toxicity.**

True. All local anesthetics have direct cardiac and peripheral vascular effects.

The dose required for cardiovascular to CNS (CVS:CNS) toxicity is lower for bupivacaine than for lidocaine. Toxic doses of lidocaine cause hypotension, bradycardia, and hypoxia while toxic doses of bupivacaine lead to cardiovascular collapse due to ventricular dysrhythmias. Cardiac resuscitation after bupivacaine toxicity is more difficult.

○ **T/F: Pregnant patients appear to be more sensitive to the cardiotoxic effect of bupivacaine than nonpregnant patients.**

True.

○ **Do ropivacaine and levobupivacaine reduce the risk of toxicity?**

Both ropivacaine and levobupivacaine have an improved safety profile compared with bupivacaine particularly with respect to cardiac toxicity. However, there are numerous recent reports of both cardiac and CNS toxicity to these agents. Commercial bupivacaine is a 50:50 racemic mixture of both the *S*- and *R*-enantiomers. Ropivacaine and levobupivacaine are the pure *S*-form of the drug that is less cardiotoxic than the *R*-isomer. All currently available LA are racemic mixtures (50:50) with the exception of lidocaine (does not have asymmetry), ropivacaine (*S*-enantiomer), and levobupivacaine (*S*-enantiomer).

○ **What are the factors that contribute to CNS and cardiotoxicity from local anesthetics?**

Amount of available drug (overdosage, decreased protein binding, speed of injection, direct inadvertent intravascular injection, site of injection, i.e., 0.25 mL into the vertebral artery = seizures) and systemic absorption. More potent agents are usually more toxic (i.e., 0.75% bupivacaine). Bupivacaine is also the most cardiotoxic because of its slow dissociation from myocardial sodium channels resulting in refractory cardiac depression. Hypoxia, hypercarbia, acidosis, and pregnancy all potentiate systemic toxicity.

○ **T/F: Local anesthetics bind more rapidly and with higher affinity to activated sodium channels.**

True. Sodium channels could be in three different states:

1. Resting – in the absence of stimulus resting or closed state.
2. Activated – sodium channel's open state or preceding the open state.
3. Inactivated – within milliseconds after opening, channels transition to inactivated state.

Local anesthetics bind more rapidly and with higher affinity to activated channels (open or preceding the open state) or the inactivated channels than to resting channels.

Order of affinity of local anesthetics for different channel states: open > inactivated > resting. Therefore, local anesthetic action is both voltage and time dependent. The effect is greatest when nerve fibers are firing rapidly. Regardless of the channel state, by its very binding the local anesthetic stabilizes that state.

○ **What feature of bupivacaine contributes to the higher cardiac toxicity?**

Two features of bupivacaine enhance cardiac toxicity:

1. Exhibits a much stronger binding affinity to resting and inactivated Na channels.
2. Local anesthetics bind to sodium channels during systole and dissociate during diastole. Because of the affinity, bupivacaine dissociates very slowly and the duration of diastole at physiologic heart rate (60–180 bpm) does not allow complete recovery and bupivacaine conduction block accumulates.

3. Bupivacaine also has a potent peripheral inhibitory effect on sympathetic reflexes. This has been observed even after uncomplicated regional blocks with bupivacaine. Bupivacaine has direct potent vasodilating properties, especially at high concentrations, and this may exacerbate the cardiovascular collapse.

○ **How does hypercarbia increase toxicity to local anesthetics?**

Hypercarbia reduces the seizure threshold to local anesthetics. Elevation of the $PaCO_2$ increases cerebral blood flow and delivery of the agent to the CNS. Decrease in pH decreases the amount of protein binding of local anesthetics increasing the free plasma fraction. Decrease in intracellular pH also causes ion trapping.

○ **Which local anesthetic is associated with a low risk of systemic toxicity?**

2-Chloroprocaine. It is rapidly metabolized by pseudocholinesterase (plasma half-life less than 30 seconds), allowing doses of up to 12 mg/kg.

○ **What is the one factor that mostly influence the onset of a local anesthetic?**

The pK_a. The closer the pK_a is to pH of 7.4, the more rapid the onset. An exception to this rule is 2-chloroprocaine. It has a pK_a of 8.1. However, it has a rapid onset because it is used in high concentrations (3%).

○ **In choosing a local anesthetic, the anesthesiologist desires a drug with a pK$_a$ closest to physiologic pH. What would be the anesthetic of choice?**

Mepivacaine with a pK_a of 7.6. Lidocaine (pK_a of 7.8) and bupivacaine (pK_a of 8.1) would be alternate choices. As the pK_a of the drug is closer to the physiologic pH (or less than the physiologic pH), especially in the case of weak bases such as local anesthetics, the percentage in the nonionized form increases at physiologic pH. It is this form that crosses the nerve cell membrane.

○ **What role does ionization play in the effect of local anesthetics?**

The concentration of the nonionized portion is significant because this is the amount available to pass through the lipophilic membrane. However, once inside the membrane, it is the ionized portion that then blocks the sodium channels.

○ **A newly discovered local anesthetic was found to have a pK$_a$ of 7.4. What percent of the anesthetic will be unionized in the plasma?**

Fifty percent. The pK_a of a drug is the pH at which 50% of the drug is ionized and 50% is nonionized.

○ **What steps can you take to make a local anesthetic more alkaline and thus have more molecules in the nonionized state?**

You can add bicarbonate to the solution. The ratio for lidocaine is 1 cm^3 bicarbonate to 9 cm^3 of lidocaine. The ratio for bupivacaine is 0.1 cm^3 of bicarbonate for each 9.9 cm^3 of bupivacaine. Also, select solutions that do not have epinephrine commercially added. These solutions typically have a starting pH of 3–5.0.

○ **What effect does sodium bicarbonate have when mixed with a local anesthetic?**

The bicarbonate raises the pH of the solution. This alkalization increases the nonionized fraction of the anesthetic and speeds onset. This relationship is defined by the Henderson–Hasselbalch equation: acidic drugs work better in an acidic environment (acetyl salicylic acid is better absorbed in the stomach) and basic drugs work better in a basic environment.

○ **Why have anesthesiologists been cautious with the intrathecal use of 2-chloroprocaine?**

2-Chloroprocaine has been associated with cauda equina syndrome. Although follow-up studies have implicated the preservatives or additives (bisulfite, ethylenediaminetetraacetic acid [EDTA]) as the true etiology of the neurotoxicity, recent animal studies have demonstrated opposite effects. Intrathecal administration of chloroprocaine induced significant functional impairment and histologic damage, whereas bisulfite did not. In addition, coadministration of bisulfite reduced injury induced by chloroprocaine (sodium bisulfite scapegoat for chloroprocaine neurotoxicity?). Regardless of the anesthetic chosen, only preservative-free solutions should be used in the intrathecal space.

It seems, at this point, additional data are needed before the use of chloroprocaine spinal in clinical practice [Drasner, 2005. See reference on page 526].

○ **A patient complains of severe back pain after 2-chloroprocaine epidural anesthesia. Is this a significant problem?**

As many as 40% of patients may complain of back pain with 2–3% solutions of chloroprocaine, especially with the use of >20 mL. This pain is time limited and is not associated with neurologic deficits. The preservative disodium EDTA is a high-affinity calcium chelator and may cause local muscle spasms by leaching calcium from paravertebral muscles. Chloroprocaine has become available in a preservative-free preparation.

○ **What are the anesthetics that can be applied topically?**

Tetracaine, lidocaine, cocaine, and eutectic mixture of local anesthetics (EMLA) cream. Attention to maximum dosages must be closely observed to avoid systemic toxicity.

○ **What are the active ingredients in EMLA topical cream?**

EMLA 5% cream is made from a 2.5% lidocaine–2.5% prilocaine mixture. Its onset time is approximately 45–60 minutes.

○ **Toxicity after the use of EMLA cream has been associated with what systemic effects?**

Because of the prilocaine present in EMLA, methemoglobinemia can occur with the use of EMLA cream. Usually there is minimal plasma absorbance, but toxic blood levels are possible with prolonged application or when applied to abnormal skin [Hahn I, et al., 2004. See reference on page 526].

○ **What are the contraindications (or precautions) to EMLA cream application?**

1. Known history of sensitivity to amide local anesthetics such as lidocaine and prilocaine (very rare).
2. Patients treated with class III antiarrhythmic drugs (amiodarone, bretylium, sotalol, dofetilide) should be under close supervision and ECG monitoring should be considered, because cardiac effects may be additive.
3. Animal studies have shown ototoxic effects when instilled into the middle ear.
4. Prilocaine metabolite O-toluidine can cause methemoglobinemia.
5. Should not be used in patients with congenital or idiopathic methemoglobinemia or infants <12 months on methemoglobin-inducing drugs.
6. Neonates and infants up to 3 months should be closely monitored for methemoglobin levels before, during, and after treatment with EMLA cream.

○ **Which topical anesthetic is associated with intense vasoconstriction?**

Cocaine is an intense vasoconstrictor and is beneficial in topicalization of the nasopharynx.

○ **Which neuronal membranes are blocked first by local anesthetics and why?**

B fibers, which are the preganglionic sympathetic fibers, are the first to be blocked. Traditional texts often state that small-diameter axons, such as C fibers, are more susceptible to local anesthetic blockade than larger-diameter fibers are. However, when careful measurements are made of single-impulse annihilation in individual nerve fibers, exactly the opposite differential susceptibility is seen. There is evidence that large myelinated fibers are more sensitive to LA blockade than the smaller unmyelinated fibers.

Nevertheless, placement of local anesthetic solutions in the subarachnoid space produces conduction blockade of small-diameter nerve fibers first, because the anatomy of the dorsal nerve root is such that small-diameter nerve fibers are close to the nerve root surface. (This shortens the diffusion distance of the local anesthetic.) The diffusion path to the large-diameter nerve fibers, which are situated deeper in the dorsal nerve roots, is longer, making it appear that the small-diameter nerve fibers are more sensitive to local anesthetic blockade than the larger-diameter nerve fibers.

○ **Are local anesthetic solutions that contain epinephrine more acidic or more alkaline when compared with similar solutions without epinephrine?**

Commercially prepared solutions containing epinephrine are more acidic. For example, lidocaine hydrochloride has a pH of 5.0–5.5, whereas premixed with epinephrine the pH is 2.0–2.5. The latter prevents the spontaneous hydrolysis of the solution. The greater acidity leads to less nonionized drug immediately available and slows onset. This is why anesthesiologists frequently add "fresh" epinephrine to local anesthetic solutions just prior to administration.

○ **Which local anesthetic's duration of action is most affected by the addition of epinephrine?**

The addition of epinephrine to the relatively short-acting lidocaine significantly increases the clinical duration of action. This enhancement is due to epinephrine's ability to counteract the vasodilatory effects of lidocaine and keeps the drug from being absorbed systemically. Epinephrine does not significantly prolong bupivacaine probably because the inherent duration of these drugs exceeds the duration of epinephrine's effect. However, epinephrine prolongs analgesia and improves quality of analgesia when added to more dilute solutions such as labor epidurals.

○ **When comparing plain solutions of lidocaine and mepivacaine, which agent has a greater duration of action?**

Mepivacaine has a greater duration of action even though other local anesthetic characteristics are similar.

○ **What is the average time to two-segment dermatome regression after placement of 20 mL of 2% lidocaine in the epidural space?**

Sixty to 90 minutes.

○ **Why does a motor block precede a sensory block when an axillary approach to a brachial plexus block is performed?**

Different fiber types are differentially sensitive to local anesthetic blockade. In vivo experiments show unequivocally [Miller, 2010]:

- Small myelinated axons (Aγ motor and Aδ sensory fibers) are the most susceptible.
- Next, large myelinated (Aα and Aβ fibers).
- The least susceptible are the small, unmyelinated C fibers.

○ **What local anesthetics provide the best differential blockade?**

Ropivacaine and bupivacaine provide the best differential blockade. Lower concentrations of these drugs can provide reliable sensory blockade with minimal motor blockade.

○ **What is the advantage of differential block?**

Dilution to very low concentration (0.08%) will result in analgesia with minimal or no motor blockade.

○ **A patient with end-stage liver disease is most susceptible to local anesthetic toxicity from which class of agents?**

Amides.

○ **An 18-month-old 12-kg child presents for hypospadias repair. A single-injection caudal blockade is planned for postoperative pain relief. What is the maximum recommended dose of bupivacaine?**

The maximum dose is 2 mg/kg. In this scenario, one could use 0.25% bupivacaine plain, 9.5 mL (24 mg) total.

○ **The anesthesiologist is preparing to perform an awake fiber-optic intubation on a 40-kg patient. How much 4% cocaine can she use to aid in topicalization of the airway?**

Three cubic centimeters or 120 mg. The maximum dose for topical cocaine is 3 mg/kg.

○ **A spinal anesthetic was placed for a cesarean section. In what order will the differential blockade occur?**

The first modality blocked is the sympathetic fibers. This is followed by loss of sensation (temperature first, and then pain, touch, and proprioception). The last nerves blocked are the motor fibers.

○ **What is the expected clinical duration of a single dose of epidural 2-chloroprocaine?**

Thirty to 45 minutes depending on the amount used.

○ **What effect does protein binding have on the duration of action of local anesthetics?**

Highly protein-bound local anesthetics have a prolonged duration of action. For example, procaine is poorly protein bound (6%) and accordingly has a very short duration of action.

○ **What is the most important property determining the potency of a local anesthetic?**

Lipophilicity. More lipophilic means greater potency. Alteration of molecular structure can also increase potency (e.g., the addition of a four-carbon chain to procaine to create tetracaine and the replacement of the methyl on the tertiary amine of mepivacaine with a butyl group to create bupivacaine).

○ **After performing a field block with 10 mL of 0.5% bupivacaine for an incision and drainage of an abscess, the surgeon notes that the patient is still very uncomfortable. What might explain this?**

Local anesthetics are less effective in acidic environments such as infected tissue. This is due to the low tissue pH increasing the ionized portion of the anesthetic, making less nonionized anesthetic base available to cross the lipophilic membrane.

○ **Which local anesthetic is associated with inhibition of norepinephrine reuptake?**

Cocaine inhibits norepinephrine reuptake, resulting in frequent episodes of hypertension and tachycardia.

○ **What are the possible reasons to avoid epinephrine in labor epidurals?**

Epinephrine, when absorbed systemically, may worsen hypertension in a preeclamptic patient. The beta-agonist effect may also cause uterine relaxation and prolong labor. Furthermore, downregulation of beta-adrenergic effects in normal pregnancy means an intravascular "test dose" injection will not reliably produce the diagnostic tachycardia indicative of intravascular injection.

○ **What is the maximum recommended dosage of epinephrine used in peripheral nerve blocks?**

Maximum recommended dosage is 200–250 μg.

○ **Do local anesthetics cross the placenta?**

Yes. More protein-bound agents (bupivacaine, etidocaine) have less delivery to the fetus. Ester local anesthetics also reach the fetus to a lesser extent because of their short plasma half-life.

○ **Does fetal acidosis affect fetal transfer of local anesthetics?**

Yes. Higher fetal concentrations of amide local anesthetic (ionized fraction) are detected during fetal acidosis (ion trapping).

Key Terms

Alkalinization of lidocaine
Bupivacaine toxicity: treatment
Cardiac toxicity of ropivacaine versus bupivacaine
Chloroprocaine metabolism
2-Chloroprocaine: onset
Chloroprocaine toxicity
Effects of epinephrine on lidocaine absorption
EMLA: contraindications
Ester hydrolysis of chloroprocaine
Ester local anesthetics: allergy

Hypercapnia and local anesthetics CNS toxicity
Local anesthetic absorption
Local anesthetic cardiotoxicity
Local anesthetic pK_a: onset and lipophilicity
Local anesthetic potency: lipid solubility
Local anesthetic toxicity: management
Local anesthetics: prolongation of action
Local anesthetics: stereochemistry
Peripheral nerves: sensory versus motor

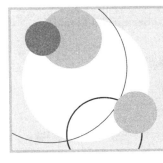

Machines

I think that anyone who comes upon a nautilus machine suddenly will agree with me that its prototype was clearly invented at some time in history when torture was considered a reasonable alternative to diplomacy.
Anna Quindlen

○ **If you are using a self-inflating resuscitation bag and mask to ventilate a patient, what will an increase in the minute ventilation do to the FiO_2 delivered?**

FiO_2 generally decreases. The exact change depends on the rate of oxygen delivery to the bag, the minute ventilation, and the specific method of oxygen delivery to the bag. The use of a reservoir combined with high oxygen flows allows 100% oxygen to be delivered irrespective of the minute ventilation. FiO_2 delivered is *directly proportional to O_2 flow rate* (usually 100% – with 10 L/min of O_2) and *inversely proportional to MV*. Use of a Venturi delivery system allows a constant FiO_2, although a lower maximal FiO_2 is achieved than with a reservoir and high-flow oxygen.

○ **If you add an oxygen reservoir tube to a self-inflating resuscitation bag, what happens to the maximal FiO_2 that can be delivered?**

The addition of an oxygen reservoir tube to a self-inflating resuscitation bag increases the maximal FiO_2 that can be delivered.

○ **What are the primary components of soda lime?**

The primary components of "wet" or "high moisture" soda lime (the most common type in use today) are calcium hydroxide (76–81%), sodium hydroxide (4%), potassium hydroxide (1%), and water (14–19%).

○ **What are the primary components of Baralyme?**

Calcium hydroxide (80%) and barium hydroxide (20%). Moisture in Baralyme is incorporated into the structure of the barium hydroxide, which exists as an octahydrate. However, Baralyme is no longer used. It was thought to be the primary absorbent responsible for fires in the breathing system when used with sevoflurane.

○ **What are the basic reactions involved in CO_2 absorption by soda lime and Baralyme?**

In both cases, CO_2 first reacts with water to form carbonic acid. The carbonic acid then combines with the various hydroxides found in the absorber chemicals to form carbonates and heat.

○ **What is the optimum size for absorbent granules?**

The optimum size for absorbent granules is four to eight mesh. Granules smaller than eight mesh cause excess resistance and tend to cake, while granules larger than four mesh offer less surface area for absorption.

○ **What volume of intergranular air must be in the carbon dioxide canister to maximize carbon dioxide absorption?**

The intergranular air space must be at least as large as the maximal tidal volume in order to trap all the CO_2 that passes through the absorber.

○ **If the canister of soda lime doesn't feel warm, what should you suspect?**

The absorption of CO_2 by either Baralyme or soda lime is exothermic. If the canister is not warm, you should suspect that CO_2 is not being absorbed.

○ **What is the maximal absorbant capacity for soda lime?**

The maximal absorbent capacity for soda lime is generally reported as about 25 L of CO_2/100 g of absorbent. With either absorber, the color indicator may revert back to its pre-exhausted color if the absorbent is rested. This does not indicate a significant recovery of absorbent capacity and the color will quickly change to its exhausted state if the absorbent is reused.

○ **How can soda lime exhaustion be detected?**

A pH-sensitive dye (usually ethyl violet) added to the granules will change color (from white to purple) in the presence of carbonic acid. Dye indicator mimosa 2 will change from pink to white when the absorbent is exhausted. Additionally, baseline CO_2 on the capnogram will increase above zero if rebreathing occurs in the presence of exhausted soda lime.

○ **What factors may cause an elevated inspired CO_2?**

Rebreathing of CO_2 results in elevated inspired CO_2. Rebreathing may be caused by a depleted, faulty, or bypassed carbon dioxide absorber, faulty unidirectional valves, and any cause of increased dead space. In a Mapleson circuit, significant rebreathing of CO_2 results from insufficient fresh gas flow (FGF). A hole in the inner tube of a coaxial circuit can allow significant rebreathing. Failure of the carbon dioxide waveform to return on the capnograph to baseline is diagnostic of rebreathing.

In some countries, anesthesia machines are equipped with CO_2 tanks and flow meters. Delivery of CO_2 from such a tank, a misfilled tank, or an incorrect connection would cause the inspired CO_2 to be elevated.

A high end-tidal CO_2 is indicative of hypercapnia usually due to inadequate alveolar ventilation. Predisposing factors may include increased CO_2 production or decreased carbon dioxide elimination.

○ **What is the significance of the desiccation of CO_2 absorbent?**

Desiccated absorbent makes the formation of compound A from sevoflurane more likely. It also increases the heat produced, and the use of sevoflurane with desiccated absorbent has been associated with fires. Desflurane is degraded into potentially significant amounts of carbon monoxide (CO) by desiccated CO_2 absorbent.

○ **What factors contribute to the generation of CO in the anesthesia circuit?**

Physical properties of the absorbent, and choice and concentration of volatile anesthetic agent.

The drier the absorbent, the more CO produced. At any given moisture content, Baralyme produces more CO than soda lime. Higher temperatures lead to greater production of CO. Increased concentration of the volatile anesthetic agent leads to greater CO production. The choice of inhaled agent influences the production rate; ranked in order of greatest to least CO production: desflurane ≥ enflurane > isoflurane >> halothane = sevoflurane.

Significant CO production from the degradation of sevoflurane is seen as the reaction temperature exceeds 80°C.

○ **What is compound A?**

It is an olefin formed by the breakdown of sevoflurane by soda lime or Baralyme. In concentrations higher than that seen in humans, it can cause renal tubular necrosis, but no case reports in humans exist. Its formation is increased in the presence of dry soda lime, low FGFs (<2 L/min), higher temperatures, and longer MAC hours of anesthesia, and is greater in the presence of Baralyme than that of soda lime.

○ **Which inhalation agent is the most unstable in soda lime? Which is the most stable?**

Most unstable: sevoflurane; most stable: desflurane.

○ **How much increase in FiO_2 occurs when the oxygen flow via nasal cannula is increased?**

FiO_2 increases approximately 4% for each L/min increase in delivered O_2, up to 6 L/min. Flow rates beyond 6 L/min do not predictably increase FiO_2 above approximately 44% and are also poorly tolerated because of drying and crusting of the nasal mucosa.

○ **What is the main advantage of Venturi (air-entrainment) face mask?**

The Venturi face mask provides a stable FiO_2 between 24% and 40%, irrespective of changes in minute ventilation and inspiratory flow rate. The performance of these masks is not appreciably affected by the patient's ventilatory pattern.

○ **Where is the dead space constituted in a properly functioning circle system?**

The dead space in a circle system with functioning unidirectional valves is limited to the area distal to the point of inspiratory and expiratory gas mixing at the Y-piece. The breathing-tube length of a circle system does not directly affect dead space.

○ **Describe one characteristic of pediatric circuits.**

They have low-compliance breathing tubes to reduce the compression volume that may cause large discrepancy between the tidal volume that is actually delivered to the patient and the tidal volume that has been preset.

○ **What are the four major functions of the breathing bag in a circle system?**

1. Reservoir of exhaled gas that allows rebreathing
2. Provides positive pressure ventilation
3. Visual and tactile monitoring of spontaneous ventilation
4. Limits the maximum pressure that can develop in the system

○ **What is the preferred order of components in a circle system?**

The unidirectional valves should be as close to the patient as possible, but not in the Y-piece as that may lead to improper orientation of the valves. Practically speaking, since the valves are not disposable, they are closer to the machine rather than closer to the patient in the flexible breathing tubes. The fresh gas inlet should be between the CO_2 absorber and the inspiratory valve, positioned upstream of the inspiratory valve. The pressure relief valve should be located immediately before the CO_2 absorber. The breathing bag should be located in the expiratory limb to reduce resistance to exhalation.

○ **What are the consequences of an inspiratory valve malfunction?**

In the unlikely event that the inspiratory valve is stuck in the closed position and the expiratory valve is competent, it would be impossible to deliver a breath to the patient. The more common scenario is failure of the inspiratory valve to properly close allowing rebreathing of expired gas containing CO_2. Hypercapnia may be tolerated or the effect slightly ameliorated by increasing the FGF rates until the valve can be replaced or an alternate breathing system employed.

○ **What are the consequences of an expiratory valve malfunction?**

Malfunction of either unidirectional valve leads to rebreathing of CO_2 resulting in hypercapnia.

Unidirectional valve problems can be detected preoperatively during the breathing system checkout using breathing method or valve tester. Some respirometers will indicate reverse flow. The capnograph will indicate inspired CO_2 greater than zero.

○ **When does rebreathing occur in a circle system?**

Rebreathing occurs with low FGF rates and requires use of a CO_2 absorber to remove carbon dioxide from the exhaled gas. Increasing FGF to greater than 5 L/min minimizes rebreathing.

○ **What are some advantages of a circle system versus a Bain (coaxial) circuit?**

The circle system allows use of a CO_2 absorber. The absorber allows CO_2 to be scrubbed from the rebreathed gases. This in turn allows rebreathing of gas without hypercapnia. Rebreathing of gas allows conservation of heat and humidity and the use of lower FGF. Lower FGF allows for reduced pollution and reduced use of agent with resultant lower cost. The downside of the circle system is that it is bigger, is less portable, is more complex, has more components, which can disconnect or fail, and has greater resistance.

○ **What is the FGF requirement of a Mapleson A circuit to prevent significant rebreathing of CO_2?**

For spontaneous ventilation, an FGF equal to the minute ventilation is sufficient. Mapleson A design is the most effective Mapleson circuit for spontaneous ventilation. For controlled ventilation, a very high and unpredictable FGF is required with Mapleson A to prevent significant rebreathing of CO_2.

○ **What is the FGF requirement to prevent significant rebreathing of CO_2 with a Mapleson D circuit?**

For spontaneous ventilation, two to three times the minute ventilation is required. For controlled ventilation, FGF of one to two times the minute ventilation is sufficient to prevent rebreathing of CO_2.

○ **Rank the Mapleson circuits in order of efficiency during spontaneous ventilation.**

A, D, E, C, B (All Doggi … Es Can Bite).

○ **Rank the Mapleson circuits in order of efficiency during controlled ventilation.**

D, E, B, C, A (DEad Bodies Can't Argue).

○ **Why are flow meters (rotameters) not interchangeable?**

Flow meters are calibrated for specific gases. Flow rate across a constriction depends on the gas's viscosity at low laminar flows and its density at high turbulent flows. Therefore, gases with similar viscosity (oxygen and helium) may read identically at low flows, while gases with similar densities (nitrous oxide [N_2O] and carbon dioxide) will read the same at high flows. Nitrous and oxygen rotameters would not read the same, having different density and viscosity.

Therefore, for calibration purposes both the density and the viscosity of the gas are important (i.e., flow meter are not interchangeable). Careful recalibration is required if a flow meter is used for a different gas than that for which it was initially designed.

○ **What effect does increased altitude has on traditional flow meters?**

Flow meters are meant to be used within a certain range of temperature and pressures (i.e., at atmospheric pressure of 760 mm Hg and room temperature of 20°C).

Practically speaking, temperature changes are slight under working environments and do not cause significant changes.

At low flow rates, flow is laminar and dependent on gas viscosity, a property that is independent of altitude.

However, at high flow rates, flow becomes turbulent and flow becomes a function of density, a property which is influenced by altitude.

Therefore, as altitude increases, barometric pressure decreases, resulting in increase in actual flow rate (i.e., flow meter will read lower than the actual flow rate).

○ **The traditional mechanical glass flow meters are described as constant-pressure, variable-orifice flow meter. Why?**

The glass tubes are tapered creating a variable orifice around the bobbin. Therefore, the pressure decrease across the bobbin stays constant.

Stated differently, the annular cross-sectional area varies (greater flow area at higher flows) while the pressure drop across the indicator remains constant for all positions inside the tube.

○ **The new anesthesia stations (Datex-Ohmeda S5/ADU, Drager Fabius GS) are equipped with virtual flow meters (no gas tubes). How are they different from traditional flow meters?**

In the virtual flow meters, the gas flows are still controlled by mechanical needle valves but flows are measured using electronic flow sensors.

The flow sensors are based on the principle of pneumotachograph. The pressure drop across a laminar flow resistor is measured using differential pressure transducer and displayed on a screen in the form of a virtual graduated flow meter with a digital display.

○ **What are some advantages of electronic flow sensors?**

1. Less expensive than rotameters.
2. Data can be used elsewhere in the work station (to record gas consumption, adjust ventilator bellows).

○ **How can you prevent a hypoxic gas mixture from being delivered to the patient, as determined by the gas flow meter settings?**

There are two systems in use in the US anesthesia machines. Ohmeda machines use a Link-25 proportioning system that is a mechanical interlink. Dräger machines use a combined pneumatic and mechanical system (oxygen ratio monitor controller), which makes it impossible to deliver more than 75% N_2O, relative to the flow of oxygen. The alarm is disabled when the "all gases" mode switch is selected, which allows the addition of a third gas.

○   **What is the significance of a circuit low-pressure alarm?**

With an anesthesia machine, mechanical ventilation is achieved by generating positive pressure in the breathing circuit. A low-pressure alarm sounds when a sufficient pressure is not generated. This alarm is also referred to as a disconnect alarm. Low-pressure alarm threshold should be set just below (<7 cm H_2O) the minimum peak pressure expected in order to detect leaks and partial disconnections.

○   **What safeguards are present to warn airway disconnections?**

A disconnect alarm that detects drop in the peak circuit pressure will be activated during controlled mechanical ventilation. A standing bellows (ascending) will fail to fill. Some machines offer an alarm that warns if insufficient expired gas is returned. Failure of the reservoir bag to inflate will occur during spontaneous ventilation and the patient may show signs of insufficient depth of anesthesia. The capnograph will record no carbon dioxide waveform and the apnea alarm will sound. Clinical signs include failure of the chest to rise and loss of breath sounds if auscultating with a precordial stethoscope. A late sign is hypoxemia as measured by a reduction in SpO_2 with pulse oximetry.

○   **What prevents positive pressure check from detecting a leak in the anesthesia machines?**

A check valve, installed to prevent the pumping effect in vaporizers, also prevents back pressure from detecting a leak.

○   **What is the purpose of a low-pressure circuit test?**

On machines equipped with a common gas outlet check valve, positive pressure is not transmitted upstream of the common gas outlet during a positive pressure check of the breathing circuit. Because of this, a leak upstream of the common gas outlet will not be detected by this test. Therefore, a negative pressure test is required. Leaks in vaporizers equipped with a check valve will go undetected by a positive pressure test only.

○   **What causes the low O_2 pressure alarm to sound?**

Low O_2 pipeline pressure, a disconnected O_2 supply hose, or a depleted or closed tank will cause this alarm to sound. This is an oxygen fail-safe valve and anything upstream of the flow meter causing low O_2 pressure will be detected by this system (except in the case of crossover in pipeline system).

○   **What is the function of the fail-safe valve?**

The fail-safe valve shuts off the flow of other gases and sounds an alarm in the event that oxygen supply pressure drops 50% below normal. It does not protect against other causes of hypoxia, especially the problems downstream of the flow meters; therefore, an oxygen analyzer is an essential monitor.

○   **What safety features does an anesthesia machine have to reduce the chance of hypoxic gas delivery?**

Oxygen, N_2O, and other anesthetic gases use the Pin Index Safety System to reduce the chance of connecting the wrong tank to a gas line. Line gas supply (wall supply) uses the Diameter Index Safety System for the same purpose. Tanks and lines are color coded. The fail-safe valve reduces or cuts off N_2O flow in the event of decreased oxygen supply pressure. An oxygen supply failure alarm sounds when oxygen pressure falls below a certain level. The flow meters are sequenced so that the oxygen meter is closest to the patient. This reduces the chances that a leak in one flow meter will cause a hypoxic mixture. The oxygen flow meter knob has a distinct feel compared with the other flow meter knobs. Some machines have a minimum oxygen flow that can be delivered even if the O_2 flow meter is off. Various methods are used to ensure at least a minimum oxygen ratio is delivered. O_2 ratio control monitor links N_2O flow to O_2 flow. Low-pressure alarms signal leaks and disconnections.

An oxygen analyzer measures the FiO_2. Using oxygen as a driving gas to power the ventilator ensures that a bellows leak leads to increased rather than decreased FiO_2.

○ **What is the significance of the "standard" sequencing of flow meters?**

The oxygen flow meter is always positioned to the right, furthest downstream, and nearest the outlet of the common manifold. The reasoning is that if a leak develops from a crack in the glass tubing of the flow meter, gas delivered upstream of the leak is lost before gas delivered downstream. This avoids the delivery of a potentially hypoxemic gas mixture. However, at high N_2O/oxygen flow ratios, a leak in the oxygen flow meter may produce a hypoxic mixture even with this arrangement.

○ **What is the effect of a ventilator bellows leak?**

In an anesthesia machine with an oxygen-powered ventilator, a leak in the bellows will allow oxygen to enter the breathing circuit and may raise the FiO_2. It may also cause barotrauma (high-pressure driving gas usually at 50 psig can enter patient circuit), and even awareness by diluting anesthetic gases with high O_2.

○ **What is the pressure at the O_2 flush valve?**

When the O_2 flush valve is activated, oxygen bypasses the flow meters and vaporizers, and is delivered directly to the common gas outlet at 35–75 L/min at a line pressure of 45–55 psig.

○ **What are the two basic types of waste gas scavenging systems?**

Passive and active.

A passive system is a simple direct line venting outside or into an air conditioning duct beyond any point of recirculation. An active system is connected to the hospital vacuum system. Components of the scavenging system include a negative pressure relief valve (protects the patient from the suction effect of the vacuum system), a positive pressure relief valve (prevents barotrauma from back pressure in the event of obstruction), and a reservoir (accommodates transient high flows).

○ **What safety features are incorporated into scavenging systems to prevent patient injury?**

Both positive and negative pressure relief valves (prevent suction effect in excess of 2.5 mm Hg or an occlusion from affecting the pressure in the breathing circuit) and a reservoir for the exhaust gas.

○ **What are the NIOSHA standards for acceptable levels of anesthetic exposure?**

NIOSHA sets the maximum acceptable level of N_2O at 25 ppm [OSHA recommendation, 1991. See reference on page 526]. The maximum acceptable level for halogenated agents is 0.5 ppm when used in combination with N_2O, and 2 ppm if used alone [NIOSHA recommended standards, 1977. See reference on page 526].

○ **How does the anesthesia ventilator generate positive airway pressure?**

The bellows in an anesthesia machine ventilator takes the place of the breathing bag. A breathing bag is compressed by hand, while the bellows is compressed by pressurized oxygen delivered to the space between the bellows and the bellows enclosure.

These are traditional bellows ventilators. The piston ventilators, classified as electrically driven, single-circuit ventilators, require no driving gas.

○ **What is the significance of plateau pressure (PP) during mechanical ventilation?**

PP is measured during a time of no gas flow (inspiratory pause) and reflects static compliance.

○ **What is the significance of peak inspiratory pressure (PIP)?**

PIP is the highest pressure generated during inspiration and reflects dynamic compliance. Increase in PIP without any change in PP signals an increase in airway resistance (bronchospasm, secretions) or inspiratory gas flow rate. Increase in both PIP and PP implies an increase in tidal volume or decrease in pulmonary compliance (i.e., pulmonary edema, pleural effusion, tension pneumothorax, ascites).

○ **What factors alter delivered tidal volume on anesthesia ventilators?**

Most anesthesia ventilators are volume preset ventilators. In a circle system, fresh gas flows continuously into the inspiratory limb of the breathing circuit. This additional volume is added to the gas delivered from the ventilator to the patient during the inspiratory phase of the breathing cycle. The positive pressure of the ventilator closes the pop-off valve, so any fresh gas delivered by the anesthesia machine while the ventilator is firing ends up going to the patient's lungs. (This is the reason why the flush valve should never be used when the ventilator is delivering a breath.) The resulting increase in tidal volume depends on the respiratory rate (higher rate = less extra volume per breath), inspiratory-to-expiratory ratio (more inspiratory phase = more extra volume per breath), and FGF rate (higher = more extra volume per breath). Long circuits can also increase the distensible volume of the circuit and decrease delivered tidal volume. In addition, malfunctions (circuit leaks, bellows leaks, etc.) can affect tidal volume.

However, in the new anesthesia workstations with the computerized compensation, the tidal volume that is delivered to the patient is precisely controlled, and therefore is not altered by increased FGF or changes in the compliance of the system. For example, once the patient's tidal volume is set by the provider, central processing unit (CPU) adjusts bellows excursion according to the FGF. If high FGF is set with a small tidal volume, bellows may move only slightly because most of the tidal volume is now provided by FGF.

During automated preuse checkout the user occludes the Y-piece and work station measures compliance of breathing system and this is also taken into account by the ventilator.

○ **How much oxygen is in a standard E cylinder when its pressure gauge reads 1,000 psi?**

For a nonliquefied gas, the pressure decreases steadily as the cylinder is emptied. Therefore, an E cylinder containing 660 L of oxygen at 2,000 psig will contain 330 L if the pressure drops to 1,000 psi.

With a liquefied gas, the pressure remains constant until all the liquid has turned to gas, and then drops as the cylinder is emptied (N_2O is three fourths empty before psig drops). Weighing the cylinder will determine the amount of liquid remaining.

○ **How long can a full E cylinder of oxygen supply oxygen flow at 10 L/min?**

To determine how long an oxygen cylinder can supply a given flow, one must determine the amount of oxygen in the cylinder. A full E cylinder of oxygen contains 660 L of oxygen at 2,000 psi. This is expected to last 66 minutes at 10 L/min.

○ **An E cylinder oxygen pressure gauge indicates 500 psig. If the oxygen flow of 10 L/min is used to ventilate a patient during transport, how long will the oxygen last?**

The time in hours can be calculated using the following formula:

$$\text{Approximate remaining time (hours)} \approx \frac{O_2 \text{ cylinder pressure (psig)}}{200 \times O_2 \text{ flow rate (L/min)}}.$$

Therefore, the answer = 500/(200 × 10) = 1/4 = 15 minutes.

(The advantage of this formula is it does not require you to remember the volume of oxygen in a full cylinder.)

○ **What is the capacity of an "E" cylinder? Does this differ for oxygen, air, N_2O, or nitrogen?**

A standard E cylinder has the capacity of 625–700 L of oxygen, air, and nitrogen gas at 1,800–2,200 psi at 20°C. There is a linear relationship for gas and pressure in these. An E cylinder of N_2O contains 1,590 L at 745 psi at 20°C. The nitrous oxide cylinder is 75% empty before the "E" cylinder pressure changes.

○ **Why is oxygen in the gas form in the E cylinder in the OR?**

At room temperature, oxygen is above its critical temperature, and therefore a gas. Above the critical temperature a gas cannot be condensed into a liquid however much pressure is applied.

○ **How is liquid oxygen stored?**

Although banks of compressed gas cylinders or oxygen concentrators may be used for the hospitals' central O_2 supply, storing O_2 as a liquid is more economical. It is stored in insulated tanks below the critical temperature of oxygen. The critical temperature is defined as temperature above which a substance cannot be converted to a liquid however much pressure is applied. The critical temperature of oxygen is −119°C. The liquid oxygen in the storage vessel is at −160°C (below the critical temperature).

○ **The N_2O E cylinder pressure reads 360 psi. Is it possible to calculate the volume of N_2O in the tank?**

The pressure of a full N_2O cylinder is 760 psi. With a liquefied gas, the pressure remains constant until all the liquid has turned to gas, and then drops as the cylinder is emptied (N_2O is three fourths empty before psi drops). The fact that the pressure is 360 psi indicates the cylinder contains no liquid N_2O.

Weighing the cylinder will determine the amount of liquid remaining.

○ **You suspect an N_2O/oxygen pipeline crossover while anesthetizing a patient. What immediate corrective actions should be taken?**

1. Backup O_2 cylinder should be turned on.
2. Pipeline supply must be disconnected. This step is mandatory; otherwise the machine will preferentially use the wrong gas coming from the 50 psig pipeline supply source instead of the lower-pressure (45 psig) oxygen cylinder source.

○ **What methods are available to add or maintain humidity of inspiratory gases?**

- Heat and moisture exchangers (artificial noses)
- Heated humidifiers
- Nebulizers
- Rebreathing circuits with low FGFs
- CO_2 absorber

○ **What is the ideal humidity in an anesthetic circuit?**

The ideal humidity level is 28–32 mg H_2O/L gas (absolute humidity) or roughly 50–75% saturated at 37°C. Dry room temperature gases have a humidity level of <10 mg H_2O/L.

Normal alveolar humidity is 44 mg H_2O/L at 37°C. Inspiration of dry gases decreases relative humidity, which can cause mucous plugging, loss of ciliary function, increased airway resistance, and atelectasis.

Excessive humidity can also injure the lung, as well as serve as a source for bacterial growth.

○   **Describe the function of a temperature-compensated variable-bypass vaporizer.**

The variable-bypass vaporizer divides incoming gas into two streams. Twenty percent or less goes through the vaporizing chamber and becomes saturated. Second portion goes through the bypass chamber. Finally, the two streams are combined to make the output of the vaporizer. Both the bimetallic strip (temperature compensation device) and the concentration dial are situated in the bypass channel and compensate for temperature changes and desired final concentration.

○   **Why are modern vaporizers temperature compensated?**

Temperature compensation is required to maintain a constant concentration of gas output from the vaporizer over a wide range of ambient temperatures and gas flows.

Vapor pressure (VP) depends on temperature. During vaporization the liquid anesthetic cools and the saturated VP decreases, as does the vaporizer output.

Mechanisms of temperature compensation include high thermal conductivity of the vaporizer (allowing rapid heat transfer to the liquid anesthetic as it cools) and a variable-bypass mechanism (which directs more gas flow to the vaporizing chamber as the vaporizer cools to compensate for decreased saturated VP).

○   **What are the unique features of the desflurane (Tec 6) vaporizer?**

Tec 6 vaporizer is an electrically heated, pressurized, electromechanically coupled, dual-circuit, constant-temperature, gas–vapor blender. Desflurane is heated to 39°C (well above its boiling point) and creates a source of pure desflurane vapor. This vapor is blended with the fresh gas near the outlet to create the vaporizer output. No fresh gas enters the vaporizing chamber. The vaporizer has an electronic display that indicates an initial warm-up period with an amber LED while the operating temperature reached is indicated with a green LED. A red LED flashes and an audible alarm sounds if the vaporizer cannot deliver the requested vapor concentration. There is an LCD desflurane liquid level meter. It uses a special filling cap (desflurane boils at room temperature, so the bottle and vaporizer interlock to prevent the loss of agent while filling).

○   **Why are conventional vaporizers unsuitable for use with desflurane?**

Because of the high VP of desflurane, carrier gas passing through the vaporizing chamber of a variable-bypass vaporizer would entrain a much larger amount of desflurane when compared with other agents (e.g., isoflurane). For example, 100 mL of carrier gas would entrain 735 mL of desflurane (VP = 669) versus 46 mL of isoflurane (VP = 238). To achieve a final concentration of 1%, the bypass flow for desflurane would have to be 86 L/min, whereas for isoflurane it is only 5 L/min. Therefore, a special vaporizer is needed for desflurane, which takes into account its high VP. In addition, the MAC of desflurane is about four times that of the other agents, so the absolute amount of desflurane that needs to be vaporized is much higher. This can cause excessive cooling of the vaporizer and hence the need for a heated vaporizer (Heated to 39°C to remain constantly vaporized).

○   **What is the VP of desflurane in the Tec 6 vaporizer?**

The sump of the Tec 6 vaporizer is heated to 39°C. At 39°C, the VP of desflurane is approximately 1,300 mm Hg absolute (2 × atmospheric pressure).

○   **What is the significance of anesthetic VP?**

Anesthetic VP determines the concentration of anesthetic vapor coming out of the vaporizing chamber of a variable-bypass vaporizer. Filling a vaporizer with an anesthetic agent with a lower VP than the agent it was meant to be used with will cause a lower concentration than is selected on the dial to be delivered. Filling a vaporizer with an anesthetic agent with a higher VP than the agent it was meant to be used with will cause a higher concentration than is selected on the dial to be delivered.

○ **Sevoflurane is added to an isoflurane vaporizer containing some isoflurane. What is the relative concentration of agents delivered to the patient?**

The relative concentrations would be 160:240, the ratio of their VPs.

○ **What would happen if you filled an isoflurane vaporizer with halothane?**

Since the saturated VPs (at 20°C) of halothane and isoflurane are almost the same, 243 and 238 mm Hg, respectively, the volume percent outputs are almost the same. However, since halothane is more potent, a higher MAC value is being administered to the patient at the same percentage delivered.

○ **An enflurane vaporizer is unknowingly and accidentally filled with halothane and is set to deliver 2% inspired concentration. What is the MAC of the halothane actually delivered to the patient?**

4 MAC.

The VP of enflurane is 175 mm Hg, and of halothane 245 mm Hg. That means the enflurane vaporizer will vaporize 1.5 times more halothane than the concentration dialed on the vaporizer, which is calibrated only for enflurane. This will result in a halothane concentration of 3%. Since the MAC of halothane is 0.75, the MAC of the halothane delivered to the patient will be 3/0.75 = 4 MAC.

○ **What is the effect of substituting sevoflurane for halothane, in a halothane vaporizer?**

The VP of halothane is 244 mm Hg and the VP of sevoflurane is 160 mm Hg. If sevoflurane was used in a halothane vaporizer, the amount of agent delivered would be 65% (160/244, the ratio of the VPs) of the dial setting. Thus, if the swap were inadvertent, the patient would be significantly underanesthetized.

○ **When a vaporizer is being changed on an anesthesia machine, it is accidentally tipped. What should you do before using the vaporizer?**

Flush the vaporizer for 20–30 minutes at high flow rates of oxygen with the vaporizer set at a low concentration. In a variable-bypass vaporizer, tipping may cause liquid anesthetic to spill from the vaporizing chamber to the bypass chamber, effectively creating two vaporizing chambers and increasing vaporizer output.

○ **What effect does changing fresh gas from 100% O_2 to 70% N_2O have on vaporizer output?**

This change will transiently lower the volatile anesthetic concentration coming out of a variable-bypass vaporizer and desflurane vaporizer.

○ **What effect does increased altitude has on the output of an anesthetic vaporizer?**

Contemporary variable-bypass vaporizers, such as isoflurane and sevoflurane vaporizers, deliver a constant partial pressure of anesthetic. Decreased barometric pressure such as found at high altitude will increase the vaporizer output because high resistance path through vapor chamber offers less resistance. Therefore, the vaporizer may require decreased dial settings at high altitude. (This however is negligible.)

When vaporizer delivery is measured as volume percent (not partial pressure), such as desflurane vaporizer (Tec 6), it requires increased dial settings at high altitudes. The required dial setting for desflurane vaporizer in this high altitude = normal dial setting at sea level × 760/atmospheric pressure at high altitude.

○ **What effects does intermittent back pressure have on the output of a variable-bypass vaporizer?**

Intermittent back pressure due to IPPV (intermittent positive pressure) or activation of oxygen flush may cause contamination of the bypass tract of the vaporizer with inhalational agents. This effect, called the pumping effect, is more likely at low flows, low dial settings, low level of liquid anesthetic, rapid respiratory rates, and high PIP. The pumping effect may be reduced by using a smaller vaporizing chamber (release of vapor to bypass less), making the inlet to the vaporizing chamber a long spiral tube, and having a check valve.

○ **Define partial pressure of gases in mixtures.**

When there is a mixture of gases in a closed container, each gas exerts a pressure proportional to its fractional volume (or mass). This is its partial pressure.

○ **What is Dalton's law of partial pressures?**

The total pressure of a gas mixture is the sum of the partial pressure of each gas:

$$P_{total} = P_{gas_1} + P_{gas_2} + \cdots + P_{gas_N}$$

The entire mixture behaves just as if it were a single gas according to the ideal gas law.

○ **What is Poiseuille's law and how does it apply to IV catheters?**

For laminar gas flow, according to Poiseuille's law, resistance $= 8NL/\pi R^4$, where R is the radius, N is the viscosity of the fluid, and L is the length of the tube. Therefore, if the radius is halved, the resistance within the tube increases 16-fold. If the length of the tube is doubled, the resistance is only doubled. Therefore, the length of the tube minimally affects resistance; however, increasing the IV cannula diameter makes a significant difference in resistance to laminar flow. (In practice, a short 16 gauge IV catheter will permit flow rates similar to a longer 14 gauge IV catheter. When you are in the middle of a tedious day in the OR, try it!)

○ **What is Reynolds number?**

The Reynolds number describes a value at which flow in a tube changes from laminar to turbulent.

Laminar flow occurs at a Reynolds number $<1,000$, and turbulent flow at $>1,500$.

Reynolds number $= 2rvd/N$, where r is the radius, v is the average velocity, d is the density, and N is the viscosity.

○ **List four conditions that change laminar flow to turbulent flow.**

(1) High gas flows, (2) sharp angles within the tube, (3) branching in the tube, and (4) change in the diameter of the tube.

○ **During turbulent gas flow, what determines the driving pressure?**

Driving pressure is directly proportional to the square of the gas flow and gas density, and inversely proportional to the fifth power of the radius of the tube.

○ **During laminar flow, the resistance is inversely proportional to gas flow rate. What happens to the resistance as the gas flow is increased during turbulent flow?**

During turbulent flow, resistance increases in proportion to the flow rate.

○ **What is the relevance of viscosity to turbulent flow?**

Turbulent flow is independent of viscosity. Viscosity is relevant under conditions of laminar flow.

○ **Will helium improve *laminar* gas flow?**

No. Helium has a low density, but its viscosity is close to that of air. Since density is directly proportional to driving pressure during turbulent flow, helium is useful when there is critical airway narrowing (subglottic edema, tracheal tumor) or abnormally high airway resistance (ventilating patients with small-diameter ETTs).

○ **What is the density of mixtures of helium and oxygen compared with pure oxygen?**

The most popular mixtures of helium, 80/20 and 70/30 helium–oxygen, have densities that are 1.805 and 1.586 times less dense, respectively, than pure oxygen.

Key Terms

Anesthesia circuits: airway humidity
Anesthetic machine low-pressure leak test
Ascending vent bellows advantages
Behavior of gas mixtures
Circle system components
Circle system: rebreathing
Circuit soda lime exhaustion
CO and inhalational anesthetics
CO from CO_2 absorber
CO_2 breathing, valve malfunction
Common gas outlet check valve
Cylinder content: weight versus pressure
Desflurane vaporizer physics/functions
Desflurane vaporizer: reason for use
E cylinder: pressure and volume relationship
Effects of misfiling vaporizer
Elevated inspiratory CO_2 causes
Factors affecting turbulent flow
Flow meter damage
Flow meter: gas properties
Flow meter, rotameter: laminar, turbulence
Fresh gas flow: Mapleson circuits
Gas flow: variable-orifice flow meter
Gas flow velocity
Gas laws: temperature/pressure changes
Gas machines: safety features
Gas mixture effect on vaporizer output
High altitude anesthesia

Incompetent expiratory valve: signs
Inhaled gas concentration: factors affecting
Intraoperative awareness: equipment malfunction
Mapleson D: rebreathing
Mechanical vent airway press patterns
Mechanical ventilator: plateau pressure
Nitrous oxide (N_2O) in tank: calculate
N_2O: gas proportioning system
O_2 and N_2O pipeline crossover
O_2 supply failure alarm
Oxygen: E cylinder volume
Peak versus plateau airway pressure
Pediatric circuits
Physical behavior of gas mixtures
Poiseuille's law
Prevention of CO_2 rebreathing
Reynolds number
Sevoflurane for halothane in vaporizer
Subglottic stenosis: helium
Vapor pressure: anesthetic concentration
Vaporizer function
Vaporizer output: altitude
Vaporizer output: calculation
Variable-bypass vaporizer: anesthetic pressure
Ventilator bellows leak/effects of ventilator bellows hole
Ventilator disconnect: detection
Wall O_2 failure: signs
Waste gas scavenging

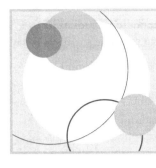

Muscle Relaxants

I'm a great believer in luck and I find the harder I work, the more I have of it.
Thomas Jefferson

○ **What are the possible deleterious effects of succinylcholine?**

- Increased intraocular (no extrusion of eye contents ever reported) and intracranial pressure (debatable).
- Hyperkalemia, after 24 hours in burns, neurologic injury, muscular dystrophies, and trauma (proliferation of extrajunctional receptors).
- Triggering malignant hyperthermia.
- Increased duration of action in patients with pseudocholinesterase deficiency (inherited pattern or liver disease, malignancies, pregnancy, and malnutrition).
- Acetylcholine-like effects (especially bradycardia and asystole) with multiple doses over a short time period or IV dose exceeding 3 mg/kg in adult patients.
- Anaphylaxis. Succinylcholine has a greater incidence than nondepolarizers.
- Phase II or desensitization block at 7–10 mg/kg in adults.

○ **Is succinylcholine contraindicated in patients who have pacemakers?**

No. Fasciculations produced by the administration of succinylcholine may be interpreted by the pacemaker sensor as an intrinsic cardiac impulse, which may then inhibit the pacemaker from firing (depending on the type of pacer). Precautions to minimize this risk include reprogramming the pacemaker to an asynchronous mode or "defasciculating" the patient with a small dose of nondepolarizing muscle relaxant prior to the administration of succinylcholine. With current bipolar pacemakers, where electrical activity is sensed between two cardiac sensors, this is less of a concern. If a patient has a unipolar pacemaker, then fasciculations should be expected to be a problem, as only one sensor is located in the myocardium and the ground sensor is outside the heart.

○ **Is succinylcholine-induced masseter muscle spasm diagnostic of malignant hyperthermia susceptibility?**

No. There is evidence that this symptom could be a harbinger of malignant hyperthermia, but all cases of masseter spasm do not progress to MH.

Masseter muscle spasm is an exaggerated contractile response causing rigidity or trismus of the jaw muscles. Clinical presentation follows the administration of succinylcholine with complete neuromuscular blockade, and then intense difficulty in opening the patient's mouth. Both myotonia and MH can cause masseter spasm, which should be differentiated from incomplete jaw relaxation, which is very common. This may be an early indicator of MH, but not consistently associated with MH (25% cases predictive of MH). Currently there is no indication to change to "nontriggering" agents in case of isolated masseter spasm. If the patient is susceptible to MH, a full-blown episode typically occurs 20–30 minutes after the onset of masseter spasm [Miller, 2010].

○ **A patient develops a fever during hernia repair under general anesthesia. He was exposed to succinylcholine, atropine, fentanyl, midazolam, propofol, isoflurane, nitrous oxide, and oxygen. What is the most likely diagnosis?**

Malignant hyperthermia until proven otherwise.

An increase in end-tidal CO_2 and unexplained tachycardia is usually the first sign. In children, in the face of normocarbia, a rise in temperature is most likely due to the anticholinergenic effect of atropine on sweat glands or overbundling.

○ **Is open globe injury of the eye a contraindication to using succinylcholine?**

Not unless the anterior chamber is open, where there is a theoretical risk (never reported clinically) of extrusion of vitreous through the wound. Succinylcholine increases IOP 5–10 mm Hg for 5–10 minutes after administration, through contracture of the extraocular muscles. Prior administration of a defasciculating dose of nondepolarizing muscle relaxant may prevent the increase in IOP.

This is nowhere near the magnitude of increase seen in IOP with "bucking" on an endotracheal tube or squinting (increases IOP 25 mm Hg). Factors that increase IOP include coughing, straining, bucking, laryngoscopy and intubation, hypercarbia, airway obstruction, "light general anesthesia," pupillary dilatation, venous congestion of the head and neck (Trendelenburg and prone positioning), pressure on the eye, retrobulbar hemorrhage, and hypertension.

○ **Does succinylcholine increase intra-gastric pressure (IGP)? Can this lead to increased risk of aspiration?**

Increased IGP is presumed to be due to abdominal muscle fasciculation and depends on the intensity of fasciculations. Normally, an IGP of more than 28 cm H_2O is required to overcome the gastroesophageal sphincter competence (less in pregnancy, hiatal hernia, or bowel obstruction). However, succinylcholine also causes increase in lower esophageal sphincter pressure. Succinylcholine does not increase IGP in children <4 years.

○ **What receptor does succinylcholine target?**

The postjunctional nicotinic cholinergic receptor.

○ **What are the most common cardiovascular effects of succinylcholine?**

Cardiac muscarinic cholinergic receptor stimulation may cause sinus bradycardia, progressing to asystole, especially in children or after a second IV dose. Elevation in heart rate and blood pressure can occur as succinylcholine mimics the effects of acetylcholine on the autonomic ganglia.

○ **What is the effect of cyclophosphamide on pseudocholinesterase?**

Cyclophosphamide is an inhibitor of pseudocholinesterase and as such may prolong the apneic response to succinylcholine. Its suppressive effect may be dose-dependent.

○ **A patient on echothiophate for treatment of glaucoma needs an emergency appendectomy. She was slow to recover from succinylcholine. Diagnosis?**

Echothiophate inactivates plasma cholinesterase, thus prolonging actions of succinylcholine.

○ **Name two common qualitative tests for plasma cholinesterase?**

Dibucaine number and fluoride number.

○ **What is the dibucaine number?**

Normal plasma cholinesterase can be effectively inhibited by dibucaine in vitro. In the presence of 10^{-5} M of dibucaine, its activity is reduced by 80%, whereas the homozygous and heterozygous atypical enzymes are inhibited by only 20% and 60%, respectively. The dibucaine numbers are then 80, 20, and 60. It is the dibucaine-susceptible enzyme that functions in vivo.

○ **How are the genotypes of the plasma cholinesterase named?**

$E_1^u E_1^u$ for typical ("usual"), $E_1^u E_1^a$ for the heterozygous, and $E_1^a E_1^a$ for the homozygous atypical enzymes.

○ **Is pseudocholinesterase a true enzyme?**

Yes, it is plasma cholinesterase. Likewise, tissue or RBC cholinesterase is also called true cholinesterase.

○ **T/F: Plasma cholinesterase is stable in banked blood.**

True.

○ **What relaxants are metabolized by the plasma cholinesterase?**

Succinylcholine and mivacurium, which are choline esters.

Mivacurium is hydrolyzed by plasma cholinesterase (pseudocholinesterase) at 80–90% of the rate of succinylcholine.

○ **What drugs or disease states can prolong the duration of action of mivacurium?**

Patients with reduced plasma cholinesterase activity: those heterozygous or homozygous for the atypical plasma cholinesterase gene, pregnancy, liver or kidney disease, malignant tumors, infection, burns, anemia, decompensated heart disease, peptic ulcer, or myxedema.

Drugs that reduce plasma cholinesterase activity include oral contraceptives, glucocorticoids, monoamine oxidase inhibitors, and irreversible inhibitors of plasma cholinesterase (e.g., echothiophate or organophosphate insecticides). Extended neuromuscular blockade with mivacurium following pancuronium has been documented, presumably due to inhibition of plasma cholinesterase.

○ **How often do you expect markedly prolonged duration of action of mivacurium?**

As is with succinylcholine, patients with homozygous atypical plasma cholinesterase (1:2,500) will remain paralyzed for about 4–6 hours, with twice the normal duration of block seen in patients who are heterozygous. In contrast to succinylcholine, with return of a twitch response to nerve stimulation, recovery from mivacurium blockade will be facilitated by the administration of cholinesterase inhibitors.

○ **Can the prolonged action of succinylcholine or mivacurium in patients with atypical or decreased levels of plasma cholinesterase be terminated?**

Yes, with IV administration of plasma cholinesterase, but the best action to take is to be patient and wait for recovery of the train-of-four (TOF). Provide ventilatory support.

○ **Will the duration of action of cisatracurium be prolonged in patients with atypical plasma cholinesterase? Why?**

No. Cisatracurium, like atracurium, does not depend on plasma cholinesterase for its breakdown. It is eliminated by Hoffmann degradation at body pH and temperature and hydrolysis by nonspecific esterases.

○ **Which relaxants are potential histamine releasers?**

D-Tubocurarine >> atracurium, mivacurium, and doxacurium (i.e., benzylisoquinoline compounds). Cisatracurium is also a benzylisoquinoline, but up to 8 × ED_{95} has no significant histamine release.

○ **Do muscle relaxants cause allergic reactions?**

Yes. Succinylcholine is the worst offender. After that, metocurine (hypersensitivity to iodide) and pancuronium (hypersensitivity to bromide) cause the most allergic reactions. The histamine-releasing side effects of muscle relaxants may cause hypotension that can confuse a diagnosis, as histamine-related effects are clinical manifestations of anaphylaxis in the anesthetized patient.

○ **What are the main differences in the mechanism of action of edrophonium and neostigmine?**

Both drugs possess positively charged quaternary ammonium groups but edrophonium lacks a carbamate and ester group and relies on noncovalent electrostatic binding to attach to the anionic site of the acetylcholinesterase enzyme. Edrophonium's onset is 2 minutes and duration of action 45–60 minutes. Neostigmine has a carbamate group that binds to the esteratic site of the enzyme and acts as a competitive substrate for acetylcholine. Onset is 7 minutes and duration of action 60–90 minutes. In equipotent doses edrophonium has less muscarinic effect, requiring only one half the amount of anticholinergic drug to prevent bradycardia. Unlike neostigmine, emetic effect is not seen with edrophonium.

Edrophonium is a less potent inhibitor of butyrylcholinesterase. Therefore, it should have less effect on metabolism of mivacurium if given as a reversal agent after mivacurium.

The anticholinergic drugs are chosen to match the onset of action of each anticholinesterase, that is, glycopyrrolate with neostigmine and atropine with edrophonium.

○ **What is the clinical dose of edrophonium?**

Usually 0.5–1 mg/kg. Maximum dose is 1–1.5 mg/kg.

○ **What is the clinical dose of neostigmine?**

Although larger doses antagonize blockade more rapidly, anticholinesterase demonstrates a ceiling effect and usually no added benefit in giving more than 0.07 mg/kg of neostigmine. Combining antagonists (giving both neostigmine and edrophonium) also has no effect in the recovery because acetylcholinesterase is already maximally inhibited.

○ **What is sugammadex?**

Sugammadex is the first selective relaxing binding agent for neuromuscular block reversal. It may be administered at any point during NDMRs, regardless of the depth.

Ring-shaped cyclodextrin engulfs rocuronium molecules to halt action.

It consists of a ring of eight sugar molecules. Outside of the ring is hydrophilic, and inside hydrophobic. The encapsulation of steroidal molecules of rocuronium within the lipophilic cavity prevents its access to nicotinic receptors leading to quick reversal.

No direct cholinergic effect, therefore no anticholinergics required.

○ **Can sugammadex reverse any type of muscle relaxant?**

Sugammadex has no ability to reverse benzylisoquinolinium-based relaxants. It is specific to rocuronium.

○ **What is the main determinant of reversibility of neuromuscular blockade?**

The main determinant is the intensity of the block.

It is recommended that reversal should not be attempted until $T1 \geq 25\%$ when all four twitches are visible. Attempted reversal at only two twitches may take 30 minutes or more to reach TOF of 0.9. There is little advantage in attempting early reversal. If neostigmine administration is timed at a TOF count of 4, then postoperative clinical problems due to residual neuromuscular blockade are unlikely.

Reversal may possibly be delayed (not hastened) if neostigmine is given when no response is present (i.e., all four twitches of TOF absent).

Other factors affecting speed of reversal include dose of antagonist (with a ceiling effect), choice of antagonist, presence of inhaled anesthetics, respiratory acidosis, electrolyte disturbances (hypokalemia, hypocalcemia, and hyponatremia), hypothermia, and antibiotics (aminoglycosides). Impairment of renal or hepatic function may significantly impact the clearance of muscle relaxants and their active metabolites [Srivastava and Hunter, 2009. See reference on page 526].

○ **How does TOF twitches correlates with the extent of blockade?**

The sequential disappearance of TOF twitches correlates with the extent of blockade (fourth twitch disappears at 70–75% block, third at 85% block, second at 94%, and the last twitch at 99%). Surgical relaxation requires 75–95% neuromuscular blockade (only one or two twitches present). A TOF count of four twitches generally correlates with clinical reversibility with any NMB. A TOF count of two or three twitches indicates reversibility, but satisfactory reversal will require more time or a larger dose of anticholinesterase drug. With the presence of a single twitch, any complicating factor in NMB metabolism or presence of potentiating drugs could prevent complete and timely reversal.

○ **How is the reversal of neuromuscular blockade assessed?**

Sustained head lift for 5 seconds, recovery of TOF, sustained tetany, and effective abdominal and intercostal muscle activity.

Clinical assessment includes the ability to maintain head lift for 5–10 seconds, hold a tongue depressor between a patient's teeth against force (tongue depressor test), arm lift for 45 seconds, ability to lift legs off the table for 5 seconds, and inspiratory effort of >40–50 cm H_2O. Adequacy of recovery of respiratory and upper airway function from nondepolarizing NMB is suggested by a TOF ratio of 0.9 or more at the adductor pollicis. Tetany (50 or 100 Hz) with a sustained contraction for 5 seconds indicates adequate, but not necessarily complete reversal [Miller, 2010; Brull, 2010. See reference on page 526].

○ **What is double-burst stimulation (DBS)? Is it better than TOF or titanic stimulation?**

DBS is more sensitive than TOF in the visual evaluation of fade (overall fade is better appreciated with DBS or tetany than with TOF).

DBS is less painful than titanic stimulation. It consists of three short bursts (0.2 milliseconds) of 50-Hz tetanic stimulation followed later (750 milliseconds) by another three bursts. Ratio of second to first impulses correlates well with TOF ratio.

However, the absent fade with DBS or TOF when manually evaluated does not exclude residual neuromuscular blockade.

○ **How does the TOF correlate with diaphragmatic paralysis?**

Different muscles have different sensitivities to muscle relaxants of which the diaphragm and vocal cords are most resistant. The adductor pollicis (ulnar nerve) is routinely used for twitch monitoring. A stimulus delivered at 2/s

(2 Hz) for a total of four stimuli is known as a TOF. Surgical relaxation usually requires a 75–95% neuromuscular blockade. When the adductor pollicis is 90% blocked by rocuronium, the diaphragm is only 25% blocked. The diaphragm has a greater ED_{50}, ED_{95}, and faster recovery of the twitch height than does the adductor pollicis when rocuronium is used. It has also been found that atracurium and vecuronium exhibit a similar degree of sparing of the diaphragm.

○ **What is "blind paralysis?"**

The term "blind paralysis" was coined for TOF ratio values in the range 0.4–0.7.

Human senses could not appreciate TOF fade if the actual measured value is between 0.4 and 0.7 (subjective monitoring).

Objective or quantitative monitoring, which involves the use of a stimulator coupled with a measuring device that displays a numerical value (accelerometer, mechanomyography, acceleromyography, kinemyography, or electromyography), can provide this information and decreases the incidence of potentially clinically significant postoperative residual paralysis.

One should make sure that the TOF ratio has returned to at least 0.9 before tracheal extubation.

However, a TOF ratio >0.9 can still have 50% of the receptors occupied.

○ **Do muscle relaxants have the same effect on the larynx, diaphragm, adductor pollicis, and orbicularis oculi muscles?**

Neuromuscular blockade at the larynx and the diaphragm is less intense than at the adductor pollicis muscle. The laryngeal adductors (vocal cords), corrugator supercilii (superciliary arch), diaphragm, and abdominal rectus are more resistant and recover from neuromuscular blockade sooner than do the thumb (adductor pollicis) and eyelid (orbicularis oculi). The masseter and pharyngeal muscles are most sensitive [Hemmerling et al., 2000; Hemmerling and Donati, 2003; Plaud et al., 2001. See reference on page 526].

○ **Does the TOF fade in myasthenic (Eaton–Lambert) syndrome, magnesium treatment, aminoglycoside overdose, or phase I depolarizing block?**

No. Instead it fades in myasthenia gravis, nondepolarizing blockade, and phase II block.

○ **How do you diagnose organophosphate poisoning?**

The effects of organophosphate poisoning are due to excess acetylcholine that results from blocking acetylcholinesterase. These effects are recalled using the mnemonic SLUDGEM or DUMBELLS.

SLUDGEM: salivation, lacrimation, urination, defecation, gastrointestinal motility, emesis, miosis.

DUMBELLS: diarrhea, urination, miosis, bradycardia, bronchospasm, emesis, lacrimation, salivation, secretion, sweating.

○ **What is the treatment of organophosphate poisoning?**

Atropine can be used as an antidote with pralidoxime or other pyridinium (such as trimedoxime or obidoxime). Atropine, a muscarinic antagonist, blocks the action of acetylcholine peripherally.

Pralidoxime attaches to the site where a cholinesterase inhibitor has attached, and then attaches to the inhibitor, removing the organophosphate from cholinesterase, allowing it to work normally again. This is known as "regenerating" or "reactivating" acetylcholinesterase. After some time, though, some inhibitors can develop a permanent bond with cholinesterase, known as aging.

○ **What is the nerve gas antidote?**

These cartridges of antidote are dispensed to the troops to counter the effects of anticholinesterase nerve gases (such as tabun and sarin). They contain only atropine, which would effectively counter the muscarinic effects of the gas. Treatment requires high-dose atropine, 35–70 mg/kg IV every 3–10 minutes until muscarinic symptoms abate. This is followed by lower doses for several days.

Atropine, however, does little to counter the high-dose nicotinic muscle paralysis or the central ventilatory depression that contributes to death from nerve gases. This requires respiratory support and specific therapy of the cholinesterase lesion. Nerve gas irreversibly inhibits cholinesterase enzyme (similar to echothiophate). Pralidoxime has been reported to reactivate cholinesterase activity by hydrolysis of the phosphate enzyme complex.

○ **If you have no IV access, how can you administer a muscle relaxant to break laryngospasm?**

IM or sublingual route. The muscle relaxant most suitable for intramuscular injection is succinylcholine.

○ **After prolonged use of muscle relaxants in the intensive care unit (1 week) how will neuromuscular transmission recover?**

The most important determinant of duration of action is depth of blockade. If the TOF indicates one or two twitches, which corresponds to an 85–95% receptor blockade, recovery will be seen within hours of discontinuing the drug. In the ICU, drug choice is important due to the impact of liver and kidney dysfunction on drug metabolism and clearance, and the possibility of accumulation of active metabolites (pancuronium and vecuronium). In addition, drugs or clinical conditions may prolong neuromuscular blockade. This includes class I antiarrhythmics, magnesium, streptomycin, polymyxin, neomycin, lithium, corticosteroids and calcium channel blockers, respiratory acidosis, metabolic alkalosis, hypothermia, and hypercalcemia. Close monitoring of neuromuscular function is essential.

○ **Explain the clinical significance of upregulation of the acetylcholine receptors?**

Any condition that significantly decreases/eliminates motor nerve activity causes a proliferation of extrajunctional neuromuscular receptors. The cell is essentially "searching" for an acetylcholine signal by putting out more receptors. These receptors are abnormal and extend beyond the normal boundary of the endplate. This immature form of receptors has different electrophysiologic characteristic with prolonged open channel time (four times longer than mature type), thus allowing long time for the potassium efflux. Hyperkalemia, predisposing to ventricular arrhythmias or cardiac arrest, may result from depolarization of these receptors by succinylcholine, which causes a massive outpouring of intracellular potassium into the plasma. Conditions include burns, muscular dystrophies, spinal cord injuries, closed head injuries, upper and lower motor neuron disease, prolonged immobility, hemiparesis, and intra-abdominal sepsis (debatable as cause but reportedly associated). It usually takes at least 24 hours for extrajunctional receptors to present.

○ **What are the EKG findings of succinylcholine-induced hyperkalemia?**

ECG abnormalities and arrhythmias typically do not appear until the serum potassium level is greater than 6.5 mEq/L. Common ECG signs include widened QRS, peaked T-waves, prolonged PR interval, loss of P waves, and atrial systole. ST-segment elevation may mimic acute myocardial infarction. First-degree block may ultimately lead to complete heart block. Late signs include prolonged QRS complex that can lead to sine-wave ventricular arrhythmia, ventricular fibrillation, or asystole.

○ **What is the treatment for succinylcholine-induced hyperkalemia?**

ECG changes with CV instability, within 2–5 minutes of succinylcholine, are diagnostic.

Usually cardiovascular instability occurs at potassium level >8 mEq/L. Treatment consists of immediate hyperventilation ($PaCO_2$ 25–30 mm Hg), 1–2 mg of calcium chloride IV, 1 mEq/kg of sodium bicarbonate, and 10 U of regular insulin in 50 mL of 50% glucose. Continue CPR as long as necessary because reversal of hyperkalemia may take longer in some patients.

○ **Does Parkinson disease predispose to hyperkalemia or malignant hyperthermia?**

No. Parkinson disease does not usually cause hyperkalemia and is not associated with malignant hyperthermia. It is a degenerative disease of the CNS characterized by loss of dopaminergic fibers in the basal ganglia. Therefore, drugs with antidopaminergic effects should be avoided.

○ **Does Guillain–Barré syndrome predispose to hyperkalemia?**

Yes. As with other lower motor neuron disorders, succinylcholine should not be used because of the risk of hyperkalemia.

○ **Immediately following burn or major nerve injury, is succinylcholine contraindicated?**

No. Risk of succinylcholine-induced hyperkalemia occurs beyond the first 24 hours postinjury and remains dangerous as long as the pathology of muscle degeneration and regeneration continues, for at least 1–2 years.

○ **What is the response of burn patients to nondepolarizing muscle relaxants?**

Resistance. Burned patients require two to five times the normal dose of nondepolarizing muscle relaxant as an increased number of extrajunctional receptors in burns patients means more receptors to block and these receptors appear to be not very sensitive to nondepolarizing muscle relaxants. Acetylcholine and succinylcholine depolarize extrajunctional receptors more easily in these patients.

○ **How do pregnant patients respond to succinylcholine?**

Normally. From the 10th week of pregnancy until 6 weeks postpartum, they have a 25–30% reduction in plasma cholinesterase activity. This decrease has little clinical significance.

○ **How do parturients differ from nonpregnant patients in dose requirements for nondepolarizing relaxants?**

Their dose–response curve is not significantly altered.

○ **How do the antibiotics potentiate the nondepolarizing muscle relaxants?**

They enhance neuromuscular blockade by inhibiting acetylcholine formation (prejunctional mechanism).

○ **How is aminoglycoside-induced paralysis best managed?**

With assisted mechanical ventilation until satisfactory recovery of neuromuscular transmission occurs. A dose ofneostigmine (maximum IV dose of 70 μg/kg, to avoid nicotinic effects) may be tried.

○ **How does stereochemistry improve therapeutic indices of anesthetic drugs?**

Different isomers have been evaluated in hopes of decreasing drug-induced toxicity. Cisatracurium causes less histamine release than atracurium. L-Bupivacaine may be less cardiotoxic than bupivacaine.

○ **Why is IV succinylcholine routinely not used for relaxation to facilitate abdominal closure after reversal of neuromuscular blockade with neostigmine?**

The duration of the subsequent block is unpredictable. Succinylcholine at intubating doses (1.5 mg/kg) normally provides 5–10 minutes of neuromuscular blockade. After administration of neostigmine, a dose of succinylcholine will cause neuromuscular blockade for up to 60 minutes. The mechanism of increased duration of neuromuscular blockade is due to the inhibition of pseudocholinesterase.

○ **What is a possible mechanism for rapacuronium-induced bronchospasm?**

M3 muscarinic receptor-mediated airway smooth muscle constriction.

Rapacuronium has a 15-fold higher affinity for M2 muscarinic receptors as compared with M3 muscarinic receptors. Blockade (antagonism) of M2 receptors could lead to the unopposed release of acetylcholine resulting in M3 muscarinic receptor-mediated airway smooth muscle constriction. These effects are reversible with α_2 agonists. Because of this side effect, this drug is no longer available for clinical use.

○ **Do all inhaled anesthetics potentiate nondepolarizing muscle relaxants?**

Yes, but to varying degrees.

Inhaled anesthetics produce CNS depression with a generalized decrease in muscle tone and decrease in sensitivity of the postjunctional membrane to depolarization. In addition, isoflurane may increase blood flow to skeletal muscle, effectively delivering more drug to the receptor sites. In general, ether-type inhaled anesthetics (isoflurane and enflurane) have a greater dose-dependent effect on augmenting the block than halothane. Halothane has a greater effect than nitrous oxide–barbiturate–narcotic or propofol anesthesia. This effect is most significant with pancuronium.

○ **How do antibiotics potentiate nondepolarizing muscle relaxants?**

Aminoglycosides (neomycin, streptomycin, gentamicin, and netilmicin) are notorious for potentiating the effects of nondepolarizing NMB. They exert their effects by inhibiting acetylcholine formation on the prejunctional side of the neuromuscular junction. Other antibiotic groups known to potentiate nondepolarizing muscle relaxants include polymyxins and lincosamines (clindamycin and lincomycin). Clindamycin prolongs the effect of pancuronium and vecuronium even in the absence of evidence of NMB. At clinically relevant doses the penicillins, cephalosporins, tetracyclines, and erythromycins are devoid of effects at the NM junction.

○ **Do local anesthetics impact the recovery from nondepolarizing neuromuscular blockade?**

Yes. Small doses can augment the blockade produced by nondepolarizing muscle relaxants, while large doses can completely block neuromuscular transmission. The mechanism for local anesthetic augmentation of blockade includes the interference with prejunctional release of acetylcholine, the stabilization of postjunctional membranes, and the direct depression of skeletal muscular fibers.

○ **What other drugs can interact with nondepolarizing muscle relaxants?**

Cardiac antidysrhythmics: lidocaine (enhance) and quinidine (enhance).

Diuretics: Lasix (enhance).

Electrolytes: calcium (antagonize) and magnesium (enhance).

Others:
- Lithium (enhance)
- Carbamazepine (antagonize)
- Phenytoin (antagonize)
- Cyclosporine (enhance)

- Azathioprine (antagonize)
- Dantrolene (enhance)
- Calcium channel blockers (enhance)
- Trimethaphan (enhance)

○ **What effect does magnesium has on the potency of nondepolarizing muscle relaxants? Depolarizing muscle relaxants?**

Magnesium increases the potency of both depolarizing (mechanism unknown) and nondepolarizing MR (decreased prejunctional release of acetylcholine and decreased sensitivity to acetylcholine).

○ **Do nondepolarizing muscle relaxants easily cross the placenta?**

Nondepolarizing muscle relaxants do not cross the placenta at detectable levels that are considered to be clinically significant due to quaternary ammonium groups that are highly ionized at physiologic pH and limit lipid solubility.

○ **Do depolarizing muscle relaxants cross the placenta?**

Depolarizing muscle relaxants do not cross the placenta at detectable levels when given in routine intubating doses. There are multiple case reports of neonatal neuromuscular blockade at birth involving either neonatal pseudocholinesterase deficiency or extremely large IV doses of succinylcholine given to the mother (300 mg).

○ **What is the definition of ED_{50}?**

The mean dose of a muscle relaxant producing a 50% suppression of the single twitch response at the adductor pollicis.

○ **What is the significance of ED_{95}?**

ED_{95} is the mean dose of a muscle relaxant producing a 95% suppression of the single twitch response at the adductor pollicis. Most commonly, it is used to describe the relative potency of neuromuscular blockers in a nitrous oxide–barbiturate–opioid anesthetic. $2 \times ED_{95}$ of a muscle relaxant is routinely used for comparison of onset and duration between different muscle relaxants.

○ **What are the characteristics of a phase I block using a peripheral nerve stimulator?**

1. Single twitch, TOF, and tetanus amplitudes are decreased in relation to the degree of blockade.
2. No fade in response to repetitive stimuli.
3. No post-tetanic facilitation.
4. Augmentation of neuromuscular blockade after administration of an anticholinesterase drug.
5. Describes depolarizing NMB.

○ **What causes a phase II block?**

A phase II block is due to ionic and conformational changes in the cell membrane after large doses or a continuous infusion of succinylcholine. It is clinically similar to the block that is present after the administration of nondepolarizing muscle relaxants. However, the response to the reversal by acetylcholinesterase inhibitors is unpredictable.

Phase II block can occur with:

- High single dose
- Cumulative doses
- Normal dose during pseudocholinesterase deficiency – relative overdose and increased concentration in the synaptic cleft

○ **What are the characteristics of a phase II block?**

1. Decreased contraction in response to a single twitch stimulation
2. Fade of the muscle response with repetitive stimulation
3. TOF ratio of <0.3
4. Post-tetanic facilitation
5. Antagonization of neuromuscular blockade after administration of an anticholinesterase drug
6. Describes nondepolarizing block

○ **Is a phase II block reversible with anticholinesterases?**

Often. However, the response of a phase II block to administration of anticholinesterases is unpredictable due to a number of factors influencing development of the block. It is best not to attempt reversal.

○ **Why is succinylcholine the ideal drug for rapid sequence induction of anesthesia?**

Succinylcholine has the fastest onset (30–60 seconds) and recovery (4–10 minutes), compared with other muscle relaxants.

○ **Which muscle relaxant is traditionally used for ECT therapy? Why?**

Succinylcholine 0.5–1 mg/kg. Muscle relaxants are routinely used during electroconvulsive therapy to prevent injury to the patient. Succinylcholine is chosen for its quick onset and short duration. Other potential options include mivacurium, atracurium, and cisatracurium.

○ **Is Na^+ an intracellular or extracellular ion at the neuromuscular junction?**

Na^+ is an extracellular ion, while K^+ is an intracellular ion. This unequal distribution of ions causes a transmembrane potential of -90 mV to exist across the membrane.

○ **What implication does myasthenia gravis have on your choice of muscle relaxants?**

Patients with myasthenia gravis are very sensitive to nondepolarizing muscle relaxants and theoretically resistant to succinylcholine. Short- or intermediate-acting muscle relaxants without active metabolites (mivacurium and cisatracurium) may be given, starting with 1/10 the normal dose, and titrating to effect.

○ **What are the main side effects of D-tubocurarine?**

Histamine release (most significant of all nondepolarizing muscle relaxants and frequently dose-related) that produces vasodilation and hypotension. Sympathetic ganglionic block occurs in animals, but not in the clinical dose range. Bradycardia has been reported.

○ **How does the pharmacokinetics of muscle relaxant drugs differ in chronic hepatorenal disease?**

There is an increased volume of distribution in renal and hepatic disease. Neuromuscular blocking drugs are polar drugs (quaternary ammonium compounds). Initially, there is increased volume of distribution (V_d) and therefore a low plasma concentration for a given dose. If dependent on hepatic/renal clearance, there will be a prolonged clearance of a given dose.

Therefore, initial greater loading dose but smaller maintenance doses are required in liver and renal disease.

○ **Are muscle relaxants contraindicated in patients with hepatorenal syndrome?**

No. Cisatracurium (and atracurium) undergoes spontaneous breakdown at physiologic temperature and pH (Hoffmann elimination) as well as ester hydrolysis. This is the ideal agent to use in patients with end-stage liver or kidney disease. However, laudanosine (metabolite) may accumulate due to prolonged elimination half-time. Cisatracurium also produces laudanosine but because of the greater potency of cisatracurium, laudanosine quantities produced by Hoffmann elimination are 5–10 times lower than in the case of atracurium.

Muscle relaxants requiring significant renal excretion should be avoided (pancuronium 40%, metocurine 43%, tubocurarine 45%, doxacurium 30%, and pipecuronium 38%). Vecuronium and pancuronium also have 3-OH metabolites that accumulate in renal failure. The 3-OH metabolite of vecuronium is 80% as potent as the parent compound and that of pancuronium has two thirds the potency of the parent compound.

Muscle relaxants that are metabolized in the liver should be avoided or administered cautiously and titrated to effect (pancuronium, vecuronium, rocuronium, and pipecuronium). Vecuronium and rocuronium also have significant biliary excretion. About 30–40% of 3-OH metabolite of vecuronium is cleared in bile. Therefore, a prolonged action may occur in patients with obstructive jaundice.

Decreased plasma cholinesterase activity seen with liver disease may prolong the effects of succinylcholine and mivacurium. However, the liver disease should be severe to prolong the duration of action of succinylcholine. Clinically evident prolongation of succinylcholine activity is seen only with 75% decrease in the level of normal pseudocholinesterase.

○ **Which relaxants are nearly totally dependent on the kidneys for excretion?**

Gallamine is excreted unchanged in urine. Pancuronium is 80% excreted renally.

Key Terms

Acetylcholine nicotinic receptor: activation
Anesthetic drugs and IOP
Anesthetic management: penetrating eye injury
Anticholinesterase poisoning treatment
Burns: effect on NM receptors
Causes of upregulation of acetylcholine receptors
Cirrhosis: NMB pharmacokinetics
Depolarizer block: characteristics
Eaton–Lambert syndrome: physiology
Ecothiopate: drug interaction
End-stage renal disease (ESRD) and nondepolarizing NMB
Factors causing prolonged NMB
Indices of NM blockade reversal

Low dibucaine number: anesthetic implications
Magnesium: side effects
Mivacurium/vecuronium interaction
Monitoring for residual NMB
Muscle relaxants/inhaled agent
Muscle relaxation: mechanism
Neostigmine: maximum dose rationale
Neostigmine: muscarinic effect
Nerve action potential termination mechanism
Nerve gas poisoning: treatment
Neuromuscular block: vecuronium
Neuromuscular disease: succinylcholine hyperkalemia
Neuromuscular physiology

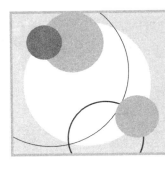

Neonatal Anesthesia

I am not young enough to know everything.
Oscar Wilde

○ **Until what age is an infant considered a neonate?**

One month.

○ **Until what age is a child considered an infant?**

One year.

○ **What are normal vital signs for a full-term neonate at birth?**

Blood pressure 65 mm Hg systolic, heart rate 130–160 beats/min (bpm), and respiratory rate 45–60 breaths/min.

○ **What are normal arterial blood gas values at birth for a healthy full-term newborn?**

The pH will be about 7.21, PaO_2 about 50 mm Hg, and the $PaCO_2$ about 40–50 mm Hg.

○ **How does the blood gas of a healthy term infant change in the first hour of life?**

The pH increases from 7.21 to 7.33 in the first hour, the $PaCO_2$ decreases to 30–40 mm Hg in the first hour, and the PaO_2 increases from 50 mm Hg at birth to 65 mm Hg at 1 hour and usually stabilizes at about 75 mm Hg by 24 hours.

○ **How does the fetal circulation differ from the extrauterine circulation?**

In the fetus, the pulmonary and systemic circulations occur in parallel and after birth, they occur in series.

○ **How does blood circulation change after birth?**

The fetal circulation essentially bypasses the lungs by shunting blood right to left: in the fetus, pulmonary vascular resistance (PVR) is relatively high because of the low PO_2 and small lung volumes, whereas the systemic vascular resistance (SVR) is low (the placenta is a low-resistance circuit). The resulting relatively higher right-sided pressures in fetal life promote blood shunting from the right atrium to the left atrium via the foramen ovale and from the pulmonary artery to the systemic circulation (aorta) via the ductus arteriosus. After birth, PVR falls rapidly as the lungs expand and clamping the umbilical cord increases SVR. As a result, right-sided pressures fall and left-sided pressures rise. Blood no longer tends to shunt right to left and blood in the pulmonary and systemic circulations is essentially separated.

○ **What features characterize persistent pulmonary hypertension of the newborn (PPHN)?**

In many ways, PPHN mimics the fetal circulation. There is increased PVR, increased pulmonary artery pressure, decreased pulmonary blood flow, and right-to-left shunting across the foramen ovale and ductus arteriosus.

○ **What causes PPHN?**

PPHN is caused by any condition that prevents the normal transition from fetal to neonatal circulation. Most commonly this is caused by conditions that increase PVR, most notably acidosis and hypoxemia.

○ **What are the common neonatal abdominal emergencies?**

Omphalocele, gastroschisis, intestinal atresia, imperforate anus, malrotation, and volvulus. Others include congenital diaphragmatic hernia (CDH), incarcerated inguinal hernia, and exstrophy of the bladder.

○ **What are the common nonabdominal neonatal emergencies?**

Myelomeningocele, tracheoesophageal fistula, and bilateral choanal atresia.

○ **What are the differences between gastroschisis and omphalocele?**

Omphalocele involves herniation of abdominal contents into an abdominal wall defect at the umbilicus. Umbilical hernia is a very mild form of omphalocele. The herniated abdominal contents (which may include abdominal organs other than bowel) are contained within a sac consisting of peritoneum that protects the organs from irritation by amniotic fluid. The peritoneal covering can rupture at birth, exposing abdominal contents to the environment. Omphalocele is often associated with other congenital anomalies.

In gastroschisis there is an abdominal wall defect to the right of the normal umbilicus through which abdominal contents herniate. Since they are not contained within a peritoneal sac, the herniated abdominal contents are exposed directly to amniotic fluid in utero. Gastroschisis outcomes may be somewhat worse than those seen with omphalocele because of the amount of time the abdominal contents spend being bathed in irritating amniotic fluid. Recovery of bowel function is slower in gastroschisis, and the bowel tends to be inflamed and edematous, often making primary closure more difficult. Gastroschisis is usually found in isolation and occurs more commonly in premature infants.

○ **When should primary closure of gastroschisis or omphalocele be attempted?**

Primary closure of omphalocele or gastroschisis may cause circulatory, ventilatory, and/or renal dysfunction, as well as bowel necrosis if the abdominal pressure is too high on closure. Primary closure should only be attempted when the intragastric pressure is <20 cm H_2O, the central venous pressure does not increase by 4 mm Hg or more, and adequate ventilation can be maintained as the abdominal viscera are replaced into the abdominal cavity.

○ **If primary closure is not attempted, how is the abdominal wall closed?**

A silastic sheet can be fashioned into a chimney or silo to contain the bowel. The silo volume is decreased over the course of a few days. Once the height of the silo is level with the rest of the abdominal wall, the infant can go to the operating room for surgical abdominal wall closure.

○ **List three major goals in the perioperative management of gastroschisis/omphalocele?**

1. Management of fluid and heat losses from exposed abdominal contents.
2. Protection of herniated organs.
3. Antibiotics to minimize the risk of sepsis.

○ **Describe the developmental history of CDH.**

Typically the abdominal viscera herniate through a defect in the left hemidiaphragm into the left hemithorax. The presence of abdominal contents in the thoracic cavity prevents adequate growth and development of both lungs, but the ipsilateral lung in particular is affected with resultant pulmonary hypoplasia. Right-sided diaphragmatic hernias occur, but are less common (10–15%).

○ **What findings are present on physical examination of neonates with CDH?**

Scaphoid abdomen, bowel sounds in the chest, displaced heart sounds, and poor air entry. At birth, these infants often exhibit the classic triad of respiratory distress, cyanosis, and apparent dextrocardia.

○ **What is the underlying cause of the respiratory failure associated with left-sided CDH?**

Left lung hypoplasia and pulmonary hypertension.

○ **What is the mortality associated with CDH?**

40–62% [Stege et al., See reference on page 526].

○ **What are the major goals in the perioperative management of neonates with CDH?**

To prevent the occurrence of hypoxemia and acidosis (which can contribute to a return to a fetal circulation pattern) by optimizing ventilation, maximizing oxygenation, and minimizing metabolic perturbations. Low-pressure, high-frequency ventilation is preferred to minimize barotrauma (and resulting pneumothorax), especially to the more compliant contralateral lung.

○ **Describe the clinical course of neonates with CDH if hypoxemia and acidosis persist despite therapy.**

Hypoxemia and acidosis induce pulmonary vasoconstriction, leading to increased PVR. Increased PVR produces an elevation in pulmonary artery, right atrial, and right ventricular pressures. Elevated right-sided pressures and resistances, in turn, induce a return to the fetal circulatory state, with reopening of the foramen ovale and the ductus arteriosus with right-to-left shunting and subsequent cyanosis. This fetal circulation pattern, usually directly due to persistent pulmonary hypertension, induces further hypoxemia and acidosis, eventually resulting in multiple organ dysfunction and death.

○ **If a fetal circulatory pattern persists in a neonate with CDH despite optimized ventilatory and pharmacologic support, what alternative therapy is available?**

Extracorporeal membrane oxygenation (ECMO).

○ **Which bowel segments are typically involved in intestinal atresias?**

Duodenum, jejunum, terminal ileum, and anus.

○ **Which bowel segment obstruction presents earliest?**

Duodenal atresia usually presents within the first few days of life. Other intestinal obstructions may not present until 2–7 days after birth, but usually occur within the first 2 weeks of life.

○ **What chromosomal anomaly is associated with duodenal atresia?**

Trisomy 21 (Down syndrome).

○ **What is meconium ileus?**

Meconium ileus is small bowel obstruction caused by inspissated meconium that was never passed. This form of bowel obstruction is pathognomonic for cystic fibrosis (although only 20% of cystic fibrosis patients have a history of meconium ileus).

○ **At what age is pyloric stenosis most commonly seen?**

The average age of onset is 3–4 weeks, with a range of 1–12 weeks.

○ **What physical findings are characteristic of pyloric stenosis?**

The "olive." This is a firm mass usually palpable just to the right of the midline in the epigastric area.

○ **What noninvasive diagnostic test can reliably confirm the diagnosis of pyloric stenosis?**

Ultrasound.

○ **What are the most common metabolic disturbances typically seen in infants with pyloric stenosis?**

Dehydration, hypokalemia, and hypochloremic metabolic alkalosis.

○ **T/F: Pyloric stenosis is a surgical emergency.**

False. Rehydration and correction of electrolyte and acid–base abnormalities should be completed first.

○ **What anesthesia-related precaution is particularly important to observe in the infant undergoing pyloromyotomy?**

These patients should always be treated as if they have a full stomach. Intravenous access should be established and the stomach should be emptied with a large-bore sump tube before induction of anesthesia. Some anesthesiologists prefer to intubate the infant awake but there is evidence that an IV induction (rapid sequence) may be better. The trachea should not be extubated at the end of the procedure until the infant's airway reflexes are intact.

○ **What is the most common form of congenital tracheoesophageal fistula?**

Proximal esophageal atresia–distal fistula. This form occurs in more than 90% of cases.

○ **Tracheoesophageal fistula is a feature of which condition?**

VATER (or VACTERL) syndrome. This invariably consists of *v*ertebral anomalies, *a*nal defects (such as atresia), *t*racheo*e*sophageal fistula or *e*sophageal atresia, and *r*enal anomalies. The term VACTERL adds *c*ardiac anomalies (most commonly ventricular septal defect [VSD] or tetralogy of Fallot) and *l*imb defects (radial defects, extra digits, syndactyly). There is a great deal of variation and not all patients will manifest all anomalies.

○ **T/F: Tracheoesophageal fistula is a surgical emergency.**

True. The stomach must be decompressed and the fistula closed in order to prevent pulmonary aspiration of stomach contents.

○ **Describe a technique for inducing anesthesia for a right thoracotomy to repair a tracheoesophageal fistula.**

(1) The proximal esophageal pouch should be emptied with a sump tube. (2) With the infant in a semi-upright position, a gas induction with sevoflurane and oxygen should be performed with the patient breathing spontaneously. (3) After airway reflexes are sufficiently obtunded, the trachea should be intubated. (4) The endotracheal tube should be advanced carefully into a mainstem bronchus, confirmed by loss of breath sounds over one hemithorax. (5) The endotracheal tube should then be pulled back slowly until breath sounds can just be heard bilaterally. (6) The endotracheal tube should be rotated so that the Murphy eye and the bevel are not facing posteriorly toward the fistula. (7) Spontaneous ventilation or gentle assist should be maintained until the chest is opened, at which time ventilation must be controlled. Until the fistula is isolated, it is best to minimize the ventilatory pressure. If the patient undergoes a decompressive gastrostomy prior to thoracotomy, the gastrostomy tube will act as a low-resistance vent that can decrease ventilation to the lungs. If this occurs, the gastrostomy tube can be partially or fully clamped. *Note:* The most likely location of the fistula is 1–2 cm above the carina on the posterior trachea.

○ **What problems do children with a history of tracheoesophageal fistula repair encounter as they grow?**

Obstructive and restrictive lung disease later in life and frequent respiratory infections. Other problems include tracheomalacia, weak tracheal wall at the fistula site, esophageal stricture, and esophageal dysmotility.

○ **What is the most significant difficulty in inducing anesthesia in an infant with myelomeningocele?**

Care must be taken to avoid direct pressure or trauma to the defect. If placed supine for induction, padding should be placed around the outside of the meningocele sac to protect it. Elevation of the occiput and shoulders should then be used to position the patient for laryngoscopy and intubation.

○ **A neonate presents with respiratory distress, cyanosis, and apnea that improves if the baby cries. What is the likely diagnosis?**

Bilateral choanal atresia, resulting in nasal obstruction. This occurs because infants are obligate nasal breathers.

○ **Until what age are infants obligate nose breathers?**

Three to 5 months.

○ **Explain why infants desaturate more quickly than adults when apneic under anesthesia.**

In infants, the cartilaginous ribcage and immature thoracic musculature result in a highly compliant chest and relatively poor outward recoil of the chest wall. The inward recoil of the lung, on the other hand, is only slightly less than in adults. As a result, the inward forces outweigh the outward forces and a reduction in functional residual capacity occurs with apnea. In addition, oxygen consumption is higher in infants than in adults. Both these phenomena contribute to a more rapid desaturation when apneic under anesthesia.

○ **T/F: The effects of opioids are more unpredictable in preterm infants and neonates compared with older children and adults.**

True. In general, the pharmacokinetics of opioids are more variable in premature infants and neonates. The plasma clearance may be reduced and the elimination half-life may be prolonged. Active metabolites of some drugs might accumulate. Also, these children may be more sensitive to the respiratory depressive effects of opioids. There is increasing evidence that even the youngest children experience pain and so analgesics should be utilized perioperatively but caution should be exercised when using opioids in premature infants and neonates due to variable effects.

○ **What is retinopathy of prematurity?**

This is a vascular disorder of the developing retinal circulation that can result in complete retinal detachment and blindness in extreme cases. The principle etiologic factor is thought to be increased PaO_2 in the developing retinal artery. Infants are thought to be at risk of retinopathy of prematurity until 44 weeks postconceptual age when the retinal vessels are mature. Until that time, the minimum oxygen tension required to maintain adequate organ perfusion should be the goal. An arterial PO_2 of 60–80 mm Hg should be adequate in most cases.

○ **What is the most common cause of bradycardia in the neonate?**

Hypoxia. Therefore, when an infant becomes bradycardic, the *first* thing to do is to ensure adequacy of ventilation and oxygenation.

○ **Why are neonates more dependent on heart rate to maintain cardiac output compared with adults?**

Cardiac output = heart rate × stroke volume. Neonatal myocardial fibers are made up of less distensible material compared with those of adults. As a result, the neonatal heart is less compliant and less able to increase stroke volume in response to an increase in preload. The relatively fixed stroke volume in neonates means that cardiac output is more dependent on heart rate compared with adults whose hearts can more readily increase stroke volume to increase cardiac output.

○ **Which neonates are at risk for hypoglycemia?**

Premature infants, small for gestational age infants, and infants of diabetic mothers.

○ **What is the definition of hypoglycemia in neonates?**

Blood glucose ≤45 mg/dL in preterm or term neonates and ≤60 mg/dL in infants and older children.

○ **T/F: Neonates experience a slower induction with *inhaled* anesthetic agents compared with older children.**

False. The ratio of minute ventilation to functional residual capacity is higher in neonates compared with older children. Therefore, the gas in the alveolar space equilibrates more quickly and induction occurs more rapidly.

○ **Does fetal hemoglobin (Hb F) have a higher or a lower P_{50} than adult hemoglobin (Hb A)?**

The P_{50} of Hb F (19 mm Hg) is lower than the P_{50} of Hb A (27 mm Hg). This represents an adaptation to intrauterine life since Hb F binds oxygen more readily than Hb A at the low oxygen tensions in utero.

○ **What is *physiologic anemia?***

Over the first few months of life, the high level of Hb F seen at birth decreases, reaching its lowest level by 2–3 months of age. A normal hematocrit at this age is 33%. The P_{50} increases rapidly during the neonatal period so that tissue oxygen delivery is still adequate despite less hemoglobin. As Hb A replaces Hb F, this anemia resolves.

○ **T/F: Beta-thalassemia is easily detectable in neonates.**

False. Normal Hb A is composed of two alpha and two beta polypeptide subunits. Beta-thalassemia is caused by a defect in one or both beta polypeptide subunits that results in abnormal Hb A. Because Hb F is made up of two alpha and two gamma polypeptide subunits (no beta), and because Hb F is the predominant hemoglobin species at birth, beta-thalassemia is rarely detected in neonates. In the first few months of life as Hb A replaces Hb F, the effects of beta-thalassemia are more likely to appear.

○ **Briefly describe the Apgar score.**

The Apgar scoring system for newborns consists of five parameters evaluated at 1 and 5 minutes following birth. Each is assigned a score from 0 to 2, for a possible total score ranging from 0 (the worst) to 10. A total score of 8–10 is normal, 4–7 indicates moderate impairment, and 0–3 indicates need for immediate resuscitation.

A-P-G-A-R:

A for appearance (color: blue both central and periphery = 0, only periphery = 1, pink all over = 2)

P for pulse (0 = 0, <100 = 1, ≥100 = 2)

G for grimace or reflex irritability when suction with catheter (none = 0, some = 1, active coughing/sneezing = 2)

A for activity or muscle tone (none or limp = 0, some = 1, active movement = 2)

R for respiration (none = 0, irregular gasping =1, robust and crying = 2)

○ **A full-term newborn is flaccid, blue, with no respiratory effort, and has a heart rate of 90 bpm after the first minute of life. What is the Apgar score?**

The Apgar score is 1.

○ **What is the *first* thing you do for this infant?**

Airway! Ventilate by bag and mask. Simply ventilating will often increase heart rate into normal range (>100 bpm).

○ **At what rate should ventilation be performed during neonatal resuscitation [Neonatal Resuscitation, 2010. See reference on page 526]?**

Forty to 60 breaths/min.

○ **What is the initial lung inflation pressure required for positive pressure ventilation in the full-term newborn infant?**

This is variable. A total of 20 cm H_2O may be sufficient but 30–40 cm H_2O may be required in some neonates. Caution should be exercised with premature infants who may be more prone to lung injury with overinflation.

○ **What are the indications for positive pressure ventilation in a neonate?**

Apnea, gasping respirations, persistent central cyanosis on 100% oxygen, and HR <100 bpm.

○ **Which clinical signs are indicative of an improvement in the neonate's status during resuscitation?**

Increasing heart rate, spontaneous respiration, and improvement in color.

○ **When should chest compressions be initiated during resuscitation of a neonate?**

When the heart rate is below 60 bpm and is not increasing after 30 seconds of positive pressure ventilation with 100% oxygen.

○ **If this infant does not clinically improve despite ventilation and chest compressions, what is the next step?**

Obtain vascular access (umbilical vein catheter) and treat with epinephrine (0.01–0.03 mg/kg) and volume expanders (10 mL/kg of isotonic crystalloid or blood). Be aware that rapid infusion of intravenous volume expanders may be associated with intraventricular hemorrhage in premature infants.

○ **Which drugs are effective when administered via the endotracheal tube during neonatal resuscitation?**

Lidocaine, epinephrine, atropine, and naloxone (L-E-A-N). Recommended intratracheal doses are approximately two times higher than intravenous doses to ensure adequate absorption. Dilution with normal saline to a volume of 1–2 mL is recommended. Surfactant may be given through the ET tube to premature neonates with respiratory distress syndrome (RDS).

Intravenous administration is the preferred route for epinephrine (i.e., given via an umbilical venous line). However, while IV access is being established, endotracheal administration may be considered if the heart rate remains less than 60 bpm after 30 seconds of adequate ventilation and chest compressions.

○ **What is the recommendation for neonatal resuscitation of a meconium-stained infant?**

If the infant is not vigorous at birth (i.e., depressed or absent respiration, heart rate less than 100 bpm, or poor muscle tone), tracheal suctioning should be performed before routine stimulation. Consider intubation, place pulse oximeter, start with room air for term infants or 40% if <37 weeks and positive pressure ventilation.

If the infant is vigorous at birth, it is not necessary to perform endotracheal suctioning even when there is thick or particulate meconium. Meconium should be removed from the mouth and nose using a bulb syringe or a suction catheter. Discourage obstetric suctioning on the perineum.

○ **At what vertebral level does the spinal cord terminate in neonates?**

The spinal cord terminates at L3 in neonates. It normally recedes to the adult level (L1) by 1 year of age.

○ **T/F: Fluid loading prior to spinal anesthesia in infants is essential in preventing hypotension.**

False. Hypotension is rarely seen in infants undergoing spinal anesthesia. Many practitioners will even place the intravenous catheter in the foot after the block has been placed.

○ **T/F: The duration of spinal anesthesia is shorter in infants compared with adults.**

True. Relatively higher cardiac output and regional blood flow result in greater uptake of drug and a shorter duration of block.

○ **What is the function of pulmonary surfactant?**

Pulmonary surfactant is produced by Type II alveolar epithelial cells in late fetal life (32–34 weeks). Phospholipid lecithin is a major constituent.

Pulmonary surfactant reduces surface tension in the lung and reduces pressure necessary to inflate the lungs. This *reduces the work of breathing*.

Surfactant promotes *alveolar stability* by decreasing surface tension in small alveoli. The Law of Laplace predicts that this will reduce the difference in pressures between alveoli of different radii and therefore allow small alveoli to exist at same pressure as large ones by decreasing surface tension ($P = 2T/R$, where P is the pressure, T is the surface tension, R is the radius).

○ **What are the effects of surfactant deficiency?**

Lung inflation is a major physiologic stimulus for the release of surfactant into the alveoli.

Preterm infants may suffer from surfactant dysfunction and deficiency and develop infant RDS. Surface tension remains high in infant RDS. Signs include tachypnea, grunting, sternal retractions, tachycardia, and cyanosis.

The stiff lungs of RDS and compliant chest wall of the newborn decrease FRC. Increased work of breathing leads to metabolic acidosis. Rapid shallow breathing pattern due to decreased lung compliance increases dead space ventilation. Abnormal surfactant also leads to hypoxemia from edema and alveolar collapse (atelectasis).

○ **T/F: The ventilatory response of premature infants to hypercapnea is equal to that of older children.**

False. Premature infants and neonates have a diminished ability to increase respiration in the face of hypercarbia compared with older children and adults. This is likely due to immaturity of respiratory control centers of the central nervous system. The slope of the CO_2-response curve increases with increasing age such that as infants age, their ventilatory response to hypercarbia improves.

○ **Which anatomic structures account for the greatest percentage of work of breathing in neonates and adults?**

In neonates, the greatest resistance to airflow occurs in the small airways and overcoming this resistance accounts for the majority of work of breathing in this age group. In adults, the nasal passages account for the greatest percentage of total airway resistance and represent the most significant impact on work of breathing.

○ **What is the most common noncyanotic congenital heart lesion?**

VSD.

○ **Why is prostaglandin given to some neonates with congenital heart disease?**

Some congenital heart lesions are "ductal-dependent," meaning that blood flow through the ductus arteriosus is critical to maintain blood flow to either the lungs or the systemic circulation. After birth when the neonate is transitioning from fetal to neonatal circulation and the ductus arteriosus closes, decompensation can occur (cyanosis, hypotension, etc.) in the setting of these specific congenital lesions. As a temporizing measure, prostaglandin (which maintains patency of the ductus arteriosus) is administered until the anatomy of the cardiac lesion can be evaluated and definitive therapy can be initiated.

○ **What is the predictive value of L/S ratio?**

As the lungs mature, the ratio of lecithin to sphingomyelin increases in the amniotic fluid. An L/S ratio of 2 or more indicates fetal lung maturity and a relatively low risk of infant RDS, and an L/S ratio of less than 1.5 is associated with a high risk of infant RDS.

○ **What factors make newborns more susceptible to hypothermia?**

- Increased heat loss due to increased surface-area-to-mass ratio.
- High respiratory water loss and thin subcutaneous tissues causing increased thermal conductance.
- Immature central thermoregulatory response.
- Diminished ability to produce endogenous heat (reduced shivering thermogenesis).
- Sedative drugs, hypoglycemia, and cerebral damage further increase heat loss.

○   **What is the advantage of neutral thermal environment?**

In utero, heat production by the fetus results in a fetal temperature 0.5°C higher than maternal temperature. Following delivery, the neonate is at risk of hypothermia. Maintaining a neutral thermal environment is thus a primary challenge for the neonate to avoid the complications of heat loss.

○   **What unique method do neonates utilize to maintain body temperature?**

Nonshivering thermogenesis, which occurs primarily through the metabolism of brown fat. It makes up about 5% of an infant's body weight. Brown fat differentiates around 26–30 weeks gestation and so may not be available to some premature infants.

Voluntary muscle activity is restricted during the perioperative period and shivering thermogenesis is not significant until the infant reaches at least 1 year of age. Vasoconstriction can occur in both full-term and premature infants, decreasing cutaneous blood flow and conductive heat loss.

○   **What are the consequences of hypothermia in neonates?**

Hypothermia can result in acidosis, hypoxemia, apnea, hypoventilation, and cardiac arrest. Pulmonary vasoconstriction may cause an increase in pulmonary artery pressure, right-to-left intracardiac shunting, and cardiopulmonary decompensation.

○   **Water accounts for what percentage of body weight in premature neonates?**

Eighty percent.

○   **Water accounts for what percentage of body weight in full-term neonates?**

Seventy percent.

○   **What is the estimated blood volume of a premature neonate?**

Ninety to 100 mL/kg.

○   **What is the estimated blood volume of a full-term neonate?**

Eighty to 90 mL/kg.

○   **What is the maximum concentration of urine possible in a neonate?**

Six hundred to 700 mOsm/L. The kidneys are not capable of concentrating to the adult maximum of 1,400 mOsm/L until the end of the first year of life.

○   **How does the immaturity of the neonatal kidney contribute to problems with the regulation of intravascular volume?**

The inability of the neonatal kidney to fully concentrate urine makes the neonate less able to protect intravascular volume in the face of hypovolemia.

○   **What size and at what depth should an oral endotracheal tube be taped in a full-term neonate?**

A 3.0–3.5 mm internal diameter tube secured at 9 cm at the lips is a good guideline. Bilateral breath sounds should always be confirmed. A depth of three times the internal diameter is a useful guideline for infants.

○ **How does the position of the larynx differ between neonates and adults?**

In premature infants, the larynx lies at the third cervical vertebra (C3). In term neonates, the larynx is usually at C3–4. In adults, the larynx has descended to C4–5.

○ **How does the shape of the epiglottis differ between neonates and adults?**

In neonates, the epiglottis is relatively long, omega-shaped, and stiff. In adults, it is often flat and short and less obstructive on laryngoscopic view.

○ **During anesthesia, a neonate's heart rate is 200 bpm. Does this indicate a problem?**

Although tachycardia may represent a response to surgical stimulation, high heart rates in neonates are often indicative of intravascular volume depletion. A fluid challenge of 10 mL/kg of crystalloid or colloid solution will often slow the heart rate.

○ **Which carries blood highest in oxygen tension and lowest in carbon dioxide tension, the umbilical vein or the umbilical artery?**

The umbilical vein.

○ **Does the ductus venosus carry oxygenated or deoxygenated blood in fetal life?**

Oxygenated blood from the placenta.

○ **What will the cardiovascular evaluation of a newborn with a patent ductus arteriosus (PDA) reveal?**

A machine-like, continuous murmur at the left upper sternal border, bounding pulses, and a widened pulse pressure.

○ **T/F: PDA is a surgical emergency.**

False. Most neonates with PDA will undergo a trial of medical therapy with indomethacin in an attempt to close the shunt. If this fails and the patient is symptomatic, surgery may be undertaken.

○ **T/F: Neonates are more sensitive to nondepolarizing neuromuscular blockers than are adults and older children.**

True. However, since infants generally have a higher volume of distribution for these drugs, clinical doses are similar to adults on a milligram per kilogram basis.

○ **T/F: Infants require less neostigmine than adults for reversal of neuromuscular blockade.**

True. The standard dose of neostigmine in infants is 30–50 μg/kg.

○ **T/F: Infants are more sensitive to the neuromuscular blocking effect of succinylcholine.**

False. Neonates and infants are more resistant to succinylcholine compared with adults and older children. Doses of 2 mg/kg are suggested for intubation of neonates.

○   **Explain the increase in succinylcholine dosing for neonatal intubation.**

The neonatal response to neuromuscular blockers is affected by immaturity of the neuromuscular junction and an increase in extracellular fluid and volume of distribution. Therefore, initial dosing of nondepolarizers is similar to that of adults. The dosage of succinylcholine, however, is increased to as much as twice the adult dosage.

○   **What IM dose of succinylcholine is used for intubation in the neonate?**

Succinylcholine 4 mg/kg.

○   **What IV dose of succinylcholine is indicated for an RSI or intubation in the neonate?**

Succinylcholine 2 mg/kg.

Key Terms

Anatomy of fetal circulation
Anesthetic management of congenital diaphragmatic hernia (CDH)
APGAR scoring/calculation
Beta-thalassemias – newborn
Congenital diaphragmatic hernia: anesthetic management
Congenital heart disease: pulmonary hypertension – treatment
Congenital lobar emphysema
Cyanosis: newborn
Gastroschisis: abdominal closure pulmonary effects
Meconium-stained delivery: management
Meningomyelocele: Arnold–Chiari association
Neonatal apnea/hypoxia: physiology
Neonatal blood gas analysis
Neonatal bradycardia: treatment
Neonatal intraventricular hemorrhage
Neonatal pharmacology
Neonatal respiratory physiology
Neonatal resuscitation and meconium
Neonatal resuscitation: steps
Neonatal surgical emergencies

Neonatal versus adult cardiac cycle
Neonate airway anatomy
Neonate: duration of postanesthesia monitoring
Newborn RDS: symptoms
Newborn dehydration: assessment
Omphalocele repair: fluid management/postoperative management
Opioid sensitivity: neonate
Patent ductus arteriosus (PDA): diagnosis
PDA ligation: circulatory effects
Persistent fetal circulation
Predictive value L/S ratio
Premature neonate: mechanical vent
Prematurity: decreased CO_2 response
Pyloric stenosis: electrolytes/fluid therapy
Pyloric stenosis: lab findings
Pyloric stenosis: metabolic abnormality
Spinal anesthetics: infants versus adults
Surfactant deficiency
Transitional circulation: effects on SpO_2
Ventricular function: neonate versus adult
Work of breathing: neonate versus adult

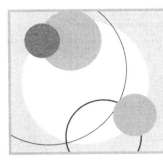

Neurosurgery

The ultimate measure of a man is not where he stands in moments of comfort and convenience, but where he stands at times of challenge and controversy.
Dr Martin Luther King, Jr.

○ **What are the main components of a somatosensory evoked potential (SSEP) signal?**

Amplitude and latency. Amplitude is the size of the recorded wave and latency is the time lag between sensory nerve stimulation and when the signal is received.

○ **What medications decrease the sensory evoked potential amplitude and/or prolong latency?**

Inhalational agents including nitrous oxide generally have a more depressant effect (increased latency and decreased amplitude) on evoked potentials than intravenous agents. Cortical evoked potentials (VEP and SSEP) are very sensitive while brain stem and spinal components (BAEP) are resistant to anesthetic influence.

Propofol and thiopental attenuate the amplitude but do not obliterate them. Therefore, even during burst suppression with these agents, SSEP (and MEP) can be monitored. BAEP recording is resistant.

However, bolus administration of any IV anesthetic agents or change in the depth of anesthetic level with inhalational agents should be avoided during the critical periods of the surgery.

Opioids and benzodiazepines have negligible effect on recording of evoked potentials.

Ketamine and etomidate have been shown to enhance the quality of signals of evoked potentials.

○ **A 15-year-old female with idiopathic thoracolumbar scoliosis is undergoing spinal instrumentation and fusion under general anesthesia with N_2O-O_2, narcotic, and muscle relaxant. What information is provided with the monitoring of SSEPs intraoperatively?**

In this case SSEPs are elicited by stimulation of the common peroneal or posterior tibial nerve (PTN) at the ankle. Characteristic electrical responses detected over the cortex indicate that the associated neural pathways along the spinal cord are intact. Baseline latency ("latency") of the response and the magnitude of the response ("amplitude") are measured preoperatively. Values for latency and amplitude are then obtained nearly continuously intraoperatively, and compared with baseline values. The amplitude of the response is considered to be a more valid indication of the status of the nervous system than is the latency of the response.

○ **How will the administration of muscle relaxants affect the SSEP signal?**

The signal would be improved due to elimination of the background "noise."

○ **An otherwise healthy 16-year-old female with severe thoracolumbar scoliosis is to undergo spinal instrumentation under general anesthesia. Monitoring of SSEPs by stimulation of the PTN (posterior tibial nerve) at the ankle is planned. During the operation, what are the likely causes for an increase in latency and decrease in amplitude of SSEPs with stimulation of the PTN?**

- Cold irrigation of the spinal cord.
- An electrode dislodged from the skin or disconnected from the computer resulting in loss of signal.
- Spinal cord stretch or pressure causing ischemia.
- Pedicle screw placement with impingement on the spinal cord or nerve root.
- Improper limb positioning causing nerve compression.
- Hypotension – mean arterial pressure (MAP) <40 mm Hg decreases amplitude.
- Hypothermia – when the body temperature falls <35°C, there is a progressive slowing of EEG activity with complete electrical silence occurring at 15–20°C.
- Hypocarbia – end-tidal CO_2 <25 mm Hg increases latency.
- Hypoxia – decreases amplitude.
- Hematocrit <15% increases latency.

○ **Describe proper SSEP electrode placement.**

SSEP signals are intended to evaluate sensory nerve signal conduction. A signal is produced in the periphery and recorded at the brain. In order to ensure a signal is propagating down a nerve, there are intermediate sites of signal recording in the periphery. For upper extremity SSEPs, the signals are normally produced at the wrist over the ulnar nerve, sensed in the brachial plexus at Erb's point, and then finally sensed in the brain by scalp electrodes. Lower extremity signals are produced at the PTN at the ankle and sensed in the popliteal fossa, as well as the brain.

○ **What parts of the spinal cord do SSEP and MEP (motor evoked potentials) signals interrogate?**

SSEP signals interrogate the posterior columns, while MEP signals interrogate the anterior horn. Therefore, SSEP signals will not detect anterior cord ischemia and cannot detect the onset of motor paralysis (unless caused by whole cord ischemia).

○ **How will the administration of muscle relaxants affect the MEP signal?**

In contrast to SSEPs, it will eliminate them. On the other hand, the same anesthetic agents that decrease SSEP signals will also decrease MEP signals to an even greater degree.

○ **Why is MEP monitoring performed during AAA repair?**

To determine if cross-clamping of the aorta reduces blood flow through the artery of Adamkiewicz sufficiently to cause ischemia of the anterior spinal cord resulting in paralysis.

○ **How are neurogenic motor evoked potentials (NMEPs) produced?**

The signal is generated at the spinal cord by direct electrode contact and then sensed at the popliteal fossa or PTN. Spinal cord stimulation must occur in a dry field or the current will be dissipated away from the motor neurons of the spinal cord. These signals are relatively resistant to suppression by anesthetic agents and are not eliminated (may actually be improved) if muscle relaxants are given.

○ **Which EEG rhythm waves correspond to various depths of anesthesia?**

Theta waves are seen during moderately deep anesthesia and delta waves during deep anesthesia. Alpha waves are predominant in the resting awake adult. Beta waves are seen during mental activity and possibly light anesthesia.

○ **What are the causes of EEG burst suppression intraoperatively?**

High-dose propofol, isoflurane (2 MAC), barbiturates, etomidate, severe hypoxia, and profound hypothermia (around 20°C).

○ **During carotid endarterectomy surgery, carotid clamping results in an ipsilateral slowing of the EEG amplitude signal. What does this mean and how should it be treated?**

This means EEG evidence of cerebral ischemia. Pharmacologically elevating the blood pressure may shunt blood from the contralateral side of the brain to the affected side. If this does not rectify the problem, then the surgeon can place a carotid bypass shunt.

○ **How does thiopental affect the brain?**

Decreases cerebral metabolic rate for oxygen ($CMRO_2$) and cerebral blood flow (CBF) until isoelectric (=maximum of 50% reduction of $CMRO_2$ at this point). Decrease in CBF is due to increased cerebral vascular resistance (coupled changes in CBF).

○ **What are the causes of decrease in basal $CMRO_2$?**

Only hypothermia decreases the basal $CMRO_2$ of the brain (energy requirement for cellular homeostasis).

○ **What is the relationship of CBF and $CMRO_2$ to body temperature changes?**

For each 1°C increase in body temperature, CBF and $CMRO_2$ increase by 7%. As body temperature cools, CBF and $CMRO_2$ decrease. At 20°C, EEG becomes isoelectric but further decrease in temperature continues to reduce CMR throughout the brain.

○ **Which anesthetic agents decrease brain $CMRO_2$?**

Propofol, etomidate, thiopental, volatile anesthetics and to a lesser extent benzodiazepines, and lidocaine decrease brain $CMRO_2$. Opioids do not decrease $CMRO_2$.

○ **Which volatile anesthetic provides the best cerebral protection?**

Isoflurane has classically been the answer. However, newer volatile anesthetics such as sevoflurane appear to have less vasodilatory effect on CBF.

○ **What is cerebral metabolic uncoupling and how is it produced?**

Normally CBF increases to areas of increased metabolic rate and decreases to areas of decreased metabolic rate. Volatile anesthetics decrease $CMRO_2$ and at the same time cause vasodilation and an increase in CBF. This uncoupling phenomenon produces luxury perfusion, or increased perfusion to brain that actually requires less nutrient delivery because of decreased neuronal activity.

○ **What inhaled anesthetic agent is recommended for use during neurosurgery and why?**

Isoflurane. The level of CBF necessary to prevent ischemic changes in CNS tissue is least with isoflurane (critical CBF is 10 mL/(100 g/min)) compared with enflurane (15 mL/(100 g/min)) and halothane (20 mL/(100 g/min)). All volatile agents depress the $CMRO_2$ and cause cerebral vasodilation. This "uncoupling" of $CMRO_2$ and CBF is most marked with halothane and least with isoflurane. In addition, to prevent an increase in intracranial pressure (ICP), CO_2 reduction should be initiated just prior to the introduction of halothane. CO_2 reactivity is generally retained with isoflurane and sevoflurane.

○ **How do propofol and isoflurane differ in their effect on CBF and CMRO$_2$?**

Propofol and isoflurane decrease cerebral metabolic rate. Isoflurane increases CBF that results in an uncoupling of CBF and CMRO$_2$. In contrast, propofol causes cerebral vasoconstriction and a decrease in CBF to the areas of decreased metabolic demand. The decrease in metabolic rate is more pronounced than the decrease in blood flow.

All inhaled drugs including N$_2$O have intrinsic cerebral vasodilatory activity due to direct effect on vascular smooth muscle. However, the CBF increase due to the newer potent volatile agents (especially sevoflurane) appears to be not that significant under 1 MAC concentration. The net effect on CBF is the balance between augmentation of CBF due to vasodilatory effect and reduction in CBF due to suppression of CMR.

For example, at 0.5 MAC, CMR suppression predominates and CBF decreases, compared with awake state.

At 1 MAC, CBF remains unchanged; suppression and vasodilatory effects are balanced.

At >1 MAC doses, vasodilatory effect predominates and CBF increases significantly even though CMR is suppressed largely as well (uncoupling of flow and metabolism).

The order of vasodilating potency: halothane (200%) >> enflurane > desflurane ≈ isoflurane (20%) > sevoflurane.

These differences disappear with hyperventilation, especially with the newer agents. Also with continued administration, blood flow begins to return to normal (3 hours after initial exposure to 1.3 MAC).

○ **What is EEG burst suppression?**

An EEG pattern of deep sedation where periods of electrical silence are interrupted by brief episodes of activity.

○ **At what CBF does cerebral ischemia become apparent on the EEG?**

Twenty millimeters per 100 g/min. Normal global CBF is 50 mL/100 g/min. Neuronal damage is thought to occur at CBF below 10 mL/100 g/min.

○ **What are the best established uses of induced mild hypothermia following neurological injury?**

Moderate hypothermia to 33–35°C has been shown to be useful in:

1. Control of refractory intracranial hypertension

2. Amelioration of neurological injury after cardiac arrest

Although clinical trials have some encouraging data, statistically significant improvement in outcome after traumatic brain injury (TBI) has not been shown.

○ **What are the guidelines for initiating mild hypothermia following cardiac arrest?**

It is commonly accepted and recommended that mild hypothermia (32–34°C) should be initiated without delay (within 4 hours) after cardiac arrest and continued 12–24 hours (surface cooling or ice-cold infusions).

Survival rate (and neurological outcome) was shown to be higher in patients who received out-of-hospital cooling treatment in cases of out-of-hospital arrests.

Efficacy of induced hypothermia as a treatment to prevent injury from global ischemia has been demonstrated [Peberdy et al., 2010. See reference on page 527].

○ **What appears to be the mechanism by which mild hypothermia improves outcome of cardiac arrest victims?**

Hypothermia reduces metabolism, CMRO$_2$. There is a decrease in reactive O$_2$ species and excitatory amino acids during hypothermia and also direct inhibition of apoptosis. Inhibition of coagulation cascade and inflammatory reactions also may help improve the cerebral reperfusion.

○ **Is deep hypothermia useful in cerebral ischemia?**

Profound hypothermia is well known for its neuroprotective effect. At <20°C, circulatory arrest up to 30 minutes appears to be well tolerated.

However, the concerns of deep hypothermia are:

1. Need for cardiopulmonary bypass during the cooling and warming portion of the procedure
2. Hypothermia-induced coagulopathy

○ **How does systemic hypertension affect cerebral autoregulation?**

Chronic uncontrolled hypertension will shift the upper and lower limits of the cerebral autoregulation curve to the right (to higher pressures). This phenomenon can be reversed by adequate blood pressure control but it will take at least a few months to shift the cerebral autoregulation limits back toward normal.

○ **Explain how hyperventilation can actually improve blood flow to the diseased area of brain in a patient with a gliobastoma tumor?**

The key is that, in general, cerebral autoregulation is not preserved in diseased areas of brain. Hyperventilation leading to a decrease in $PaCO_2$ will cause cerebral vasoconstriction in normal vessels and preferential shunting of blood flow toward the diseased area of brain. This is the "reverse steal phenomenon."

○ **Describe intracranial compliance in terms of the volume–pressure relationship.**

The cranial cavity is a fixed space. Initially, increases in intracranial volume are well compensated for with minimal increases in pressure. However, when the capacity to compensate for volume expansion is exhausted, even a small further increase in volume will dramatically increase pressure. Intracranial compliance ($\Delta V/\Delta P$) has been exhausted when intraventricular injection of 1 mL saline results in a 4 mm Hg increase in ICP.

○ **What are the different ways in which ICP can be measured?**

A bolt (extradural pressure monitor), subdural catheter or bolt, ventriculostomy catheter (usually lateral ventricular placement), and intraparenchymal fiber-optic catheter.

○ **Name the three components of intracranial volume.**

Brain (1,400 mL, 85%), blood (150 mL, 10%), and CSF (75–100 mL, 5%).

○ **What is Cushing's triad?**

Elevated ICP, hypertension, and bradycardia. Reduce ICP to break the reflex.

○ **The surgeon reports that the patient's brain is tight. What are the treatment choices?**

Hyperventilate to a $PaCO_2$ of about 30 mm Hg, elevate the patient's head, administer thiopental (cerebral vasoconstrictor and decreases $CMRO_2$), make sure there is no obstruction to cranial venous outflow (check head position), and reduce ICP by opening the CSF drain, if this is an option.

○ **Is the ICP-lowering effect sustained with prolonged hyperventilation?**

The CBF- and ICP-lowering effect of hyperventilation is not sustained. The duration of effectiveness for lowering ICP may be as short as 4–6 hours. Although the decreased $PaCO_2$ and systemic alkalosis persist for the duration of the period of hyperventilation, the pH of the brain and CBF return toward normal over a period of 8–12 hours and vessel caliber returns to baseline.

○ **How does mannitol influence ICP?**

Intracranial volume is reduced by the increased osmolality caused by mannitol in the blood, pulling water out of the brain compartment. Mannitol is also a weak vasodilator and causes a transient increase in cerebral blood volume. The overall effect of mannitol is to decrease ICP.

○ **What effect does $PaCO_2$ have on ICP?**

$PaCO_2$ causes cerebral vasodilation and increases CBF 2–4% per mm Hg increase in $PaCO_2$ within the range of 20 and 80 mm Hg. The increased CBF leads to increased intracranial blood volume resulting in an increase in ICP.

○ **What are the possible side effects of nitroprusside used to induce deliberate hypotension?**

Sodium nitroprusside is a nonselective potent vasodilator. It results in both systemic (hypotension) and pulmonary vasodilation (loss of hypoxic pulmonary vasoconstriction, shunting, hypoxemia). Nitroprusside is metabolized by a liver-based enzyme, rhodonase, to thiocyanate, which is renally excreted. Prolonged infusions in patients with liver or renal impairment may predispose the patient to cyanide toxicity and hypoxemia. Rebound hypertension is possible with discontinuation of a sodium nitroprusside infusion.

○ **How does induced deliberate hypotension affect ICP?**

All vasodilators cause an increase in intracranial blood volume and hence increase ICP.

○ **Should anxiolytics be given preoperatively to a patient with a brain tumor?**

This decision can only be made on an individual patient basis. In patients with documented or suspected elevation in ICP it is prudent to avoid sedatives. Hypoventilation leading to elevated $PaCO_2$ and increased CBF can worsen elevated ICP. In addition, preoperative sedation may preclude immediate postoperative neurological assessment.

○ **A 26-year-old patient with multiple trauma is admitted to the intensive care unit postoperatively. He developed polyuria, hypotension, low urine sodium excretion, and high serum osmolality. What is the diagnosis?**

Posterior pituitary dysfunction (DI) occurs more frequently after head injury. Urine Sp G of ≤1.005 is confirmative. If patient cannot maintain fluid balance, treatment is exogenous vasopressin.

○ **Can a head injury patient develop the syndrome of inappropriate antidiuretic hormone (SIADH)?**

Yes, SIADH usually begins 3–15 days after trauma and the treatment is water restriction and diuretics. (DI develops earlier than SIADH)

○ **What is Glasgow Coma Scale (GCS)? What are its components?**

The GCS provides a reproducible method of assessing the seriousness of brain injury and for following the neurological status. GCS less than 8 points indicates severe injury.

Components are:

1. Eye open (never, to pain, to speech, spontaneously), 1–4
2. Best verbal response (none, incomprehensible sounds, inappropriate words, confused but converse, oriented), 1–5
3. Best motor response (none, extension, abnormal flexion, withdrawal, localize pain, obey commands), 1–6

○ **Describe initial management priorities of a head injury patient.**

Major goals: optimize cerebral perfusion and oxygenation:

1. Immobilization of the cervical spine.

2. Establishment of a patent airway and protection of lungs from aspiration of gastric contents as in the case of Glasgow Coma Score <9.

   Blind nasal intubation is contraindicated in the presence of a basilar skull fracture, suggested by CSF rhinorrhea or otorrhea, hemotympanum, or ecchymosis into periorbital tissues (raccoon sign) or behind the ear (Battle's sign).

3. Associated lung injuries may impair oxygenation and ventilation and necessitate mechanical support of ventilation (check neurological status). Use any IV agent except ketamine.

4. Stabilization of the circulation. Maintain cerebral perfusion pressure (CPP) 50–70 mm Hg.

   Avoid or correct immediately hypotension (SBP <90) and hypoxia (SaO_2 <90% or PaO_2 <60).

5. Indications for ICP monitoring – GCS 3–8 with abnormal CT or two or more of the following:

   Age >40 years, motor posturing, and SBP <90.

   Initiate treatment for ICP >20 mm Hg.

   Avoid prophylactic hyperventilation ($PaCO_2$ <25) during first 24 hours.

   Mannitol 0.25–1 mg/kg effective for control of ICP.

○ **Define CPP.**

CPP is defined as MAP minus ICP or central venous pressure (CVP), whichever is higher. Target goals for CPP and ICP are >60 and <20 mm Hg, respectively.

○ **T/F: Maintenance of CPP is very important after TBI.**

True. Hypotension is profoundly detrimental in TBI and may lead to secondary brain injury. Some areas of the brain have very low CBF after an acute insult and also the autoregulatory responses may not be intact.

○ **Describe different types of edema seen in the brain after injury.**

Brain edema is classified as cytotoxic or vasogenic.

Cytotoxic edema is due to neuronal damage (trauma related), which leads to increased sodium and water in the brain cells (increased intracellular volume).

Vasogenic edema is caused by a breakdown of the blood brain barrier (BBB) and the movement of protein from the blood into the extracellular space of the brain (increased extracellular fluid in the brain).

In patients with a Glasgow Coma Score of <8, the risk of increased ICP is greater than 50%.

○ **Is barbiturate coma indicated in head injury patients?**

A small subset of severe head injury patients may benefit from barbiturate coma (thiopental 4–10 mg/(kg h)).

In these patients management is targeted at efforts to:

1. Optimize CPPs
2. Minimize cerebral ischemia
3. Avoid drugs and techniques that increase ICP

○ **Which substances freely penetrate the BBB?**

Lipid-soluble substances such as CO_2, O_2, volatile agents, and water pass BBB rapidly.

BBB impedes the flow of:

Ions such as K, Ca, Mg, and Na

Polar substances such as glucose, amino acids, and mannitol

Macromolecules such as proteins

They may use active or passive (facilitated diffusion – concentration dependent) transport to go across the BBB.

○ **Describe the clinical manifestations of subarachnoid hemorrhage (SAH).**

Headache, loss of consciousness, pulmonary edema, and decreased ventricular wall motion. The pulmonary and cardiac manifestations are thought to be secondary to norepinephrine release [Delbert et al., 2000. See reference on page 527].

○ **When does cerebral vasospasm usually occur relative to the onset of SAH?**

It usually occurs 4 days to 2 weeks after the initial bleed.

○ **How do you prevent cerebral vasospasm?**

Anticipate and treat it before it happens. Two currently accepted therapeutic interventions, calcium channel blockers and triple H therapy, may decrease the incidence or severity of vasospasm.

○ **How is the diagnosis of cerebral vasospasm made?**

Clinical signs and symptoms of cerebral ischemia to the areas supplied by the constricted cerebral artery raise the possibility of cerebral vasospasm. The diagnosis can be confirmed by transcranial Doppler, contrast CT, MRA, or cerebral angiography.

○ **A 55-year-old patient with SAH undergoes clipping of a cerebral aneurysm and is treated in the neurointensive care unit for cerebral vasospasm. What therapy has been shown to improve outcome?**

The goal is to improve cerebral perfusion and minimize neurological injury in the setting of ischemia. Generally treated with nimodipine (controversial, probably works as a neuroprotectant, not by dilating vessels) and "triple H therapy" (hypertension, hypervolemia, and hemodilution, also controversial).

Triple H therapy may incur significant medical morbidity, including pulmonary edema, myocardial ischemia, hyponatremia, renal medullary washout, indwelling catheter-related complications, cerebral hemorrhage, and cerebral edema.

In the aftermath of SAH, when nimodipine and triple H therapy fail to avert cerebral vasospasm, balloon angioplasty may be performed to forcibly dilate constricted vessels and restore perfusion to the affected (ischemic) brain regions. In addition to mechanical angioplasty, vasodilating agents such as papaverine, verapamil or milrinone can be infused directly intraarterially (chemical angioplasty) and has been shown to be effective and safe to reverse vasospasm secondary to aneurysmal SAH [Fraticelli et al., 2008. See reference on page 527].

○ **What is the classification of intraventricular hemorrhage?**

Grade I: Bleeding in just a small area of the ventricles.

Grade II: Bleeding also inside the ventricles.

Grade III: Ventricles are enlarged by blood.

Grade IV: Bleeding extends into brain parenchyma around the ventricles.

○ **What are the EKG findings of SAH?**

The EKG changes originate from the centrally mediated norepinephrine surge associated with SAH and range from ST segment changes and T wave abnormalities to prolonged QT intervals, presence of U waves, and P wave abnormalities.

○ **What factors have been implicated in the development of delayed ischemic deficits from cerebral vasospasm following SAH?**

Blood in the basilar cistern, hypovolemia, and hyponatremia.

○ **A 45-year-old patient with SAH secondary to intracranial aneurysm leak develops hyponatremia. What is the most likely cause?**

Two main causes are cerebral salt-wasting (CSW) syndrome (more common, probably due to brain natriuretic peptide release) and SIADH (less common). CSW is characterized by the triad of hyponatremia, volume contraction, and high urine sodium concentrations (>50 mmol/L). The distinction between CSW and SIADH is important and is based on *volume status*. SIADH, which is characterized by normovolemia or mild hypervolemia, is treated by volume restriction. Fluid restriction and further volume contraction may be deleterious in a patient after SAH in the presence of CSW and should be avoided.

○ **Describe the important factors in the anesthetic management of cerebral aneurysm clipping.**

  a. Avoiding aneurysmal rupture.

  Maintain transmural aneurysm pressure.

  Transmural pressure (TP) = MAP − ICP; increased TP (by increased MAP or decreased ICP) leads to aneurysm rupture.

  b. Avoiding factors that promote cerebral ischemia. Maintain CPP at high to normal range, and slack brain to minimize retraction pressure.

  Slack brain can be achieved by hyperventilation, diuretics, spinal drainage, and head position.

  (However, hyperventilation may decrease CBF, especially in patients with vasospasm.)

  c. Be prepared to perform manipulation of MAP during attempts to clip the aneurysm or to control bleeding from a ruptured aneurysm, including temporary vessel occlusion.

○ **Describe the arterial blood supply to the spinal cord.**

A single anterior spinal artery supplies blood to the anterior two thirds of the spinal cord. Paired posterior spinal arteries supply blood to the posterior one third of the spinal cord.

○ **What are the determinants of the spinal cord blood flow?**

Spinal cord blood flow = MAP − CVP (or ICP, if ICP is greater than CVP). Autoregulation is intact and drug effects on spinal cord blood flow mimic those changes seen in CBF. Mass effect (or stretch) can decrease spinal cord blood flow just as it does CBF.

○ **In an elderly patient undergoing elective abdominal aortic aneurysm repair, what techniques can be employed to minimize the potential for anterior spinal artery syndrome?**

The goal is to minimize the potential for spinal cord ischemia by maximizing blood flow to the spinal cord and decreasing metabolic rate. Spinal cord blood flow is determined by MAP minus ICP; therefore, a lumbar drain would allow for lowering ICP and improving blood flow. Moderate hypothermia is advantageous as it decreases metabolic rate. Hyperglycemia can worsen ischemia-induced neurological injury, so monitoring and tight control of serum glucose is essential.

○ **A patient is positioned at a 45° incline for sitting craniotomy. Monitoring includes an arterial line with the transducer placed at wrist level (20 cm below the earlobe) and central line with the catheter tip at the SVC/RA junction. The surgeon has just opened the dura. BP 110/50 mm Hg and CVP 10 mm Hg. What is this patient's CPP?**

CPP = MAP − CVP, or ICP whichever is greater. In this problem CVP is greater since ICP is zero with the dura open.

MAP is calculated by ((2 × DBP) + SBP)/3, or 210/3; therefore, MAP = 70 mm Hg. However, the MAP at the earlobe is used for CPP calculation. The transducer is 20 cm H_2O lower than the earlobe. 1 cm H_2O = 0.74 mm Hg. Therefore, three quarters of 20 is 15 and the MAP at the ear is 15 mm Hg less than 70, or 55 mm Hg. The calculation then is: 55 mm Hg (MAP) − 10 mm Hg (CVP) = 45 mm Hg. The CPP is 45 mm Hg.

○ **What is the neurological prognosis of victims with traumatic spinal cord injury?**

Cervical spinal cord injuries are more common than thoracic, thoracolumbar, or lumbar injuries. Approximately one third of patients with an upper cervical spinal cord injury die at the scene. Of those who make it to the hospital, most are neurologically intact. At least 5% of spine injury patients experience onset of neurological symptoms, or worsening of preexisting symptoms, after arrival to the hospital [van Middendorp et al., 2011. See reference on page 527].

○ **What level of cervical spine injury results in dependence on mechanical ventilation?**

C4 or higher [Rao and Tetzlaff, 2000. See reference on page 527].

○ **What is the correct technique to intubate a trauma patient with suspected cervical spine injury using direct laryngoscopy?**

Care must be taken to avoid neck traction as it may worsen neurological damage.

Administer hypnotic and relaxant, and intubate with in-line axial stabilization (occiput held firmly to the backboard positioning hands along the side of the head with fingertips on the mastoid holding occiput down) and cricoid pressure; posterior portion of cervical collar remains in place that discourages atlantoaxial extension.

○ **What are the cardiovascular effects of a cervical spinal cord injury?**

Spinal shock due to loss of sympathetic tone leading to vasodilation, relative hypovolemia, and hypotension. Unfortunately, because the cardiac accelerator fibers (T1–T4) are located below the level of injury, the normal tachycardic response to hypovolemia will be absent. The patient will not likely be able to compensate for the lowered SVR and will require pressor support.

○ **Describe the management of acute spinal cord injury.**

Immobilization of the spinal cord and maintenance of spinal cord perfusion.

Most authorities recommend a MAP of 85 mm Hg or higher, achieved with fluid and pressors, as necessary.

High-dose corticosteroids are *highly controversial* and are based on data from the NASCIS II and III trials (2000). Dosing recommendations include methylprednisolone 30 mg/kg followed by a 5.4 mg/(kg h) infusion, if started within 8 hours of the injury [Coleman et al., 2000. See reference on page 527].

○ **What is the treatment for patients in acute neurogenic shock?**

Lack of sympathetic tone produces relative hypovolemia and hypotension. Fluids are the first line of therapy followed by a vasoconstrictor such as norepinephrine. Lesions above the cardiac accelerator fibers (T1–T4) may be associated with bradycardia that can be treated with atropine, dopamine, isoproterenol, or epinephrine.

○ **What postoperative complications might you expect after resection of a fourth ventricle tumor?**

Brain stem swelling may cause central apnea (compression of the respiratory center) or difficulties swallowing (ninth cranial nerve nucleus). Of note, fixed and dilated pupils would not be seen with brain stem swelling. The nucleus of the third cranial nerve lies above the tentorium cerebelli and supratentorial pressure is required to cause uncal herniation compressing pupilloconstrictor fibers of the occulomotor nerve producing a fixed and dilated pupil.

○ **What methods are employed for detection of venous air embolism (VAE) during a sitting craniotomy?**

Precordial Doppler is the most common method employed and is as sensitive as TEE.

The monitors for VAE from most sensitive to least sensitive are TEE, precordial Doppler, $\uparrow$ PA pressure, $\downarrow$ $ETCO_2$, and $\uparrow$ ETN_2.

○ **What methods are used for prevention/treatment of VAE during a sitting craniotomy?**

VAE is possible whenever the operative field is elevated $\geqslant$5 cm above the right atrial level.

CVP catheter placement for aspiration of air: optimal position for the tip of a single-orifice catheter is 3.0 cm above the superior vena cava right atrium junction (multi-orifice catheter is more effective than single orifice). The proper position of the catheter can be determined using a saline-filled catheter as an intracardiac ECG (biphasic P waves indicate midatrial position and catheter should be withdrawn until inverted P waves are seen).

The pulmonary artery catheter lumen is poorly designed for air aspiration.

A Doppler in conjunction with either a capnography or a PA catheter usually detects air before physiological alteration begins.

Treatment is directed at preventing further influx of air.

Surgeon is notified immediately. The surgical field flooded with saline and packed, and bone edges are waxed.

N_2O if used is discontinued.

Neck veins are compressed as a means of increasing JVP, which prevents further air entry and helps to localize the source of air.

Aspiration of air from the right atrial catheter is attempted. With significant air embolism, patient's position should be changed to lower the head to heart level when possible.

Vasopressors and volume infusion are administered to treat hypotension.

PEEP and Valsalva maneuver are avoided because they increase the right atrial pressure and the likelihood of paradoxical air embolism.

○ **A 70-year-old man does not regain consciousness after a 4-hour resection of a large meningioma. What could be the cause of delayed emergence?**

The possibilities are pharmacologic, endocrine/metabolic, or structural causes. Common pharmacologic causes include residual effect of volatile agents, opioids, benzodiazepines, or muscle relaxants. Metabolic causes include hypothermia, hypocapnea (which raises the pH and decreases ionized calcium), hypoxia, hyponatremia, acidosis, and hypoglycemia. Unrecognized hypothyroidism might also be a culprit. Structural causes are related to the surgical site with bleeding or swelling leading to elevated ICP or a postictal state following seizures.

○ **What are the effects of anterior cerebral artery stroke?**

Paralysis or weakness of the contralateral foot and leg, sensory loss in the contralateral foot and leg, motor aphasia due to left-sided strokes, gait apraxia, and urinary incontinence may be present.

○   **Intracranial bleeding can occur from what vessels during the transsphenoidal approach to pituitary tumor resection?**

The transsphenoidal approach has many advantages (lower morbidity and mortality, lower incidence of diabetes insipidus, no need for brain retraction) but does not allow the same degree of peripituitary structural visualization as the transcranial approach. Significant bleeding can occur from the cavernous sinuses or carotid arteries.

○   **Immediately prior to induction of anesthesia, a patient scheduled for resection of a brain tumor begins to have seizures. How should this be managed?**

ABCs and stop the seizure activity (thiopental or benzodiazepine) with subsequent EEG monitoring to evaluate for continuing seizure activity. Seizures result in increased metabolic demand on the brain and increased CBF. The additional volume of blood within the cranial vault may further increase ICP.

○   **What are the anesthetic considerations of posterior fossa craniotomy?**

Hemodynamic effects of the sitting position: Measures to avoid hypotension include prehydration, wrapping of legs, and slow positioning.

MAP should be measured at the head level and minimum CPP value of 60 mm Hg is recommended. The lower limit of CPP should be increased in elderly and patients with cerebrovascular diseases.

Quadriplegia: Rarely may occur probably due to neck flexion resulting in stretching or compression of cervical spinal cord.

Macroglossia: Flexion of the neck reduces anterior–posterior diameter of the hypopharynx. Avoid unnecessary foreign body in the oral cavity. Use a rolled gauze bite block to prevent tongue getting trapped between teeth.

It is advisable to maintain at least two fingerbreadths of distance between the chin and the sternum in the sitting position to prevent excessive reduction in anteroposterior diameter of the oropharynx.

Pneumocephalus and air embolism: Tension pneumocephalus may cause delayed awakening and severe headache (=mass lesion).

Diagnosis – brow-up lateral x-ray or CT.

Treatment – twist drill hole followed by needle puncture of dura.

Hemodynamic effects of brain stem or cranial nerve manipulation: Neurosurgical procedures often do not require deep anesthesia because they are not very stimulatory. However, sudden arousal (with cranial nerve irritation or traction) and blood pressure responses (irritation or traction involving brain stem) are likely particularly with posterior fossa surgery. The cardiovascular responses may include bradycardia, hypotension, tachycardia, hypertension, and ventricular dysrhythmias. One should be constantly aware of this (meticulous attention to ECG, invasive BP) and inform the surgeon immediately because of possible traction or compression of cranial nerve nuclei or respiratory center. When planning on extubation at the end, possible cranial nerve dysfunction affecting patency and control of airway (cranial nerve IX, X, XII) and swelling of brain stem affecting respiratory drive should be taken into account.

Difficulties with swallowing (ninth cranial nerve nucleus) also may occur.

○   **Describe general guidelines for intraoperative fluid management of a patient undergoing neurosurgery.**

The preoperative intravascular volume deficit may be estimated similar to that used for patients undergoing other types of surgical procedures. Hyperglycemia before or during an episode of ischemia worsens neurological outcome. Therefore, hypo-osmolar solutions and dextrose-containing solutions should be avoided. Iso-osmolar crystalloids (0.9% NS or LR) are given at a rate sufficient to replace the patient's urine output and insensible losses (1:1 ratio). Blood loss is replaced at about a 3:1 ratio (crystalloid/blood) down to a hematocrit value of approximately 25–30%, depending on the patient's general medical condition.

Overall goal in the intraoperative fluid management in the adult neurosurgical patients is to maintain a mild negative balance than a positive balance. However, maintenance of a reasonable MAP is important.

Key Terms

Acute spinal cord injury

Air embolism diagnosis/prevention

Anesthetic effects: cerebral perfusion

Anesthetic effects on EEG

Anterior cerebral artery stroke effects

Ascending, descending spinal columns

Barbiturate coma: indications

Blood brain barrier (BBB): fluid transfer

Bradycardia during neurosurgery: causes

Brain injury and edema

Cardiac arrest: induced hypothermia

CBF: temperature effect

Cerebral aneurysm clipping: anesthetic management

Cerebral aneurysm: determinants of rupture

Cerebral autoregulation

Cerebral blood flow (CBF): anesthetic and ventilatory effects

Cerebral blood flow: interventions

Cerebral ischemia: deep hypothermia

Cerebral salt-wasting syndrome: diagnosis

Cerebral vasospasm: treatment

Cervical cord injury: physiological effects

Cervical fracture: intubation techniques

CNS trauma: increased ICP diagnosis

CNS trauma: systemic effects

Craniotomy: lumbar CSF drainage

CSF: sustained hyperventilation

Determinants of intracranial pressure (ICP)

DI: intracranial surgery

EEG burst suppression: anesthetic drugs

Evoked potentials: anesthetic effects

Glasgow Coma Scale: definition/components

Head injury: acute management

Hypertension: brain stem surgery

Intracranial hypertension: treatment and acute treatment

Motor evoked potential: spinal cord

Neuroanesthesia intraoperative fluid

Nimodipine and subarachnoid hemorrhage

Sitting position: blood pressure measurement

SSEP intraoperative changes

SSEP: physiological effects

Subarachnoid hemorrhage: nimodipine/ECG effect

Traumatic brain injury: cerebral perfusion pressure (CPP)

Treatment: seizures

Vasodilators: cerebral vasospasm

Vasopressin treatment in DI

Venous air embolism: detection/treatment

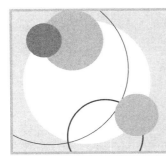

Nonopioid Intravenous Anesthetics

It is the tragedy of the world that no one knows what he doesn't know -- and the less a man knows, the more sure he is he knows everything.
Joyce Cary

○ **Which nonopioid intravenous anesthetic agents possess analgesic properties?**

Ketamine.

Ketamine produces profound dose-dependent analgesia and at higher doses a dissociative state. The general anesthetic effect, as well as the analgesia properties of ketamine, may be mediated by the *N*-methyl-D-aspartate (NMDA) receptor.

○ **On what receptors does ketamine act to mediate its effects?**

Ketamine is classified as NMDA receptor antagonist. At high or anesthetic doses, ketamine has also been found to bind to opioid mu and kappa receptors in brain and spinal cord. Ketamine also interacts with muscarinic receptors, descending monoaminergic pain pathways, and voltage-gated calcium channels.

○ **What are the effects of nonopioid intravenous anesthetic agents on somatosensory evoked potentials (SSEP)?**

A dose-dependent increase in latency and a (minimal) reduction in amplitude of SSEP (with the exception of ketamine and etomidate). These changes are similar to those seen with spinal cord ischemia but do not necessarily preclude the use of nonopioid intravenous anesthetics during SSEP monitoring. Intravenous agents have significantly less effect than equipotent doses of inhaled anesthetics. In general, however, to obtain satisfactory intraoperative sensory evoked potential, it is important to maintain a constant anesthetic level. Avoid bolus IV agents, especially when injury might occur (or during critical stages of surgery). An induction dose of thiopental (4 mg/kg) will produce a maximum effect in 4–6 minutes, with a return to baseline occurring after 12 minutes. When these changes are taken into account, adequate monitoring of SSEP is possible even during infusions. Infusions of propofol have a similar effect on SSEP. Diazepam, 20 mg intravenously, has no effect on SSEP and midazolam 0.2 mg/kg IV bolus followed by a 5 mg/h infusion has no clinically significant effect on SSEP.

Etomidate (and ketamine) produces an increase in amplitude of SSEP and has been used to enhance SSEP recording in cases where reproducible responses were difficult to obtain.

○ **What is the duration and mechanism of action of thiopental?**

Thiopental induces central nervous system (CNS) depression by an effect on the GABA receptor complex. Barbiturates both enhance and mimic the action of GABA. At low concentrations binding to the barbiturate site (one of five protein subunits) decreases the rate of dissociation of GABA from its receptor and increases the duration of GABA-activated chloride conductance through the ion channel, hyperpolarizing and reducing the

315

excitability of the postsynaptic neuron. This results in a sedative–hypnotic effect and amnesia. At slightly higher concentrations, barbiturates directly activate chloride channels, even in the absence of GABA, which may be responsible for "barbiturate anesthesia."

○   **What are the effects of barbiturates on the CNS?**

Barbiturates produce a dose-dependent depression of the CNS, decrease in cerebral metabolic requirement for oxygen ($CMRO_2$; similar to other CNS depressants), and progressive slowing of EEG. The EEG will evolve to burst suppression and finally become isoelectric. A maximum decrease in $CMRO_2$ (50% from baseline) is seen at isoelectric EEG, which can be maintained with 4–6 mg/(kg h) infusion rate of thiopental. This reflects a depression of neuronal rather than metabolic activity. A further decrease in $CMRO_2$ can only be achieved with hypothermia. There is parallel reduction in cerebral blood flow (CBF) with the reduction in $CMRO_2$. An increase in cerebral vascular resistance occurs while CBF and intracranial pressure (ICP) decrease.

Thiopental is an effective anticonvulsant. It does not provide analgesia and may also be hyperalgesic in subanesthetic concentration. Methohexital has a proconvulsant activity and is currently being used to induce anesthesia during electroconvulsive therapy (ECT).

○   **What are the effects of ketamine on the CNS?**

Excitatory, with an increase in CMR, CBF, and ICP.

Ketamine has an excitatory effect on the CNS, thus increasing cerebral metabolism (CMR), and CBF which, in turn, produces an increase in the ICP. Ketamine is also a cerebral vasodilator, which will further increase the CBF and ICP. The increase in CMR and CBF can be blocked by diazepam and thiopental. The increase in ICP can be attenuated by hyperventilation as the cerebrovascular response to CO_2 is preserved with ketamine.

Ketamine can produce undesirable psychological reactions during emergence (bad dreams and multisensorial illusions), which may progress to delirium.

Ketamine doses that create unresponsiveness may not change BIS. BIS may not have clinical utility when used with ketamine alone or ketamine with other anesthetic drugs.

○   **What are the effects of etomidate on the CNS?**

Hypnosis, with a reduction in CMR, CBF, and ICP.

Etomidate produces hypnosis with no analgesic effect through a mechanism that is not fully understood. Since it can be reversed by a GABA antagonist, etomidate's action may be related to the GABA-adrenergic system. Induction doses of etomidate reduce $CMRO_2$ and CBF without decreasing mean arterial pressure. Etomidate also decreases ICP by up to 50% in patients with intracranial hypertension. The possibility of a neuroprotective effect is controversial.

Etomidate increases EEG electrical activity and has a proconvulsant effect that has been proven useful for intraoperative mapping of seizures. It can also cause myoclonic movements not associated with seizure activity.

○   **What are the effects of propofol on the CNS?**

Propofol is an anesthetic agent used for sedation or for induction and maintenance of anesthesia. It had gained popularity for use in surgical procedures requiring a prompt wake-up (rapid recovery profile) and early assessment of neurologic function.

Propofol may be a neuroprotective drug as it preserves cerebral autoregulation and reduces CBF, $CMRO_2$, and ICP. It can be used to achieve EEG burst suppression, which may reduce neuronal injury following incomplete cerebral ischemia. Data concerning the effects of propofol on epileptogenic EEG activity are controversial. Propofol has been reported to both induce and treat seizure-like activity. It is similar to thiopental for anticonvulsant properties, but is not antianalgesic.

○ **What are the effects of benzodiazepines on the CNS?**

They have anxiolytic, hypnotic, anterograde amnesic, muscle relaxant, and anticonvulsant effects.

Benzodiazepines exert their effect mainly by GABA receptor activation and potentiation of the effects of GABA throughout the nervous system. They may also have other sites of action.

Benzodiazepines produce a dose-dependent reduction in $CMRO_2$ and CBF. However, there is a ceiling effect on decreasing of $CMRO_2$ and they do not produce burst suppression or isoelectric EEG. Benzodiazepines are not considered neuroprotective.

○ **What are the pharmacodynamics of midazolam?**

Profound anterograde amnesia, anxiolysis, central respiratory depression, anticonvulsant, and enhance GABA by acting on specific benzodiazepine receptors on GABAa receptor complex. Decreases $CMRO_2$ and CBF, but unable to produce isoelectric EEG. Preserves vasomotor responsiveness to CO_2.

○ **What are some important ways in which diazepam differs from midazolam?**

Diazepam	Midazolam
Water insoluble	Water soluble
Long acting (T$\beta_{1/2}$ = age in years)	Short acting (T$\beta_{1/2}$ = 1–4 hours)
Less potent	Two to four times more potent
Pain on injection and venous thrombosis	No local irritation (propylene glycol and sodium benzoate)
Liver metabolized to active metabolites (prolonged by H_2 blockers)	Liver metabolized to active metabolites (not altered by H_2 blockers)
Protein binding + +	Protein binding + +

○ **What are the effects of ketamine on the respiratory system?**

- Minimal effect on the respiratory drive and maintenance of spontaneous ventilation.
- Bronchodilator.
- Hypersalivation.
- Although upper respiratory reflexes (swallow, cough, gag) are relatively intact, silent aspiration can occur under ketamine anesthesia.

The response to carbon dioxide is unaltered and arterial blood gases are usually preserved when ketamine is used alone. Rarely, apnea may follow with high-dose administration. In children, ketamine should be considered a respiratory depressant. It improves pulmonary compliance in patients with reactive airway diseases or bronchospasm. Bronchodilatory effects are secondary to the release of endogenous catecholamines with β_2-agonist action and a direct relaxant effect on smooth muscle of lesser significance. Pretreatment with an antisialagogue is recommended (glycopyrrolate) for hypersalivation.

○ **What are the effects of benzodiazepines on the respiratory system?**

Benzodiazepines produce dose-dependent central respiratory depression resulting in a depressed ventilatory response to carbon dioxide, reduced respiratory rate, smaller tidal volumes, and decreased minute ventilation. Benzodiazepines and opioids may have synergistic effects. The risk and severity of apnea following benzodiazepine administration is increased in patients with chronic obstructive pulmonary disease and the elderly or debilitated.

○ **Describe sedative effects of midazolam and apneic potential of the drug.**

Midazolam enhances the inhibitory tone of GABA receptors in the CNS producing sedation. It can be given IV and PO, and is the only benzodiazepine with reliable IM absorption. Produces dose-dependent decrease in respiratory rate and tidal volume. Big dose and rapid injection can cause transient apnea (>0.15 mg/kg IV); the effect is more pronounced in the presence of opioids.

○ **What are the times of peak serum concentration of midazolam after IM, rectal, and oral routes?**

The times are 15, 30, and 53 minutes, respectively.

○ **What is the bioavailability of midazolam when given IM, rectal, and oral?**

There is lower bioavailability via rectal and oral routes. The bioavailability is 87% when given IM, 18% via rectal, and 27% via oral. Lower bioavailability requires higher dosing when given via oral or rectal routes. Oral dose of midazolam is usually 0.5 mg/kg, five times the IV dose.

○ **Can you reverse the effects of benzodiazepines?**

Flumazenil (Romazicon, Anexate) is a competitive antagonist at benzodiazepine receptor with high affinity, great specificity, and minimal intrinsic activity.

Flumazenil produces dependable reversal of unconsciousness, respiratory depression, sedation, amnesia, psychomotor dysfunction, muscle relaxation, and EEG changes.

It may be given in incremental dose of 0.2–0.5 mg up to 3 mg. The reversal is rapid, with peak effect in 1–3 minutes.

○ **What is the duration of action of flumazenil?**

Onset: 1–2 minutes after IV injection; peak effect: 6–10 minutes; elimination: brain, 20–30 minutes and plasma, 54 minutes. Reversal of benzodiazepines depends on the dose and plasma concentration of both drugs.

The duration of action for reversal of: sedation, 30 minutes; psychomotor deficits, 45 minutes; anterograde amnesia, 60 minutes. Flumazenil also improves respiratory function by increasing tidal volume.

○ **Is resedation possible after flumazenil?**

Yes. Flumazenil is metabolized in the liver, and rapidly cleared with a plasma half-life of 1 hour. Therefore, resedation is possible and depending on the benzodiazepine being reversed, continuous infusion should be considered (0.5–1 μg/(kg min)).

○ **Is reversal with flumazenil associated with any side effects?**

The reversal is free of cardiovascular effects, unlike naloxone.

Flumazenil may precipitate withdrawal symptoms including seizures in those dependent on benzodiazepines.

There is no current contraindication for flumazenil. It has been given oral and IV.

It does not appear to change CBF or $CMRO_2$, but acute increase in ICP has been reported in head-injured patients.

○ **What are the effects of etomidate on the respiratory system?**

Etomidate produces minimal effects on ventilation. The incidence of apnea is lower with etomidate when compared with equivalent doses of thiopental. Depression of ventilatory response to carbon dioxide is less with etomidate when compared with equivalent doses of methohexital.

○ **What are the effects of barbiturates on the respiratory system?**

Barbiturates produce dose-dependent central respiratory depression resulting in a diminished ventilatory response to hypoxemia, reduced respiratory rate, smaller tidal volumes, and decreased minute ventilation. Apnea occurs at higher doses. Thiopental does not completely depress the noxious airway reflexes and may cause bronchospasm and laryngospasm with airway manipulation. Laryngeal reflexes are more active with thiopental than with equivalent dose of propofol. Blunting laryngeal reflexes may require large doses of barbiturates or the use of adjuvant agents to achieve a sufficient depth of anesthesia.

○ **What are the effects of propofol on the respiratory system?**

Propofol produces respiratory depression similar to barbiturates, and only mild bronchodilation (or no significant effect on airway tone) in patients with chronic obstructive airways disease. Upper airway reflexes are depressed more than thiopental.

○ **What are the effects of barbiturates on the cardiovascular system?**

Direct venodilation and depression of myocardial contractility.

The main effect is venodilation. The myocardial depressant effect is less than that produced by volatile anesthetics. During normal induction doses systemic vascular resistance is usually unaffected, and cardiac output is reduced despite an increase in heart rate. Hypertensive patients (treated and untreated) exhibit greater hypotension for a given dose than normotensive patients.

○ **What are the effects of ketamine on the cardiovascular system?**

Increase in blood pressure, heart rate, and cardiac output, which are independent of dosing.

Ketamine causes central sympathetic stimulation producing increases in blood pressure, heart rate, and cardiac output, all of which are desirable during acute hypovolemic shock. This offsets ketamine's direct effects of myocardial depression and vasodilation, which are seen in patients with spinal cord transection (sympathetic blockade) or severe end-stage shock where catecholamine stores are depleted. Ketamine should be avoided in patients at risk for myocardial ischemia or right and/or left heart failure due to the indirect hemodynamic effects described. It causes increases in pulmonary vascular resistance and myocardial oxygen demands (in excess of increases in coronary blood flow). It may increase the arrythmogenic potential of epinephrine.

○ **What are the effects of etomidate on the cardiovascular system?**

Minimal. Approximately, 10% reduction in mean arterial blood pressure and peripheral vascular resistance and 10% increase in heart rate and cardiac index. Minimal changes are also observed in patients with myocardial disease. Contrary to ketamine, etomidate does not have a direct myocardial depression effect. Hemodynamic stability may be due to lack of effect on sympathetic nervous system or baroreceptors, and lack of histamine release.

○ **What are the effects of propofol on the cardiovascular system?**

Induction doses of propofol produce a moderate decrease (15–25%) in cardiac output, stroke volume, and systemic vascular resistance. The resulting 40% decrease in systemic blood pressure is caused by myocardial depression and vasodilation (direct effect on smooth muscle and reduction in sympathetic activity). Interestingly, the heart rate does not change significantly during induction. These effects are more pronounced in elderly patients.

○ **What happens to the dose requirement of propofol when an opioid is used in conjunction with it?**

The concomitant use of an opioid reduces propofol requirements significantly.

○ **What are the effects of benzodiazepines on the cardiovascular system?**

Benzodiazepines when used alone produce a mild decrease in arterial blood pressure. Midazolam causes significantly more hypotension than other benzodiazepines, but has been reported to be safe for induction (<0.2 mg/kg) in patients with severe aortic stenosis. A combination of benzodiazepines and narcotics may produce an exaggerated hypotensive response due to a reduction of sympathetic tone.

○ **What is the mechanism for rapid onset and short duration of action of thiopental?**

Thiopental given as an IV bolus (3–5 mg/kg) for induction produces a loss of consciousness within 15 seconds and maximal effect within 1 minute. Duration of action is 20–30 minutes with termination of the effect of an induction dose (5–8 minutes). Due to high lipid solubility and low ionization at physiological pH, it quickly crosses lipid membranes into the brain producing hypnosis. Thiopental has a long elimination half-life (6–12 hours) but a rapid initial redistribution from the central compartment to the peripheral tissues (vessel rich, muscle or lean tissues and then fat) causing the plasma concentration to quickly decline below the effective concentration. Within 1 or 2 minutes the vessel-rich group (VRG) will reach its peak concentration first, which will rapidly decline thereafter; the lean tissues will follow with a peak concentration between 15 and 30 minutes, and finally the fat will reach its peak around 300 minutes. At the same time, the thiopental concentration at the effect site will rapidly decrease and the drug action will be terminated. Multiple doses, very large initial doses, or a continuous infusion of thiopental will result in redistribution sites reaching equilibrium with the blood and saturation of drug-metabolizing enzymes in the liver and prolonged drug action.

○ **Does age affect IV induction dose requirements of thiopental?**

Yes, if the calculation is based on actual body weight. Doses based on lean body mass compensate for age, gender, and body habitus differences. Induction doses: healthy adult 2.5–4.5 mg/kg; children 5–6 mg/kg; infants 7–8 mg/kg; premedicated geriatric patient 30–35% reduction in dose compared with younger patients.

○ **What are the determinants of the volume of distribution for barbiturates?**

Lipid solubility is the main determinant followed by protein binding and degree of ionization. The rate of delivery of the barbiturates is dependent on blood flow.

○ **Where are barbiturates metabolized?**

Liver (10–15% per hour). Less than 1% is excreted unchanged by the kidneys.

○ **One of your colleagues suggests that you use the same induction dose of sodium thiopental in patients with renal failure as you would in healthy patients, as the termination of clinical effect is due to redistribution and not metabolism or excretion. Your clinical experience does not support this. Why?**

Sodium thiopental is 75–85% protein bound to albumin and due to low plasma protein levels in renal failure one would expect greater free drug available to cross the blood brain barrier. Sodium thiopental also has weakly acidic properties with a pK_a in the physiological range, making greater unionized levels available in the typically acidemic chronic renal failure patient. These changes may increase free drug availability from 15% in healthy patients to 28% in renal failure patients.

○ **When should the calculated dose of thiopental be adjusted?**

Increased sensitivity to thiopental has been demonstrated in neonates, women, the elderly, and patients with renal failure or those suffering from hypovolemia.

This increased sensitivity is due to a change either in pharmacodynamics or in early distribution pharmacokinetics.

For example, neonates and patients with renal failure have decreased protein binding of thiopental, which results in an increase in the free fraction available to diffuse into the brain.

Lower induction dose is required in elderly (30–40% less) due to:

1. Decreased volume of the central compartment: this leads to higher initial drug concentration (decreased initial V_d).
2. Slower redistribution from the VRG to intermediate compartment (muscles).

○ **List factors affecting speed of IV induction.**

Following IV administration, drugs mix rapidly within a central blood pool and are distributed by blood flow and molecular diffusion throughout the tissues of the body according to their rate of perfusion (cardiac output), affinity for the drug (lipid solubility), and the relative concentration of drug in the tissues and blood (drug concentration and protein binding).

○ **In drug elimination process what is meant by the first-order kinetics?**

Most drugs follow *first-order kinetics*, that is, the rate of elimination of the drug is proportional to the drug concentration that is present in the plasma. The result is that the drug's concentration in plasma decreases *exponentially* with time; stated differently, half-life of elimination is a constant regardless of the amount in the body.

○ **What are the measures of an exponential process?**

These are half-life and time constant.

○ **What is a half-life?**

This is the time taken for the quantity (Q) to fall to 1/2 its initial value.

In 2 × half-life the quantity will fall to 1/4 initial.

In 3 × half-life the quantity will fall to 1/8 initial.

About 5 × half-lives are required for nearly total (96.9%) completion of a process.

○ **What is time constant?**

Time at which the process would have been completed had the initial rate of change continued.

After one time constant the Q (quantity) has fallen to 37% of its value.

Therefore, time constant (37% left) is bigger than half-life (50% left).

Three time constants are required to complete a process.

○ **What is the elimination half-life of diazepam, lorazepam, and midazolam?**

Diazepam: 20–50 hours.

Lorazepam: 11–22 hours.

Midazolam: 1.7–2.6 hours.

○ **Define clearance, volume of distribution, and elimination half-life.**

Clearance is defined as a unit of volume being completely cleared of drug per unit of time. Volume of distribution is a concept designed to describe an observed plasma drug concentration after a known amount of drug has been given. If an amount of drug is diluted in a volume, the resulting concentration will be:

$$\text{Plasma drug concentration} = \frac{\text{amout of drug in the body}}{\text{volume}}.$$

Volume of distribution can be defined as:

$$\text{Volume } (V_d) = \frac{\text{amount of drug in the body}}{\text{plasma drug concentration}}.$$

Factors, such as lipid solubility, that will affect the measured plasma concentration of a drug will effectively change the volume of distribution.

The elimination half-life is the time required for the plasma concentration to decrease by 50% due to the elimination of the drug (as opposed to the decay of the plasma concentration due to redistribution). The elimination half-life is related to the volume of distribution and clearance according to the following equation:

$$\text{Elimination half-life } (T_{1/2}) = 0.693 \times \left(\frac{\text{volume of distribution}}{\text{clearance}}\right).$$

○ **What is context-sensitive half-time?**

Elimination half-time does not provide insight into the rate of decrease in plasma concentration after discontinuation of IV drug administration, especially with certain drugs that accumulate.

Context-sensitive half-time is the time necessary for the *effect compartment (i.e., effect site)* concentration to decrease by 50% in relation to the duration of the infusion.

○ **Which nonopioid intravenous anesthetic drug does not reduce the intraocular pressure (IOP)?**

Ketamine.

In general, nonopioid intravenous anesthetics reduce IOP by relaxing extraocular muscle tone, improving outflow of aqueous humor, and lowering arterial and venous blood pressure. Ketamine has been reported as either having no effect or increasing IOP. It may decrease IOP in children. Although not an anesthetic, succinylcholine transiently increases IOP and it is usually avoided in open eye injuries, although no adverse events have ever been reported in such circumstances.

○ **Which nonopioid intravenous anesthetic has muscle relaxant properties?**

Midazolam has muscle relaxant properties mediated by the GABA receptor. Propofol does not have intrinsic muscle relaxant properties; however, good intubating conditions have been reported with propofol.

○ **Which intravenous anesthetic agents cause myoclonus?**

Etomidate, propofol, and methohexital.

○ **What are the undesirable side effects of barbiturates?**

- *Direct venodilation* and depression of *myocardial contractility.*
- *Hyperalgesia.*
- *Histamine release,* which is rarely of clinical importance.
- *Enzyme induction* increasing liver microsomal protein content occurs after 2–7 days of sustained drug administration, of which phenobarbital is the most potent. It may persist for up to 30 days after drug discontinuation.

- *Acute tolerance* may occur faster than enzyme induction and the required effective dose of barbiturate may increase 6-fold.
- *Intra-arterial injection* of thiopental results in immediate severe vasoconstriction and excruciating pain. Gangrene and permanent nerve damage may occur especially with high concentrations such as 5% solution (not used anymore). Treatment must be immediate and includes leaving the intra-arterial catheter or needle in place, dilution of barbiturates by injection of saline, and injection of lidocaine, papaverine, or phenoxybenzamine to produce vasodilation. If the catheter has been removed, injection of vasodilators may be attempted proximally. Direct injection of heparin has also been advocated. Other possible treatments include sympathectomy of the upper extremity with a stellate ganglion block or a brachial plexus block and urokinase. However, the current concentration (2.5%) causes pain and is unlikely to cause major problems
- *Anaphylactic or anaphylactoid response.* The estimated incidence of allergic reaction to thiopental is 1 per 30,000 patients [Hepner and Castells, 2003. See reference on page 527].
- *Acute intermittent porphyria.* Barbiturates can induce delta-aminolevulinic acid synthetase, which catalyzes the rate-limiting step in the synthesis of porphyrins, which may result in paralysis and death.

○ **Which nonopioid intravenous anesthetic can cause a transient suppression of adrenocortical function?**

Etomidate.

Etomidate causes a dose-dependent reversible inhibition of the enzyme 11-β-hydroxylase, which results in decreased production of cortisol and aldosterone. Cortisol can be restored to normal levels with vitamin C supplementation. Long-term (5 days or longer) sedative infusion of etomidate was identified as the causative factor for an increased mortality in mechanically ventilated ICU patients. However, following a single induction dose of etomidate, the adrenocortical suppression is not clinically significant. There is no case report of a negative clinical outcome related to a single dose of etomidate or a short-term infusion. Many studies have consistently shown that cortisol levels are only slightly depressed following a single induction dose of etomidate and return to normal within 20 hours. Patients having high-stress surgery have been shown to be able to overcome the temporary adrenocortical suppression caused by etomidate.

○ **What are the other side effects of etomidate?**

Nausea and vomiting, thrombophlebitis, pain during injection, myoclonus and hiccups, and enhanced neuromuscular blockade of nondepolarizing muscle relaxants.

Etomidate is associated with a high (30–40%) incidence of postoperative nausea and vomiting that is further increased by the addition of fentanyl. Thrombophlebitis of the vein used may occur 48–72 hours after etomidate injection. Pain during injection is similar to that with propofol and can be eliminated by injecting lidocaine prior to etomidate. The reported incidence of myoclonus and hiccups is variable (0–70%). Myoclonus may be reduced by premedication with either a narcotic or a benzodiazepine. Etomidate enhances neuromuscular blockade of nondepolarizing neuromuscular blockers.

○ **What is propofol infusion syndrome?**

This is a rare, but lethal syndrome usually seen in pediatric intensive care patients (PICU) receiving propofol sedation due to lipid accumulation (may occur in adult patients also) [Kam and Cardone, 2007. See reference on page 527].

○ **How do you diagnose propofol infusion syndrome?**

Patients may present with rhabdomyolysis, metabolic acidosis, acute treatment-resistant bradycardia that progresses to cardiac failure, asystole, and renal failure.

Laboratory findings that strongly support the diagnosis are lipidemic serum, fatty liver enlargement, and severe metabolic acidosis.

Therefore, patients receiving propofol sedation should be monitored for unexplained metabolic acidosis or arrhythmias.

○ **Are there any risk factors for developing propofol infusion syndrome?**

Analysis of cases suggests the following risk factors in adults:

1. Propofol infusion exceeding 5 mg/(kg h)

2. Infusion lasting more than 48 hours (some case reports with >10 hours)

Monitoring serum free fatty acid and lactic acid concentrations may help early diagnosis.

○ **Compare the uses of propofol and ketamine.**

Propofol: IV hypnotic agent used routinely for induction and maintenance of anesthesia as well as sedation for monitored anesthetic care. Approved for neurologic and cardiac anesthesia but caution should be exercised for use in hypovolemic patients due to arterial and venous vasodilation and mild negative inotropic effects that may cause hypotension. Unlike barbiturates, it is not antianalgesic. It tends to produce a state of well-being, but hallucinations, sexual fantasies, and opisthotonos have been reported. Ideal agent for ambulatory surgery patients due to antiemetic properties with more rapid recovery in cases of <1 hour duration than barbiturates.

Ketamine: IV induction agent producing CNS depression with hypnosis, sedation, amnesia, and analgesia. Ketamine is not used as a routine induction agent primarily due to its unwanted emergent reactions. Sympathomimetic activity and bronchodilating properties are unique. It stimulates the cardiovascular system, increasing heart rate, blood pressure, and cardiac output. Recommended for selective use for induction in ASA IV patients with respiratory (bronchospasm) and CV disorders (cardiomyopathy, cardiac tamponade and restrictive pericarditis, right-to-left shunt congenital heart disease, sepsis, or hypovolemia, excluding ischemic heart disease). However, in patients with increased pulmonary artery pressure ketamine causes more pronounced increase in pulmonary artery pressure.

Ketamine increases ICP and cerebral metabolism, therefore it is contraindicated in patients with elevated ICP. EEG-based monitors are not accurate if ketamine is used as the primary anesthetic.

May interact with tricyclic antidepressants causing hypertension and dysrhythmias. In addition, low-dose ketamine is used as an analgesic, for sedation during off-site procedural cases in pediatric patients, and as an adjunct to regional anesthesia.

Key Terms

Barbiturate pharmacology in renal failure
Barbiturates: CNS effects
Barbiturates: mechanism of action
Benzodiazepine antagonism/respiratory effects
Context-sensitive half-times
Etomidate: CNS effects
Etomidate: side effects/adrenal suppression
First-order kinetics
Flumazenil use
IV agents: ketamine, BIS
Ketamine: analgesic mechanism/receptors
Ketamine: CV effects
Ketamine: pharmacodynamics

Ketamine: receptor effects
Midazolam: bioavailability versus route
Muscle relaxation; anesthetic agents
Myoclonus caused by IV agents
Pharmacokinetics of intravenous drugs
Pharmacology: flumazenil
Propofol: CNS effects
Propofol: CV effects
Propofol infusion syndrome: diagnosis
Propofol: mechanism of action
Thiopental: CV effects
Thiopental: termination of action
Time constant: definition

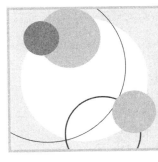

Obstetrics

The difference between genius and stupidity, is genius has its limits.
Albert Einstein

○ **What are the determinants of uterine blood flow (UBF) in pregnant women?**

UBF is directly proportional to the change in blood pressure across the organ (mean arterial pressure minus central venous pressure) and inversely proportional to uterine vascular resistance (UVR). Flow = (UAP − UVP)/UVR, where UAP is the uterine arterial pressure and UVP is the uterine venous pressure. For example, during a contraction, uterine muscle tone increases, increasing UVR and decreasing flow.

○ **Describe the autoregulatory curve for UBF.**

UBF is not autoregulated but linearly proportional to mean arterial blood pressure.

○ **How do uterine contractions during labor affect UBF?**

UBF is approximately 700 mL/min at term. Approximately 70–90% of UBF passes through the intervillous space. The uterine vascular bed is almost maximally dilated under normal conditions.

Uterine contractions decrease UBF secondary to increased UVP brought about by increased intramural pressure of the uterus. There may also be a decrease in UAP with contractions. Therefore, correction of maternal hypotension and decrease of excessive uterine activity are useful means of increasing UBF when fetal late decelerations occur during labor.

In the case of maternal hypertension, it is likely that the UVR is also increased. This will result in decrease in UBF (according to the above equation). In the preeclamptic patients, epidural analgesia increases the UBF and improves the maternal blood pressure control during painful contractions.

○ **What are the effects of regional anesthesia on UBF during labor?**

Regional anesthesia can increase UBF by reducing maternal pain and stress during labor, which decreases uterine tone and vascular resistance. However, Chen et al., showed that continuous lower dose (0.05–0.1%) infusion of epidural analgesia increases the resistance of uterine artery and therefore possibly reduces the uterine blood flow [Chen et al., 2006. See reference on page 527]. In contrast, hypotension caused by regional anesthesia can decrease UBF. In the setting of severe preeclampsia (PE), epidural anesthesia may increase intervillous blood flow [Jouppila et al., 1982. See reference on page 527].

○ **What is the effect of ketamine on UBF?**

Ketamine, in intravenous doses up to 1 mg/kg, is unlikely to alter UBF. Higher doses of ketamine (>2 mg/kg) may decrease UBF due to increased uterine tone (UVR); however, in the setting of decreased intravascular volume, ketamine may help to maintain systemic blood pressure and thus maintain UBF.

○ **What effect do the following agents have on uterine tone?**

Volatile anesthetics: At 0.2 MAC minimal effect and beyond that dose-dependent reduction in uterine tone. Below 1 MAC uterine response to oxytocin is preserved.

Local anesthetics (LA): Clinically insignificant effect at normal serum concentration. Direct myometrial injection may cause uterine hyperstimulation.

Ketamine: Dose-dependent increase in uterine tone. Clinically insignificant effect with normal induction dose.

Opioids: No effect.

Nondepolarizing NMBs: No effect on smooth muscle.

Succinylcholine: No effect on smooth muscle.

○ **What are the determinants of placental transfer?**

- Maternal drug concentration
- Fetal drug concentration
- Placental factors (surface area, membrane thickness, and metabolism)
- Drug factors (lipid solubility, protein binding, molecular weight, and ionization)
- Placental blood flow

○ **Describe drug factors that favor drug transfer across the placenta.**

- Low molecular weight. A molecular weight of 1,000 Da (Dalton) is a rough dividing line between those substances that cross the placenta by diffusion and those that are relatively impermeable by diffusion.
- Low protein binding.
- High lipid solubility.
- Low degree of ionization.

○ **What factors affect the placental transfer of oxygen to the fetus?**

Oxygen transfer across the placenta depends on the maternal-to-fetal blood oxygen partial pressure gradient. There are several factors that affect transfer of O_2 to the fetus:

1. The parallel arrangement of maternal and fetal blood flow appears to have a key role in human placenta.
2. The difference in oxyhemoglobin dissociation curves of maternal and fetal blood: The fetal curve is positioned to the left of maternal curve and this arrangement promotes transfer of oxygen across placenta.
3. The Bohr effect: The fetal-to-maternal transfer of carbon dioxide makes maternal blood more acidic and fetal blood more alkalotic. This difference causes right and left shifts of maternal and fetal O_2 dissociation curves and further enhances transplacental O_2 transfer to the fetus.

○ **What is the P_{50} in the fetus and mother at term? (And what *is* a P_{50}?)**

P_{50} is the partial pressure of O_2 at which hemoglobin molecules are 50% saturated with oxygen. P_{50} values are 19 and 30 mm Hg in the fetus and mother at term, respectively. P_{50} is 27 mm Hg in normal adults.

○ **Why is this difference in P_{50} important?**

The maternal–fetal P_{50} gap indicates that fetal hemoglobin has a greater affinity for oxygen than does maternal hemoglobin, encouraging maternal–fetal oxygen transfer.

○ **Fetal PaO_2 is never more than 50–60 mm Hg even when mother is on 100% oxygen. Why?**

This is due to several reasons:

1. Placenta functions as a venous rather than arterial equilibrator. Because of the shape of the O_2 dissociation curve, maternal PaO_2 above 100 mm Hg does not provide significant increase in arterial O_2 content.

2. Placenta consumes a large amount of oxygen (20–30%) and this reduces the amount of O_2 available to transfer to the fetus.

3. Fetal arterial blood represents a mixture of umbilical venous blood (oxygenated) and inferior vena cava (IVC) blood (deoxygenated).

○ **What factors affect the placental transfer of thiopental administered to the mother?**

Following maternal administration, thiopental quickly appears in the umbilical venous blood with mean F/M (Fetal: Maternal ratio) ratios between 0.4 and 1.1. This suggests thiopental is freely diffusible. However, a wide intersubject variability in umbilical cord blood concentration at delivery suggests factors other than simple diffusion may play a role. Maternal and fetal protein concentration strongly influences both maternal-to-fetal and fetal-to-maternal transfer of thiopental.

○ **What is the placental transfer rate of anticholinergics?**

This directly correlates with the drugs' ability to cross the blood–brain barrier. Drugs such as atropine and scopolamine cross the placenta easily and have high F/M ratios. Glycopyrrolate is poorly transferred, has a low F/M ratio, and therefore does not result in fetal hemodynamic changes.

○ **How does pregnancy affect ventilatory parameters?**

During pregnancy respiratory rate and pattern remains somewhat unchanged. However, the resting minute ventilation increases primarily due to increase in tidal volume (TV). This change occurs due to hormonal changes (respiratory stimulant effect of progesterone) and increased carbon dioxide production.

○ **What is the normal $PaCO_2$ in pregnancy?**

About 30 mm Hg. Chronic mild hyperventilation is presumably a result of a progesterone effect and causes increase in the TV and minute ventilation. The $PaCO_2$ declines to about 30 mm Hg by 12 weeks gestation and remains at that level for the rest of the pregnancy.

○ **What is the predominant change in the lung volumes in pregnancy?**

TV increases by 45%, with approximately half of the change occurring in the first trimester.

Decrease in functional residual capacity (FRC), by as much as 15–25%. This change is caused by the reduction in expiratory reserve volume (ERV) and residual volume (RV).

Inspiratory capacity increases by 15% during third trimester (increased TV and IRV).

○ **T/F: The elevated diaphragm reduces TV.**

False. TV actually increases and accounts for the increased minute ventilation and mild respiratory alkalosis.

○   **Why is inhalation induction of anesthesia faster in pregnant women than in nonpregnant women?**

Decreased FRC and increased minute ventilation result in a more rapid rise in alveolar concentration of anesthetic agent. Elevated cardiac output counteracts this effect somewhat, but the net effect remains that of faster inhalational induction in pregnancy.

○   **What effect does pregnancy has on the MAC of inhaled anesthetic agents?**

MAC is reduced by 30% during early pregnancy and returns to normal within the first 3 days following delivery.

○   **When does the cardiac output maximally increase in the parturient?**

In the immediate postpartum period, cardiac output can increase up to 75% above prelabor values.

○   **What happens to cardiac output during pregnancy? When do you see the maximum increase?**

Cardiac output increases during the first and the second trimester until it reaches a level of about 50% greater than that of nonpregnant state. There is no further change seen during the third trimester. Increase in cardiac output occurs due to increase in heart rate (15–25% increase) and stroke volume (20–30% increase).

Central venous and pulmonary capillary wedge pressures (PCWPs) remain within normal nonpregnant levels.

○   **What is "autotransfusion" during labor?**

Three hundred to 500 mL of blood will enter into the maternal circulation with each uterine contraction during labor. This "autotransfusion" can increase cardiac output and central blood volume by an additional 15–25%. When parturients receive effective analgesia, cardiac output and stroke volume are augmented to a lesser degree.

○   **Why is left uterine displacement (LUD) important in pregnant women in the supine position?**

In most term parturients, lying supine results in compression of the aorta and IVC by the gravid uterus. This may result in elevated venous pressure in the lower extremities and decreased venous return to the heart, causing hypotension and reduced uteroplacental perfusion. When positioned in the left lateral position (15–30° tilt), the weight of the uterus shifts off of the IVC and aorta. Adverse hemodynamic effects of aortocaval compression are reduced once the fetal head is engaged.

○   **When does LUD become important?**

Supine aortocaval compression can be identified as early as the end of the first trimester and is universally present by the 28th week.

○   **What is "supine hypotension syndrome?"**

Near term, approximately 8% of parturients experience hypotension when lying supine – the so-called supine hypotension syndrome. Profound aortocaval compression causes a significant reduction in venous return to the heart resulting in hypotension that is not corrected by a compensatory increase in heart rate and SVR. If left untreated, bradycardia will develop and the patient will develop signs of shock – including hypotension, pallor, sweating, nausea, vomiting, and changes in mental status.

○   **What size of endotracheal tube should be used in obstetric patients?**

A 6.5 mm endotracheal tube is a good choice for most pregnant women. Small size cuffed endotracheal tubes (6.0 –7.0 mm ID) should be available. Nasotracheal intubation should be avoided and may lead to severe epistaxis.

○ **What physiologic factors predispose the parturient to hypoxemia during intubation?**

Decreased FRC results in a diminished volume of alveolar oxygen available for absorption. Increased metabolic activity causes higher oxygen consumption and carbon dioxide production. With the respiratory quotient unchanged, the net effect is a more rapid fall in PaO_2 during apnea.

○ **What are normal arterial blood gas (ABG) values in the parturient at term?**

pH = 7.44, $PaCO_2$ = 30 mm Hg, PaO_2 = 103 mm Hg, and bicarbonate = 20 mEq/mL; of course, the normal nonpregnant values are pH = 7.40, $PaCO_2$ = 40 mm Hg, PaO_2 = 100 mm Hg, and bicarbonate = 24 mEq/mL. One can deduce that in the parturient there is a respiratory alkalosis with metabolic compensation.

○ **What is the normal hematocrit value at term gestation?**

About 35%.

○ **What is the reason for drop in hematocrit value during pregnancy?**

During pregnancy there is plasma volume expansion (+55%) that exceeds the red blood cell volume increase (+30%). This results in physiologic anemia of pregnancy.

○ **Is the physiologic anemia beneficial to the pregnancy?**

The decrease in blood viscosity lowers resistance to blood flow, possibly an essential component of maintaining uteroplacental blood flow.

○ **When does the plasma volume expansion occur in pregnancy?**

This begins as early as 6 weeks gestation and continues until about 34 weeks.

○ **Is there a change in plasma proteins during pregnancy?**

Yes, both the albumin concentration and the albumin to globulin ratio decrease. Maternal colloid osmotic pressure decreases by about 5 mm Hg.

○ **Why pregnancy is considered a hypercoagulable state?**

The concentration of most coagulation factors increases during pregnancy and the PT and PTT values are shortened. Thromboelastographic changes in pregnancy also suggest hypercoagulable state. There is enhanced platelet turnover, clotting, and fibrinolysis during pregnancy. Therefore, pregnancy represents an accelerated but compensated state of intravascular coagulation.

○ **When should a parturient be considered to have a full stomach?**

Precautions against aspiration should be taken from as early as 12 weeks. After the first trimester, every parturient should be managed as a patient with a full stomach.

○ **What are the factors in pregnancy increasing the risk of aspiration of stomach contents?**

Increased intragastric pressure from the gravid uterus, progesterone-induced relaxation of the lower esophageal sphincter, delayed gastric emptying in labor, and depressed mental status from analgesia.

○ **How does plasma cholinesterase activity change during pregnancy?**

The plasma cholinesterase activity is reduced about 25%. After delivery there is a further reduction to less than 60% of the nonpregnant value. However, there is no clinically significant prolongation of action of succinylcholine or ester-type LA in the dosages generally given.

○ **When is the critical period of organogenesis?**

Between 15 and 60 days of gestation; however, the CNS does not fully develop until after birth.

○ **Is pain sensation different between the first stage and the second stage of labor?**

Yes. During the first stage of labor, pain results from stretching of the uterus and cervix. Pain signals are transmitted through visceral afferents to T10–L1 nerve roots. This pain is often described as dull, aching, and cramping, and is poorly localized. During the second stage of labor, pain results from stretching of the vagina and perineum as the fetal head descends. This pain is transmitted through somatosensory afferents to S2–S4 nerve roots and is described as sharp and well localized.

○ **What peripheral afferent or neuraxial block techniques can be used to ameliorate pain of the first stage of labor?**

Amelioration of pain should occur with:

* Paracervical block
* Paravertebral sympathetic nerve block
* Epidural block from T10 to L1
* Intrathecal injection of an LA with or without opioid

○ **What peripheral nerve block techniques (non-neuraxial) can be used to provide analgesia during the second stage of labor?**

Pudendal nerve block is an effective non-neuraxial technique for analgesia during the second stage. It is not effective, however, for midforceps deliveries, uterine manipulation, or repair of cervical lacerations. Paracervical and lumbar sympathetic blocks provide analgesia only for the first stage of labor.

○ **What are the concerns of performing regional analgesia/anesthesia for parturients?**

The main concern is maintaining UBF and fetal well-being. Avoid maternal hypotension and treat it aggressively. Remember the absolute contraindications to regional analgesia: marked hypovolemia, coagulopathy, generalized sepsis, infection over the injection site, true allergy to LA drugs, and the patient's refusal of or inability to cooperate with regional anesthesia.

○ **Does epidural analgesia affect the course of labor?**

Studies have shown epidural analgesia does not slow the progress of labor in the first stage; however, the second stage of labor may be prolonged slightly (about 25 minutes). There is no evidence that this prolongation is harmful to the fetus [Wong et al., 2005. See reference on page 527].

○ **Why should an epidural be placed early in the morbidly obese pregnant patient?**

Lumbar epidural anesthesia is an excellent choice for labor and vaginal delivery. More than 50% of morbidly obese patients need cesarean section [Edwards et al., 1996. See reference on page 527]. Early epidural placement during labor decreases the likelihood of requiring general anesthesia for cesarean section. Epidural anesthesia reduces oxygen consumption and attenuates increases in cardiac output that occur during labor and delivery.

○ **A vaginal birth after cesarean section (VBAC) patient with a well-functioning labor epidural infusion complains of persistent breakthrough pain. What are you concerned about?**

Uterine rupture. Always consider this possibility in patients with persistent breakthrough pain with epidural analgesia. Diaphragmatic irritation from uterine rupture may be referred to the shoulder. Abdominal ultrasound may confirm the diagnosis.

○ **Is an epidural contraindicated for VBAC?**

No. The main concern is that the epidural may mask the pain of uterine rupture; however, pain from uterine rupture usually is sharp and unrelenting, not associated with contractions, in an unusual location for labor pains, and not relieved with additional epidural LA administration.

○ **What is the most common presenting sign of uterine rupture?**

Fetal distress is the most reliable sign of uterine rupture. In fact, abdominal pain has been shown to occur in only 10% of patients with uterine dehiscence or true uterine rupture. Other signs include vaginal bleeding, maternal hypotension, and cessation of labor.

○ **What are risk factors for uterine rupture?**

Risk factors include grand multiparity, fetal malpresentation, bicornuate uterus, previous myomectomy, and use of oxytocin or prostaglandin to augment labor. Uterine rupture is rare in the absence of previous uterine surgery, and hemorrhage from rupture of a classical scar is more severe than that of a low transverse scar. This is because the anterior uterine wall is highly vascular, may include the area of placental implantation. Also the lateral extension of rupture can lead to massive bleeding from the involvement of major uterine vessels.

○ **Is major regional anesthesia for cesarean section contraindicated in patients with aortic stenosis?**

Single-injection spinal anesthesia is contraindicated. Epidural anesthesia can be used if administered slowly with appropriate hemodynamic monitoring to preserve preload, blood pressure, and SVR. It is best not to include epinephrine with test or therapeutic doses of LA.

○ **What is the major disadvantage of paracervical block?**

Fetal bradycardia (up to 33%). It may be related to decreased UBF secondary to uterine vasoconstriction from the LA applied closely to the uterine artery and direct cardiac toxicity due to high fetal blood levels of LA.

○ **What is the relationship between the site of administration of LA drugs and maternal peak blood levels?**

For the various anesthetic techniques used in obstetrics, maternal peak blood levels from highest to lowest are as follows: intravenous > intercostals > caudal > paracervical block > epidural > subarachnoid block.

○ **How does the requirement for LA used in regional anesthesia change during pregnancy?**

It decreases. Pregnant women need 25–30% less LA for regional anesthesia than do nonpregnant women. Distention of the epidural veins may decrease the epidural and intrathecal spaces and facilitate spread of epidural and spinal LA. Exaggerated lumbar lordosis may enhance cephalad spread of spinal LA. Increased progesterone during pregnancy may increase nerve sensitivity to LA or may enhance diffusion of the LA to the membrane receptor site.

○ **What is the placental transfer rate of LA?**

LA agents readily cross the placenta. Fetal plasma protein binding is about 50% that of maternal plasma. Therefore, at any given plasma concentration, there is greater amount of free drug in the fetus than in the mother.

○ **What happens to the LA distribution in fetal acidosis and hypoxemia?**

The circulatory adaptation that results in increased blood flow to vital organs causes higher concentration of LA in these organs than in healthy fetus.

○ **What is "ion trapping" of LA?**

Decreased fetal pH will increase the concentration of ionized LA in the fetal circulation. The ionization of the LA prevents diffusion across the placenta back to the maternal circulation. The unionized LA continue to move to the fetus down its concentration gradient. Thus, LA can accumulate in fetal blood. This phenomenon is called "ion trapping" and explains the higher concentration of lidocaine in the fetus in the presence of fetal acidosis.

○ **Which LA may be a good choice for epidural anesthesia and fetal distress? Why?**

2-Chloroprocaine (ester LA). It is fast in onset and rapidly hydrolyzed by the mother and the fetus. Fetal acidosis less likely to promote fetal accumulation of the LA.

○ **What are the major disadvantages of using 2-chloroprocaine?**

The duration of drug action is approximately 45 minutes, depending on the length of the case, so the epidural may need to be topped up with a longer-acting LA. Chloroprocaine may also antagonize the activity of neuraxial morphine used for postoperative epidural analgesia.

○ **What techniques can be used to facilitate uterine relaxation following vaginal delivery?**

The obstetrician may request uterine relaxation for a patient with retained placenta or uterine inversion. Nitroglycerin can be administered either sublingually (400 μg spray) or intravenously (100–200 μg), while monitoring for accompanying hypotension. If relaxation is not sufficient, rapid sequence induction, endotracheal intubation, and high concentrations of volatile anesthetic agents will provide profound uterine relaxation.

○ **What techniques are used in the treatment of uterine atony?**

The first line of treatment for uterine atony is drug therapy. Oxytocin is routinely administered intravenously following vaginal and cesarean deliveries. In nonpreeclamptic patients, methylergonovine (Methergine®) is administered *intramuscularly* for continued atony. The third drug of choice is 15-methyl prostaglandin $F_{2\text{-alpha}}$. Obstetricians may administer prostaglandin E_2 rectal or vaginal suppositories as the last noninvasive measure. The second line of treatment involves invasive techniques such as uterine artery embolization or ligation, with hysterectomy as a possible last resort.

○ **What is the mechanism of action of oxytocin?**

Oxytocin binds to a G protein on the surface of the uterine myocytes and leads to release of calcium from sarcoplasmic reticulum. There is stimulation of prostaglandin synthesis during this pathway as well as via activation of COX-2. The amount of myometrial receptors increases as gestation advances increasing sensitivity to oxytocin.

The half-life of oxytocin is only 10–15 minutes.

○ **What is the most common side effect of oxytocin?**

Systemic hypotension caused by peripheral vasodilatation. This occurs probably via calcium-dependent stimulation of nitric oxide pathway.

Other side effects of oxytocin include:

Oxytocin also causes release of atrial and brain natriuretic peptide.

In humans oxytocin may have some negative inotropic effect due to the presence of chlorbutanol on atrial myocytes, a commercial preservative.

Pulmonary artery pressure is shown to markedly increase and stay increased for at least 10 minutes after a bolus of 10 IU during GA.

A recent investigator using the technique of vectorcardiography showed considerable ST segment changes following 10 IU oxytocin IV during spinal anesthesia for CS in volunteers. These changes were more marked than those following IV ergometrine 0.2 mg [Dyer et al., 2010. See reference on page 527].

○ **What electrolyte disturbances may occur with oxytocin administration?**

Prolonged infusion of large doses may result in water retention, hyponatremia, seizure, and coma.

○ **What is the mechanism of action of Methergine® (methylergonovine)?**

Little is known about the mechanism of action. This may occur via calcium channel, or alpha-adrenergic receptors in the inner myometrial layer.

The half-life of ergometrine is 120 minutes.

○ **What are the side effects of methylergonovine?**

Ergot alkaloids such as methylergonovine may cause nausea, vomiting, pulmonary hypertension, coronary artery vasoconstriction, and systemic hypertension (especially in patients with preeclampsia).

○ **What is the mechanism of action of Hemabate?**

Hemabate® (15-methyl prostaglandin $F_{2\text{-alpha}}$) increases uterine tone by increasing myometrial intracellular calcium concentration.

○ **What are the side effects of Hemabate®?**

Side effects of Hemabate® administration include bronchospasm, nausea, vomiting, and diarrhea. Increased pulmonary vascular resistance may lead to pulmonary hypertension, increased intrapulmonary shunting, and hypoxemia. The recommended dose is 250 μg administered IM or intramyometrial (however, intramyometrial route is not licensed). The dose may be repeated every 15–30 minutes (total dose 2 mg).

○ **Can methylergonovine be given intravenously for postpartum hemorrhage?**

Bolus intravenous administration is not recommended. If hemorrhage is profound and life threatening, 0.2 mg may be diluted in 250 mL of intravenous fluid and administered with close attention to blood pressure and ECG.

○ **How could general anesthesia for emergent cesarean section be administered without intravenous access?**

At least one case report has described using a sevoflurane inhalational induction by mask with cricoid pressure applied in a patient with no IV access and fetal distress. Placement of an intravenous catheter, either peripheral or central, is essential.

○ **Why should excessive mechanical hyperventilation ($P_{ET}CO_2$ <24 mm Hg) be avoided?**

Hypocapnia may reduce maternal cardiac output and UBF, resulting in fetal hypoxemia and acidosis.

○ **How quickly should the baby be delivered under general anesthesia?**

Prolonged skin incision to delivery time (>8 minutes?) can redistribute general anesthetic agents from the neonatal fat to the circulation and cause secondary neonatal ventilatory depression. Therefore, the neonatologist should be present until a normal breathing pattern is established in the newborn. However, a significant neonatal depression is unlikely following maternal administration of a single, normal dose of an induction agent.

A uterine incision to delivery time longer than 180 minutes can result in lower Apgar scores and greater fetal acidosis. However, this is more likely due to difficulty in delivering the baby rather than a direct effect of the anesthetics.

○ **Does the parturient's height determine the requirement of LA for spinal anesthesia for cesarean section?**

Most clinicians use 10–15 mg of bupivacaine with opioids for single-shot spinal anesthesia for cesarean delivery. Studies have demonstrated that the spread of hyperbaric spinal bupivacaine administered for cesarean section is unaffected by the parturient's age, height, weight, or body mass index (weight/height in m^2). For most patients, except the very short (<5-ft/150-cm) or very tall (>6-ft/180-cm), 15 mg of bupivacaine will achieve a T4–T6 level, which is necessary to ensure adequate anesthesia for cesarean section [Norris, 1990. See reference on page 527].

○ **What is the average anticipated blood loss for vaginal delivery and cesarean section?**

Five hundred to 600 mL for vaginal delivery and 1,000 mL for cesarean section.

○ **What are the features of fetal heart rate (FHR) pattern in normal labor?**

FHR pattern can be monitored using Doppler ultrasonography (abdominal) or fetal scalp ECG.
The features that are assessed include:

1. Baseline FHR: 110–160 bpm is normal.
2. FHR variability: normal variability reflects presence of intact pathways from – and within – the fetal cortex, midbrain, vagus nerve, and cardiac conduction system. FHR variability can be affected by maternally administered medications.
3. Periodic changes: in normal labor early decelerations are seen as a result of reflex vagal activity due to fetal head compression.

○ **What other supplemental methods of fetal assessment are used during the intrapartum period?**

1. Fetal scalp blood pH determination: pH of >7.25 is acceptable. pH 7.20–7.25 warrants a second determination.
2. Fetal scalp stimulation: The heart rate should accelerate in response to scalp stimulation.
3. ST waveform analysis: This is a new technology that is proposed to enhance fetal assessment. Fetal hypoxia induces changes in ST and T waves of ECG.

○ **Explain the causes of fetal deceleration patterns.**

Early – benign: due to fetal head compression during uterine contractions.

Late – indicates uteroplacental insufficiency.

Variable – usually benign: caused by cord compression.

○ **What are normal values for fetal blood gases?**

In the fetus, the umbilical artery (UA) is traveling to the placenta. It therefore carries with it the metabolic waste products of the fetus. Hence, it has low PaO_2, SpO_2, and pH values, and high $PaCO_2$ values.

Conversely, the umbilical vein (UV) is returning blood from the placenta. It therefore has higher values for PO_2, SpO_2, and pH, and low values for PCO_2. See the values below.

○ **At birth normal fetal cord blood gas values are as follows.**

UV:

  pH 7.25–7.35

  PO_2 28–32 mm Hg

  PCO_2 40–50 mm Hg

  BE 0–5 mEq/L

UA:

  pH 7.28

  PO_2 16–20 mm Hg

  PCO_2 40–50 mm Hg

  BE 0–10 mEq/L

○ **What fetal scalp blood gas values indicate that the fetus is in distress?**

In general, there will be a low pH and a low PaO_2 with high $PaCO_2$ for the fetus. Considering the normal fetal scalp blood gas values, you could expect a pH less than 7.20, a PaO_2 less than 25 mm Hg, and a $PaCO_2$ greater than 60 mm Hg.

Fetal scalp pH values of 7.25 or more are classified as normal and indicate that a patient may continue with labor. If the pH is <7.20, delivery should be expedited.

○ **What is EXIT procedure?**

Ex utero intrapartum therapy. This procedure is most often employed to:

1. Secure an airway by intubation/bronchoscopy/tracheostomy

2. Perform a procedure while gas exchange continues in the placenta

○ **What anesthetic techniques may be used for EXIT procedure?**

Anesthesia can be provided with general anesthesia or neuraxial anesthesia. Uterine relaxation during the procedure can be achieved with volatile agents during general anesthesia; during neuraxial blocks, nitroglycerin can be used.

○ **After performing EXIT procedure under general anesthesia with volatile agents, what steps should be taken to reduce postpartum uterine atony?**

Volatile agents should be discontinued and general anesthesia continued with nitrous oxide 70% with opioid. Ventilation should be increased to facilitate elimination of volatile agents.

Oxytocin infusion should be started immediately.

○ **What is twin-to-twin transfusion syndrome (TTTS)?**

This is a syndrome that usually manifests in the second trimester of monochorionic twin gestation. There is abnormal vascular communication between the twins that results in imbalanced twin-to-twin transfusion and TTTS. The recipient demonstrates polyhydramnios, polyuria, polycythemia, and hypertrophic cardiomyopathy (HOCM). This twin is at risk of hydrops fetalis and death. The donor twin typically has oligohydramnios, hypovolemia, oliguria, and growth retardation and is stuck against the endometrium ("stuck twin"). This twin is at risk of neonatal renal failure.

○ **What is the treatment of TTTS?**

If TTTS occurs before 25 weeks of gestation and untreated, fetal mortality is very high [ACOG Practice Bulletin, 2004. See reference on page 527]. Treatment options include:

1. Serial amnioreduction to control polyhydramnios

2. Surgical septostomy of amnios to equalize amniotic pressure

3. Selective feticide to allow other fetus to survive

4. Selective fetoscopic laser photocoagulation (SFLP) of vascular anastomosis

○ **What type of anesthesia is usually provided for TTTS surgery?**

In most cases local anesthetic infiltration of the abdominal wall is sufficient to reduce maternal discomfort during the percutaneous procedure. Supplemental maternal analgesia and anxiolysis can be achieved by maternal administration of benzodiazepines, opioids, or low-dose propofol infusion. This may provide fetal analgesia and immobility via placental transfer. Continuous infusion of remifentanil also has been used to improve fetal immobility and effective maternal sedation [Van de Velde et al., 2005. See reference on page 527].

○ **What are the differences in cardiopulmonary resuscitation (CPR) between pregnant and nonpregnant patients?**

Avoid aortocaval compression by maintaining left lateral uterine displacement during CPR. If CPR is ineffective to resuscitate the mother, it may be necessary to deliver the baby by emergent cesarean section. Maternal and fetal outcomes are best when cesarean section is performed within 5 minutes of maternal arrest. If cardiac arrest occurs before 24 weeks gestation (onset of fetal viability), the only concern should be saving the mother. Beginning at 18–20 weeks, maintain LUD while placing the patient on a hard surface [Kundra et al., 2007. See reference on page 527].

○ **Why is rapid cesarean delivery an important part of maternal resuscitation?**

Delivery of the fetus relieves aortocaval compression. With uterine contraction after delivery, autotransfusion may help increase venous return. Cardiac output produced by chest compression may be more effective without the fetus.

○ **What factors should be taken into consideration during intubation of a pregnant patient?**

Anatomic and physiologic changes of pregnancy increase the risk of failed intubation. Always observe full stomach precautions.

○ **How does management of the difficult airway differ for the pregnant patient?**

Two main concerns in establishing a difficult airway in obstetric patients are: (1) fetal considerations – with failed intubation and fetal distress, if we can ventilate, maintain cricoid pressure and deliver the fetus; if no fetal distress, wake the patient up; and (2) full stomach precautions must be observed with all parturients regardless of NPO status.

○ **If one encounters difficult intubation during an emergency cesarean delivery, what is the management?**

Initial management:

Reposition the patient; try to achieve proper sniffing position.

Use of different laryngoscopy blades, gum elastic bougie, and smaller-diameter ETT.

Laryngoscopy attempts should be limited to no more than three. However, if grade IV view is identified, immediate attention should be directed to ensure oxygenation and ventilation with mask (with continued cricoid pressure). Assistance should be requested. Oral airway placement or two-person technique should be employed if difficulty encountered.

If mask ventilation is adequate and mother or the fetus is in danger, one may consider proceeding with surgery after carefully weighing the benefit of prompt delivery versus the risks of unsecured airway.

If mask ventilation is inadequate, following rescue options should be considered (according to ASA difficult airway algorithm): laryngeal mask airway, Combitube, cricothyrotomy with transtracheal jet ventilation, and emergency cricothyrotomy or tracheostomy. Risks and benefits of proceeding with surgery should be discussed with the team. Ideally a more definitive airway should be established before proceeding with surgery.

○ **What is the treatment of supraventricular tachycardia (SVT) in pregnancy?**

SVT seems to be the most common arrhythmia in pregnancy.

Adenosine is primarily indicated for SVT. It has a short plasma half-life and the onset of action is rapid. It is unlikely to affect the fetus adversely.

Verapamil also may be used during pregnancy and crosses the placenta to a limited degree. Beta-adrenergic receptors, although widely used in pregnancy, readily cross the placenta and may cause fetal bradycardia and hypoglycemia.

○ **What are the fetal effects of maternal cardioversion?**

Direct current cardioversion may be necessary when tachyarrhythmia is serious and causing maternal hemodynamic instability or refractory to pharmacological interventions.

Direct current cardioversion is reported as a safe procedure during pregnancy. However, sustained fetal bradycardia has occurred during or after cardioversion. Therefore, the procedure should be carried out in a facility where FHR can be monitored and be able to do an emergency CS if necessary. It was thought that the direct cardioversion may lead to sustained uterine contractions, causing fetal compromise [Barnes et al., 2002. See reference on page 527].

○ **How does cocaine use during pregnancy affect the fetus?**

Cocaine use during pregnancy can cause (1) uterine contractions resulting in preterm labor, (2) placental abruption, (3) intrauterine growth retardation, and (4) fetal death. Cocaine can directly affect the fetus by (1) cerebral vasoconstriction, (2) teratogenic and developmental disturbances, (3) neurobehavioral abnormalities, and (4) subarachnoid and intraventricular hemorrhage.

○ **When is the best time to perform elective surgery during pregnancy?**

All elective surgeries should be postponed until after delivery. Urgent surgeries are best deferred until the second or third trimester unless maternal health is in danger.

○ **At what gestational age is continuous FHR monitoring feasible during surgery in the pregnant patient?**

Eighteen to 20 weeks gestational age. Technical problems may limit the use of continuous FHR monitoring early on and accurate interpretation of the tracing is essential.

○ **What are the indications for FHR monitoring in pregnant women undergoing nonobstetric surgery?**

FHR monitoring should be carried out during surgery whenever possible. The obstetrician should be involved in the decision making and trained personnel should be available to interpret the tracing.

The greatest value of intraoperative FHR monitoring is that it identifies a need to improve fetal oxygenation if the fetus shows signs of compromise. A change in FHR mandates evaluation of maternal position, blood pressure, oxygenation, acid–base status, and inspection of the surgical field.

FHR variability, a good indicator of fetal well-being, is present from 25 to 27 weeks gestation.

FHR and FHR variability changes that occur due to anesthetic agents and other medications must be distinguished from changes that occur due to true fetal compromise. Persistent severe fetal bradycardia typically indicates true compromise.

○ **What strategies may prevent fetal compromise during nonobstetric surgery?**

Maintain uteroplacental perfusion and fetal oxygenation by: (1) LUD, (2) administration of a higher inspired concentration of oxygen, (3) maintaining normal PaO_2 and $PaCO_2$, (4) augmentation of maternal circulating blood volume, and (5) pharmacological treatment of hypotension.

○ **For nonobstetric surgery during pregnancy, what is the best anesthetic technique?**

No study has documented that any anesthetic agent or technique is associated with a higher or lower incidence of preterm labor or improved fetal outcome. The anesthetic management of the parturient during surgery should focus on avoidance of hypoxemia, hypotension, acidosis, and hyperventilation. The type and location of the operation are the only factors that correlate with preterm labor.

○ **Can laparoscopic procedures be done during pregnancy?**

Yes. The Society of American Gastrointestinal Endoscopic Surgeons has issued *Guidelines for Laparoscopic Surgery during Pregnancy*, which recommends the following: (1) deferring surgery until the second trimester, (2) using intermittent pneumatic compression devices to prevent thrombosis resulting from lower extremity venous stasis, (3) monitoring fetal and uterine status and maternal end-tidal CO_2 and ABG measurements, (4) using an open technique to enter the abdomen, (5) avoiding aortocaval compression, (6) maintaining low pneumoperitoneum pressures (not to exceed 15 mm Hg), and (7) obtaining preoperative obstetric consultation.

○ **What are the adverse effects of CO_2 pneumoperitoneum on a pregnant patient?**

(1) Uterine or fetal trauma, (2) fetal acidosis from systemic absorption of carbon dioxide, and (3) decreased maternal cardiac output and uteroplacental perfusion.

○ **What anesthetic techniques are used for cervical cerclage?**

Transvaginal cervical cerclage is usually performed under spinal, epidural, or general anesthesia.

○ **If neuraxial anesthesia is chosen, what level of sensory blockade is required?**

Sensory blockade from T10 through the sacral dermatomes is required.

○ **When is general anesthesia preferred over neuraxial anesthesia for cervical cerclage?**

In patients with dilated cervix and bulging membranes general anesthesia may be preferred. (However, spinal anesthesia can be placed safely in the lateral position.)

Under general anesthesia, volatile anesthetics cause relaxation of uterine smooth muscles and decrease intrauterine pressure. This facilitates replacement of the bulging membranes and placement of the cerclage.

○ **What precautions should be taken during induction of general anesthesia in cases with bulging membranes?**

Coughing should be avoided during laryngoscopy and intubation. Vomiting also raises intrauterine pressure significantly.

○ **Is anesthesia required for removal of cerclage?**

Removal of McDonald cerclage often requires no anesthesia. Anesthesia is usually required for removal of Shirodkar cerclage. Removal is usually done at 37–38 weeks and neuraxial block may be performed.

○ **What effect does preeclampsia has on the intravascular volume status?**

Although parturients with preeclampsia are edematous and have elevated total body water, the intravascular volume is often diminished. PCWP in preeclampsia is often in the range of 1–5 mm Hg, compared with 6–12 mm Hg in normal parturients. In preeclampsia the vasculature is constricted and porous.

○ **Hypertension in pregnancy includes what disorders?**

Hypertension in pregnancy includes many disorders. In the year 2000, the National High Blood Pressure Education Program (NHBPEP) published a classification scheme establishing a definition for hypertensive disorders in pregnancy [See reference on page 527]. According to this definition this disorder includes:

Gestational hypertension (GH)

Preeclampsia – mild and severe

Chronic hypertension (CH)

CH with superimposed preeclampsia

○ **How is the diagnosis of chronic (or essential) hypertension made in pregnancy?**

CH is differentiated from preeclampsia or GH from the following clinical features:

1. Time of onset – CH is present before the 20th week of gestation while preeclampsia usually appears after the 20th week. GH typically occurs in the third trimester.
2. GH presents with mild hypertension. CH or preeclampsia may have mild or severe hypertension.
3. Proteinuria is absent in CH and GH. Preeclampsia typically presents with proteinuria.
4. Elevated serum uric acid (>5.5 mg/dL) is rare in CH and absent in GH but present in almost all cases of preeclampsia.
5. Signs of hemoconcentration, thrombocytopenia, and hepatic dysfunction are absent in CH and GH but present in severe preeclampsia.

○ **What is known to be the pathophysiology of preeclampsia?**

The pathogenic mechanism of this disorder is still unknown. The pathogenic focus appears to be the placenta. The remodeling of the spiral arteries that occurs in normal pregnancy due to trophoblast invasion is incomplete and only occurs in the superficial decidual segments in preeclamptic woman. This superficial placentation leads to decreased placental perfusion, infarcts, and intrauterine growth retardation. This first stage of reduced perfusion of the intervillous area may go on to the symptomatic second stage in some women. The second stage is characterized by widespread maternal endothelial dysfunction and symptoms such as hypertension, proteinuria, and risk for other severe manifestation of this disorder.

○ **What laboratory tests are abnormal in preeclampsia?**

1. Hemoglobin and hematocrit – elevated; hemoconcentration is an indicator of severity.
2. Platelet count – decreased and indicates severe preeclampsia.
3. Urine protein – increased to more than 300 mg per 24 hours.
4. Serum creatinine – rising.
5. Serum transaminase – rising; suggests liver involvement.
6. Serum uric acid – increased; suggests the diagnosis of preeclampsia.

○ **How should oliguria be treated in the parturient with preeclampsia?**

Oliguria in most patients with preeclampsia is caused by low intravascular volume and can be treated with cautious administration of intravenous crystalloid or colloid. Oliguria is a late manifestation of severe preeclampsia and parallels the severity of disease. Invasive central monitoring may be rarely needed to monitor response to fluid administration.

○ **What are the indications for insertion of a pulmonary artery catheter (PAC) in severe preeclampsia?**

The use of PAC in obstetrics is very low. The presence of severe preeclampsia per se is not an indication for invasive central monitoring. Most patients get better following delivery. Therefore, one should plan for immediate transfer to the operating room and delivery rather than delaying for central line placement. However, if central monitoring is required, in most cases CVP is adequate to guide fluid administration and as a route for venous drug administration.

In a variety of populations, the use of PAC has not been demonstrated to improve outcome. The placements of central catheters (CVP, PAC) are not benign procedures and should be performed only after careful consideration of the risks and benefits.

Hemodynamic monitoring and measurement of mixed venous oxygen saturation may be considered in the following clinical settings:

- Sepsis with refractory hypotension or oliguria
- Unexplained or refractory pulmonary edema, heart failure, or oliguria
- Cardiovascular decompensation
- Massive blood and volume loss or replacement
- ARDS

○ **What are the side effects of magnesium sulfate?**

Therapeutic serum levels are considered to be 6–8 mg/dL. Side effects of magnesium administration may include chest pain and tightness, palpitations, nausea, transient hypotension, blurred vision, sedation, pulmonary edema, respiratory depression, cardiac conduction defects (widened QRS, increased PR interval), and cardiac arrest. Neonatal side effects include hypotonia, drowsiness, decreased gastric motility, and hypocalcemia.

○ **What is the management of retained placenta?**

The incidence of retained placenta is approximately 1% of all vaginal deliveries. Most cases require anesthesia or analgesia for removal of the retained products. Assess and estimate the quantity of blood already lost. Blood should be available and a good intravenous access should be established. If there is no evidence of major blood loss or evidence of coagulopathy, the procedure can be carried out under regional anesthesia technique. If the parturient received a labor epidural, T10 to S4 level block can be established using the existing epidural catheter for painless manual exploration of the retained placenta.

If general anesthesia is used, rapid sequence induction with cricoid pressure, preoxygenation, and intubation using suxamethonium should be chosen. Nonparticulate antacid should be given before induction.

In addition to providing anesthesia or analgesia, uterine (cervical) relaxation is required in some cases to facilitate removal of the placenta. Intravenous administration of 50–100 µg of nitroglycerin results in relaxation sufficient to remove the placenta. Although hypotension is possible, because of the short duration of the drug it is easily treatable.

○ **What are the risk factors for placenta accreta?**

Placenta accreta is an abnormally adhered placenta.

The presence of placenta previa greatly increases the risk of placenta accreta. There is about 3% incidence of placenta accreta when placenta previa occurred in unscarred uterus. This incidence increases to 11% with one previous cesarean delivery and to 40% with two previous cesarean deliveries [Miller et al., 1997. See reference on page 527].

○ **Why is the incidence of thromboembolic events increased in pregnancy?**

The risk is five to six times greater than that for nonpregnant patients. The mechanism is venous stasis from uterine pressure on the IVC, vascular injury during delivery, and an increase in clotting factors. There is elevated platelet activation, clotting, and fibrinolysis representing a state of accelerated but compensated intravascular coagulation.

○ **What are some additional risk factors for thromboembolism in pregnancy?**

Previous embolus in pregnancy, underlying genetic hypercoagulable states, cesarean section, multiparity, bed rest, obesity, increased maternal age, and surgical procedures.

○ **Which anticoagulant is safe for use in pregnancy?**

Heparin. Risks of heparin administration include maternal thrombocytopenia, osteoporosis, hemorrhage, abruptio placentae, and spontaneous abortion. A plan for discontinuation is essential when epidural anesthesia is planned. Warfarin is usually avoided, especially during the first trimester owing to teratogenicity. Low-molecular-weight heparin (LMWH) has been used safely, as it does not cross the placenta. Careful coordination of epidural placement/removal and anticoagulant dosing is necessary to minimize the risk of epidural hematoma.

○ **What is antiphospholipid syndrome?**

It is a prothrombotic disorder that is characterized by the presence of two autoantibodies, lupus anticoagulant and anticardiolipin antibody.

○ **How is it antiphospholipid syndrome diagnosed in pregnancy?**

Unexplained clinical history of recurrent venous/arterial thrombosis and/or pregnancy loss as well as the presence of two antibodies described above makes the diagnosis.

○ **What is the obstetric management of antiphospholipid syndrome?**

ACOG recommends:

1. Women with antiphospholipid syndrome and no thrombotic history should receive prophylactic doses of heparin and low-dose aspirin during pregnancy and 6–8 weeks postpartum.

2. Women with antiphospholipid syndrome and a previous history of thrombosis should receive full anticoagulation throughout pregnancy and the postpartum period.

○ **What is the anesthetic management of a patient with antiphospholipid syndrome?**

Lupus anticoagulant (which may cause prolonged aPTT in vitro) does not suggest bleeding disorder. However, rarely, antiphospholipid antibodies can cause coagulation factor deficiency.

Aspirin alone is not a contraindication for neuraxial anesthesia. However, if she has received thromboprophylaxis with standard unfractionated heparin and uninterrupted aspirin therapy, a 4-hour wait after the last heparin dose is recommended before neuraxial anesthesia. Administration of LMWH thromboprophylaxis requires a 12-hour wait; prophylactic dose of LMWH requires a 24-hour wait before neuraxial anesthesia.

If there is fetal compromise secondary to multi-infarct in placenta in these patients, gradual onset of epidural anesthesia or modified CSE should be considered to avoid sudden hypotension.

○ **How does amniotic fluid enter the maternal circulation?**

Through uterine tears or injury and endocervical veins.

○ **What are the major consequences of amniotic fluid embolism?**

Hypotension, cardiac arrest, pulmonary edema, ARDS, and disseminated intravascular coagulation are all common sequelae.

○ **What are the potential mechanisms of cardiorespiratory collapse following amniotic fluid embolism?**

The early phase consists of transient (but intense) pulmonary vasospasm. This may account for the right heart dysfunction that is often fatal. Low cardiac output leads to increased V/Q mismatch, hypoxemia, and hypotension. A second phase of left ventricular failure and pulmonary edema occurs in those women who survive the initial insult.

○ **How can amniotic fluid embolism be diagnosed?**

The diagnosis of AFE is one of exclusion. In the past, it was thought by demonstrating fetal squamous cells in the maternal pulmonary circulation or lanugo and mucin in pulmonary arterial blood was pathognomonic of AFE. However, these tests lack specificity. Obstetricians have detected fetal squamous cells in pulmonary circulation of otherwise healthy antepartum and postpartum women. A search for more sensitive markers is ongoing.

○ **What is the treatment of amniotic fluid embolism?**

Supportive care. The differential diagnosis includes venous air embolism (VAE), thromboembolism, concealed placental abruption, LA toxicity, septic shock, and complications of severe PE.

○ **What is the mortality rate in amniotic fluid embolism?**

First-hour maternal mortality may be as high as 65%, and overall maternal mortality rate is 60–80%.

○ **What is the classic presentation of VAE (venous air embolism)?**

Chest pain or dyspnea and sudden onset of hypotension with a mill wheel murmur audible over the precordium. Other features include cyanosis, low SpO_2, low end-tidal CO_2, and cardiac dysrhythmias.

○ **What is the incidence of VAE during cesarean section?**

According to one study, subclinical VAE can be detected during cesarean delivery in up to 97% of patients receiving general anesthesia or 67% performed under neuraxial anesthesia, using precordial Doppler monitoring [Lew et al., 1993. See reference on page 527]. These are hemodynamically significant in only 0.7–2% of cesarean sections. Clinical suspicion of VAE should be high in the case of cardiopulmonary collapse during or immediately following cesarean section.

○ **What factors increase the risk of VAE during cesarean section?**

Steep Trendelenburg (head-down) position that places the operative site above the heart and low central venous pressure.

○ **What is the general outcome of asthma in pregnancy?**

The course of asthma in pregnancy may be the same, worse, or better.

○ **Is the medical management of asthma different during pregnancy?**

It is not different. Perinatal outcome studies suggest that the risks of uncontrolled asthma are significantly higher than medication-associated risks. Medications used during asthma fall into two main categories, bronchodilators (beta-adrenergic agonists) and anti-inflammatory agents (inhaled corticosteroids, cromolyn sodium). These agents are shown to be safe for the fetus.

○ **T/F: An arterial $PaCO_2$ of 36 mm Hg does not represent severe asthma.**

False. When interpreting ABG, remember that a normal $PaCO_2$ during pregnancy ranges from 32 to 34 mm Hg. This benign-looking $PaCO_2$ may actually indicate that the patient is getting tired.

○ **What is the treatment of preterm labor?**

Bed rest and hydration

Tocolytic therapy

Administration of corticosteroids when there is a significant risk of preterm delivery between 24 and 34 weeks of gestation

○ **What are the side effects of beta-adrenergic receptor agonists?**

There are maternal, fetal, and neonatal side effects.

Maternal cardiopulmonary effects include arrhythmias, tachycardia, hypotension, pulmonary edema, and myocardial ischemia.

Maternal metabolic effects include hyperglycemia, hyperinsulinemia, and hypokalemia.

Other maternal effects include tremor, palpitation, and nervousness.

Fetal side effects include tachycardia, hyperglycemia, hyperinsulinemia, and myocardial ischemia.

Neonatal side effects include tachycardia, hypoglycemia, hypotension, IVH, and hypocalcemia.

○ **What is the major pulmonary complication of tocolytic therapy?**

Tocolytic-induced pulmonary edema.

○ **Which agents are associated with this syndrome?**

Terbutaline, ritodrine, and magnesium sulfate.

○ **What are the proposed mechanisms for tocolytic-induced pulmonary edema?**

Fluid overload, myocardial toxicity, cardiac failure secondary to tachycardia, and increased pulmonary vascular permeability probably due to infection (reason for preterm labor?) and release of endotoxins have been suggested.

○ **What is the therapy for terbutaline-induced pulmonary edema?**

Stop the tocolytics and provide supportive care, restrict fluids, administer oxygen, diurese, and intubate as needed.

○ **What concerns you may have when using tocolytic medications in a cocaine abuse patient?**

Cocaine potentiates the effects of adrenergic stimulation by inhibiting the reuptake of norepinephrine after its release. Maternal complications linked to cocaine abuse include placental abruption, preterm labor, and cardiac dysrhythmias with infarction. Morbidity associated with these cardiac sequelae may be increased, since pregnancy results in an increased sensitivity to the cardiovascular effects of cocaine.

The beta agonists potentiate the cardiac effects of cocaine by further increasing catecholamine levels and severe hypertension and arrhythmias can be expected when used as a tocolytic agent.

○ **How can the anesthesiologist help facilitate breech vaginal delivery complicated by fetal head entrapment?**

Breech vaginal delivery is not performed in the United States due to the possibility of shoulder dystocia, fetal head entrapment, and trauma.

The goals here are (1) relaxation of cervical smooth and skeletal muscle and (2) analgesia for forceps delivery with external suprapubic pressure. Cervical smooth muscle relaxation is achieved with sublingual or intravenous nitroglycerin. General endotracheal intubation and administration of inhalational agents may be required.

○ **What is the treatment for acute fatty liver of pregnancy (AFLP)?**

AFLP is a medical emergency. It may lead to hepatic failure and fetal death within few days. As soon as the diagnosis is made, plans should be made for delivery by cesarean or expeditious vaginal delivery. Treatment consists of stabilization of electrolyte, treatment of hypoglycemia, and coagulation abnormalities, followed by delivery of the fetus. Maternal condition improves within 24 hours of delivery, and there are no long-term hepatic sequelae in most cases. The most common anesthetic concern is management of significant peripartum hemorrhage that frequently occurs as a result of coagulopathy.

○ **Which nerves are most frequently injured as a result of obstetric rather than anesthetic complications during vaginal delivery?**

Obstetric injuries usually involve compression injuries to the lumbosacral plexus, obturator, femoral, and lateral femoral cutaneous nerves. These injuries are typically unilateral, have a dermatomal distribution corresponding to a peripheral nerve, and may involve sensory and motor deficits (i.e., foot drop).

○ **T/F: Anesthesia is the cause of 15% of the 7.5 maternal deaths per 100,000 live births each year in the United States.**

False. Anesthesia-related maternal mortality (1998–2005) is 1.3 per million live births (representing 1.2% of the total), according to the latest report [Berg et al., 2010. See reference on page 527].

Other important causes of maternal mortality (10–13% contribution) include hemorrhage (12.5%), emboli (thrombotic 10.2% or amniotic fluid 7.5%), hypertensive disorders (12.3%), infection (10.7%), cardiomyopathy (11.5%), noncardiovascular conditions (13.2%), and cardiovascular conditions (12.4%). According to this latest report, indirect causes such as cardiovascular conditions appear to play a major role in maternal mortality than direct obstetric causes such as hypertensive disorders and hemorrhage.

○ **What is the incidence of peripartum cardiomyopathy?**

The incidence is 1 in 3,000 to 1 in 15,000 live births in the United States.

○ **How is peripartum cardiomyopathy diagnosed?**

The diagnosis is made by ruling out the other causes of cardiomyopathy.

Diagnostic criteria are congestive heart failure in the last months of pregnancy or the first 5 months postpartum in a woman with:

No history of cardiac disease

No identifiable cause

Impaired left ventricular function on echo – ejection fraction <45% and/or decreased shortening fraction <30%, and end-diastolic dimension >2.7 cm/m^2 [Karaye and Henein, 2011. See reference on page 527].

○ **Describe the management of HOCM during pregnancy.**

The outflow tract obstruction is worsened by decreased SVR, decreased volume, and increased contractility.

Although the plasma volume is increased, pregnancy may have negative effects due to decreased SVR, increased heart rate, contractility, and decreased preload due to aortocaval compression.

Although epidural block relieves pain (decreasing catecholamine), sudden drop in SVR may not be tolerated. Very dilute solutions of bupivacaine may be used for labor with slow titration.

General anesthesia is safe for cesarean delivery.

Oxytocin should be administered with caution.

○ **How is von Willebrand disease managed during pregnancy?**

Patients with von Willebrand disease have variable levels of both von Willebrand factor and F VIII (see chapter "Hemostasis" for more details). von Willebrand disease can be divided into several subtypes depending on the quantitative or qualitative defect in von Willebrand factor.

F VIII levels should be checked periodically during the antenatal period and prophylactic treatment is reserved for patients with F VIII level below 25%. 1-Deamino-8-D-arginine vasopressin (DDAVP) should be used in type I and IIa as labor begins. A dose of 0.3 mg/kg (maximum 25 μg) is administered over 30 minutes, and the dose is repeated every 12 hours. If there is no response to DDAVP, FFP or cryoprecipitate (500–1,500 U of F VIII activity) should be administered.

During labor, F VIII levels should be maintained at 50% of normal. For cesarean delivery F VIII level should be 80% of normal. F VIII level should be checked daily during the postpartum period. Treatment may be required if level falls below 25% or symptomatic bleeding occurs.

○ **How should you manage labor in a patient with a history of autonomic hyperreflexia?**

Regional techniques can offer adequate levels of anesthesia to prevent sympathetic hyperreflexia. Regional analgesia eliminates noxious signals from the lower sacral nerve roots, thereby preventing the reflex. However, one must always be prepared to treat a hypertensive crisis.

○ **What is the management of traumatic placental abruption?**

Trauma due to motor vehicle accidents may present with placental abruption. Uterine tenderness and pain, and nonreassuring fetal heart tracing are the common presenting symptoms. Although ultrasonography is not very sensitive (24%) for abruption, it is highly specific (96%). The major complications are hemorrhagic shock, coagulopathy, acute renal failure, and fetal compromise or demise.

Bleeding may be concealed, and severity of vaginal bleeding therefore has no correlation to the severity of abruption. Therefore, place two large-bore IVs and crossmatch at least 4 U of blood. If the patient is unstable, activate massive transfusion protocol (institutional) and transfer to the operating room for cesarean delivery under general anesthesia. Ketamine or etomidate should be used for induction for the patient with decreased intravascular volume. Neonatologist should be available for potential newborn resuscitation. The patient may develop DIC secondary to abruption. Aggressive fluid resuscitation is critical. Apart from the vital signs and urine output, frequent blood gases (A-line) should be used to assess the adequacy of fluid resuscitation. The patient should be kept warm using fluid warmers and forced air warming device.

Key Terms

Amniotic fluid embolism: diagnosis
Anesthesia: uterine muscle tone
Anesthetic techniques: first-stage labor
Antiphospholipid syndrome
Arterial blood gases (ABG) in pregnancy
Asthma: postpartum hemorrhage treatment
Autonomic hyperreflexia: labor epidural
Autotransfusion: complications
Cervical cerclage: anesthetic management
Chloroprocaine placental transfer
Drugs crossing the placenta
Emergency cesarean: difficult airway
Epidural: labor/delivery
Essential hypertension: pregnancy
EXIT procedure: uterine atony
Fetal barbiturate metabolism
Fetal blood gas values
Fetal disposition of drugs
Fetal heart rate: maternal hypotension
Fetal heart rate pattern: normal labor
Fetal heart rate variability
Fetal monitoring
Fetal oxygenation
Fetal transfer of local anesthetics
Fetal uptake of drugs: factors
FRC reduction in pregnancy: hypoxemia

GI physiology in pregnancy
Inhaled agents: uterine tone
Lung volumes in pregnancy
Magnesium effects on ECG
Management of retained placenta
Maternal cardioversion: fetal effects
Maternal congenital heart disease in obstetric anesthesia
Maternal mortality causes
Maternal physiology: electrolyte changes
Maternal physiology: hematology
Methods: uterine relaxation
Nitroglycerin: uterine relaxation
Nonobstetric surgery during pregnancy
Oliguria in preeclampsia: treatment
Oxygen delivery to fetus in labor
Oxygen transfer to fetus
Oxytocin: electrolyte effects
Peripartum changes in CO
Placenta accrete: risk factors
Placental oxygen transport
Placental transfer: anticholinergic
Placental transfer: local anesthetics
Placental transfer of anesthetic agents
Postpartum cardiomyopathy: TEE
Preeclampsia: lab abnormalities
Preeclampsia: pathophysiology

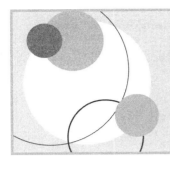

Opioids and Substance Abuse

Everyone wants to live on top of the mountain, but all the happiness and growth occurs while you're climbing it.
Andy Rooney

○ **What side effects are associated with epidural or spinal opioids?**

Respiratory depression, urinary retention, pruritus, nausea, vomiting, and sedation.

○ **What is the incidence of side effects with intraspinal narcotics [Miller, 2010]?**

	Spinal	Epidural
Respiratory depression (%)	5–7	0.1–2
Pruritus (%)	60	1–100
Nausea (%)	20–50	20–30
Urinary retention (%)	50	15–25

○ **When is respiratory depression seen with spinal opioids?**

Early respiratory depression (within 30 minutes of administration) can be seen with lipophilic opioids, while delayed respiratory depression (more likely 3–10 hours after administration) is more commonly seen with hydrophilic opioids such as morphine.

○ **What seems to be the mechanism of early respiratory depression?**

Early respiratory depression is due to rapid vascular uptake (plasma level = IM or IV) and rapid brain penetration of lipophilic opioids. The risk is dose related.

○ **What seems to be the mechanism of late respiratory depression?**

This occurs due to the rostral spread of opioids in the cerebrospinal fluid (CSF) and reaching medullary respiratory center to cause direct depression hours later. Therefore, late-onset respiratory depression is potentially more dangerous and may occur unexpectedly hours after opioid injection. It is more likely with hydrophilic opioids such as morphine. In these cases the plasma level of morphine is relatively low and the CSF level is several hundred times higher.

○ **Is respiratory depression after neuraxial opioids more likely in the pregnant patients compared with nonpregnant patients?**

Because of highly vascular epidural space, this risk should be increased in pregnancy. However, in general it is a minor problem (progesterone is a respiratory stimulant). There is considerable evidence that healthy obstetric population is not a high-risk group (incidence 0–0.25%) [Carvalho, 2008. See reference on page 528].

○ **What are the differences between epidural fentanyl and morphine?**

Agent	Onset (Minutes)	Peak CSF	Duration (Hours)
Morphine	60	1–4 hours	12–24
Fentanyl	5–10	20 minutes	3–5

○ **What factors increase the incidence and magnitude of respiratory depression after spinal opioids?**

1. Advanced age.
2. Neonates have a greater respiratory depression because of immature blood–brain barrier. This permits higher concentration of hydrophilic morphine molecules to reach the brain.
3. Concomitant use of parenteral opioids and/or sedatives such as benzodiazepines, inhalational agents, and barbiturates. Droperidol, scopolamine, and clonidine are exceptions in that they do not enhance respiratory depressant effect of opioids.
4. Use of large doses of opioids.
5. Renal insufficiency. For example, morphing metabolite M6G accumulates in patients with renal insufficiency.
6. Opioid-naïve patient due to lack of tolerance.

○ **Which epidurally administered opioid has the fewest side effects?**

Fentanyl.

○ **What are the major advantages of epidural opioid administration?**

Improved pain relief, steady pain relief, decreased postoperative morbidity, and shortened hospital stays. Improved pulmonary function has also been demonstrated.

○ **What are the signs of impending epidural opioid toxicity?**

Altered mental status, decreased level of consciousness, respiratory depression (decreased pulse oximetry readings, decreased respiratory rate, apnea, and increased end-tidal CO_2 levels), and miosis.

○ **Is the anatomic location of an epidural catheter important when using *hydrophilic* opioids?**

No. Once the hydrophilic opioid (i.e., morphine and hydromorphone) reaches the CSF through direct intrathecal injection or gradual migration from the epidural space, it tends to remain within the CSF and produce a delayed but longer duration of analgesia, along with a larger dermatomal spread because of the cephalic or supraspinal spread of these compounds. Therefore, it is not necessary to place the catheter in a near-dermatomal distribution of the patient's pain pattern.

○ **Is the anatomic location of an epidural catheter important when using *lipophilic* opioids?**

Using lipophilic opioids (fentanyl) it is hypothesized that there is a band-like distribution of the agent within several dermatomes. Therefore, it is generally felt that placing the catheter in the middle of the surgical dermatomal pattern affords better analgesia with the concomitant need for a reduced amount of opioid.

○ **What is the proposed site of action of neuraxial opioids?**

Mu opioid receptors in the substantia gelatinosa of the dorsal horn of the spinal cord.

○ **What is the proposed mechanism of action of epidural opioids?**

Epidural opioids diffuse directly across the dura and bind to opioid receptors of the substantia gelatinosa, situated within the lamina II of the dorsal horn of the spinal cord. Activation of the enkephalinergic interneurons of substantia gelatinosa by opioids reduces the amount of substance P released by the action potential in the primary afferent fibers of the pain pathways leading to the spinothalamic tract. (Substance P is the neurotransmitter of the nociceptive primary afferent neurons.)

However, the analgesic effect of highly lipophilic agents after epidural administration (prolonged administration) is mostly due to systemic absorption. With bolus or brief infusions, there is evidence of spinal effect.

The uptake via the epidural vasculature promotes a systemic spread of the agent. Systemic opioids stimulate μ_1 receptors in the supraspinal brain regions to cause activation of the descending modulatory systems and affect neural transmission in the substantia gelatinosa of the dorsal horn of the spinal cord.

○ **What is the physiology of intrathecal opioids?**

Once the drug enters the CSF (diffused across meninges or given spinally):

1. The drug molecules may leave CSF to enter the epidural fat, and thereafter slowly absorbed into circulation (happens with majority of sufentanil due to high lipid solubility).
2. Diffuse within CSF, cranially and caudad (rapid).
3. Penetrate spinal cord to reach the dorsal horn gray matter. The efficiency of penetration depends on the lipid solubility of the drug.

At the dorsal horn, extremely lipid-soluble drugs such as sufentanil may partition into axon-rich white matter on the surface. Once in the dorsal horn, more hydrophilic morphine appears to be the best in penetrating gray matter.

○ **Describe the receptors where opioids demonstrate effects.**

Opioid receptor classification is continually being expanded/revised:

Mu_1: Analgesia (somatic and visceral pain)

Mu_2: Respiratory depression, bradycardia, physical dependence, euphoria, and ileus

Delta: Modulates the activity at the mu receptor

Kappa: Analgesia (visceral pain), sedation, dysphoria, and psychomimetic effects

Sigma: Dysphoria, hypertonia, tachycardia, tachypnea, and mydriasis

○ **How does the binding of an opioid agonist with an opioid receptor produce an intracellular effect?**

Opioid receptors belong to the G protein–coupled receptor family and they signal via a secondary messenger (cyclic AMP) or an ion channel (K^+).

○ **What are the cellular effects of opioids?**

Opioids decrease calcium ion entry resulting in a decrease in presynaptic neurotransmitter release (e.g., substance P release from primary afferents in the spinal cord dorsal horn). They also enhance potassium ion efflux resulting in the hyperpolarization of postsynaptic neurons causing a decrease in synaptic transmission. A third mode of action is in the inhibition of GABAergic transmission in a local circuit having the net effect of exciting an inhibitory circuit.

○ **What is the time to maximal respiratory depression after an IV dose of fentanyl or morphine?**

Fentanyl, 5–7 minutes; and morphine, approximately 20–30 minutes.

○ **How do opioids affect the respiratory pattern?**

Decrease in rate, tidal volume, minute ventilation, and apnea at higher doses. Opioid causes a greater reduction in respiratory rate than in tidal volume with prolonged expiratory time in the respiratory cycle.

The pattern may also be irregular (periodic breathing or Cheyne–Stokes).

○ **How do opioids affect the CO_2 response curve?**

The CO_2 response curve is shifted to the right. The slope of the CO_2 response curve is decreased.

○ **How do opioids affect hypoxic respiratory drive?**

Opioids blunt this drive.

○ **Will respiratory acidosis increase or decrease opioid respiratory depression?**

Increase. Respiratory acidosis increases the ionized fraction at the receptor site.

○ **How do you treat opioid-induced biliary spasm?**

Both naloxone in titrated doses and glucagon (1–3 mg IV) are effective treatments.

○ **You suggest the possibility of epidural narcotics after caesarian section to the obstetrician, but he expresses concern about urinary retention. What can you tell him?**

Urinary retention occurs in up to 40% of patients receiving epidural narcotics [Baldini et al., 2009. See reference on page 528]. The incidence is probably lower with lipid-soluble opioids than with morphine. If the plan is to have an indwelling urinary catheter, this is probably not an issue.

○ **Which opioid should not be used in patients on MAO inhibitors?**

Meperidine. This combination can lead to serotonin syndrome, which includes autonomic hyperactivity, excitation, convulsions, and lethal hyperpyrexia. The mechanism of this interaction is unclear, but may be due to increased brain serotonin levels.

○ **Why is a continuous meperidine PCA infusion not recommended?**

Accumulation of its renally excreted metabolite normeperidine can cause seizures and myoclonus.

○ **If the potency of morphine is 1, what are the relative potencies of meperidine, codeine, methadone, butorphanol, hydromorphone, nalbuphine, alfentanil, fentanyl, and sufentanil?**

Meperidine 0.1, codeine 0.05–0.1, methadone 1, butorphanol 5, hydromorphone 10, nalbuphine 1, alfentanil 10, fentanyl 100, and sufentanil 1,000. This is easily remembered as "the multiples of tens."

○ **At physiological pH, do opioids exist mainly in the ionized or unionized form?**

Ionized. The pK_a values for morphine, meperidine, fentanyl, and sufentanil are 8.0, 8.5, 8.4, and 8.0, respectively. Alfentanil, with a pK_a of 6.5, is the only commonly used opioid that is predominantly unionized. Plasma levels of morphine have the poorest correlation with analgesic effect because it is the least lipid soluble of the opioid drugs.

○ **Morphine is an agonist for which class of opioid receptors?**

Mu_1 receptors.

○ **What are the most prominent CNS side effects of opioids?**

Respiratory depression, nausea, vomiting, sedation, constipation, pruritus, pupillary constriction, and cough suppression.

○ **To which side effects of opioid administration are patients least likely to develop tolerance?**

Constipation and pupillary constriction.

○ **How does high-dose opioid affect EEG?**

High-dose opioid does not cause burst suppression. Opioids characteristically produce only a monophasic (decreased frequency and increased amplitude), dose-dependent depression of EEG.

○ **Do opioids affect somatosensory evoked potentials?**

Opioids have a minimal effect. There is increase in the latency with minimal or no effect on the amplitude. However, these changes remain stable and do *not* interfere with intraoperative monitoring.

○ **How do opioids affect cerebral blood flow?**

If ventilation is controlled, they cause a slight decrease. There is some controversy with sufentanil, with some studies showing an increase in CBF and others demonstrating no effect.

○ **What are the effects of opioids on cerebral metabolic rate?**

In general, opioids may cause a minor reduction or no effect on CBF and CMR. However, occasionally opioid-induced neuroexcitation can cause focal increases in CMR.

○ **Describe the pharmacogenetics of codeine.**

Codeine is primarily metabolized by glucoronidation, but also undergoes *N*-demethylation to norcodeine and *O*-demethylation to morphine. The latter pathway depends on a genetically polymorphic enzyme that is absent in 7% of the white population. Therefore, the analgesic effects of codeine may be somewhat reduced in people who lack this enzyme.

O **What are the clinical effects of nalbuphine?**

It is an agonist–antagonist opioid. Equal in analgesic potential to morphine but one fourth potent as nalorphine as an antagonist.

Clinical effects are analgesia, sedation, respiratory depression, and dysphoria. It is free of CVS side effects. Abrupt withdrawal can cause withdrawal symptoms milder than morphine. Antagonist effects are due to its action at mu receptors. This is useful in the postoperative period to reverse the pruritus caused by morphine or fentanyl while still maintaining analgesia.

O **What is the plateau effect mechanism of nalbuphine?**

The plateau (ceiling) effect mechanism is due to nalbuphine's partial agonist/antagonist properties. Partial agonists produce a shallower dose–response curve and a lower maximal effect than a full agonist. This holds true for all major opiate effects including euphoria and respiratory depression. For this reason nalbuphine is considered to have a reduced addiction liability.

However, it can precipitate withdrawal symptoms in those physically dependent on opioids.

O **What are the characteristic withdrawal symptoms when opioids are discontinued?**

Withdrawal symptoms include excessive sympathetic nervous system activity.

In order of increasing severity:

1. Anxiety, irritability, and craving for the drug
2. Watery eyes, runny nose, salivation, and yawning
3. Dilated pupils, loss of appetite, gooseflesh, shakes, hot and cold flashes, and muscle aches
4. Severe tremors, fever, high blood pressure, fast pulse, and rapid breathing
5. Diarrhea, vomiting, low blood pressure, sweating, confusion, and dehydration

O **Does methadone produce a more severe or less severe withdrawal syndrome than morphine?**

Less severe. Methadone has a longer half-life, so symptoms develop more slowly and tend to be less intense.

O **What are the advantages and disadvantages of methadone administration?**

Advantages are a long drug half-life ($T_{1/2\beta} = 35$ hours), an elixir formulation, high bioavailability (it is well absorbed orally with bioavailability 90%), and no active metabolites.

Disadvantages are accumulation and longer time to reach steady state than other opioids. Urinary acidifiers may increase elimination and potentially precipitate an acute withdrawal syndrome.

O **Can methadone cause QTc prolongation?**

Recently reports have associated methadone administration with prolongation of the QTc interval and development of torsade de pointes tachycardia and even sudden death [Krantz et al., 2002. See reference on page 528]. Although there are no current guidelines, ECG evaluation may be warranted if methadone dose over 100 mg, additional risk factors for QTc prolongation (such as hypokalemia, other QTc-prolonging drugs, cytochrome P450 inhibitors), or structural heart disease present.

O **What problems may be encountered in methadone-maintained patients during anesthesia for surgery?**

These patients should have methadone maintained during the perioperative period.

They are likely to require larger doses of opioids. Therefore, there is no advantage in trying to maintain anesthesia with opioids.

Chronic opioid usage leads to cross-tolerance to other central nervous system depressants also. Therefore, they may have decreased analgesic response to nitrous oxide.

These patients could develop perioperative hypotension due to inadequate intravascular fluid volume secondary to chronic infections, malnutrition, or adrenocortical insufficiency.

Opioid addicts experience exaggerated postoperative pain. Methadone alone provides poor analgesic activity. Addition of meperidine or other opioid to the usual maintenance dose of methadone is usually required.

How does opioid tolerance manifest?

Tolerance is a pharmacologic phenomenon in which repeated exposure to a drug results in a decreased therapeutic effect or the need for a higher dose to maintain the same effect.

Tolerance may develop rapidly to depressant effects of opioids (analgesia, sedation, emesis, euphoria, hypoventilation) but slowly to stimulant effects (miosis, constipation).

Fortunately, as tolerance increases, so does the lethal dose of opioids.

Acute opioid tolerance manifests as tachyphylaxis. Chronic tolerance takes time to develop and lasts longer. Opioid tolerance can occur without physical dependence, where withdrawal symptoms occur when opioids are abruptly stopped or reversed.

Describe the methods and effects of opioid reversal.

Naloxone, a pure antagonist at μ, κ, and δ receptors with the greatest affinity for μ receptors, is usually used for reversal of opioid effects such as respiratory depression or pruritus. Nalbuphine, a partial antagonist at μ receptor, also can be used to reverse pruritus. However, it has been shown that the potency ratio between naloxone and nalbuphine for reversal of pruritus following epidural morphine is 40:1.

Sudden complete antagonism of opioid effects with naloxone may cause severe hypertension, tachycardia, ventricular dysrhythmia, and fatal pulmonary edema (centrally mediated catecholamine release).

Antagonist may also precipitate opioid withdrawal in addicts.

Careful slow titration (IV 20–40 μg administered every 2–3 minutes) can restore adequate ventilation without reversal of analgesia.

Naloxone has a half-life of about 30–60 minutes. Therefore, the respiratory depression may recur. The initial loading dose should be followed by an infusion at 4–5 μg/kg/h.

How is morphine metabolized?

Glucuronidation in the liver followed by renal excretion of an active metabolite.

Which morphine metabolite is active?

Morphine-6-glucuronide. The duration of action of M6G is similar to morphine and may accumulate in patients with renal failure, leading to prolonged ventilatory depression.

Compared with parenteral administration, how potent is oral morphine?

One sixth as potent. This is because of the first-pass effect in the liver, with only 20–30% reaching the systemic circulation.

What are the times to peak analgesic effect of IV, IM, and PO morphine?

Approximately 20–30, 45, and 90 minutes, respectively.

O   **Do spinal or parenteral opioids alter uterine blood flow?**

No. However, meperidine may increase uterine contractility.

O   **Which opioids release histamine?**

Morphine, codeine, and meperidine. Fentanyl, sufentanil, and alfentanil do not stimulate histamine release.

O   **What are the mechanisms of opioid-induced hypotension?**

Histamine release causing vasodilation, dose-dependent bradycardia, negative inotropic effects (meperidine), and decreased sympathetic tone.

O   **What is the mechanism of opioid-induced bradycardia?**

The dose-dependent bradycardia seen with most opioids is likely an effect secondary to direct, central stimulation of the vagal nucleus.

O   **Which opioid is a cardiac depressant and increases heart rate?**

There is no significant myocardial depression at therapeutic levels of opioids except with high-dose meperidine, which is due to its local anesthetic effect.

Meperidine may also elicit tachycardia due to its structural similarity to atropine.

Opioids preserve cardiovascular responses to circulating catecholamines, which is good for critically ill patients.

O   **Do opioids interfere with hypoxic pulmonary vasoconstriction?**

No.

O   **How should opioid-induced seizures be treated?**

With barbiturates and benzodiazepines. Naloxone will generally not reverse seizure activity, especially when induced by normeperidine.

O   **Which opioid is effective in treating shivering?**

Meperidine. It is effective in treating postoperative, transfusion-related, or epidural anesthesia-related shivering.

O   **How do parenteral opioids affect the surgical stress response?**

They decrease the response, with the fentanyl class of drugs apparently more effective than morphine. Blood glucose, catecholamine, cortisol, ACTH, and growth hormone levels are all decreased. This effect appears to be short-lived, and may require sustained administration to maintain this response. Effects on postoperative outcome remain controversial.

O   **What are the effects of opioids on intraocular pressure?**

They can decrease IOP and prevent increases in IOP due to succinylcholine and intubation.

O   **Do opioids cross the placenta?**

Yes. Impaired metabolism and excretion may result in opioid effects lasting up to 3 days in the neonate.

○ **Which opioid should be used with caution in neonates?**

Morphine. The blood–brain barrier is immature in neonates, which permits higher concentrations of the polar morphine molecule to reach the brain.

○ **How is opioid pharmacokinetics altered in neonates?**

Clearance is decreased, and elimination half-life is increased. Decreased protein binding may lead to enhanced effects. Intraoperative clearance of fentanyl can be quite variable in newborns.

○ **How is opioid pharmacokinetics altered in the elderly?**

Decreased clearance and increased elimination half-life. Volume of distribution and protein binding can also be less, leading to a greater opioid effect for a given dose.

○ **What is the impact of liver disease on opioid pharmacokinetics?**

Decreased clearance and longer elimination half-life. Hyperbilirubinemia and hypoalbuminemia accompany liver disease, which may render patients more sensitive to opioids.

○ **The nephrologist cautions you against using morphine intraoperatively for a patient with chronic renal failure (CRF). What are the issues that need to be considered? What are your alternate choices for analgesia?**

Morphine is a prototypical example of an opioid with active metabolites that are dependent on renal clearance mechanisms for elimination. It is principally metabolized by conjugation in the liver and is eliminated via renal excretion of water-soluble glucuronides (morphine-6-glucuronide, morphine-3-glucuronide). The kidney also plays a role in the conjugation of morphine, accounting for nearly 40% of its metabolism. M3G is the major metabolite but does not bind to opioid receptors and has little or no analgesic activity. Morphine-6-glucuronide (approximately 10% of the morphine's metabolite) is a mu agonist with greater potency than morphine and similar duration. Patients with renal failure can develop very high levels of morphine-6-glucuronide and life-threatening respiratory depression.

Like morphine, meperidine is metabolized in the liver to several metabolites that are eventually excreted by the kidney. Normeperidine, the chief metabolite, with one half the analgesic potency, has CNS excitatory effects including seizures at high levels.

In contrast to morphine and meperidine, the clinical pharmacology of the fentanyl congeners is not grossly altered by kidney failure, and their large volume of distribution minimizes any effect that decreased plasma protein binding may potentially play. Sufentanil pharmacokinetics is not altered in any consistent fashion by renal disease, although greater variability exists in its clearance and elimination half-life. No delay in recovery after alfentanil administration should be expected in patients with renal failure. Neither the pharmacokinetics nor the pharmacodynamics of remifentanil is altered by impaired renal function.

○ **How is remifentanil metabolized?**

Nonspecific plasma esterases.

○ **What are the consequences of administering remifentanil to patients with pseudocholinesterase deficiency?**

The circulating esterases responsible for remifentanil metabolism are distinct from those enzymes that metabolize succinylcholine or acetylcholine, and the short duration of remifentanil may even be preserved in patients with deficiency of pseudocholinesterase activity or in patients taking medications that inhibit plasma pseudocholinesterases (e.g., echothiophate). In fact, the pharmacokinetics of remifentanil in patients with impaired hepatic or renal function appears to be unchanged.

○ **What are the toxicities of propoxyphene (Darvon)?**

Hallucinations, convulsions, and cardiotoxicity. The cardiotoxicity may be partly due to the metabolite norpropoxyphene, and not entirely reversible by naloxone. Propoxyphene is a mu agonist.

○ **What is the potency of oral propoxyphene (Darvon) compared with oral codeine?**

Propoxyphene is one half as potent as codeine.

○ **Which anesthetics when combined with opioids can lead to cardiovascular depression?**

Nitrous oxide, volatile anesthetics, barbiturates, and propofol. Opioids have a synergistic effect with all general anesthetics.

○ **After continuous infusion, which opioid drug level decreases most slowly: alfentanil, fentanyl, or sufentanil?**

Fentanyl.

○ **How do opioids interact with local anesthetics?**

Coadministration of opioids (fentanyl, morphine) with most local anesthetics epidurally or intrathecally produces synergistic analgesia; makes the local anesthetic onset faster and duration of action longer with improved quality of the block. However, 2-chloroprocaine appears to decrease the effectiveness of epidural opioids.

Combining local anesthetics with opioids for peripheral nerve blocks or for intra-articular administration appears to be ineffective.

○ **Which opioid is most suitable for the transdermal route of administration?**

Fentanyl. It has a relatively high lipid solubility compared with morphine.

○ **Describe the pharmacokinetics of transdermal fentanyl.**

The transdermal route creates a skin reservoir that results in a 12-hour delay in onset and offset. Factors that affect skin perfusion will affect the rate of absorption. The transdermal route circumvents the first-pass metabolism of fentanyl in the liver.

○ **What is iontophoresis?**

The transcutaneous absorption is passive and the onset time is delayed. This can be overcome by using an electric current to "drive" ionized drugs into the skin, a method called *iontophoresis.*

○ **Which opioid is most suitable for continuous infusion when a rapid offset of effect is required?**

Remifentanil. The drug is extensively bound to plasma proteins (70%) and has a low volume of distribution compared with other opioids. The clearance is much greater than that of other similar drugs; as such, remifentanil has a very short elimination half-life (3–10 minutes). The offset of activity following continuous infusion of remifentanil is considerably more rapid than with fentanyl or alfentanil. This can be attributed to a context-sensitive half-time of 3–5 minutes.

○ **Order the hydrophilicity of opioids from most to least.**

Morphine > meperidine > methadone > alfentanil > fentanyl > sufentanil.

○ **What is the onset of action of fentanyl after an intravenous injection?**

One arm–brain circulation (45 seconds to 1 minute), after IV administration.

○ **What is the duration of analgesia of fentanyl?**

Approximately 45 minutes. Despite its short duration of action, recovery and discharge times have been reported to be no different using fentanyl or morphine for postoperative analgesia after ambulatory surgical procedures.

○ **Describe the pharmacokinetics of alfentanil.**

Alfentanil has a context-sensitive half-life of 58 minutes and depends on its small volume of distribution for short elimination half-life.

○ **What are some of the common side effects of opiates and their treatments?**

Side Effect	Treatment
Nausea	Ondansetron, phenothiazines, metoclopramide, scopolamine
Sedation	Naloxone
Constipation	Laxatives, stool softeners
Urinary retention	Reduction of dosage, catheterization
Pruritus	Low-dose naloxone, nalbuphine, ondansetron
Respiratory depression	Naloxone

○ **Mention one method to reduce the postoperative opioid usage.**

Use of NSAIDs such as ketorolac.

It has been shown that ketorolac 30 mg has a potency similar to about 5–10 mg of parenteral morphine.

○ **Describe the pharmacokinetic properties of cocaine.**

Cocaine is readily absorbed from all mucous membranes. Due to its local vasoconstrictive effect, measurable quantities have been reported to remain in the nasal mucosa for 3 hours after application. There is a significant risk of systemic toxicity due to rapid absorption with an onset of action in less than 1 minute, 5 minutes to peak effect, and elimination half-life of 1–1.5 hours. Duration of action is approximately 30–60 minutes (average 20–40 minutes). Cocaine is hydrolyzed by plasma and hepatic cholinesterases. The primary metabolites (benzoylecgonine and ecgonine methyl ester) and 10–20% of the unchanged drug are renally eliminated.

○ **What is the mechanism of action of cocaine?**

Cocaine facilitates catecholaminergic action by blocking the reuptake of norepinephrine, epinephrine, and especially dopamine. Reuptake process normally removes many of these transmitters from synapses, thereby preventing overstimulation of postsynaptic neurons. Cocaine blocks this and produces the characteristic "cocaine high."

Cocaine is highly addictive and its use is associated with life-threatening side effects. Overwhelming sympathetic stimulation of cardiovascular system causes uncontrolled hypertension leading to pulmonary and cerebral edema. Increased circulating catecholamines may cause coronary artery vasoconstriction and platelet aggregation.

○ **What are the manifestations of acute cocaine toxicity?**

Tachycardia (increase in heart rate of 20–50%), hypertension, ventricular arrhythmias, and fever due to excessive sympathetic stimulation. When low doses are administered, tachycardia may initially be preceded by bradycardia due to central vagal stimulation. Signs and symptoms of systemic toxicity occur in three phases: early stimulation (cardiovascular; CNS: agitation, excitement, dysphoria, headache; abdominal pain, nausea, sweating; unusually large pupils), advanced stimulation (ventricular arrhythmias, CNS hemorrhage, CHF, convulsions, myocardial ischemia), and depression (loss of reflexes, flaccid paralysis, fixed dilated pupils, loss of consciousness, pulmonary edema, cardiac arrest).

Myocardial ischemia and hypotension lasting as long as 6 weeks can occur after discontinuing cocaine use.

Cocaine may be administered intranasally, orally, or intravenously or by inhalation. Death due to cocaine use has occurred with all routes and is usually due to apnea, seizures, or cardiac dysrhythmias.

Cocaine use during pregnancy is associated with spontaneous abortion, abruption placenta, and fetal malformations. Cocaine decreases uterine blood flow. Hyperpyrexia caused by cocaine can contribute to seizures.

Cocaine is metabolized by plasma cholinesterase. Those who have decreased levels (elderly, severe liver disease, parturients) are at increased risk of sudden death when using cocaine.

○ **What are the manifestations of chronic cocaine abuse?**

After long-term exposure to cocaine, there is excessive sensitivity of coronary vasculature to catecholamines. This may be due to depletion of dopamine stores. Smoking of cocaine causes lung damage and pulmonary edema.

Long-term use is also associated with nasal septal atrophy, heightened reflexes, agitation, and paranoid thinking. Cocaine withdrawal causes symptoms such as depression, fatigue, and increased appetite.

○ **How is acute cocaine toxicity treated?**

Nitroglycerine and alpha-adrenergic blockade to treat coronary vasoconstriction and hypertension. Benzodiazepines to control seizures. Active cooling if hyperpyrexia is present.

○ **What are the anesthetic interactions of methamphetamine?**

Methamphetamine taken acutely increases anesthetic requirements. This probably reflects the acute release of norepinephrine, epinephrine, and dopamine and blocking their uptake.

Conversely, chronic administration depletes the nerve endings of these neurotransmitters and decreases CNS stores, and therefore the anesthetic requirement may be decreased.

○ **What is the definition of addiction?**

Addiction is a physical or psychological need for a habit-forming substance, such as a drug or alcohol. In physical addiction, the body adapts to the substance being used and gradually requires increasing amounts to reproduce the effects.

○ **What is the definition of substance abuse?**

Substance abuse is self-administration of drugs deviating from accepted social or medical use. When sustained, this behavior can lead to physical and psychological dependence (presence of the drug in the body is necessary for normal physiological function and to prevent withdrawal symptoms).

○ **What is the prevalence of substance abuse among anesthesiologists compared with other physician groups?**

It has been shown that in the United States anesthesiologists show a higher incidence of substance abuse problem (numbers attending the addictive programs three times higher compared with other physician groups). Currently, 12–15% of all physicians in treatment are anesthesiologists. High-risk groups are <35 years old, residents, male, white, and academic departments.

○ **What is the most commonly abused drug?**

Seventy-six to 90% use opiates as the drug of choice; especially fentanyl and sufentanil are accessible drugs and have highly addictive potentials [Bryson and Silverstein, 2008. See reference on page 528].

○ **What is the risk of relapse with an addictive disease?**

The risk of relapse is greatest in the first 5 years. The relapse rate for anesthesiologists is the highest of all physicians and, unfortunately, the death is the primary presenting sign of relapse in opiate-addicted anesthesiologists.

○ **What is the best way to manage postoperative pain in the patient with a concurrent problem of opioid addiction (psychological dependence)?**

The risk of iatrogenic addition is less than 0.1%. The psychological dependence seen with addiction is characterized by a compulsive behavior pattern involved in acquiring opioids for nonmedical psychic effects as opposed to pain relief. Abuse potential of narcotics is related to their relative μ-receptor activity.

Before surgery there should be a thorough and frank discussion about the pain and expectations about pain relief. An addict's maintenance treatment of methadone should be continued up to the day of surgery and restarted postoperatively. A fentanyl patch should be kept on throughout the perioperative period. Narcotic antagonists should be avoided. "PRN" injections should be avoided. Following surgery the patient should receive IV PCA for pain, specifically including a basal infusion, and be restarted on his or her scheduled oral opioid. Methadone is probably the best choice for an oral opioid. Continuous regional and neuraxial techniques as alternatives or adjunctive treatment should be used if possible, as these can be continued postoperatively. Acetaminophen and NSAIDs should also be given. For general anesthesia low-dose ketamine infusion intraoperatively has been used as an adjunctive pain therapy. Consideration must be made for the patient's tolerance to "usual" doses of opioids, as higher doses of opioid may be needed to produce the same pharmacologic effect.

For addicts already withdrawn from narcotics prior to surgery, do not premedicate with a narcotic. General, regional, and neuraxial anesthesia is appropriate. Narcotic antagonists butorphanol and nalbuphine are good analgesics. Adjunct analgesics such as clonidine and NSAIDs should be given if not otherwise contraindicated.

Key Terms

Acute cocaine toxicity
Addiction: definition
Adding local anesthetics to epidural opioid infusion; effects
Anesthesiologist drug abuse: fentanyl
Anesthesiologist: substance abuse
Catecholamine: chronic cocaine abuse
Cellular mechanisms of opioid action
Cocaine: mechanism of action

Codeine-active metabolite
Codeine: pharmacogenetics
Complications of fentanyl
Drug interactions: cocaine
ECG: high-dose opioids
Epidural morphine: respiratory depression
Epidural opioid analgesics: mechanism
Intrathecal versus epidural morphine
Meperidine toxicity

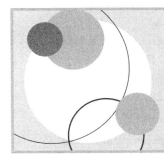

Orthopedic Surgery

*Sticks and stones may break my bones, but words will make me go in a
corner and cry by myself for hours.*
Eric Idle

○ **During which orthopedic procedures is there a risk of venous air embolism?**

Air embolism can occur whenever a blood vessel is open and a pressure gradient exists favoring entry of gas. This may occur during any procedure where the operative field is above the level of the heart, especially if the distance is >5 cm (cervical spine surgery in the sitting position, shoulder surgery in the beach chair position, spine surgery in the prone position, and hip surgery in the lateral position), when sinuses are open (after bone cement removal during revision of total hip arthroplasty), with a large gravitational gradient and low central venous filling pressure and from the pressurization of the cement when it is placed at a site without protection of the circulation by pneumatic tourniquet (endoprosthesis insertions into the femur), and use of hydrogen peroxide for the irrigation of open wounds, especially in closed spaces. Only 10 mL of 6% hydrogen peroxide irrigant can produce 200 mL of gas.

○ **A 45-year-old male patient is scheduled for lumbar discectomy in the prone position. After irrigation of the surgical wound with 25 mL 3% hydrogen peroxide the patient suddenly develops hypoxia with a decrease in end-tidal carbon dioxide and a "mill-wheel" murmur on cardiac auscultation. What is the most likely diagnosis?**

Oxygen venous embolism. Hydrogen peroxide is degraded by catalase from human tissues into gaseous oxygen.

○ **Describe the EKG findings of venous air embolism.**

Sinus tachycardia, right axis deviation, right ventricular strain, and ST depression. In healthy humans, 5–8 mL/kg of air is needed to obstruct the right ventricle and pulmonary artery. Venous air may move paradoxically from the pulmonary artery to the systemic circulation (cardiac defects with right-to-left shunting or transpulmonary passage). As little as 0.5 mL of air may cause coronary artery occlusion with ST elevation.

○ **What is the management of acute venous air embolism?**

Prevent further air entry:
- Notify surgeon to flood or pack the field or terminate central line placement and clamp the line.
- Apply jugular compression.
- Lower the patient's head into the Trendelenburg position.
- If feasible, rotate the patient toward the left lateral decubitus position.

Remove intravascular air and treat hemodynamic consequences:

- Aspirate the right heart catheter from the distal port of the central line and attempt to remove air.
- Administer 100% oxygen and intubate for respiratory distress or hypoxemia.
- Discontinue nitrous oxide.
- Circulatory collapse: external chest compressions and fluids/pressors/inotropes.
- Hyperbaric oxygen therapy.

○ **During repair of a femur fracture in a 60-year-old woman, the patient suddenly develops profound hypotension, unresponsive to 5 mg and then 10 mg of IV ephedrine. Her heart rate increases from 72 to 150 bpm accompanied by a new intraventricular conduction delay in lead II and a decrease in end-tidal CO_2. Hypotension persists with the development of severe central cyanosis of the upper thorax and head. What is the most likely diagnosis and what are your treatment options?**

Right ventricular dysfunction from acute pulmonary embolism. Hemodynamic support (fluids, 100% oxygen, inotropic vasoactive agents: dobutamine, milrinone, norepinephrine), invasive monitoring, TEE diagnosis (acute right atrial and ventricular dilation and hypokinesis; systolic septal flattening; clot in the superior vena cava, RV, and PA; altered flow through the PA; normal LV function with decreased filling; tricuspid regurgitation; changes in the right to left ventricular end-diastolic area ratio), heparin IV, centrally administered thrombolytic drugs, Greenfield filter, embolectomy by catheter or surgery.

○ **Describe the clinical manifestations and treatment of fat embolism associated with closed long bone fractures.**

Classic presentation consists of an asymptomatic interval of 12–48 hours followed by pulmonary and neurologic manifestations combined with a petechial rash that appears on the upper anterior portion of the body (pathognomonic sign). A fulminant form may present as acute cor pulmonale, respiratory failure, and/or embolic phenomena leading to death within a few hours of injury. Laboratory tests are nonspecific. Chest x-ray may show a snow storm appearance with increased pulmonary markings and dilatation of the right heart.

Fat embolism syndrome is clinically not so apparent and remains a diagnosis of exclusion.

Treatment is supportive and may be prevented by early fixation of long bone fractures.

○ **What is the predominant cause of mortality following total joint replacement [Horlocker, 2011. See reference on page 528; Geerts et al., 2008. See reference on page 528]?**

Fatal pulmonary embolism; rates as high as 3–5% have been reported.

○ **List signs of intraoperative pulmonary embolism.**

Increased pulmonary arterial pressure, increased central venous pressure, right ventricular strain, decreased cardiac output with decreased PCWP and decreased end-tidal PCO_2, increased arterial PCO_2 due to hypoventilation (increased dead space), hypoxemia, pulmonary edema, and bronchoconstriction with wheezing. Signs may be subtle or can present with cardiocirculatory collapse depending on size and location of pulmonary embolus.

○ **Does echocardiography have a role in the diagnosis of pulmonary embolism?**

Echocardiography can be helpful in the diagnosis of pulmonary embolism, although the gold standard is still pulmonary angiography. TEE findings may include evidence of acute right ventricular pressure overload with right ventricular dilation and hypokinesis, pulmonary hypertension, and the paradoxical motion of the interventricular septum due to a shift by a dilated right ventricle or direct identification of thrombotic masses in the pulmonary arteries or floating intracavitary thrombi. Results of TEE are highly dependent on the expertise of the echocardiographer.

The technetium–xenon lung scan, which attempts to identify mismatches between the lung ventilation and perfusion, is still widely utilized. A negative scan can effectively exclude the diagnosis and a high probability scan does carry a very good predictive value, but an intermediate probability scan carries a 30% chance of pulmonary embolism. Contrast spiral computerized tomography (CT) is now the preferred method of diagnosis of acute pulmonary embolism and it carries greater than 90% positive and negative predictive values. Although it is not the gold standard, it is much easier to obtain and does not require an angiography suite as pulmonary angiography would require. The adjunct blood test D-dimer enzyme-linked immunosorbent assay has a very high negative predictive value (greater than 99%) and can help exclude pulmonary embolism as a diagnosis, especially in patients with low or moderate pretest probability. However, in patients with a high pretest probability, imagine should be performed instead of D-dimer testing [Tapson, 2008. See reference on page 528].

○ **What clinical findings would you expect to find with a pulmonary embolism following deflation of a pneumatic tourniquet placed on the thigh? What is the mechanism?**

Sudden, unexplained hypotension, hypoxemia, and/or bronchospasm (wheeze, increase in peak airway pressures, decrease in SpO_2).

A decrease in end-tidal CO_2 from increased dead space ventilation is suggestive, but not specific. Should invasive monitoring be in place, an elevation of the central venous pressure and pulmonary artery pressure may be observed from mechanical obstruction of the right ventricle, pulmonary hypertension, acute ischemia from coronary embolization, or combinations thereof.

Significant pulmonary embolism is rare, but has been reported with pneumatic tourniquet inflation (preexisting clot) and deflation (decreased fibrinolysis or release of plasminogen activators secondary to the inflated tourniquet or the metabolic conditions distal to it). Patients at risk for upper leg and pelvic DVT include advanced age, bed rest, prior DVT or pulmonary embolism, morbid obesity, venous insufficiency, oral contraceptive use among young female patients, and malignancy. The risk of embolism from immobilization increases with time. Embolization of fat, marrow, or air may occur from high-volume and pressurized cement use, especially in the femoral canal.

○ **In general, what tourniquet pressures are required to prevent bleeding during orthopedic surgery?**

A cuff pressure 100 mm Hg above a patient's measured systolic pressure is adequate for the thigh, while 50 mm Hg above systolic pressure is adequate for the arm.

Arbitrary numbers such as 250 and 300 mm Hg are often selected. Should hypertensive episodes occur, cuff pressure should be increased accordingly. A general rule is to select a pressure between 1.5 and 2 times the average anticipated systolic pressure. If the patient's systolic pressure exceeds the inflation pressure of the tourniquet, obstruction to venous outflow will occur (venous tourniquet). Inflation to very high pressures may create a bloodless field but cause disruption of the microvascular anatomy of the underlying muscle.

○ **What are the risks of using tourniquets for extremity surgery?**

Neurologic injury resulting from inflation of a tourniquet is a function of tourniquet pressure and the duration of inflation. The recommended pressure is 100 mm Hg above systolic pressure or a tourniquet pressure of 250 mm Hg while maintaining the systolic pressure at 90–100 mm Hg. Tourniquet time should be less than 2 hours in the upper extremity and 4 hours in the lower extremity to avoid ischemic tissue damage.

○ **What are contraindications of tourniquet use?**

Absolute contraindications:
- Sickle cell disease or other hemoglobinopathies that change configuration in response to acidosis or hypoxia
- Severe peripheral vascular disease with arterial spasm or vasculitis
- Ongoing ischemia in the operative limb

Relative contraindications:

- Existing peripheral neuropathy
- Chronic vascular insufficiency of the limb
- Synthetic or venous vascular graft for dialysis (thrombosis risk)
- Existing venous insufficiency from either lymph node dissection (mastectomy) or vein harvest for revascularization or radiation therapy
- Proven infection in the operative extremity, as both acute pulmonary edema and cardiac arrest have been reported after tourniquet release
- An extremity with a tumor where tumor cells may be introduced into the systemic circulation

○   **What are the systemic effects of tourniquet release during limb surgery under general anesthesia?**

Depending on the duration of tourniquet inflation (especially longer than 30 minutes), and whether an upper or lower limb is isolated (the effect is significantly greater in the lower extremity), the following hemodynamic and metabolic effects may be noted:

- Transient drop in mean arterial pressure and CVP that may remain significantly depressed up to 15 minutes postrelease caused by volume shift back to the limb on deflation of the tourniquet, postischemic reactive vasodilation with decrease in SVR, myocardial depression, and bleeding from nonligated vessels.
- Increase in heart rate 6–12 bpm.
- Transient increase in cerebral blood flow and decrease in cerebral perfusion pressure.
- Decrease in core body temperature of 0.7°C within 90 seconds of deflation of lower limb tourniquet.
- Release of vasoactive substances (lactate, prostaglandin, and bradykinin).
- Reduction in pH and serum bicarbonate.
- Elevation of potassium, lactic acid, lactic acid dehydrogenase, and creatinine kinase.
- Transient decrease in central venous oxygen tension, but systemic hypoxemia is unusual.
- Acute rise in end-tidal CO_2, with peak levels observed within 1 minute, persisting for 10 minutes.
- Changes in arterial pH, PaO_2, $PaCO_2$, lactate, and potassium normalize within 30 minutes.

○   **Prior to tourniquet deflation in a trauma patient who may have associated blunt head injury, what considerations should be given to prevent secondary injury to the brain?**

Intravenous fluid administration with hyperventilation and vasopressor agents, as needed, just before and for 10–15 minutes following tourniquet deflation may ameliorate the associated hypotension and hypercarbia that could produce an increase in cerebral blood flow and ICP, with a decrease in cerebral perfusion pressure that would worsen the cerebral injury.

○   **How does recovery of transient hypotension and hypercapnia after release of a pneumatic thigh tourniquet differ in general anesthesia with mechanically controlled ventilation (CMV) when compared with regional anesthesia (epidural or spinal) with conscious spontaneous respiration?**

The recovery of hypotension is faster in general anesthesia with CMV than regional anesthesia with conscious spontaneous respiration. The reverse is true for recovery from hypercapnia.

○   **What is the explanation for a gradual increase in blood pressure during application of a pneumatic tourniquet for limb surgery?**

The mechanism is not completely understood. It has been suggested increased blood pressure represent activation of sympathetic nervous system in response to development of tourniquet pain. Plasma norepinephrine levels increase in parallel with arterial pressure during tourniquet inflation. [Deloughry and Griffiths, 2009. See reference on page 528].

○ **Describe tourniquet pain. What modalities of treatment have been proposed?**

Tourniquet pain is described as dull, burning, deep, poorly localized, and aching pain that increases steadily until it becomes unbearable. It develops in up to 66% of patients during limb surgery under regional anesthesia, 30–60 minutes after cuff inflation. Tourniquet pain is hypothesized to be due to impulse propagation by small, unmyelinated, slow-conduction C nerve fibers and pain from tissue damage due to capillary and muscle injury secondary to tissue acidosis. Suggested treatments includes addition of IV analgesia and sedation, addition of nitrous oxide analgesia, addition of adjuvants (ketamine, clonidine, opioids) to local anesthetics has been investigated with positive results, double cuff with distal cuff over anesthetized area, intercostobrachial and musculocutaneous block for the upper arm, sympathetic block, EMLA, choice of bupivacaine versus tetracaine for neuraxial anesthesia, and addition of morphine to local anesthetics that may increase tolerance to tourniquet pain. When tourniquet pain occurs, most interventions are ineffective. Deflation of the cuff is the definitive treatment.

○ **What advantage may regional anesthesia provide over general anesthesia for total hip replacement [Buckley, 1993. See reference on page 528]?**

- Lower total blood loss.
- Less risk of transfusion-related morbidity and cost.
- Lower incidence of deep venous thrombosis.
- Less acute postoperative confusion (not significant at 3 months postoperatively).
- Hypotensive epidural anesthesia may improve the quality of the interface between methylmethacrylate and bone.
- May improve neutrophil activity.

○ **How does hypotensive anesthesia affect the quality of cement–bone fixation during total hip replacement?**

Hypotensive anesthesia has radiographically been demonstrated to improve the quality of cement–bone fixation, as the quality of fixation at the cement–bone interface is improved if there is an absence of blood across the cancellous bone during application of the cement.

○ **How may profound hypotension and hypoxia result from the employment of polymethylmethacrylate cement and the insertion of a cemented femoral prosthesis during total hip replacement?**

Profound hypotension and circulatory collapse occurs in less than 5% of long stem and revision total hip arthroplasties [Kassim et al., 2002. See reference on page 528]. This occurrence may result from the solubilization of fat and embolization of fat, air, or bone marrow following relocation of the hip joint and the unkinking of femoral vein. Also possible but unproven is a direct action of the cement (monomer, and to a lesser extent the small-chain polymer), which may cause vasodilation and/or direct myocardial depression, degranulation of mast cells, and the release of histamine.

○ **Anterior atlantoaxial subluxation is a common finding in patients with rheumatoid arthritis (25%). Are there additional airway structures that may be affected?**

Yes. Subaxial subluxation, ankylosis of the cervical spine causing a fixed flexion deformity, osteoporosis (chronic steroid usage), cricoarytenoid involvement (dyspnea, SOB, hoarseness, obstruction), temporomandibular (TM) joint involvement, and obstruction from laryngeal amyloidosis and rheumatoid nodules.

○   **What are the considerations in securing the airway in a patient with rheumatoid arthritis who is to undergo general anesthesia for total knee replacement?**

Ankylosis of the TM joint, if present, leads to limited mouth opening. Ankylosis and fixation of the cervical vertebrae will result in severely limited range of motion of the neck. Laxity or disruption of the cruciform ligament of the axis leads to mobility of the odontoid process within the spinal canal. Anterior atlantoaxial subluxation occurs in approximately 20–40% of patients. Posterior subluxation, occurring during neck flexion, is far less common, and can result in severe neurologic injury, including quadriplegia [Chang and Paget, 1993. See reference on page 528]. Arthritis of the cricoarytenoid joint is fairly common, which can present with a foreign body feeling and painful swallowing or speaking. It can progress to hoarseness and stridor, which may occur because of swelling and fixation of the vocal cords.

○   **An 8-year-old male suffered a fractured right forearm and femur during a motor vehicle accident. His past medical history includes severe juvenile rheumatoid arthritis. What anesthetic considerations must be made for his medical condition?**

These pediatric patients are apt to develop fusion of the cervical spine and perichondrium of epiphyseal plates. Endotracheal intubation may therefore be complicated by a fixed neck and hypoplastic mandible. Axillary brachial plexus block may be difficult if this patient is unable to abduct his injured upper extremity. Conduction blockade may be technically difficult if he is frozen in a characteristic lumbar lordosis. Exaggerated neck flexion and inability of the patient to rotate his head may make placement of a central line via an internal jugular approach difficult to achieve.

○   **How can postoperative ulnar neuropathy be avoided in a patient undergoing hand surgery?**

Padding and proper positioning of both the operative and nonoperative upper extremity are important so that direct compression of the ulnar nerve immediately above the elbow and in the olecranon notch does not occur. Supination, as opposed to pronation of the forearm, is desirable. Ongoing vigilance is mandatory, as movement caused by the surgery may alter correct positioning. However, all postoperative ulnar neuropathies are not preventable, and may occur without any evident cause.

○   **What is the concentration of epinephrine that corresponds to a 1:200,000 dilution?**

5 μg/mL. 1 g/mL = 1,000,000 μg/mL. Divide 1,000,000 μg by dilution factor of 1:200,000 (1,000,000/200,000) = 5. (Or 1:200,000 = 1 G in 200,000 mL; therefore, 5 μg in 1 mL.)

○   **A 35-year-old male is scheduled to undergo the removal of a protruding right fibular screw, originally placed 8 months prior, during an open reduction and internal fixation of the right ankle following a skiing accident. The area surrounding the protruding screw appears to be infected. Why is the injection of bupivacaine 0.25% around this area unlikely to produce an effective infiltrative nerve block?**

Local anesthetics are weak bases and cross nerve membranes to provide local anesthesia when in a lipid-soluble, nonionized form at physiological pH. An injection into an acidic, infected area will provide poor-quality anesthesia, as the predominant fraction of the anesthetic will exist in an ionized form that will not cross membranes.

○ **An active and otherwise healthy 80-year-old female with osteoarthritis is to undergo general anesthesia with propofol, rocuronium, sevoflurane, air, and O_2, for left hip replacement. Following induction and endotracheal intubation, the lungs are easily ventilated bilaterally. After she is placed in the right lateral decubitus position, however, lung inflation requires high peak airway pressures. On auscultation, breath sounds are faint; wheezing is heard. What diagnoses do you entertain, and what immediate action(s) is (are) appropriate?**

Consider light anesthesia versus migration or mechanical obstruction of the endotracheal tube. The patient may also have underlying hyperactive airways disease.

Visually inspect whether the airway is patent as this is most likely from the description of little airway movement (breath sounds are faint). Listen to breath sounds bilaterally. If an obstruction/mainstem intubation is not immediately apparent, note the vital signs, and deepen the patient's anesthesia with the thought that bronchospasm is the result of light anesthesia. If that is insufficient, reposition the patient supine, reauscultate, and ensure patency and proper positioning of the endotracheal tube (fiber-optic inspection or extubate and reintubate).

○ **An 8-year old male with severe cerebral palsy presents for bilateral, femoral flexor tendon releases under general anesthesia. What are the pertinent anesthetic considerations?**

- Chronic malnutrition and dehydration.
- Mild renal impairment.
- Intravenous access may be difficult if contractures are severe, or if the patient is uncooperative.
- An agitated or uncooperative patient may be dangerous to the health care team.
- Positioning may be challenging.
- Aspiration is a risk due to chronic gastroesophageal reflux, agitation, and bulbar palsy with incompetent airway reflexes.
- Chronic aspiration may lead to pulmonary dysfunction.
- Succinylcholine in this case is not contraindicated.
- Postoperative risk of respiratory depression from narcotics and residual anesthetic effects.
- Nursing considerations related to limb spasticity.

○ **A 4-year-old boy with osteogenesis imperfecta and multiple long bone fractures is to undergo placement of bilateral femoral and tibial Sheffield expanding rods under general anesthesia. What are the considerations in securing this patient's airway?**

Head positioning for mask ventilation and intubation may be complicated by iatrogenic cervical fractures. Positioning of the head is furthermore made difficult by the likelihood that the patient may have an enlarged head and atlantoaxial instability. As these patients present with brittle teeth, placement of an oral airway, performance of laryngoscopy, and endotracheal intubation must be accomplished with great care, as teeth are easily broken.

○ **T/F: Neurologic complications after regional anesthesia for total knee arthroplasty (TKA) are greater than in patients having general anesthesia.**

Controversial. Peripheral nerve injury (PNI) is associated with TKA, occurring in 0.01–10% of patients. One 20-year cohort study [Jacob et al., 2011. See reference on page 528] reported that type of anesthesia, specifically neuraxial anesthesia or peripheral nerve blockade (RA), was not associated with PNI in patients undergoing TKA. However, patients undergoing peripheral nerve blockade and experiencing PNI may be less likely to have complete neurologic recovery than patients not undergoing RA. Age, bilateral procedures, and total tourniquet time were independent variables associated with risk for PNI.

○   **Describe the major risk factors for, diagnosis, and treatment of compartment syndrome.**

Compartment syndrome can occur wherever a compartment is present. This includes lower extremity, upper extremity, abdomen, and buttock. Almost any injury can cause this.

The major risk factor is orthopedic trauma, particularly tibial fractures. Clinical diagnosis is based on the presence of the "Five P's"—palpable pulse, pallor, paralysis, paresthesia, and pain. Only the latter two are reliable in the diagnosis of compartment syndrome. To confirm the diagnosis, compartment pressures can be measured using a pressure transducer module with a simple intravenous catheter and needle. Treatment is fasciotomy to relieve the pressure, usually attempted when the intracompartmental pressure is >30 cm H_2O.

Anterior compartment syndrome occurs in front of the shin when the tibialis anterior muscle becomes too big for the sheath.

If left untreated, tissue necrosis, permanent functional impairment, renal failure, and death may occur.

Key Terms

Anterior compartment syndrome
Compartment syndrome: diagnosis
Hip fracture: fat embolism diagnosis/management
Orthopedic surgery: risk of air embolism
Pulmonary embolism: diagnosis/tests

Total knee replacement: regional anesthesia technique
Tourniquet deflation: physiological effect
Tourniquet: metabolic effects
Tourniquet pain: management
Treatment of intraoperative pulmonary embolism

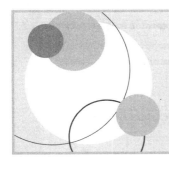

Outpatient Surgery

*We are made wise not by the recollection of our past,
but by the responsibility for our future.*
George Bernard Shaw

○ **What role might oral clonidine play in the preoperative period?**

As an alpha-2-adrenergic agonist, oral clonidine (3 μg/kg) can reduce anesthetic requirements by virtue of its analgesic effects, and has been used to provide sedation and anxiolysis while reducing the lability of intraoperative blood pressure.

○ **List types of medications that generally should be discontinued or withheld before general anesthesia.**

Oral hypoglycemic agents (1 day), all anticoagulants (coumadin 3–5 days, heparin 4 hours, Lovenox – low-molecular-weight heparin – 24 hours), and antiplatelet drugs such as Plavix (clopidogrel bisulfate) 5–7 days, depending on the surgery, and the reason for its administration. Amiodarone, angiotensin-converting enzyme inhibitors (ACEI, e.g., enalapril), and angiotensin II receptor antagonists (ARA, e.g., irbesartan) are still controversial issues.

After warfarin therapy is stopped, it takes about 4 days for the international normalized ratio (INR) to reach 1.5 in almost all patients. If a patient's INR is between 2.0 and 3.0, four scheduled doses of warfarin should be withheld to allow the INR to fall spontaneously to 1.5 or less before surgery. Warfarin should be withheld for a longer period if the INR is normally maintained above 3.0 or if it is necessary to keep it at a lower level (i.e., <1.3). The INR should be measured a day before surgery to ensure adequate progress in the reversal of anticoagulation [Horlocker, 2010. See reference on page 528].

○ **Why is history alone a poor method of assessing coronary artery disease in diabetic patients?**

There is a high incidence of silent (painless) myocardial ischemia and infarction in diabetic patients with hypertension and diabetic autonomic neuropathy (early satiety, lack of sweating, reduced sinus arrhythmia and beat-to-beat variability of the heart rate, orthostatic hypotension, impotence, resting tachycardia, nocturnal diarrhea, peripheral neuropathy). The type II diabetic patient has the same risk of fatal or nonfatal MI and death from cardiovascular causes as a nondiabetic with prior MI.

○ **What is the best anesthetic technique for a high-risk cardiac ambulatory patient undergoing noncardiac surgery: general or regional?**

There are no randomized prospective data comparing the two types of anesthesia in the high-risk cardiac patient undergoing noncardiac surgery that have ever shown a significant outcome difference [Rodgers, 2000. See reference on page 528].

○ **How would you attenuate the hemodynamic response to intubation in high-risk cardiac ambulatory patients?**

Attenuation of this pressor response may be achieved by avoiding prolonged laryngoscopy and blunting the stimulation of airway instrumentation with ultrashort acting opiates, beta-blockers, and IV or endotracheal lidocaine. 0.5 mg/kg of esmolol is an excellent choice.

○ **What important actions of nitroglycerin are beneficial in treating myocardial ischemia or elevated pulmonary artery pressures?**

For ischemia: coronary vasodilation (redistributes blood flow from epicardial to subendocardial vessels and relieves abnormal coronary artery vasoconstriction) and venodilation, thereby reducing preload and subendocardial wall tension. The latter is thought to be most important. For increased PA pressures, decreased RV preload, and pulmonary venous dilation, are helpful.

○ **What is the adverse effect of tachycardia in a patient with mitral stenosis?**

Tachycardia decreases left ventricular diastolic filling leading to increased left atrial pressure, with an increased risk of developing pulmonary edema.

○ **What are the anesthetic goals of patients with mitral regurgitation?**

Anesthetic management should aim to decrease the regurgitant fraction by promoting forward flow and decreasing stretch of the mitral valve annulus:

Maintain or increase heart rate (avoid bradycardia).

Maintain contractility—dobutamine is the choice if an inotrope is required.

Control atrial fibrillation—a common associated problem.

Decrease SVR.

Decrease pulmonary vascular resistance (avoid hypercapnia, hypoxia, nitrous oxide, and pulmonary vasoconstrictors).

Maintain preload based on clinical response to fluid challenge but do not overfill the heart as this will stretch the annulus and increase regurgitation.

○ **What is the most common form of valvular heart disease in ambulatory surgical patients?**

Mitral valve prolapse.

○ **What is the purpose of preoperative screening in the ambulatory pediatric patient?**

To ensure that the child has no active respiratory tract infection or other preexisting condition that requires additional investigation or treatment.

○ **What are some adverse effects of extended fasting times prior to elective surgery?**

Long fasting prior to an elective operation not only is uncomfortable for the patient but also has detrimental effects. It causes thirst, hunger, irritability, noncompliance, and resentment in adult patients. Prolonged fasting is especially deleterious in children since it may also produce dehydration, hypovolemia, and hypoglycemia.

○ **Are patients who take clear liquids closer to their surgery at greater risk of aspiration syndrome?**

No, it appears that patients who have been drinking are at no greater risk of aspiration syndrome should regurgitation occur [ASA Practice Guidelines for Preoperative Fasting, 2011. See reference on page 528].

○ **What advantages might there be to maintaining anesthesia with propofol instead of volatile agents in pediatric ambulatory patients?**

Propofol induction and maintenance of anesthesia in pediatric outpatients has been shown to be associated with less postoperative emesis. Not only is this drug safe in children, but it also appears to be associated with a decreased incidence of airway obstruction. Thus, propofol is a useful alternative to volatile agent anesthetics in pediatric anesthesia.

○ **What are the advantages of using propofol instead of thiopental for induction and/or maintenance in pediatric patients undergoing ambulatory surgery?**

It has been shown that the continuous infusion of propofol is a well-tolerated anesthetic technique in children. The speed and quality of recovery after propofol is superior to that observed after thiopental and/or halothane administration, and is associated with an extremely low incidence of vomiting.

○ **What are three reasons for such widespread popularity of propofol in ambulatory anesthesia?**

(1) Propofol has the shortest time to recovery of all IV induction agents. (2) It has a lower incidence of postoperative nausea and vomiting. (3) It has a high degree of patient satisfaction, due to the rapid return to a clear-headed state, minimal side effects, and elation produced by the drug.

○ **What is a reliable alternative induction technique in a 5-year-old struggling child who refuses the mask and cannot be managed by an IV induction because of lack of accessible veins?**

Ketamine 4–8 mg/kg IM has been shown to be a useful drug for induction of the uncooperative child (2–4 mg/kg IM is the sedation and analgesia dose). The onset time is short, and the recovery time is not prolonged unless larger doses of ketamine (>5 mg/kg) are combined with a volatile anesthetic. Recurrent illusions, vivid dreams, and flashbacks have been reported several weeks after ketamine administration in children. However, dysphoric symptoms are less common in pediatric compared with adult patients. (Pediatric IV induction dose of ketamine: 1–2 mg/kg.)

○ **What type of patients may be best suited for oral ketamine?**

The oral administration of ketamine (or IM) either for analgesia or to induce anesthesia is a recognized technique in situations that may be hazardous for staff to approach a patient or when the patient is distressed (i.e., severely mentally handicapped individuals who are frightened, unruly, and uncooperative). The use of small volumes of attractive fluid to camouflage ketamine (10 mg/kg) may help to overcome the problem, especially with thirsty patients who have been fasting.

○ **Which nondepolarizing neuromuscular blocking agent might be best in an ambulatory patient who might be particularly sensitive to blood pressure changes?**

Vecuronium and cisatracurium are the only neuromuscular blocking agents essentially devoid of cardiovascular side effects.

○ **What are the benefits of intraoperative analgesics?**

The intraoperative use of analgesic drugs improves hemodynamic stability, decreases the anesthetic requirement, provides for a more rapid emergence from anesthesia, and decreases postoperative pain and discomfort. Adequate pain control achieved prior to entry to PACU decreases discharge times.

○ **Are there advantages in administering morphine instead of fentanyl for postoperative pain in ambulatory patients?**

Morphine has been shown to produce a better quality of analgesia (lower pain scores and less oral analgesic use) than fentanyl in ambulatory surgical patients, with no difference in recovery times or discharge times. It is associated with increased nausea and vomiting, especially after discharge.

○ **What is usually the etiology for serious reactions to local anesthetics?**

Inadvertent intravascular injections of large volumes causing CNS and rarely cardiac toxicity.

○ **How can you decrease the incidence of toxic symptoms and increase the percentage of successful blocks while performing intravenous regional anesthesia?**

A successful block can be achieved by elevating the arm and exsanguinating with an elastic Esmarch bandage applied from distal to proximal, inflating the upper arm tourniquet to a pressure of at least 300 mm Hg, and then injecting a low concentration and high volume of local anesthetic (e.g., 0.5% lidocaine at 3 mg/kg) over at least 90 seconds, into a vein on the distal dorsum of the hand.

Patient safety depends on the integrity of the pneumatic tourniquet, which must be inflated and maintained for a safe interval (>30 minutes), regardless of the duration of the surgery (usually 1 hour or less). Use of a double tourniquet is ideal. Care must be taken in deflating the tourniquet to minimize the CNS toxicity from a bolus release of local anesthetic into the venous system. For short surgeries, the tourniquet should be deflated for 1–2 seconds and then reinflated, checking for CNS signs between each deflation–inflation sequence (only if done less than 30–40 minutes due to lack of time for diffusion to occur out of vasculature). Drug choice is usually 0.5% lidocaine, avoiding the more cardiotoxic agents, that is, bupivacaine. Lidocaine 0.5% should be prepared from a 1% solution by dilution with normal saline, avoiding dextrose-containing solutions which increase the incidence of thrombophlebitis. Midazolam IV should be used as a sedative given its anxiolytic and anticonvulsant properties that raise the seizure threshold.

○ **What is the best tourniquet deflation technique after intravenous regional anesthesia to minimize the peak blood level of local anesthetics?**

Cyclic deflation–reinflation techniques have been shown to be superior to single deflation in minimizing local anesthetic toxicity. Although cyclic techniques do not reduce the peak plasma concentration of local anesthetics, they significantly prolong the time to reach peak concentration. If the cuff is released after 10 minutes, about 30% of the dose is released immediately in the first flush. After 45 minutes, drug release is much slower; 30% of the total dose release takes almost 4 minutes. Drugs released must first pass through lungs, protecting the CNS and heart (extravascular pH of lung < plasma causing ion trapping).

○ **What are the advantages of using intravenous regional anesthesia (Bier block)?**

Advantages include that it is easily performed, is reliable and safe, has a high degree of patient satisfaction, and rapidly resolves with tourniquet release.

○ **What type of procedures would a Bier block be appropriate for?**

Procedures distal to the elbow requiring an arm tourniquet time of less than 60 minutes, and surgical time not exceeding 90 minutes.

○ **What are contraindications to the use of an intravenous regional anesthetic?**

All contraindications and relative contraindications to the use of pneumatic tourniquets.

Intravenous regional anesthesia should be avoided in patients with severe peripheral vascular disease, and Raynaud's disease, where extended peripheral ischemia may occur. Sickle cell disease or trait is of concern, where sickling is promoted in acidic, hypoxemic, cold, or ischemic environments. Patients with significant systolic hypertension, heart block, seizure disorder, hepatic disease, or cellulitis at the tourniquet site should also not be considered candidates for intravenous regional anesthesia.

○ **What is the mechanism of action of IV regional anesthesia (Bier block)?**

The exact mechanism of action for intravenous regional anesthesia is not clear. There may be multiple mechanisms responsible for producing analgesia and anesthesia. A large volume of dilute anesthetic injected into the extremity is required to produce the block.

○ **List at least three advantages of spinal anesthesia over lumbar epidural anesthesia in the outpatient setting.**

It is technically easier and more rapidly performed, has a faster onset time, has a higher success rate, is less likely to be associated with intravascular injection and toxicity, and is more reliable in achieving complete sensory block, especially sacral segments.

○ **Why are medications such as pilocarpine beneficial in patients with glaucoma?**

Pilocarpine causes miosis that enlarges the radius of the spaces of Fontana thereby facilitating aqueous humor outflow.

○ **How do vomiting, straining, and coughing increase IOP?**

All three maneuvers increase systemic venous pressure that reduces outflow of aqueous humor, which can increase IOP 40 mm Hg or more.

○ **What effect do CNS depressant drugs have on IOP?**

Virtually all CNS depressants, including barbiturates, neuroleptics, narcotics, tranquilizers, and hypnotics, lower IOP in both normal and glaucomatous eyes.

○ **What effect does respiratory acidosis have on IOP?**

Respiratory acidosis increases both choroidal blood volume and IOP, presumably by retinal vasodilation occurring in conjunction with cerebral vasodilation.

○ **What effect does hypothermia have on IOP?**

Hypothermia lowers IOP by reducing aqueous humor production and vasoconstriction.

○ **Describe the oculocardiac reflex arc.**

Trigeminal–vagal reflex, described by Aschner and Dagnini (1908).

This reflex arc consists of a trigeminal afferent (ciliary branch of the ophthalmic division) and vagal efferent limb. It can be elicited by direct pressure on the globe and traction on all extraocular muscles (the medial rectus was initially observed to be the most potent, now questionable) as well as ocular manipulation and ocular pain. The reflex may also be triggered by a retrobulbar block, by ocular trauma, and by direct pressure on tissue remaining in the orbital apex. Sinus bradycardia is the most common manifestation, followed by a potpourri of arrhythmias.

○ **What are potential maneuvers to obtund or abolish the oculocardiac reflex?**

Inclusion of IM anticholinergic drug (atropine or glycopyrrolate) in the premedication regimen for oculocardiac prophylaxis is ineffective. (Near-complete vagal block in the adult requires 2–3 mg of atropine or 0.03–0.05 mg/kg and peak action occurs 30 minutes after administration.) During pediatric strabismus surgery, current popular practice favors administration of atropine 0.02 mg/kg IV before commencing surgery. Ask the surgeon to stop ocular manipulation immediately and deepen the level of anesthesia (pain stimulus). The OCR tends to fatigue, but if the arrhythmia is malignant, the patient is unstable, or the reflex persists, IV atropine should be given. Atropine may cause more serious and refractory arrhythmias than the reflex itself. Local infiltration of the recti muscle may successfully block the reflex.

○ **What is the most likely cause of bradycardia seen during eye surgery?**

Always suspect the oculocardiac reflex—a trigeminal vagal reflex. Never forget possible hypoxia though.

○ **Describe the afferent limb of the oculocardiac reflex.**

Transmission occurs via the trigeminal nerve, through the ciliary ganglion to the ophthalmic division of the trigeminal nerve and from there the gasserian ganglion to the sensory nucleus of the fourth ventricle.

○ **Describe the efferent limb of the oculocardiac reflex.**

The vagus nerve carries output from the sensory nucleus of the fourth ventricle.

○ **Stimulation of the oculocardiac reflex causes what cardiovascular perturbations?**

Bradycardia, nodal rhythm, premature ventricular contractions, ventricular fibrillation, or asystole.

○ **What is the most important therapy for bradycardia due to the oculocardiac reflex?**

Stop the stimulus!

○ **After you stop the stimulus how do you treat persistent bradycardia and prevent further episodes?**

Give atropine (or other anticholinergic), ventilate and oxygenate, and deepen the level of anesthesia.

○ **What are some intraoperative and postoperative problems associated with strabismus surgery?**

Oculocardiac reflex-induced dysrhythmias, postoperative nausea and vomiting, masseter spasm, and malignant hyperthermia (MH-susceptible persons often have localized areas of skeletal muscle weakness or other musculoskeletal abnormalities).

○ **What are some anesthetic considerations for pediatric cases in remote locations of the hospital?**

(1) The anesthetic technique must provide predictable, brief anesthesia of adequate depth and an immobile patient; (2) the anesthetics must be able to be safely given repeatedly with portable equipment; (3) a rapid awakening with short recovery time is desirable; (4) maintenance of a patent airway in a variety of body positions and during transport is mandatory; (5) provisions for standard monitoring are required for general anesthesia remote from the patient; and (6) minimizing psychological and physical trauma during the repeated procedures is desirable.

○ **Which radiological procedure has more scatter radiation, fluoroscopy or CT?**

Fluoroscopy.

○ **What safety precautions can anesthesiologists take to prevent excessive radiation exposure?**

Lead aprons, thyroid collars, lead glass screens, and treated glasses and goggles.

○ **What distance away from a radiation source is a bystander considered safe?**

Six feet of distance, equivalent to 2.5 mm of lead.

○ **What signs and symptoms might you see after contrast media administration?**

These hyperosmolar solutions may cause flushing, tachycardia, and nausea by releasing vasoactive substances.

During cerebral angiography – neurotoxic reactions: dizziness, convulsions, coma, hemiplegia, blindness, and aphasia. Allergic reactions: pruritus, burning on injection, mild skin rashes, wheezing, dyspnea, syncope, and cardiovascular collapse.

During coronary angiography – myocardial depression, coronary vasodilation, decrease in blood pH, and increase in serum osmolarity and allergic reactions (limit to 5 mL/kg).

Contrast agents may also cause osmotic diuresis, volume contraction, high urine osmolality, and nephropathy.

○ **How safe are patients with spinal fusion rods and limb prostheses in the magnetic resonance imaging (MRI) scanner?**

The concern would be attraction of ferromagnetic objects to the magnet (aluminum, titanium OK).

Generally these types of implants are not a problem, although temperature increases may be noted around metallic implants. Detailed lists of each manufacturer's implantable devices and their ferromagnetic properties have been published and should be consulted.

○ **What effect do magnetic fields have on pacemakers?**

The effects are variable. Potential problems include possible reed switch closure or damage, pacemaker inhibition, or reversion to an asynchronous mode. Programming changes, torque on the pacemaker itself, or development of voltage across the pacemaker inhibiting its discharge may also occur. MRI may deactivate implanted automatic cardiac defibrillators.

○ **Where should the pulse oximetry probe be placed in a patient having an MRI scan?**

The extremity as far as possible from the scanner (usually the foot) with the cable in a straight line and wrapped with aluminum to minimize RF artifact in the MRI image. Metal parts of the sensor have been known to cause patient burns, especially if the cable is wrapped around an extremity, increasing the strength of the magnetic field. All leads must be properly insulated, not permitted to loop within the magnetic core and separated from the patient's skin by thermal insulating padding. Pulse oximetry manufacturers have incorporated RF filters, ECG-locking facilities, and fiber-optic signal linking between the sensor and the monitor.

○ **Is it possible to monitor ECG during MRI scan?**

ECG telemetry and capnography systems cause minimal distortion of MRI signal. However, ECG cables must be shielded to prevent interference with the scanning. RF signals can induce voltage in the wire lead of unshielded electrodes and cause electrical shock hazards and burns to the patient.

○ **What are some advantages to the use of total intravenous anesthesia in remote locations?**

The difficulty of transporting an anesthesia machine to multiple locations is eliminated as there is no need to scavenge anesthetic gases, and a rapid emergence for prompt recovery and discharge can be anticipated.

○ **What anesthetic techniques are appropriate for a patient receiving liposuction (ultrasound-assisted lipoplasty [UAL])?**

Patients can receive general anesthesia, neuraxial anesthesia (although this is rarely used), or MAC with local infiltration of lidocaine (tumescent lidocaine injection technique).

○ **What dose of lidocaine is used during the tumescent technique?**

The original description of the technique documented the use of a dilute mixture of lidocaine (0.05–0.2%) and epinephrine (1:100,000); the dose of lidocaine was limited to 35 mg/kg.

○ **What is considered a toxic dose of lidocaine during the tumescent technique?**

The American Society for Dermatologic Surgery has issued a statement that lidocaine should not be used in doses greater than 55 mg/kg. However, individual patients may manifest symptoms of lidocaine overdose at significantly smaller doses [Gordley and Basu, 2006. See reference on page 528].

○ **What are the complications of the tumescent technique?**

The chief complication seen is lidocaine toxicity secondary to overdose. This typically manifests first with CNS symptoms such as dizziness, perioral numbness, and eventually seizures. Larger doses may precipitate cardiac arrhythmias or asystole. Other complications include allergic reactions (rare when amide local anesthetics are used), pulmonary edema (if there is too much absorption of the dilute lidocaine solution), or circulatory collapse (if too much volume is removed from the patient).

○ **What are major anesthetic challenges for UAL?**

Estimating blood loss, fluid and electrolyte imbalances, pulmonary edema, pulmonary embolism, and determining the appropriate time for discharge home or to a 23-hour observation unit. With tumescent and superwet techniques 30–35 mg/kg of tissue can be safely removed.

○ **How might spinal or epidural anesthesia be disadvantageous to patients having liposuction?**

When the anticipated volume of aspirate exceeds 1 L, an estimation of the patient's volume status is essential and inadequate volume status may be complicated by the sympathetic blockade. However, with adequate fluid loading, epidural anesthesia may be the anesthesia of choice for patients undergoing UAL as the incidence of nausea and vomiting is reduced and discharge is facilitated by a return of motor and sensory functions within 30–45 minutes of completion of the surgery if 1.5% lidocaine and 3% chloroprocaine are the local anesthetics used.

○ **Clinically how would vocal cord edema present differently than croup?**

Vocal cord edema is characterized by inspiratory stridor, whereas croup is characterized by expiratory or biphasic stridor.

○ **What are some factors implicated in producing postextubation croup?**

Tight-fitting endotracheal tube, traumatic or repeated intubations, coughing while intubated, passive head repositioning, a previous history of postextubation croup, prolonged intubation and high-pressure–low-volume cuffs, patient age 1–4 years, and nonhumidified gases.

○ **What is the treatment for edema induced by partial glottic or subglottic airway obstruction?**

Therapy consists of humidified oxygen, adequate hydration, and if necessary corticosteroids alone or in combination with nebulized racemic epinephrine.

○ **What type of sedation should children with sleep apnea be given preoperatively?**

None. No sedative premedication should be given to children with a history of sleep apnea, intermittent airway obstruction, or extremely hypertrophied tonsils.

○ **What are the physiologic effects of electroconvulsive therapy (ECT) on the cardiovascular system?**

The immediate response is parasympathetic discharge potentially resulting in bradycardia, asystole, hypotension, and PVCs. Sympathetic discharge then follows immediately with tachycardia, severe hypertension, dysrhythmias, and increased myocardial oxygen consumption.

Usually, ECG changes may include ST-segment depression and T-wave inversion without changes in cardiac enzymes consistent with myocardial infarction.

Venous return to the heart is decreased by the increased intrathoracic pressure that accompanies the seizure and/or positive pressure ventilation.

○ **What are the physiologic effects of ECT on the cerebrovascular system?**

Electrically induced seizures (brief tonic and then clonic phase for 30–50 seconds) transiently result in increased cerebral oxygen consumption. Initial constriction of cerebral blood vessels is followed by an increase in cerebral blood flow, and an increase in intracranial pressure. Cerebral blood flow increases up to 7-fold, reflecting increased oxygen consumption due to seizure activity. (Although increase in intracranial pressure is transient, it may prohibit ECT in patients with space-occupying lesions or head injury.)

Elevated intraocular pressure may prohibit ECT in glaucoma patients.

○ **What are contraindications to ECT from the standpoint of the anesthesiologist?**

Pheochromocytoma and increased intracranial pressure must be treated prior to ECT. Unless a patient is deemed extremely suicidal, recent MI or CVA within the last 3 months are patients who are almost always postponed. Although the tachycardia is self-limiting, peaking at 2 minutes, these may be undesirable in patients with ischemic heart disease. Myocardial infarctions and dysrhythmias are the most common cause of death following ECT.

○ **What effect does ECT have on the parturient?**

Anesthetic considerations include aortocaval compression, fetal hypoxia, pulmonary aspiration, and specific drugs for anesthesia. ECT may be used safely in all three trimesters. Although it appears that ECT has minimal effect on fetal heart rate, noninvasive monitoring of fetal heart rate and uterine contractions is recommended after 20 weeks gestation. Anticholinergic medications should be discontinued. The patient should be wedged to the left to avoid aortocaval compression and anticipating the increase in intragastric pressure, and lowered pH of the gastric contents, aspiration prophylaxis, and tracheal intubation after the first trimester are mandatory. Severe respiratory alkalosis must be avoided. The patient should be observed for contractions and bleeding post-ECT.

○ **What is the muscle relaxant of choice for ECT?**

Succinylcholine.

○ **What are the most common adverse effects of lithium?**

The most common adverse effects are gastric distress, weight gain, tremor, fatigue, and mild cognitive impairment. Other potential side effects include reversible T-wave EKG changes, mild leukocytosis, and hypothyroidism or vasopressin-resistant diabetes insipidus-like syndrome. At toxic levels the patient may become confused, sedated, and weak and develop tremor or slurred speech and then develop EKG changes including widening of the QRS complex and AV dissociation with hypotension and seizure activity.

○ **What are specific anesthetic ramifications of lithium?**

Lithium has been reported to potentiate depolarizing and nondepolarizing muscle relaxants as well as decrease MAC and prolong drowsiness following general anesthesia. Clinically these effects are minor.

○ **Why should lithium be discontinued, if possible, before ECT?**

Lithium may limit the therapeutic effect of the ECT. Patients receiving lithium may show delayed awakening, memory loss, postictal confusion, acute organic brain syndrome, delirium, and other atypical neurologic findings.

○ **What are the cardiovascular side effects of tricyclic antidepressants (TCAs)?**

Orthostatic hypotension is the most common cardiovascular side effect of TCAs. Quinidine-like cardiac effects include tachycardia, T-wave flattening or inversion, and prolongation of the PR, QRS, and QT intervals. Exaggerated responses to indirect-acting vasopressors and sympathetic stimulation should be anticipated. With chronic use and resulting depletion of cardiac catecholamines, the patient may be at risk for the cardiodepressant action of anesthetic agents.

○ **During diagnostic laparoscopy for primary infertility, the patient suddenly develops hypotension and hypoxemia, and then arrests. What is the problem?**

There are many possible etiologies for the arrest. The most likely problem due to the described "sudden" onset is CO_2 embolus. Possibilities specific to this procedure include CO_2 gas embolus, massive hemorrhage, and pneumothorax or pneumomediastinum. One must attempt to diagnose the problem quickly and provide supportive care and resuscitation in the interim.

○ **What are the signs of venous gas embolism during laparoscopy?**

Venous gas embolism is a rare but potentially lethal complication of laparoscopic surgery. Profound hypotension, hypoxemia, cyanosis, tachycardia, or other dysrhythmias can occur. EKG changes may indicate right heart strain. A "mill wheel" murmur may be auscultated with an esophageal or precordial stethoscope.

○ **Describe what happens to the end-tidal CO_2 during venous embolization of the insufflating gas.**

An initial increase in $ETCO_2$ due to pulmonary excretion of absorbed CO_2 is followed by a sudden decrease due to fall in cardiac output.

○ **By what route does CO_2 enter the bloodstream during laparoscopy?**

Gas embolism can occur through a tear in a vessel in the abdominal wall or peritoneum. The risk of embolic episodes is highest during induction of the pneumoperitoneum. The risk decreases after completion of the pneumoperitoneum because increased intra-abdominal pressure causes the injured vessel to collapse. Embolism resulting in sudden CV collapse can also occur due to inadvertent placement of the Veress needle or trocar directly into a vein or parenchymal organ.

○ **What is the immediate course of action should CO_2 embolism occur?**

Release of CO_2 pneumoperitoneum, ventilate with 100% O_2, check vital signs, position the patient in steep head down, and left lateral decubitus and hemodynamic support.

○ **List the potential complications of laparoscopy.**

Nausea, vomiting, shoulder tip pain, hypoventilation, hypotension, subcutaneous emphysema, pneumothorax, pneumopericardium, pneumomediastinum, hemorrhage, perforated viscera, electrical burns, and neuropathy. Hypercarbia will produce hypertension and tachycardia.

○ **What is the most common complication of pelvic laparoscopy?**

Nausea and vomiting that may occur in up to 50% of patients following a general anesthetic for the procedure [Miller, 2010].

○ **What is a safe insufflation pressure for laparoscopy?**

There is no truly safe pressure limit for laparoscopy. However, keeping pressures at or below 10–15 mm Hg is usually well tolerated, though tolerated less well in the obese, sicker ASA II or III patients.

○ **What are the hemodynamic effects of pneumoperitoneum?**

Significant alterations can occur at insufflation pressures over 10 mm Hg. As a result of increased intra-abdominal pressure during pneumoperitoneum, mean arterial blood pressure, systemic vascular resistance (afterload), and pulmonary vascular resistance are all increased while venous return (preload) is decreased. Heart rate remains unchanged or slightly increased. Cardiac output usually decreases by 10–30%. However, transient elevations in cardiac output have been reported and are thought to be a result of surgical stress.

○ **How does CO_2 insufflation affect total peripheral resistance during laparoscopy?**

Total peripheral resistance is increased because of compression of the abdominal aorta directly, and an indirect sympathomimetic effect of hypercarbia increases tone of arterioles, and venous resistance.

○ **What is the mechanism for decreased cardiac output as a result of pneumoperitoneum?**

The mechanism is multifactorial including decreased venous return (caval compression, pooling in lower extremities), increased venous resistance, and increased systemic vascular resistance.

At low intra-abdominal pressures less than 10 mm Hg, venous return may actually increase transiently. As peritoneal insufflations increases, caval compression and pooling of blood in the lower extremities ensue leading to a decrease in preload.

○ **How are myocardial filling pressures affected by abdominal insufflation and is this significant?**

Transesophageal echocardiogram has been used to demonstrate decrease in left ventricular end-diastolic volume. Increases in cardiac filling pressures are also seen as a result of increased intrathoracic pressure from insufflation.

Despite the decrease in venous return, there is a paradoxical increase in right atrial and pulmonary capillary wedge pressure presumably secondary to increased intrathoracic pressure as a result of pneumoperitoneum. Therefore, with regards to actual cardiac filling during pneumoperitoneum, CVP and PCWP may not be accurate measures.

○ **Are the cardiovascular effects of pneumoperitoneum clinically significant?**

At the typical insufflation pressures of 10–15 mm Hg, the small decrease in cardiac output is of little significance in healthy patients. However, in patients with limited cardiac reserve, or the institution of high insufflations pressures, the increase in afterload coupled with decreased preload may result in myocardial ischemia and significant decreases in cardiac output. These reductions in venous return and cardiac output can be attenuated by adequate fluid loading or prevention of peripheral blood pooling with SCDs or wrapping of the legs with elastic bandages [Miller, 2010].

○ **What are the principal concerns for the cardiac patient undergoing laparoscopic surgery?**

Hemodynamic alterations induced by laparoscopy are well documented and most pronounced in individuals with preexisting low cardiac output, low CVP, and high SVR. Intraoperative risks imposed by these hemodynamic alterations should be carefully weighed against the postoperative benefits of laparoscopy, particularly in patients with CHF, ischemic heart disease, cardiomyopathy, and/or significant valvular disease.

○ **What precautions can be taken to attenuate hemodynamic changes in the cardiac patient undergoing laparoscopy?**

Invasive monitoring (arterial catheter, pulmonary artery catheter, TEE) should be strongly considered. Hypovolemia should be corrected prior to surgery. Slow insufflation of CO_2 and low intra-abdominal pressures (10 mm Hg) may attenuate some of the changes.

○ **What is the etiology of severe bradycardia and cardiac arrest during laparoscopy?**

These phenomena are presumed to be due to vagal stimulation secondary to peritoneal stimulation. They are rare but serious complications.

○ **What are the hormonal effects of insufflation with carbon dioxide?**

Peritoneal insufflation results in a significant reduction of cardiac output and increases in mean arterial pressure and systemic and pulmonary vascular resistances. Laparoscopy results in progressive and significant increases in plasma concentrations of cortisol, epinephrine, norepinephrine, and renin. Vasopressin plasma concentrations markedly increase immediately after the beginning of insufflations.

○ **What are the principal respiratory complications of abdominal CO_2 insufflation for laparoscopy?**

The creation of a pneumoperitoneum is routinely achieved by intraperitoneal insufflation of CO_2.

This results in decreased pulmonary compliance by 30–50%, reductions in FRC and subsequent atelectasis, increased airway pressures, and V/Q mismatching. Respiratory complications include subcutaneous emphysema, pneumothorax, endobronchial intubation, and gas embolism. Pneumomediastinum and pneumopericardium can also occur.

○ **What are the causes of increased (end-tidal CO₂ or) PaCO₂ during laparoscopy?**

At institution of abdominal insufflations, $PaCO_2$ will increase by 15–25% due to increased vascular absorption of the gas and will generally plateau after 15–30 minutes. During an otherwise uncomplicated laparoscopy, $PaCO_2$ can be normalized by increasing alveolar ventilation by 10–25%.

Other causes of elevated $PaCO_2$ include:

a. V/Q mismatch (increased physiologic dead space). Decreased diaphragmatic excursion after pneumoperitoneum results in decreased tidal volumes unless the mechanical ventilation settings are changed.

b. Light/insufficient anesthesia (increased metabolism).

c. Depression of ventilation from anesthetics (spontaneously breathing patient).

d. Accidental events such as endobronchial intubation, capnothorax, CO_2 emphysema, or gas embolism.

○ **T/F: Endobronchial intubation does not occur during laparoscopic cholecystectomy because the patient is in reverse Trendelenburg (head-up) position.**

False. The upward displacement of the diaphragm during pneumoperitoneum also causes cephalad displacement of the carina. Endobronchial intubation has been reported despite head-up positioning of the patient.

○ **Describe the necessary action in the case of CO₂ pneumothorax in the absence of any cardiopulmonary compromise.**

Because CO_2 is highly diffusible, spontaneous resolution will occur within 30–60 minutes of exsufflation. In this scenario, thoracentesis may be avoided.

Guidelines suggest to stop N_2O, correct hypoxemia, apply PEEP, and minimize intra-abdominal pressure. These guidelines do not hold true if pneumothorax is secondary to ruptured bullae in which case PEEP should not be applied and thoracentesis is mandatory.

○ **What are the anesthetic contraindications for laparoscopy?**

Absolute anesthetic contraindications to laparoscopy have yet to be defined. Because of the physiologic alterations that occur, laparoscopy is undesirable in patients with elevated ICP, V-P or peritoneojugular shunts, severe cardiac disease, child's grade 3 cirrhosis, and hypovolemia. Special care should be taken in patients with renal insufficiency to avoid nephrotoxic drugs and optimize hemodynamics during pneumoperitoneum.

○ **Can laparoscopy be performed on individuals with V-P or peritoneojugular shunts?**

Yes. However, these shunts should be clamped prior to initiation of pneumoperitoneum.

○ **Can laparoscopy be performed in pregnancy?**

Yes. An open technique, an optical trocar, or a Veress needle should be used for abdominal entry to avoid damage to the gravid uterus. Left uterine displacement should be utilized to avoid aortocaval compression. Although CO_2 insufflation can lead to fetal respiratory acidosis and a subsequent increase in fetal heart rate and arterial pressure, these changes have been found to be minimal and of no clinical significance. Lower insufflations pressures should be used whenever possible. Placental perfusion pressure, blood flow, and pH remain unaffected if the physiologic maternal respiratory alkalosis that occurs in pregnancy is maintained. Fetal monitoring can still be achieved using transvaginal ultrasound. To avoid the effects of CO_2 pnuemoperitoneum, gasless laparoscopy can be considered [Chestnut et al., 2009; Miller, 2010].

○   **At what diastolic blood pressure would it be reasonable to delay an elective surgical case?**

The answer to this question is dictated by the patient, surgical procedure, and surgeon's and anesthesiologist's preference. A reasonable cutoff would be a diastolic pressure of greater than 110 mm Hg, in a patient previously undiagnosed or not well medically managed. Old studies suggest an increased risk of severe cardiopulmonary complications.

If the patient is normally well controlled but suffering from "white coat anxiety," treatment may be as simple as IV anxiolytics and reevaluation. Checking several serial blood pressures is appropriate. Clonidine will reduce lability of intraoperative blood pressure and anesthetic requirements. Diastolic hypertension is associated with an increase in SVR and is thought to be the major contributor to hypertensive morbidity (coronary artery disease, intracranial hemorrhage, and renal failure). Cardiac complications include myocardial ischemia, congestive heart failure, intraoperative lability in blood pressure, or death.

○   **What is the ideal intraoperative blood pressure for the hypertensive patient?**

The blood pressure and heart rate should be maintained near baseline values if the patient is medically well controlled (fluctuation in a range of 20%, with a target systolic blood pressure of 150 mm Hg).

○   **List at least five secondary causes of hypertension.**

Preexisting causes (excluding essential hypertension):

Renal disease: renal parenchymal diseases, renal artery stenosis, polycystic kidney disease, and chronic pyelonephritis

Endocrine disorders: adrenocortical dysfunction, pheochromocytoma, myxedema, acromegaly, and thyrotoxicosis

Coarctation of the aorta

Neurogenic: autonomic hyperreflexia, familial dysautonomia, polyneuritis, and increased intracranial pressure

Obesity

Tumors (carcinoid, Wilms tumor)

Preeclampsia

Drugs: cyclosporine A or FK506, amphetamines, oral contraceptives, estrogens, and steroids

Perioperative-specific:

Hypoxia

Hypercarbia (MH, CO_2 insufflation for laparoscopy)

Pain

Anxiety

Light anesthesia

Increased intravascular volume

Shivering

Intravenous indigo carmine dye

Drugs: anesthetic agents (ketamine, cocaine), vasopressors (epinephrine, ephedrine, phenylephrine), and withdrawal or rebound hypertension (antihypertensive medication, alcohol, narcotics)

Surgery-specific: aortic cross-clamping, tourniquet pain, drug-induced hypertension, postcarotid endarterectomy, and trigeminal nerve stimulation

Bladder distension, hypothermia, and hypoglycemia

○ **How does EKG evidence of LVH and strain affect perioperative outcome?**

Patients with EKG evidence of LVH and strain have been shown to have an 8-fold increase in cardiovascular deaths.

○ **What diagnostic test is more sensitive in diagnosing LVH, EKG or echocardiography?**

Echocardiography.

○ **When in the perioperative period is myocardial ischemia most likely to occur?**

Newer studies report perioperative MIs occur in the first 24–48 hours after surgery (not third postoperative day as earlier thought) [Le manach et al., 2005. See reference on page 528].

These MIs are preceded by tachycardia and ST depression, are often silent, and present as NSTEMI.

These observations support the hypothesis that perioperative myocardial injury develops as a consequence of increased myocardial oxygen demand (increased BP and HR) in the context of compromised myocardial oxygen supply.

○ **What are the relative contraindications to using a laryngeal mask airway (LMA)?**

(1) When pulmonary aspiration of gastric contents is probable and (2) where controlled ventilation is likely to require a high inflation pressure (>20 cm H_2O).

○ **What type of economic benefits are there for using an MAC (propofol sedation with an ilioinguinal–hypogastric nerve block) technique versus general (LMA, propofol, sevoflurane, nitrous oxide/oxygen) or spinal (bupivacaine–fentanyl) anesthesia in ambulatory patients having unilateral inguinal herniorrhaphy?**

The use of peripheral nerve block with propofol sedation results in shorter time-to-home readiness, lower pain scores at discharge, greater patient satisfaction, and lower associated anesthetic-related institutional costs compared with general and spinal anesthesia.

○ **What discharge criteria should be met for patients undergoing outpatient surgery?**

Discharge criteria are hospital-specific, and while different scoring systems are available (e.g., the modified Aldrete score), each institution sets its own criteria, as no single set has been proven to be more effective. In general, the following conditions are monitored prior to discharging a patient home after outpatient surgery:

- Stable vital signs for at least 1 hour
- Controlled bleeding, and acceptable wound drainage
- Fully awake and orientated
- Able to drink
- Able to pass urine
- Able to ambulate
- Pain and nausea well controlled
- Relevant social care in place
- Written and verbal discharge information given, including follow-up visits and emergency information

Key Terms

Anesthesia for electroconvulsive therapy (ECT): lidocaine effect

Anesthesia for liposuction

ECT and heart disease: anesthetic consideration

ECT and hemodynamic management

ECT: side effects

Elevated $ETCO_2$: differential diagnosis

Hemodynamic responses: ECT

Hemodynamics of laparoscopy

Induction for ECT: seizure duration

IV regional anesthesia: complications

IV regional: mechanism

Laparoscopy: $ETCO_2$

Liposuction: lidocaine toxic dose

Lithium and NMB

Magnetic resonance imaging (MRI): ECG complications

MRI suite: O_2 delivery

Oculocardiac reflex: management/afferent path

Outpatient surgery: discharge criteria

Pneumoperitoneum: vagal arrest

Radiation exposure versus distance

Retrobulbar block: oculocardiac reflex

Seizure activation by anesthetics

Tourniquet management: IV regional anesthesia

Tumescent liposuction complications

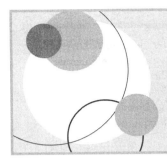

Patient Monitors

*One should always play fair when one
has the winning cards.*
Oscar Wilde

○ **What is the theoretical basis for infrared (IR) gas analysis?**

Molecules containing at least two dissimilar atoms have unique IR absorption spectra. For this reason, IR analysis can be used for nitrous oxide and the halogenated agents, but not for oxygen as it does not absorb IR light.

○ **What are the four phases of the capnography?**

Phase I: Initial phase of expiration. Dead space gases, no CO_2.

Phase II: Sharp upstroke, slope determined by evenness of ventilation and alveolar emptying. Consists of mixture of alveolar and dead space gases.

Phase III: Alveolar plateau. Consists of alveolar gas and normally horizontal. The peak represents end-expiratory CO_2 (P_{ETCO_2}).

Phase IV: Inspiratory phase. Steep downstroke.

Generally $PaCO_2$ to P_{ETCO_2} difference is 1–5 mm Hg due to small amount of alveolar dead space. Factors that increase alveolar dead space will widen this gradient.

○ **What are the standard American Society of Anesthesiology (ASA) basic monitors?**

Inspired O_2, pulse oximeter, ECG, BP, body temperature, and expired CO_2.

○ **List factors that increase $PaCO_2$ to P_{ETCO_2} gradient.**

1. *Increase in dead space*—such as altered volume or distribution of blood flow:

   a. Pulmonary embolism (PE)
   b. Pulmonary stenosis (PS)
   c. Occlusion of pulmonary artery
   d. Decreased cardiac output
   e. Pulmonary hypotension

2. *Venous admixture (R to L shunt)*—effect is less dramatic and causes minimal change in the gradient:

   a. Atelectasis
   b. Endobronchial intubation
   c. Certain cyanotic congenital heart diseases

○   **What information is available from the analysis of the CO_2 waveform using capnography?**

Confirmation of tracheal placement of the endotracheal tube, adequacy of ventilation, detection of rebreathing of CO_2 (baseline >0), evidence of obstructive lung disease or spontaneous breathing during mechanical ventilation, and circuit disconnect or partial disconnection of the capnograph sampling hose. The capnometer gives a numerical value of the end-tidal CO_2, which can be used to approximate and follow the $PaCO_2$, although discrepancies exist between end-tidal and arterial CO_2. Early detection of increased CO_2 production from malignant hyperthermia or thyrotoxicosis or during carbon dioxide insufflation with laparoscopic procedures is possible.

○   **What changes occur on the capnogram during bronchospasm?**

The slope of phase III can be increased (linear upslope) in obstructive airway disease or during prolonged expiration.

○   **Which monitors are based on Beer–Lambert law?**

Pulse oximetry and IR analyzer.

○   **Based on the Beer–Lambert law, how does pulse oximetry work?**

$A = \mathring{a}bc$ (A is the absorbance value at specific wavelength, $\mathring{a}$ is the absorptivity coefficient of the material at that wavelength, b is the pathlength through the sample, c is the concentration of the compound in solution).

Beer–Lambert law states that at a constant light intensity and hemoglobin (Hb) concentration, intensity of light transmitted through tissues is a logarithmic function of oxygen saturation of Hb.

The first pulse oximeters manufactured in the early 1980s used the Beer–Lambert law to calculate the values of arterial SaO_2. Pulse oximeters measure the absorption of red (deoxyhemoglobin) and IR light (oxyhemoglobin [HbO_2]). LEDs are used as a light source, which passes through a patient's finger and is detected by light sensors. During an arterial pulse there is an increase in blood volume and this increase in absorption differentiates arterial from venous and other tissues. From these data (plethysmographic analysis) the pulse oximeter determines the percent oxygen saturation of the arterial blood using the Beer–Lambert law. Measurements for SaO_2 values below 85% are often erroneous, as the effect of scattering of light by the red blood cell is not taken into consideration in this formula. Most pulse oximeters now use look-up tables derived from calibration studies of healthy volunteers whose oxygen saturation is measured invasively.

Pulse oximetry combines the technology of spectrophotometry and plethysmography.

○   **How many wavelengths of light are required to distinguish HbO_2 from reduced Hb?**

Two different wavelengths, in the red (600–700 nm) and near-IR (800–940 nm) spectrum.

○   **What is the difference between the SpO_2 measured by pulse oximetry and the SaO_2 measured by the laboratory co-oximeter?**

Adult blood usually contains four species of Hb: HbO_2, reduced Hb, methemoglobin (metHb), and carboxyhemoglobin (COHb). Each of these Hbs has a different light absorption profile and therefore requires four wavelengths of light to measure them.

SpO_2 uses two wavelengths and measures the "functional" saturation, which is given by the following equation:

$$\text{Functional } SaO_2 = \frac{O_2Hb}{O_2Hb + \text{reduced Hb}} \times 100$$

Laboratory co-oximeters use multiple wavelengths and measure the "fractional" saturation, which is given by the following equation:

$$\text{Fractional SaO}_2 = \frac{\text{O}_2\text{Hb}}{\text{O}_2\text{Hb} + \text{reduced Hb} + \text{COHb} + \text{metHb}} \times 100$$

○ **What effect will COHb and metHb have on the SpO₂ measurement?**

At 940 nm, COHb has an extremely low absorbance and does not contribute to total absorbance. However, at 660 nm, COHb has an absorbance very similar to that of O_2Hb; therefore, SpO_2 will read falsely high. In the presence of high metHb, SpO_2 reads 85%, independent of the actual arterial oxygenation.

○ **What factors can cause errors in measuring SpO₂?**

- Methylene blue IV results in a severe decrease, indigo carmine a small decrease, and indocyanine green an intermediate effect in measured SpO_2.
- Blue, black, and green nail polish with absorbance near 660 nm may cause an artifactual decrease in SpO_2 reading.
- Ambient light, especially fluorescent light, can falsely elevate SpO_2 reading, especially if the flicker frequency of the light is close to the harmonic of the diode switching frequency.
- Vasoconstriction or hypotension can cause loss of SpO_2 signal.
- Delayed detection of hypoxic events may be seen due to a significant delay between a change in the alveolar oxygen tension and a change in the oximeter reading.
- Erratic performance with irregular rhythms, electrical interference, and motion artifacts.
- COHb is interpreted as HbO_2 and the SpO_2 is artifactually raised toward 100%. MetHb causes the SpO_2 to trend toward 85%. Fetal and sickle Hbs have little effect.
- Pulsatile veins (i.e., tricuspid regurgitation) cannot be distinguished from pulsatile arteries and can cause falsely low SpO_2 readings.

○ **Since isoflurane and enflurane are isomers, having the same charge to mass ratio, how does a mass spectrometer delineate between the two?**

The high energies involved in a mass spectrometer actually break the covalent bonds in the anesthetic molecules into components that have different charge to mass ratios. These fractions are the ones sampled to determine the percentage of gas present in the system.

○ **You notice the anesthesia machine you are about to use does not have a functioning oxygen analyzer. What should you do?**

There are several possible equipment problems that could cause a hypoxic gas mixture to be delivered to the patient that can only be detected by an oxygen analyzer. ASA practice guidelines for monitoring require routine use of an oxygen analyzer.

○ **How does the oxygen analyzer on an anesthesia machine work?**

Two methods are used in the modern anesthesia workstation:

1. Electrochemical oxygen analysis: It uses an electrochemical sensor (galvanic or fuel cell). Oxygen reacts with the electrodes (anode: lead; cathode: silver or gold), generating a current that is proportional to the oxygen partial pressure in the sample gas. The polarographic method uses a Clark electrode (anode: silver; cathode: platinum or gold), battery power source, and KCl electrolyte solution.

2. Paramagnetic oxygen analysis: Oxygen is paramagnetic and therefore gets attracted into a magnetic field. In fact, oxygen is the only paramagnetic gas that is important in anesthesia. Most other gases, for example, N_2, are weakly diamagnetic and are repelled from a magnetic field. When a gas that contains oxygen is passed through a magnetic

field, it will cause pressure wave that is proportional to the oxygen partial pressure. These changes are detected by the transducer and converted to electrical signal that is displayed on a screen as oxygen partial pressure or volume percent. They have a fast response time and can differentiate between inspired and expired oxygen concentrations.

○ **Where should the arterial line transducer be located during intracranial surgery?**

At the level of the head, preferably auditory meatus = circle of Willis.

A key concern during intracranial surgery is the cerebral perfusion pressure, which is mean arterial pressure minus central venous pressure or intracranial pressure, whichever is greater. Whenever the head is above the heart, the actual mean arterial pressure to the head is lower by the hydrostatic pressure of the column of blood. The simplest method to correct for this is to zero the arterial transducer at the level of the head, rather than the right atrium.

○ **How can the natural frequency of a catheter–stopcock–transducer system be measured?**

Natural frequency is the frequency at which the monitoring system resonates and amplifies the signals it receives. Apply a 300 mm Hg square wave pulse to the system by activating the flush. The system will "ring" with a number of oscillations. Take the reciprocal of the time between peaks. (Resonant frequency is measured in hertz, which is oscillations per second.)

○ **List two reasons for overshoot in the systolic upstroke of the invasive intra-arterial pressure waveform.**

1. If the monitoring system has a natural frequency that is too low, frequencies in the monitored pressure waveform will approach the natural frequency of the measurement system. This will cause the system to resonate and the pressure waveform will be exaggerated or amplified. This will be displayed as overshoot, ringing, or resonance.

2. The monitoring system should have an adequate damping coefficient for accurate reproduction of the arterial waveform. The underdamped pressure waveforms display systolic pressure overshoot.

○ **What does underdamping do to the systolic, mean, and diastolic pressures measured by direct arterial pressure monitoring?**

Underdamping will overestimate the systolic and underestimate the diastolic blood pressure, with little change in mean pressure. These changes are usually worse with tachycardia.

○ **T/F: Compared with central aortic pressure, peripheral arterial waveforms have higher systolic pressure, lower diastolic pressure, and wider pulse pressure.**

True. This is due to the physiologic amplification of the waveform from the aorta to the peripheral arteries.

The arterial waveform becomes narrower and increases in amplitude in peripheral arteries. Therefore, SBP tends to increase and DBP tends to decrease as the location of the catheter becomes more peripheral (wider pulse pressure). The arterial upstroke becomes steeper, dicrotic notch appears later, diastolic wave becomes prominent, and end-diastolic pressure becomes lower when traveling from central aorta to the periphery.

For example, SBP in the dorsalis pedis artery is higher than in the aorta. This change is caused by the change in diameter of the vessels and their elasticity and possibly also because of the reflection of the wave pattern from the vessel walls.

○ **Mention some other conditions that produce arterial pressure gradients.**

Vascular disease and vasoconstriction decreases both SBP and DBP in proportion to the severity of disease (common to note an error of 50 mm Hg or more in cold, severely vasoconstricted patients).

○ **Describe the normal arterial waveform.**

Normal arterial waveform has the following:

1. Systolic upstroke
2. Systolic peak pressure
3. Systolic decline
4. Dicrotic notch
5. Diastolic runoff
6. End-diastolic pressure

Slope of the upstroke correlates with dp/dt, which gives a rough indication of *myocardial contractility*.

Increase in systemic vascular resistance (SVR) will result in both an increase in the slope of the upstroke and a decrease in the slope of the downstroke.

○ **How does hypovolemia manifest on the arterial pressure waveform?**

Hypovolemia is suggested when a large respiratory variation and a narrowed pulse pressure are observed.

During positive pressure ventilation there is a cyclic variation in systemic arterial pressure, and this may be quantified as the systolic pressure variation (SPV). The normal SPV is 7–10 mm Hg. Hypovolemia causes a significant increase in SPV and may be used as a diagnostic tool. A large SPV of >15 mm Hg was shown to be highly predictive of low pulmonary capillary wedge pressure (PCWP) of <10 mm Hg.

○ **In aortic stenosis, the arterial pressure waveform appears overdamped. Why?**

In aortic stenosis, there is a fixed obstruction to left ventricular ejection. This results in a reduced stroke volume and a small-amplitude arterial pressure waveform that rises slowly and peaks late in systole.

○ **Bisferiens pulse is diagnostic of which valvular cardiac lesion?**

Aortic regurgitation. Because of the large stroke volume ejected from the left ventricle, there is a wide pulse pressure and the pulse may have two systolic peaks.

○ **How can you avoid artifacts in the invasive arterial pressure monitoring system?**

1. Use appropriate size cannula (20 gauge for radial, 18 gauge for axillary and femoral).
2. Use a connecting tube that is rigid, internal diameter 1.5–3.0 mm, and maximal length 120 cm.
3. Use only one stopcock per line and the line should be free of bubbles, clots, and kinks.
4. Use a continuous flushing system and slow 1–3 mL/h infusion of saline to prevent thrombus formation (heparinized saline increases the risk of HITT; use normal saline).
5. Use a transducer with the highest frequency response.
6. Ensure proper zeroing/leveling of transducer at the heart level in supine patient (error of 1.36 cm H_2O = 1 mm Hg).

○ **What are some major complications of brachial artery cannulation?**

Compartment syndrome and median nerve damage are some of the possible complications. A slightly longer catheter is preferred and may accommodate 18 gauge cannulae.

○ **What are the contraindications to placing a pulmonary artery catheter (PAC)?**

Absolute contraindications:

1. Tricuspid stenosis/pulmonic stenosis, where PAC may worsen the obstruction to flow.

2. Right atrial/right ventricular masses (tumor, thrombus). Catheter may dislodge the mass causing pulmonary or paradoxical embolization.

3. Tetralogy of Fallot, where PAC may cause "tet spell."

Relative contraindications:

Complete LBBB, WPW, and Ebstein malformation (causes tachyarrhythmia). Use catheter with pacing abilities. Newly inserted pacemaker wires (before 4–6 weeks) may get dislodged.

○ **How accurate is the thermodilution cardiac output measurement in the face of a large left-to-right or right-to-left shunt?**

The thermodilution technique measures right ventricular output and pulmonary artery blood flow. In those situations, right ventricular and left ventricular outputs will not be equal.

○ **What will happen if the constant entered in the cardiac output computer was 10 mL injectate, but only a 5 mL injectate was used in determining cardiac output?**

The area under the thermodilution curve would be approximately one half the expected value. The computed cardiac output would overestimate the true cardiac output by a factor of two.

○ **How does right-sided valvular regurgitation (severe tricuspid regurgitation) affect cardiac output as measured by thermodilution?**

In patients with tricuspid regurgitation, recirculation of the thermal signal occurs between the right atrium and right ventricle, resulting in an abnormally prolonged decay time and inaccurate measurement of cardiac output (usually underestimated, but may be overestimated depending on the severity of valvular regurgitation and the magnitude of the cardiac output).

○ **List four situations that will give rise to low-amplitude curves during the thermodilutional cardiac output measurements.**

1. The injectate volume is too small (less than volume entered in the computer).

2. The temperature differential between injectate and blood temperature is small.

3. When the thermistor is improperly positioned. If there is an undamped pulmonary artery waveform, one may assume acceptable thermistor position.

4. Partly or completely wedged PAC will reduce flow past the thermistor. Therefore, the thermistor should be located in the center of the flowing blood.

○ **Why doesn't the PCWP always correlate with LV volume?**

Ideally, the changes in LVEDP (hence, left ventricular volume) are reflected by all the proximal pressures (left atrial, pulmonary artery end-diastolic pressure [PAEDP], and PCWP) because at end diastole, there is cessation of forward blood flow, and a static fluid column is presumed to exist from the left ventricle to the PAC tip.

Factors that alter the premise that PAOP is a consistent, accurate reflection of LVEDP/V are:

1. Airway pressure

2. Pulmonary hypertension

3. Mitral stenosis

4. Ventricular compliance

○ **Why is it important to position the PAC in west Zone III?**

Location in a low-flow area of the lung exposes the tracing and PAOP to greater influences of airway pressure changes. Ideally the PAC should be in Zone III (Pa > Pv > PA) of the lung. This can be confirmed by x-ray, but typically occurs spontaneously since these are "flow-directed" catheters.

○ **List some characteristics that suggest the PAC tip is not in Zone III.**

a. PCWP > PAEDP

b. Nonphasic PCWP tracing

c. Inability to aspirate blood from the distal port when the catheter is wedged

○ **How does PEEP affect the PCWP reading?**

The effect of PEEP is minimal if the level of PEEP is low (<10 cm) or the PAC is located in Zone III. (When PEEP is above 10 cm H_2O, subtracting 1–2 mm Hg from the displayed "wedge" pressure for each 5 cm H_2O of PEEP gives an estimate.)

○ **List some conditions that increase the gradient between PCWP and PADP.**

- Chronic lung disease.
- PE.
- Alveolar hypoxia.
- Acidosis.
- Hypoxemia.
- Vasoactive drugs that increase pulmonary vascular resistance (PVR).
- Tachycardia shortens ventricular diastole and also increases PVR.

○ **What are the causes of large "v" wave on the PCWP tracing?**

Mitral regurgitation (MR)

LV diastolic noncompliance

Episode of myocardial ischemia (decreases ventricular compliance, papillary muscle dysfunction)

○ **When tall "v" waves are present (as in MR), how does it change the morphology of the pulmonary artery pressure (PAP) waveform?**

Prominent regurgitant "v" wave changes the morphology of the PAP waveform giving it a bifid appearance and obscuring normal dicrotic notch.

It is important to differentiate wedge pressure waveform from unwedged PAP waveform, because wedge trace with a tall systolic "v" *resembles a typical unwedged PAP trace* (could be disastrous if not recognizing inflate the balloon).

Therefore, in this situation look for differences between wedge pressure and PAP, which include:

1. PAP upstroke is steeper and slightly precedes systemic arterial pressure upstroke.

2. Wedge wave peaks after the ECG T wave.

○ **Shortly after placing a PAC, you notice bright red blood in the endotracheal tube. What is wrong?**

Your worst clinical nightmare, pulmonary artery rupture.

The incidence is between 0.064% and 0.20% and mortality is high. Risk factors for PA rupture include advanced age, female sex, pulmonary hypertension, and coagulopathy. Iatrogenic factors include inflation of the balloon when the catheter tip is positioned distally, overinflation of the balloon, and prolonged wedging of the catheter. Treatment for PA rupture is initially to protect the patient from asphyxiation with bronchoscopy, suctioning, oxygen, positive pressure ventilation, and lung isolation. Surgery may be necessary. Whether to deflate the balloon and pull the PAC back or to leave it in place to retard bleeding and to provide a route for administration of fibrin glue is controversial.

○ **You are attempting to remove a PAC in the PACU and encounter resistance. What should you do?**

Do not forcibly remove the catheter. Verify that the balloon is deflated. The catheter may be knotted, possibly around the chordae tendineae. Forcible removal could cause cardiac or vascular injury. Radiologic evaluation is necessary.

○ **The relationship between oxygen consumption, oxygen content, and cardiac output is expressed by which equation?**

Fick equation: oxygen delivery = cardiac output $\times$ ($CaO_2 - CvO_2$).

With a normal oxygen consumption of 250 mL and a cardiac output of 5,000 mL/min, the normal arteriovenous difference by this equation calculates to be about 5 mL O_2/dL blood.

Arteriovenous O_2 difference is a good measure of the overall oxygen delivery.

○ **How does a Doppler flow probe work?**

The Doppler technique utilizes the Doppler effect, which is the reflection of sound waves off a moving object causing an apparent frequency shift.

A Doppler probe emits an ultrasonic signal that is reflected by underlying tissue. A Doppler frequency shift is caused by red blood cells moving through the artery. The difference between the transmitted and received frequencies indicates blood flow, which is characterized by a swishing sound (systolic blood pressure). Use of a piezoelectric crystal will detect lateral arterial wall movement, measuring systolic and diastolic pressures.

○ **In what four ways does a patient lose heat in the operating room?**

By conduction, convection, evaporation, and radiation.

○ **What is the difference between a thermistor, a resistance thermometer, and a thermocouple?**

A resistance thermometer uses increases in resistance of a metal (conductor) as temperature increases to measure temperature (the detector is part of a Wheatstone bridge). A thermistor is a semiconductor that decreases its resistance as temperature increases. A thermocouple uses dissimilar metals; one junction is kept at a reference temperature, the other acts as a sensor, and the voltage between the two is measured.

○ **If a blood sample is obtained from a hypothermic patient for ABG analysis, is it important to correct for temperature?**

Yes. The PO_2 and PCO_2 derived from a 37°C electrode are overestimated in this hypothermic patient.

○ **If temperature correction is not applied, what is the percentage of error in PO_2 derived from a 37°C electrode?**

At high PO_2 values (>400 mm Hg) the effect is small because Hb is fully saturated in this region. However, at PO_2 values below 100 mm Hg, the degree of overestimation may be severe. For example, at a patient temperature of 30°C and PO_2 below 80 mm Hg, the true PO_2 is overestimated by about 60%.

○ **A patient is undergoing surgery with field block and sedation. List two ways of monitoring his sedation level.**

1. Observer's Assessment of Alertness/Sedation (OAA/S) Scale
2. BIS index

○ **How does the BIS index correlate with OAA/S?**

In volunteers the BIS index has been shown to correlate with OAA/S scores during propofol-induced sedation. An increasing depth of sedation was associated with a predictable decrease in BIS index and absence of recall with BIS values below 80.

○ **Which monitoring method (BIS or OAA/S) appears to be superior?**

OAA/S involves patient stimulation at frequent intervals to determine the level of consciousness, requires patient cooperation, and is subject to testing fatigue. Although the potential to titrate drugs more accurately using BIS values is appealing, conventional assessment of sedation is important to maintain continuous patient contact. Therefore, BIS monitoring should be employed as an adjunct to clinical evaluation rather than as the primary monitor of consciousness. ASA recommends using BIS in combination with other modalities (checking for purposeful movement and conventional monitoring – HR, BP, ECG, CO_2).

○ **List the two main factors that determine the central venous pressure.**

Intravascular blood volume and intrinsic vascular tone of the capacitance vessels.

○ **How does ventilation affect the CVP?**

There will be alterations in the intrathoracic pressure and juxtacardiac pressure during the respiratory cycle depending on whether the patient is breathing spontaneously or receiving positive pressure ventilation.

○ **What is the best time to monitor cardiac filling pressures?**

At the end of expiration, when intrathoracic and juxtacardiac pressures approach atmospheric pressures, depending on whether the patient is breathing spontaneously or receiving positive pressure ventilation.

○ **What causes the sequence of waves seen in a typical CVP trace?**

Normal mechanical events of the cardiac cycle are responsible for the three peaks and two descents.
Waves:
"a" wave due to atrial kick
"c" wave due to contraction of the ventricle (isovolemic)
"v" wave with atrial filling
Descents:
"x" descent due to relaxation of atrium
"y" descent with ventricular filling

○ **What causes cannon waves on CVP tracing?**

Giant "a" or tall "cannon" waves occur when right atrium contracts while tricuspid valve remains closed, such as in complete heart block, junctional (nodal) rhythm, or ventricular pacing.

○ **What changes are seen in constrictive pericarditis on the CVP tracing?**

Tall "a" and "v" waves, and steep "x" and "y" descent with M or W configuration.

○ **What steps should be taken to prevent infections associated with central venous catheters [ASA Practice Guidelines for Central Venous Access, 2012. See reference on page 528]?**

Aseptic precautions, which include basic sterile precautions (include mask, cap, sterile gloves, gown, and a large drape) and skin disinfection (2% chlorhexidine gluconate with 70% alcohol), are mandatory when placing central venous catheters. Remove all jewelry items (rings, watches) and wash hands with a disinfectant agent before wearing sterile gloves prior to catheter insertion and during catheter care.

Transparent adhesive dressings (which are now semipermeable) are commonly used around the central venous catheter sites. The Biopatch, a foam dressing impregnated with chlorhexidine gluconate, should be used at the catheter insertion site.

Studies suggest that topical antibiotic ointments or creams should not be applied routinely on catheter insertion sites because of the high likelihood of promoting resistance. Although bacteria also become resistant to antiseptic agents, this occurs far less frequently than resistance to antibiotics.

Whenever possible, routine parenteral fluids should be prepared in the pharmacy with laminar flow hood using aseptic technique.

In order to reduce the risk of contamination, a central venous catheter hub has been engineered by incorporating an antiseptic solution that is pierced by a blunt needle.

Current recommendations are for replacement of administration sets, including secondary sets and add-on devices, no more frequently than at 72-hour intervals, unless catheter-related infection is suspected.

The CDC recommends the use of antimicrobial/antiseptic-impregnated catheters in adults whose catheter is expected to remain in place for >5 days.

The subclavian (SC) approach is associated with lower risks of thrombosis and infection and may therefore be the preferred site when the risk of infection is high.

○ **What surface lead is best for monitoring atrial activity?**

Lead II. It is the best surface lead for monitoring atrial activity as it displays the greatest P wave voltage.

○ **Describe the ECG interpretation and analysis.**

ECG interpretation involves:

- Heart rate.
- P waves. Inverted P waves indicate an abnormal pathway for the conduction of the cardiac impulse or ectopic pacemaker sites.
- The duration of the PR interval. Normally, 0.12–0.2 second when the heart rate is normal, prolongation occurs with delayed conduction through the AV node and shortening with a junctional rhythm.
- The duration of the QRS complex. This normally is 0.05–0.1 second. Prolongation suggests abnormal intraventricular conduction. A pathologic Q wave is one greater than 0.04 second.

- Regularity of the ventricular rhythm.
- Early cardiac beats or abnormal pauses after the QRS complex.
- The ST segment. This is normally isoelectric but may be elevated up to 1 mm in the absence of an abnormality. It is not normally depressed.
- T waves. These are in the same direction as the QRS and should not exceed 5 mm amplitude in standard leads or 10 mm in precordial leads.
- The Q–T interval must be corrected for heart rate but normally should be less than one half the preceding R–R interval.

Key Terms

Abnormal PAD/LVEDP gradient: causes
Arterial pressure monitoring artifacts
Arterial pulse waveform
Arterial waveform: peripheral versus central
Arterial waveform: reason for shape
ASA basic monitoring standards
Brachial artery catheter: complications
Calculation: pulmonary versus systemic resistance
Cannon a wave on CVP trace
Capnogram: bronchospasm
Capnogram waveform; obstruction
Central line: infection prevention
Constrictive pericarditis: venous waveform
CVP trace: interpretation
Infrared gas analyzer: theory
ECG: atrial activity

ECG interpretation
ECG: P wave detection
Errors in pulse oximetry
HbCO detection: oximetry
Inaccuracies of cardiac output measurement
Interpretation of pulmonary artery occlusion pressure
Intra-arterial SBP amplification mechanism
MAP decrease in arteries
Mitral regurgitation: PA monitoring
PA catheter risk with LBBB
PA monitoring: cause of V-waves
Pulmonary artery catheter (PAC): interpretation
Pulse pressure changes in arteries
SpO_2 effect of metHb
Systolic blood pressure changes in arteries
Thermodilution CO (Tco), errors

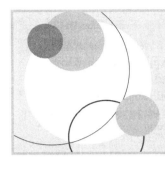

Patient Positioning

Facts do not cease to exist because they are ignored.
Aldous Huxley

○ **A patient develops brachial plexus nerve palsy after vaginal hysterectomy. What are the relevant positioning concerns?**

Typically the patient would be in lithotomy position with arms placed outstretched on arm boards. Care must be exercised to avoid arm adduction beyond 90°, which may be exacerbated in steep Trendelenburg. The patient's head should be in a neutral position. Turning it to one side causes the brachial plexus on the contralateral side to be stretched. Flexion of the arms at the elbow will tend to relieve tension on the brachial plexus.

○ **With supine positioning, what is the ideal placement of the arms?**

The goal is to avoid stretching the brachial plexus and compression of the ulnar nerve. The arms should be abducted less than 90°, and supinated with palms up, elbows padded, and the head held in the neutral position (avoid rotation and flexion, especially to the contralateral side of the "out" arm, if the other is tucked). The arms should be properly secured to prevent them from falling off the arm board, causing translocation of the humerus below the horizontal plane of the scapula. If the arms are suspended overhead, extremely abducted, or in anterior flexion, which tenses the arcuate ligament at the elbow, ulnar nerve compression is possible.

○ **What is the most frequent site of anesthesia-related peripheral nerve injury?**

Ulnar nerve [Cheney et al., 1999. See reference on page 528].

○ **What are the most common sites and signs of ulnar nerve injury?**

Ulnar nerve injury commonly occurs with nerve compression at the elbow where the nerve passes posterior to the medial epicondyle of the humerus. Pronated arm position can increase the risk of ulnar nerve injury in a supine patient. Symptoms include numbness and tingling of the medial part of the palm and the fourth and fifth digits. Patients have difficulty making a fist because they cannot flex their fourth and fifth fingers at the distal interphalangeal joints. This gives the appearance of a "claw hand" when the patient attempts to straighten the fingers.

○ **Which of the three major nerves in the arm (radial, median, and ulnar) is *least* likely to be damaged from improper positioning?**

Median nerve. Injury is usually due to entrapment (pronator syndrome due to compression between the two heads of the pronator teres) or laceration at the elbow or just proximal to the flexor retinaculum due to wrist slashing in an attempted suicide.

○ **What is the most likely mechanism of radial nerve injury?**

External compression causing ischemia.

The radial nerve courses unprotected in the spiral groove on the lateral aspect of the humerus about three fingerbreadths above the lateral epicondyle. The most common site of entrapment of the radial nerve is in the middle of the arm seen with too frequent cycling of the automatic blood pressure monitoring cuff for long periods or too prolonged use of a tourniquet set at high pressure. In addition, resting the lateral portion of the upper arm against a vertical bar (either screen or surgical retraction system such as the Kent retractor during upper abdominal surgery or the self-retractor for the dissection of the left internal mammary artery with coronary artery surgery) can also cause a compression injury.

○ **What are the signs of radial nerve injury?**

Injury occurring *proximal to the origin of the radial branches to the triceps muscle* (i.e., "Saturday night palsy," with the arm thrown over the back of a chair to hold an intoxicated patient upright) results in injury to the posterior cord of the brachial plexus and an inability to extend at the elbow joint.

With nerve injury *in the middle of the humerus* there is paralysis of the extensor muscles of the forearm and digits causing wrist drop, with normal strength of the triceps muscle. Sensory loss is variable, and usually limited to a patch on the dorsum of the hand between the first and second digits.

Selected injury of the *posterior interosseous nerve* on the dorsal aspect of the forearm from insufficient padding of the dependent arm with the patient positioned lateral will also cause wrist drop.

If the *deep branch of the radial nerve* is severed, the patient will be unable to extend the thumb and the metacarpophalangeal joints of the other digits. There is no loss of sensation.

Selective injury of the *superficial branch of the radial nerve* may result in loss of sensation on the posterior surface of the forearm, hand, and proximal phalanges of the lateral three and one-half digits.

○ **How does steep Trendelenburg (head-down) positioning used during laparoscopic surgery cause hypoxemia?**

Trendelenburg position causes the abdominal viscera to move cephalad impairing diaphragmatic excursion and lung expansion, resulting in decreased thoracopulmonary compliance and functional residual capacity. This is more exaggerated in the morbidly obese patient. There is also the potential for right mainstem bronchial intubation and an increased risk of pulmonary aspiration, particularly in a nonintubated patient.

○ **Why are axillary rolls used in lateral decubitus positioning of the patient?**

To prevent compression of the dependent arm's axillary neurovascular bundle (arterial insufficiency, venous stasis and/or thrombosis, brachial plexus nerve injury) and allow better chest excursion. The wedge may also prevent circumduction of the "down" shoulder, which could result in stretching of the suprascapular nerve. Additional useful techniques that complement axillary rolls include placing the pulse oximeter probe, inserting arterial line, or checking the radial pulse on the dependent arm to detect arterial insufficiency; placing the NIBP cuff on the upper arm, with frequent checks for cyanosis or mottling of the skin on the dependent arm; being cognizant of the fact that a surgical resident leaning on and swinging the arm board upwards could contribute to stretch injury of the brachial plexus.

○ **What happens to the distribution of V/Q ratios of the two lungs when an awake patient breathing spontaneously assumes lateral decubitus position?**

Not much; V/Q is maintained. Preferential ventilation to the dependent lung (R > L) is matched by an increase in perfusion, so the V/Q ratio decreases from the nondependent to the dependent lung, just as it does in upright and supine lungs.

○ **Are there any special considerations in positioning a patient with rib fractures in the lateral position?**

The injured side should not be placed dependent. The weight of the patient may displace the rib fracture, causing trauma to the pleura or lung. If there is an associated underlying lung contusion, V/Q mismatch is minimized with the fractured rib in the nondependent position as preferential perfusion to the dependent lung will move blood flow away from the contused and poorly ventilated alveoli.

○ **Why are chest rolls needed for positioning a patient prone?**

To reduce intra-abdominal and intrathoracic pressure.

Abdominal compression will impair diaphragmatic excursion, resulting in an acute restrictive pattern of ventilation. Compression of the vena cava will cause venous congestion and increased bleeding during back surgery from blood shunted to the epidural venous plexus and may preclude venous return to the heart. Direct pressure on the aorta may raise the blood pressure causing vascular insufficiency distally. The increase in intra-abdominal pressure may contribute to the development of vision deficits postoperatively. Elevated support for the pelvis and chest with chest rolls minimizes the number of pressure points, especially to the breasts and genitalia, which could result in skin pressure necrosis. The head may then be able to assume a more neutral position. Note that the positioning devices may also injure the patient by direct pressure-induced ischemia, as well as stretch injury (brachial plexus or ulnar nerve).

○ **What are the other potential complications of prone positioning [Edgecombe et al., 2008. See reference on page 529]?**

- Postoperative visual loss (POVL): 67% of POVL occurs during prone spinal surgery, mostly due to perioperative ischemic optic neuropathy (PO-ION), involving the posterior optic nerve [Roth, 2009. See reference on page 529].
- Corneal abrasion or pressure injury to eyes.
- Cervical spine injury or occlusion of the carotid/vertebral arteries due to extension or rotation of the neck.
- Pressure injury to breasts or genitals.
- Pressure (direct and indirect) or stretch injury.
- Hypotension due to hip or knee flexion and venous pooling in the lower extremities.
- Displacement of venous lines and indwelling catheters.
- Brachial plexopathy.
- Compression of the lateral femoral cutaneous nerve (meralgia paresthetica).
- Hemodynamics: decrease in cardiac index; obstruction of the IVC (increased bleeding, venous stasis, thrombotic complications).

○ **What is midcervical paraplegia?**

This is unexplained postoperative paraplegia, which is rare, from stretching or compression of the cervical spinal cord causing ischemic injury in the midcervical segment (C5) due to neck flexion with the patient in the sitting position. There is potential loss of function at the shoulders and biceps, and complete loss of function at the wrists and hands. Patients considered at risk include those with significant degenerative disease of the cervical spine, cervical spinal stenosis, and/or cerebral vascular disease. Cerebral perfusion pressure (CPP) should be maintained at a minimum of 60 mm Hg, with the MAP transduced at the level of the head.

○ **What are the potential complications associated with the sitting position?**

- Hypotension, especially on initial assumption of the position.
- Venous air embolism.
- Pneumocephalus and tension pneumocephalus.
- Flexed position of the neck causes midcervical paraplegia, macroglossia, facial edema, and venous bleeding.
- Brachial plexus injury.
- Peripheral nerve injury: common peroneal nerve and recurrent laryngeal nerve palsy.

○ **Where should the mean arterial pressure be transduced in a sitting patient?**

Mean arterial pressure should be measured with the transducer of the arterial line placed at or corrected to the level of the head (Circle of Willis). The auditory meatus is an external landmark. This will give a meaningful measurement of CPP (CPP = MAP − cerebral venous pressure).

○ **What is the most common ophthalmologic diagnosis for POVL?**

ION (ischemic optic neuropathy).

○ **According to the POVL Registry of the ASA Closed Claims Study Group, what is the most common cause of postoperative blindness [Lee, 2003. See reference on page 529]?**

The majority of cases are associated with prone operations (67%) followed by cardiac bypass procedures (10%). The remaining 23% of cases are composed of liver transplants, thoracoabdominal aneurysm resections, peripheral vascular procedures, head and neck operations, and prostatectomies. Of the 53 cases of POVL associated with spine surgery in the registry, ophthalmologic diagnoses included ION ($n = 43$, 81%), central retinal artery occlusion ($n = 7$, 13%), and unknown diagnosis ($n = 3$, 6%).

○ **List possible causes of postoperative unilateral blindness after nonocular surgery.**

- ION is the commonest diagnosis. It has been documented in a wide variety of procedures, the most common of which are cardiopulmonary bypass, head and neck operations, and prone spine operations.
- Retinal artery occlusion.
- Cortical blindness from hemorrhagic or embolic occipital lobe infarction.
- Stretch or compression of optic nerve in prone patient.

○ **What are the risk factors associated with ION?**

In a case controlled study of 80 patients with ION, compared with 315 matched controlled subjects, independent risk factors were male sex, obesity, Wilson frame use, longer anesthetic duration, greater estimated blood loss, and lower percent colloid administration [Postoperative Visual Loss Study Group, 2012. See reference on page 529].

○ **How does ION differ from central retinal artery occlusion as a cause for visual loss following surgery?**

ION is associated with larger blood loss (>2 L), hypotension, anemia (median lowest Hct of 25), longer duration (median time 9 hours) in the prone position, and/or vaso-occlusive disease. The high percentage of patients with bilateral disease and reported cases occurring in patients whose heads are suspended in Mayfield tongs makes direct globe pressure an unlikely etiology. Recovery of vision is reported in 56% of cases.

The etiology of central retinal artery occlusion is thought to be direct pressure on the globe, emboli, or low perfusion pressure in the retina. Supporting evidence includes low estimated blood loss, lack of anemia, shorter duration of prone position, unilateral disease, and no recovery of vision. Direct pressure on the globe may also cause unilateral periorbital bruising, proptosis, paresis of extraocular eye muscles, and/or supraorbital paresthesias.

○ **What are the recommendations for major spine surgery cases with high risk for POVL?**

1. Consider consenting patients for risk of POVL [ASA Practice Advisory for Perioperative Visual Loss Associated with Spine Surgery, 2012. See reference on page 528].
2. Arterial line to monitor BP, and consider CVP.
3. Use colloids along with crystalloid for volume replacement.
4. Position the head so that it is equal to or above the level of the heart. Position the patient to reduce intra-abdominal pressure.
5. Consider staging the procedure (cases lasting >5 hours and median blood loss 2 L are risk factors).

○ **List the risks of lithotomy positioning.**

- Common peroneal nerve injury
- Venous stasis in the lower legs, with the risk of phlebitis
- Arterial vascular insufficiency
- Compartment syndrome
- Compression or stretching of sciatic (exaggerated hip flexion), femoral (kinked at the hip), saphenous (medial tibial condyle against the leg support), obturator (stretch), or posterior tibial nerve
- Back pain (especially with a history of herniated disc)
- Hip dislocation
- Lower extremity tendon and ligament injuries
- Crush injury to the fingers if they are caught when the leg section of the table is raised back to support a supine position

○ **A patient develops foot drop following vaginal hysterectomy. Her ankles were placed in candy cane stirrups to assume the classic lithotomy position. What happened?**

Injury to the common peroneal nerve due to improper positioning or padding.

Common peroneal nerve compression may occur where the nerve is most superficial and sweeps over the head of the fibula just below the lateral aspect of the knee. Compression against the leg support device or insufficient padding will cause nerve injury and weakness or paralysis in the dorsiflexion muscles of the foot and ankle.

○ **Explain the mechanism of femoral neuropathy following lithotomy positioning.**

Positional compression and stretch injury.

Flexion of the hip can compress the femoral nerve beneath the inguinal ligament and within the body of the psoas muscle, at the iliopsoas groove. Excessive hip abduction and external rotation causes additional stretch on the nerve. Direct trauma or retraction compression to the nerve and retroperitoneal hematoma during surgery or delivery should also be considered.

○ **Can median sternotomy and sternal retraction cause brachial plexus injuries?**

Yes. Excessive sternal retraction may result in fracture of the first rib and injury to the brachial neurovascular bundle.

○ **A patient complains of paresthesia in his left little finger after CABG. What is wrong?**

The incidence of postoperative brachial plexus injury is about 21% in these patients. These injuries are probably due to excessive chest retraction stretching the brachial plexus, hyperextension of the arms [Canbaz et al., 2005. See refernce on page 528], or direct nerve compression. Ischemic injury is compounded by a decrease in temperature and perfusion pressure during cardiopulmonary bypass.

○ **Which nerve injury associated with anesthesia is reported to have the highest median litigation-related payment?**

Spinal cord injury associated with delayed diagnosis of epidural hematoma.

Key Terms

Anesthesia complications: nerve injury
Head-down position: hypoxemia
Lithotomy position: nerve injury
Postoperative blindness: causes

Prone position: complications
Sitting position: blood pressure measurement
Unilateral blindness: etiology

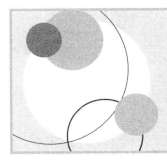

Pediatric Anesthesia

Great spirits have always found violent opposition from mediocre minds.
Albert Einstein

○ **For healthy children undergoing elective procedures, what are appropriate fasting guidelines?**

According to the American Society of Anesthesiologists, regardless of age, the appropriate minimum fasting times are 2 hours for clear liquids, 4 hours for breast milk, and 6 hours for a light meal, formula or nonhuman milk.

○ **How do infant formula and breast milk affect gastric emptying?**

Both have a high fat content and will result in delayed emptying. Hence the recommendation of no breast milk within 4 hours of surgery.

○ **T/F: Breast milk is not considered a solid food.**

False. Breast milk should be regarded as similar to a solid.

The 2011 ASA practice guidelines, updated in 2010, recommend a minimum fasting period for nonhuman milk and infant formula of 6 hours and for breast milk 4 hours [Practice Guidelines for Preoperative Fasting, 2011. See reference on page 529].

○ **What are two adverse medical consequences of prolonged fasting in children?**

Hypoglycemia and/or hypovolemia.

○ **Children may have unlimited clear liquids up to how many hours prior to scheduled anesthetic induction?**

Two hours.

○ **Calculate maintenance fluids in a 35-kg child.**

Maintenance is 75 mL/h. Calculation: 4 mL/kg for the first 10 kg, 2 mL/kg for the next 10, and 1 mL/kg thereafter.

○ **How does minimum alveolar concentration (MAC) change with age?**

MAC is highest in infants at term to 6 months of age and decreases with both increasing age and prematurity.

○ **Why is sevoflurane favored for use in pediatric anesthesia?**

Sevoflurane has a low blood solubility (blood:gas partition coefficient 0.68, at 37°C), which provides for a rapid inhalational induction and awakening. It is nonpungent and less irritating, so better tolerated by children. Also, it has excellent cardiovascular stability by primarily decreasing SVR while tending to support cardiac output.

○ **Compare and contrast the cardiovascular effects of sevoflurane and halothane.**

Sevoflurane tends to maintain blood pressure with an increase in heart rate, whereas halothane maintains or lowers heart rate with a fall in systolic blood pressure.

○ **What is the most common cardiovascular side effect of succinylcholine in children?**

Bradycardia, especially with a second dose. Atropine administration (20 μg/kg) may help to minimize this side effect.

○ **What is the first sign of hypovolemia in children under general anesthesia?**

Tachycardia. Hypotension usually does not occur in children until there is about a 20% loss of circulating blood volume.

○ **What is the leading cause of death in children over age 1 in the United States?**

Trauma. Motor vehicle accidents represent the most frequent cause. Serious head injury is the most common injury leading to death.

○ **Acute renal failure, hemolytic anemia, and thrombocytopenia comprise the triad for which syndrome?**

Hemolytic uremic syndrome (HUS).

○ **What is the most common cause of superior vena cava syndrome in children?**

Mediastinal malignancies, most commonly lymphomas.

○ **The most feared complication associated with extracorporeal membrane oxygenation (ECMO) is?**

Intracranial hemorrhage (ICH).

○ **What are the hemodynamic findings of decompensated shock?**

Hypotension and low cardiac output. Tachycardia is often present. Bradycardia, if present, is an ominous sign and suggests impending cardiac arrest.

○ **The lower limit of systolic blood pressure for a child older than 1 year of age can be estimated by using which formula?**

70 mm Hg + (2 × age in years).

○ **What is the most common cause of shock in children?**

Hypovolemic shock. It is usually associated with dehydration or hemorrhage but can also occur due to massive extravascular fluid shifts such as those seen in sepsis or extensive burns.

○ **When should epinephrine or atropine be used for the treatment of bradycardia in children?**

Only after adequate ventilation and oxygenation have been established, since hypoxemia is a common cause of bradycardia, and usually only if the child is symptomatic with cardiorespiratory compromise.

○ **Which drugs are contraindicated for infusion through an intraosseous route?**

None. The intraosseous route can safely be used to administer any intravenous drug or fluid required during the resuscitation of children.

○ **What is the major cause of intracerebral hemorrhage in children?**

Congenital abnormalities of the cerebral blood vessels. The most common of these are arteriovenous malformations.

○ **Acute myocardial infarction in children is associated with which pediatric diseases?**

Kawasaki disease and anomalous origin of the left coronary artery.

○ **Aplastic crisis in sickle cell disease is associated with what infectious agent?**

Parvovirus (the causative agent in fifth disease). The primary erythropoietic failure during aplastic crisis can result in a life-threatening anemia in these patients with a significantly decreased RBC life span.

○ **A 2-year-old sickle cell patient presents with pallor, weakness, tachycardia, and abdominal fullness. What diagnosis should you suspect?**

Acute splenic sequestration. This disorder is caused by acute and massive splenic enlargement due to sequestration of a large portion of the sickle cell patient's blood volume. This is an emergency since acute hypovolemia can result from so much blood being trapped within the spleen.

○ **What should the treatment plan for this patient include?**

Fluid and blood transfusions to correct hypovolemia and anemia.

○ **A child with hemoglobin SS disease (sickle cell anemia) is scheduled for cholecystectomy. His hematocrit is 20%. Is transfusion necessary?**

These children are at increased risk for perioperative sickling and stroke in the presence of hypoxemia, hypothermia, hypovolemia, and acidosis. Steps should be taken both to minimize these triggers and to reduce the concentration of hemoglobin S (HbS) either through exchange transfusion or by simple transfusion of packed red blood cells. A target goal for HbS concentration is less than 30–50%, with the hematocrit approximately 30%. Hemoglobin electrophoresis measuring HbS should be performed to follow response to therapy [Josephson et al., 2007. See reference on page 529].

○ **What is the most common age range for esophageal foreign bodies?**

One to 6 years of age.

○ **What are the most common esophageal foreign bodies?**

Coins.

○   **What complications can occur when hypotonic maintenance fluids are used for volume resuscitation?**

Hyponatremia and hyperglycemia.

○   **The end-tidal CO_2 in a T-piece breathing circuit depends on what factors?**

The fresh gas flow and the minute ventilation.

○   **Why are T-piece breathing systems considered useful in pediatric anesthesia?**

They have minimal dead space and no valves, which reduces the resistance to breathing.

○   **What are the disadvantages of a T-piece breathing system?**

They require high fresh gas flows (to prevent rebreathing) and large volumes of volatile anesthetics. They conserve heat and humidity poorly.

○   **Are T-piece breathing systems classified as semi-open or semiclosed?**

Semi-open, because rebreathing of alveolar gas with CO_2 occurs if fresh gas flow is decreased. In a semiclosed system, rebreathing of CO_2 does not occur due to the presence of a CO_2 absorber and valves separating the inspiratory from the expiratory limbs.

○   **What are the causes of inspiratory stridor in infants?**

Upper airway obstruction including obstruction from enlarged tonsils and/or adenoids, midface hypoplasia, laryngomalacia, or other congenital laryngeal anomalies and infectious processes such as croup. All of these abnormalities occur above the thoracic inlet.

○   **A 4-year-old child presents to the emergency department. The child was well 6 hours earlier but has since developed a fever and dyspnea. The child is leaning forward, drooling, and complaining of a sore throat. How should this child be managed?**

This is a classic presentation of epiglottitis.

The diagnosis of acute epiglottitis must be considered until ruled out. In general, epiglottitis involves the acute onset (6–24 hours) of a bacterial inflammation of the epiglottis that can rapidly lead to airway obstruction. Although a lateral x-ray of the neck may confirm epiglottic enlargement, if the diagnosis is suspected, immediate intubation for airway control is the first priority. The child should be kept calm and transported immediately to the operating room.

Routine pediatric vaccination for *Haemophilus influenzae* type b (Hib) has dramatically decreased the incidence of acute epiglottitis.

○   **How does one induce anesthesia in a child with epiglottitis?**

On a nurse or parent's lap the child is preoxygenated. Ventilation is not assisted during inhalational induction. An IV is established only after the patient is deeply anesthetized with the subsequent administration of 0.01–0.02 mg/kg IV atropine. Muscle relaxants should be avoided. A gentle laryngoscopy should be performed by an individual who is most experienced; the endotracheal tube should be at least one size (0.5 mm) smaller than would normally be used and preloaded with a stylet.

Patient should be immediately started on intravenous antibiotic treatment.

○ **Is an intravenous induction or an inhalation induction preferred in a child with epiglottitis?**

Children with epiglottitis are at risk for acute airway obstruction as the inflamed epiglottis and surrounding supraglottic tissues occlude the laryngeal inlet. Inhalation induction with maintenance of spontaneous respiration may be preferred to maintain airway patency, even if an intravenous line is in place. Efforts should be made to avoid upsetting the child and promoting airway obstruction with crying.

○ **Should a rapid sequence induction be performed in a child with epiglottitis?**

No. Laryngoscopy should be performed under deep general anesthesia without muscle relaxants to minimize the possibility of complete loss of the airway. Complications from aspiration have been rare.

○ **Why do children with epiglottitis have altered airway dynamics and stridor?**

Inspiration past a significant obstruction at the level of the epiglottis results in an exaggerated negative intrathoracic pressure during inspiration and a dynamic collapse of the trachea below the level of the obstruction, resulting in inspiratory stridor.

○ **Five minutes after intubating a child with epiglottitis frothy secretions are suctioned from the endotracheal tube; why?**

Patients with epiglottitis are known to develop negative pressure pulmonary edema as a complication. This is due to generation of high negative inspiratory pressures against an obstructed laryngeal inlet. It occurs only after relief of airway obstruction, which facilitates increased venous return and thus extravasation of fluid from damaged alveolar capillaries.

○ **How is negative pressure pulmonary edema treated?**

It usually requires supportive care and is generally self-limited; it may be improved with PEEP/CPAP.

○ **How long should an epiglottitis patient remain intubated?**

Inflammation resolves in 24–72 hours. The patient is usually ready for extubation within 36–72 hours of starting antibiotic therapy. Some anesthesiologists recommend revisualization of the epiglottis prior to extubation. Others believe this is unnecessary and that leak around the endotracheal tube can be used safely as a guide to readiness for extubation.

○ **At what age does laryngotracheobronchitis (croup) occur?**

It occurs at ages 6 months to 6 years and typically lasts less than 5 days. This is in contrast to children with epiglottitis, a disease that typically occurs in older children aged 2–6, but may occur into adulthood.

○ **What is the treatment for croup?**

Treatment begins with humidified oxygen. If tachypnea and cyanosis are present, aerosolized racemic epinephrine may be helpful. The use of corticosteroids is controversial. If symptoms persist for more than 7 days, or the child is less than 4 months of age, laryngoscopy should be considered to rule out other causes.

○ **How can croup and epiglottitis be clinically differentiated?**

Croup is more common in infants, whereas epiglottis tends to occur in 2- to 6-year-old children. Epiglottitis is associated with a high fever, toxic appearance, and abrupt onset of respiratory distress and stridor. Croup, however, is usually more subacute in onset with lower fevers and is characterized by a barking cough.

○ **How can croup and epiglottitis be radiologically differentiated?**

X-ray of the neck shows enlarged epiglottis in epiglottitis and narrow epiglottis in croup. The A-P neck film shows tracheal narrowing in epiglottitis and subglottic narrowing (Steeple sign) in croup.

○ **What are the laboratory findings in epiglottitis versus croup?**

WBC:

Marked elevation with left shift in epiglottitis

Variable in croup

Bacteriology:

H. influenzae, type b isolated from throat and blood culture in epiglottitis

Viral etiology, parainfluenza usually in croup

○ **What is the differential diagnosis of partial airway obstruction in children?**

Extrinsic pathology: hypertrophied tonsils/adenoids, infection, cystic hygroma, vascular abnormalities, and neoplasm.

Intrinsic pathology: epiglottitis, croup, subglottic stenosis, vocal cord paralysis, and laryngeal stricture anomalies.

○ **What is the narrowest point in the airway of a child less than 10 years of age?**

The cricoid cartilage.

○ **What is resistance to airflow in the airway inversely proportional to?**

The fourth power of the radius of the airway (when laminar airflow is present during quiet breathing). A smaller radius means higher resistance. This is Poiseuille's law.

○ **What is the formula to estimate uncuffed endotracheal tube size?**

Endotracheal tube size = (age in years/4) + 4.

○ **What is the average endotracheal tube length (measured at the lips) appropriate for a 2- and a 5-year-old child?**

Twelve and 15 cm, respectively.

○ **Why is it recommended to administer a vagolytic drug prior to laryngoscopy in infants?**

Infants have a higher resting vagal tone, and laryngoscopy excites the vagal nerve, leading to potential vasovagal symptoms such as complete heart block or sinus arrest. Intravenous atropine 10 μg/kg is given to prevent bradycardia and hypotension. The effect of atropine also helps with bradycardia and hypotension seen with the inhaled anesthetic halothane. Atropine increases cardiac output by increasing heart rate.

○ **Why is a "leak test" often performed after placement of uncuffed endotracheal tubes in young children?**

A leak around an uncuffed endotracheal tube suggests that the tube is not too tight and therefore not exerting excessive pressure on the mucosa of the airway, especially at the level of the circumferential cricoid cartilage (the narrowest part of the airway in young children). A leak heard at less than an inspiratory pressure of 30 cm H_2O

is generally considered safe. This is an approximation of the capillary pressure of the airway mucosa. Higher pressures exerted for extended periods of time could potentially cause tissue damage and result in acute edema that might result in postextubation stridor or long-term problems such as scarring and subglottic stenosis.

○ **Are cuffed endotracheal tubes safe in children?**

Recent studies suggest that when used properly, cuffed endotracheal tubes can be safely used in children. Generally speaking, a half-size smaller tube should be utilized (compared with uncuffed size calculated using the standard formula) to account for the added bulk of the cuff itself. One must be vigilant to make sure the cuff lies below the vocal cords and the tip of the tube rests above the carina. It may be useful to measure the pressure in the endotracheal tube cuff to minimize the pressure exerted on the airway mucosa.

○ **At what age are infants no longer obligate nose breathers?**

Three to 5 months.

○ **Describe the unique characteristics of the infant airway.**

Infants have soft, easily collapsible tissue in the airway. The larynx is located more anterior and cephalad (C_{3-4}). The epiglottis is large, omega shaped and tends to obscure the view of the glottis opening on laryngoscopic view.

○ **How often do neonates with cleft lip and palate have associated anomalies?**

Associated congenital anomalies occur 30 times more frequently. Ten to 25% have anomalies of other organs.

○ **When should a child with cleft lip or palate have it repaired?**

The lip is usually repaired at 3 months of age provided there are no associated anomalies. Many surgeons have adopted "Musgrave's" rule of 10 to determine appropriate timing of lip closure (hemoglobin >10 g, >10 weeks of age, weight ≥10 kg, and WBC <10,000). The palate can be closed up to 4 years of age, but speech development is optimized if repair is before 18 months of age.

○ **A child presents with wheezing and is using accessory muscles to breathe. The child appears otherwise well. Examination shows hyperlucency in the right upper lobe. What is your presumptive diagnosis?**

Aspiration of a foreign body should be strongly suspected. It is the most common cause of wheezing refractory to medical treatment in children. Death by asphyxiation due to aspiration is the leading cause of death in children <1 year old, followed by motor vehicle accidents. Children present with wheezing, coughing, and gagging. Cyanosis, hemoptysis, intercostal muscle retractions, and use of the accessory respiratory muscles may be observed. Most foreign bodies are radiolucent but a chest x-ray may demonstrate atelectasis or obstructive emphysema.

○ **What are the classic findings on physical examination for a foreign body aspiration?**

The classic symptoms include the sudden onset of coughing, with stridor, localized wheezing, and/or diminished breath sounds. If obstruction is severe, cyanosis may occur. Patients may be asymptomatic and physical findings may not be present.

Lower airway: localized wheezing, dyspnea, fever, and cough. Upper airway: dyspnea, stridor, cough, and cyanosis.

○ **What are the most common objects aspirated by children?**

Food items such as peanuts, popcorn, and carrots. Less common are plastic and metal parts of toys.

○   **T/F: Most airway foreign bodies are radiopaque.**

False. Airway foreign bodies are usually radiolucent, making the diagnosis more difficult.

○   **What types of airway foreign bodies typically produce the greatest inflammatory response?**

Food items, peanuts in particular.

○   **Why do peanuts pose a special risk when aspirated?**

During bronchoscopy and extraction, the peanut may break apart, spreading particles into distal lung segments or the contralateral lung. The oil in peanuts can also cause a local tissue reaction.

○   **How is anesthesia induced in a child who has aspirated a foreign body?**

An inhalational induction is the safest method. Avoid assisting ventilation since this may drive the foreign body further into the airway causing complete obstruction or contribute to air trapping distal to the object. Rectally administered medication may be used to assist with induction in the uncooperative patient.

○   **During airway foreign body extraction, at what point is complete immobility of the patient crucial?**

As the endoscopist is delivering the foreign body across the glottis. If the patient coughs or moves during this phase of the procedure, the foreign body can be dislodged and fall into the airway.

○   **Why does a patient often not improve immediately after removal of an airway foreign body?**

Depending on the type of foreign body and the duration of impaction, the airway mounts an inflammatory response that may persist well beyond the point of removal. Local swelling may decrease the cross-sectional area of the airway lumen and continue to limit airflow. Systemic inflammatory mediators may increase airway smooth muscle reactivity causing generalized bronchospasm.

○   **Children, particularly infants, have larger volumes of distribution for many drugs compared with adults. Why?**

Infants, especially neonates, have lower protein binding to act as a drug reservoir. Also, total body water, extracellular fluid volume, and blood volume are relatively higher in young children compared with adults.

○   **How does a larger volume of distribution affect the pharmacokinetics of a drug?**

More drug may be required (on a milligram per kilogram of weight basis) to achieve the desired clinical effect.

○   **List any features of concern for an anesthesia care provider in patients with Trisomy 21 (Down syndrome).**

Developmental delay, cervical spine instability (primarily due to ligamentous laxity), hypotonia, cardiac disease (occurring in 40–60% of individuals) [Freeman et al., 1998. See reference on page 529], gastrointestinal disease (including duodenal atresia), eye disorders (cataracts, strabismus), leukemias, hypothyroidism, subglotttic narrowing, large tongue, and adenotonsillar hypertrophy (causing upper airway obstruction). These patients may be prone to bradycardia when exposed to halogenated anesthetics such as sevoflurane.

○   **What is the most common congenital heart defect associated with Trisomy 21 (Down syndrome)?**

Endocardial cushion defect (also known as A-V canal or atrioventricular septal defect).

○ **What are the four classic cardiac features of tetralogy of Fallot (TOF)?**

Right ventricular hypertrophy, ventriculoseptal defect (VSD), infundibular pulmonary stenosis, and an overriding aorta.

○ **What is a "tet spell"?**

In a patient with TOF, a hypercyanotic or "tet spell" results from spasm of the subpulmonary infundibulum causing increased resistance to blood flow into the right ventricular outflow tract. This results in decreased pulmonary blood flow and an increased right-to-left shunt across the VSD with subsequent cyanosis.

○ **What is the cause and treatment of a "tet spell"?**

Patients with TOF have a fixed stenosis caused by the hypertrophy of the right ventricular outflow tract musculature. This fixed stenosis can be augmented by dynamic stenosis caused by spasm of the right ventricular outflow tract muscle under conditions of stress and excess catecholamines, hypothermia, hypovolemia, hypoxia, hypercarbia, and metabolic acidosis. These conditions can cause a sudden decrease in pulmonary blood flow and hypoxia, known as a "tet spell". Squatting in order to increase preload and afterload is a well-known method by which a patient can force more blood through the lungs. Pharmacologically, the increase in afterload can be produced by the use of a bolus of the alpha-agonist phenylephrine, followed by a drip. This drug has the advantage of raising systemic vascular resistance (thereby augmenting left-to-right shunt through the ventricular defect and increasing pulmonary blood flow) without also increasing contractility and augmenting right ventricular outflow tract obstruction. Increasing preload and pulmonary blood flow with a bolus of crystalloid and/or colloid is also extremely useful. If these initial maneuvers are not adequate, then a beta-blocker can be employed to relieve the hypercontractile state of the muscle of the right ventricular outflow tract. If these treatments are not enough to raise pulmonary blood flow and arterial oxygen saturation, then an attempt to reopen the ductus arteriosus by employing a drip of prostaglandin E1 should be tried.

○ **During general anesthesia, how do you treat a hypercyanotic spell in a patient with TOF?**

Management is aimed at reducing right-to-left shunting by increasing SVR and decreasing resistance in the pulmonary outflow tract. Methods of treatment include administration of intravenous volume (boluses of 10 mL/kg), ventilation with 100% oxygen, and boluses (1–10 μg/kg) or an infusion (0.05–0.2 μg/kg/min) of phenylephrine to increase systemic vascular resistance. The primary reason for hypoxemic spells under general anesthesia is hypovolemia. Fasting should be minimized and IV fluids should be administered preoperatively whenever possible.

○ **Why is succinylcholine contraindicated in children with muscular dystrophy?**

It can cause an exaggerated hyperkalemic response and cardiac arrest.

○ **Should succinylcholine be used for routine intubation in pediatric patients?**

This is a controversial issue. The "black box warning" indicates that there are rare reports of ventricular dysrhythmias and cardiac arrest secondary to acute rhabdomyolysis with hyperkalemia in apparently healthy children who received succinylcholine. Many of these children were subsequently found to have a skeletal muscle myopathy whose clinical signs were not obvious. Since it is difficult to identify which patients are at risk, it is recommended that the use of succinylcholine in children should be reserved for emergency intubation or where immediate securing of an airway is necessary.

○ **T/F: Children with cerebral palsy are at increased risk for hyperkalemia after succinylcholine.**

False.

○ **T/F: Every child with a runny nose should be canceled for surgery.**

False [Tait and Malyiya, 2005. See reference on page 529]. The child who has a fever, rhonchi that do not clear with coughing, wheeze, abnormal chest x-ray, elevated white count, purulent productive cough and/or nasal secretions, or decreased level of activity or is "off his or her feeds" should be rescheduled. Most anesthesiologists would proceed with surgery with a child if the upper respiratory tract infection is uncomplicated and resolving, unless the child has a history of asthma or other significant pulmonary disease. Chronic nasal discharge is usually noninfectious in origin and caused by allergy or vasomotor rhinitis.

○ **What are the effects of viral upper respiratory infections (URIs) on lung function?**

The risk of pulmonary complications is 9–11 times greater up to 2 weeks after an upper respiratory tract infection, especially if the patient is intubated. Studies in adults evaluating PFTs before and following a URI have shown changes in small airway hyperreactivity that persist up to 7 weeks and general respiratory muscle weakness up to 12 days. Similar PFT changes have been demonstrated in children aged 6 and older with a URI. Underlying abnormalities include increased airway reactivity with wheeze (decreased PEFR and MMEF), decreased diffusion capacity for oxygen, decreased compliance and resistance, decreased closing volumes (decreased FEV_1 and FVC), increased shunting, and increased incidence of hypoxemia.

○ **How does the decision to intubate influence the perioperative risk of respiratory problems in an infant with a mild URI?**

Infants with URIs who undergo *intubation* are at significant risk of developing major adverse respiratory events (i.e., postoperative croup) versus children. The reason is that edema secondary to intubation results in a greater reduction in cross-sectional area of the trachea.

○ **What are some systemic symptoms that are considered contraindications to elective surgery by most anesthesiologists?**

Fever, purulent rhinorrhea, wheeze, and productive cough.

○ **A 5-year-old presents for tonsillectomy. He has a runny nose and a cough, but no fever. Is a general anesthetic safe for this patient?**

There is no true consensus regarding the safety of anesthetizing children who have a URI. Most of the literature does suggest an increased risk of perioperative pulmonary complications in the setting of a URI. However, most of these complications are mild and do not usually result in significant morbidity. Importantly, children with reactive airways disease and those requiring an endotracheal tube have a greater risk than otherwise healthy children. The type of procedure, necessity of intubation, and general health of the child should all be considered in deciding whether to delay elective surgery.

○ **According to the American Heart Association (AHA), which children are at risk for infective endocarditis and require antibiotic prophylaxis for dental procedures?**

AHA Guidelines for Prevention of Infective Endocarditis, 2007 [See reference on page 529] include:
- Prosthetic cardiac valve or prosthetic material used for cardiac valve repair
- Cardiac transplantation recipients who develop cardiac valvulopathy

- Previous infective endocarditis
- Congenital heart disease (CHD):
  - Unrepaired cyanotic CHD, including palliative shunts and conduits
  - Completely repaired congenital heart defect with prosthetic material or device, whether placed by surgery or by catheter intervention, during the first 6 months after the procedure
  - Repaired CHD with residual defects at the site or adjacent to the site of a prosthetic patch or prosthetic device (which inhibit endothelialization)

○ **A child is having outpatient strabismus surgery. What is the risk of postoperative nausea and vomiting (PONV)?**

The incidence of significant PONV is 50–80% [Oh et al., 2010. See reference on page 529].

○ **Which procedures are most closely associated with PONV in children?**

PONV is more common after surgeries of the head (e.g., strabismus, tonsillectomy, middle ear procedures) and genitals (e.g., penile procedures, orchiopexy, inguinal hernia repair). Use of narcotics and a history of motion sickness are also associated with this complication.

○ **T/F: Intraoperative use of nitrous oxide is associated with PONV.**

True. Eliminating nitrous oxide has been associated with less PONV. This issue is still debated.

○ **T/F: In children, the incidence of postoperative vomiting (POV) increases with age?**

True. Nausea is a subjective sensation and therefore difficult to assess in young children. POV, however, is easier to assess. It is known to be uncommon in infants and young children but increases in incidence during childhood. Vomiting in children aged 3 and older is actually more common than it is in adults after surgery! This propensity to vomit decreases after puberty.

○ **T/F: Teenage girls are more likely to experience PONV compared with boys.**

True. Gender differences in the incidence of PONV are not seen until after puberty when girls tend to be more affected, just as female gender is associated with a greater incidence of PONV in adults.

○ **T/F: Infants and children have a longer induction time with inhaled anesthetic agents compared with adults.**

False. Although tidal volume per unit of body weight is constant (6 mL/kg) throughout life, infants and children have a relatively higher alveolar ventilation compared with adults and a lower relative functional residual capacity (FRC). This increased ratio of minute ventilation to FRC results in a more rapid uptake of inhaled anesthetics. The effect is less pronounced for less blood-soluble agents.

○ **T/F: Infants and children with cyanotic CHD (right-to-left shunt) have a longer induction time with *inhaled* anesthetic agents compared with children with normal hearts.**

True. With right-to-left shunt, a portion of the blood returning to the heart bypasses the lung and therefore is not exposed to anesthetic, slowing the induction of anesthesia. A large shunt will slow induction more than a smaller shunt. This effect is more pronounced with less soluble agents.

○ **T/F: Infants and children with cyanotic CHD (right-to-left shunt) have a longer induction time with *intravenous* drugs compared with children with normal hearts.**

False. Intravenous induction actually occurs slightly more quickly in children with cyanotic CHD since venous blood containing drug returns to the right atrium and a portion is shunted directly to the left heart and carried to the brain, bypassing the pulmonary circulation. With fast-acting induction agents, the clinical relevance of this effect is questionable though.

○ **T/F: Infants and children with left-to-right shunt have a slower induction with *inhalation* anesthetics.**

Unless the shunt is very large (>80%), left-to-right shunt produces negligible change in the induction time with inhaled anesthetics.

○ **List some possible complications of caudal anesthesia in children.**

Intravascular injection, dural puncture, intraosseous injection of anesthetic agents, muscle weakness, and urinary retention.

○ **What is laryngospasm?**

Laryngospasm represents the involuntary closure of the glottis by intrinsic laryngeal muscles that bring the vocal cords to the midline. It is a normal, protective reflex to prevent pulmonary aspiration.

○ **How is laryngospasm managed in pediatric patients?**

Initial therapy includes initiation of positive pressure to the airway by mask with 100% oxygen. The spasm often ceases with this maneuver within 30–45 seconds. If spasm continues and oxygen saturation falls, muscle relaxant can be administered. Succinylcholine is classically used, although nondepolarizing agents such as rocuronium can be considered. A full intubating dose is not normally required to break laryngospasm. Since bradycardia often accompanies hypoxemia in children, atropine use should be strongly considered when the laryngospasm does not resolve quickly.

○ **A surgeon wishes to repair an inguinal hernia in a 2-month-old baby as outpatient surgery. Is this appropriate?**

There is a concern that infants may develop apnea following general anesthesia. It is recommended that all former preterm infants younger than 55 weeks postconceptual age and all anemic former preterm infants be admitted to monitor their recovery.

○ **Define prematurity.**

Gestational age less than 37 weeks or weight less than 2,500 g at birth.

○ **Define gestational age.**

Number of weeks from conception to the time of birth.

○ **Define postnatal age.**

The age from birth to the present.

○ **Define postconceptual age.**

The sum of gestational age and postnatal age (weeks).

○ **How should a patient history of prematurity change postoperative care in the ambulatory setting?**

Premature infants younger than 60 postconceptual weeks should be monitored continuously for at least 12 hours to prevent apnea-related complications.

○ **How does age affect postoperative apnea in the premature infant?**

As the postconceptual age of the premature infant increases, postoperative apnea decreases proportionately.

○ **In general, what types of problems are common in premature babies?**

Neurological: intraventricular hemorrhage, hydrocephalus, retinopathy of prematurity, seizures, delayed development, and impaired temperature regulation.

Respiratory: apnea and bradycardia, bronchopulmonary dysplasia, respiratory distress syndrome, bullae, pneumonia, reactive pulmonary vasculature, subglottic stenosis, and tracheomalacia.

Cardiac: patent ductus arteriosus (PDA) and cardiomyopathy.

Endocrine: hypoglycemia, metabolic acidosis, and malnutrition.

Gastrointestinal: necrotizing enterocolitis, GE reflux, and poor gag reflex.

Genitourinary: chronic renal failure and renal tubular acidosis.

○ **Until what age are premature infants at increased risk for postoperative apnea?**

The answer to this question is somewhat controversial. The available literature suggests that postoperative apnea may be a risk in infants of 44–55 weeks postconceptual age or younger. The implication of this risk is that elective procedures requiring general anesthesia should be delayed, if possible, until these age criteria are met. If surgery is necessary before then, the infants should be admitted and monitored overnight.

○ **What conditions are associated with postoperative apnea in infants?**

Premature infants (defined as born at less than 37 weeks gestation) are most prone to apnea, especially those who receive general anesthesia (or any sedatives), have ongoing apnea, or are anemic.

○ **What is the preferred method of anesthesia for premature infants?**

There is no consensus that one anesthetic technique is better than another. Although regional anesthesia has been recommended in the past, there is no conclusive evidence that it is "safer." Even those premature infants who have regional anesthesia should be monitored in the hospital postoperatively.

○ **What drug may be effective in the prevention of postoperative apnea in premature infants?**

Intravenous caffeine (5–10 mg/kg) may have beneficial effects that can last several days.

○ **Is fusion of the cervical spines a feature of Pierre Robin syndrome?**

No. Pierre Robin syndrome is characterized by small mouth, mandibular hypoplasia, and large tongue.

○ **Describe the anesthetic implications of Pierre Robin syndrome.**

Children with Pierre Robin syndrome can be difficult to intubate due to facial anomalies. These include mandibular hypoplasia and cleft palate.

○ **What signs would you expect to find on examination of a child with a PDA?**

Tachycardia, systolic murmur, bounding peripheral pulses, widened pulse pressure, and radiographic evidence of increased pulmonary blood flow.

○ **Do most infants with PDA require surgery?**

No. Ductal closure is usually accomplished with medical therapy using indomethacin. Surgery occurs if this fails and the patient remains symptomatic.

○ **T/F: Cyanosis is a common feature of PDA.**

False. The pulmonary vasculature usually has a lower resistance than the systemic circulation, so flow across the ductus arteriosus is usually left to right.

○ **What are the implications of left-to-right shunt in infants with PDA?**

These infants usually have low pulmonary vascular resistance (PVR) and are therefore prone to excessive pulmonary circulation. They may have congestive heart failure on that basis. Neonates and premature infants may have diastolic runoff from the aorta into the ductus arteriosus that can lead to coronary hypoperfusion. Oxygenation and maintenance of ventilation (without hyperventilation) are keys to management.

○ **During surgery, a 12-kg child becomes acidotic with a pH of 7.0, serum bicarbonate 15 mEq/L, and a base deficit −10. How much bicarbonate would you need to give to correct this deficit?**

Bicarbonate deficit is calculated by the following formula: weight (kg) × 0.3 × base deficit. You should give half the calculated amount and recheck the arterial blood gas pH in 20–30 minutes.

○ **What are the possible side effects of bicarbonate administration?**

Bicarbonate can cause paradoxical acidosis when it is converted to carbon dioxide. It can also cause hypernatremia, hyperosmolality (which may contribute to intraventricular hemorrhage in premature infants), and a left shift of the oxygen hemoglobin dissociation curve secondary to alkalosis.

○ **A 3-year-old in the PACU shows signs of upper airway obstruction shortly after general anesthesia. The nurse suggests a nasal airway. Is this appropriate?**

No. Small children have abundant, friable lymphoid tissue in the nasopharynx, which is a contraindication to nasal airways or blind nasal intubation.

○ **What is the most common initial sign of respiratory distress in an infant?**

Tachypnea. Neonates (both full-term and premature) respond to hypoxemia with an initial increase in respiratory rate followed by sustained respiratory depression. By 3 weeks of age, full-term infants respond to hypoxemia with sustained hyperventilation (as do older children and adults). Newborn infants respond to hypercapnea with increased ventilation as well, although this effect is less pronounced compared with older children and adults.

○ **In premature babies or neonates, why is the pulse oximeter probe preferentially placed on the right hand or ear lobe?**

Placement of the probe on the right hand or ear lobe will accurately reflect preductal (coronary, cerebral) oxygenation. During the first several weeks of life these patients may develop persistent fetal circulation with stress (hypoxia, hypothermia, acidosis). In this case, if right atrial pressure exceeds left atrial pressure, there may be a right-to-left shunting of blood through the ductus arteriosus (and possibly foramen ovale).

○ **Describe the differences between pediatric and adult lung function.**

The pediatric lung is less compliant. Chest wall compliance, on the other hand, is greater in children due to the cartilaginous structure of the ribcage. Airway resistance is also greater in children due to smaller airway diameters (Poiseuille's law). FRC is smaller and alveolar ventilation is higher in infants and small children compared with adults. Resting tidal volume is the same on a per kilogram basis for both adults and children.

○ **T/F: Body surface area to mass ratio is greater in children compared with adults.**

True.

○ **Why is an infant at risk for hypothermia?**

Their losses are greater because infants have poor central thermoregulation, higher minute ventilation, thin insulating fat, and increased body surface area to mass ratio. Shivering is an ineffective mechanism for heat production because of limited muscle mass and nonshivering thermogenesis significantly increases oxygen consumption. A cold-stressed infant is at risk for developing cardiovascular depression and lactic acidosis.

○ **What are the effects of hypothermia in infants?**

- Apnea and bradycardia
- Respiratory depression
- Coagulopathy
- Vasoconstriction
- Altered drug clearance

○ **What factors put infants at greater risk of toxicity from local anesthetics?**

Amide local anesthetics bind to serum proteins, primarily alpha-1-acid glycoprotein and albumin. This binding decreases the free fraction of drug that can cause signs and symptoms of local anesthetic toxicity. The concentration of these binding proteins is reduced in neonates and infants, leading to a higher free fraction and a greater risk of toxicity. In addition, infants have a decreased clearance of local anesthetics through hepatic mechanisms.

○ **What are the signs of local anesthetic toxicity in infants?**

Central nervous system (CNS) and cardiovascular effects are the most worrisome problems with local anesthetic toxicity. Infants may be less likely to manifest CNS signs of local anesthetic toxicity compared with adults. General anesthesia may also mask the signs. Infants cannot express neurological symptoms (dizziness, perioral numbness) and so seizures may be a first sign of CNS toxicity in nonanesthetized infants. Arrhythmias are a more common sign and may include bradycardia or ST/T-wave changes or more serious rhythm problems such as ventricular tachycardia, ventricular fibrillation, or asystole. These rhythm disturbances are likely related to local anesthetic blockade of ion channels (particularly sodium channels) in the heart.

○ **What therapies can be used for children with pulmonary hypertension associated with CHD?**

Acute treatments aim to reduce pulmonary artery pressure and PVR. This can be accomplished with hyperventilation (while keeping airway pressures low), avoiding hypoxia, and treatment of acidosis. Inotropes to improve right ventricular function can be utilized as well as pulmonary vasodilators such as inhaled nitric oxide.

○ **What are some advantages of parental presence at induction of anesthesia?**

Less anxiety in the child through avoidance of separation from his or her parent and decreased need for premedication.

○ **After a dose of oral midazolam (0.5 mg/kg) for premedication, when is it appropriate to separate children from their parents?**

Within 10–20 minutes.

○ **Describe bronchopulmonary dysplasia (BPD) in infants.**

BPD or chronic lung disease is seen in children who need supplemental O_2 and have abnormal chest x-ray findings at 36 weeks of postconceptual age. This is most often seen in premature infants who are subjected to prolonged ventilation with both high inspiratory pressures and O_2. Other aggravating factors include persistence of a PDA. Patients with BPD have abnormalities in lung compliance and airway resistance and this may persist for years after initial injury, leading to hypercarbia, chronic hypoxia, and restrictive lung disease. Exogenous surfactant therapy does not appear to prevent development of BPD.

Key Terms

Bronchopulmonary dysplasia
Congenital heart disease: pulmonary hypertension
   treatment
Croup: radiographic diagnosis
Diagnosis of croup
Down syndrome: abnormalities/anesthetic implications
Epiglottitis and airway dynamics
Epiglottitis: anesthetic management
Epiglottitis: diagnosis
Epiglottitis: inhalation induction
Ex-premature pulmonary complications
Fluid replacement in pediatrics
Hypoplastic left heart physiology
Hypotension/tachycardia in infants: treatment
Hypovolemia signs: pediatric patient
Infant: NPO guidelines
Infant preoperative fasting: breast milk
Infants' inspiratory stridor causes
Intraoperative hypothermia in infants
Intubation/management in Pierre Robin syndrome
Local anesthetic toxicity in infants: signs
MAC: pediatric, inhalational agent

Midazolam: pediatric dose oral
Neuromuscular reversal in infants
Parenteral presence: indications
Pediatric circuits
Pediatric contraindications to succinylcholine
Pediatric sleep apnea risk factors
Postoperative apnea in preterm infant
Postoperative apnea: postconceptual age
Postoperative nausea and vomiting (PONV) after
   pediatric surgery
Postoperative vomiting: pediatric versus adults
Preoperative anxiolysis in children
Prevent hypothermia in infant
Temperature regulation: infants versus adults
Tet spells: pharmacological treatment
Tetralogy: management of cyanosis
Tetralogy of Fallot (TOF): other abnormalities/
   pathophysiology/anesthetic considerations
Tetralogy of Fallot treatment
Uncuffed ETT: maximum leak pressure
Uptake versus distribution: infants versus adults

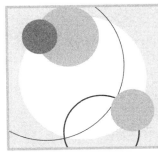

Peripheral Nerve Blocks

Continuous efforts, not strength or intelligence, is the key to unlocking our potential.
Winston Churchill

○ **What is the origin of the brachial plexus?**

It arises from the anterior primary divisions of the fifth cervical through first thoracic nerves.

○ **Name the components of the brachial plexus.**

Starting from their origin and progressing distally they are named *r*oots, *t*runks, *d*ivisions, *c*ords, and *b*ranches (*R*andy *T*ravis *D*rinks *C*old *B*eer). Between the anterior and middle scalene muscles, the roots of C5/C6 unite to form the *superior* (upper) trunk, C7 continues and forms the *middle* trunk, and C8/T1 merge to form the *inferior* (lower) trunk. At the lateral border of the first rib, each trunk bifurcates into anterior and posterior divisions [Barash et al., 2009; Miller, 2010].

○ **Where are the cords formed and how are they named?**

The divisions form three cords within the axilla: lateral, posterior, and medial. They are named for their relationship with the second part of the axillary artery. The lateral cord is formed from the anterior divisions of the upper and middle trunks (C5–C7). The middle cord is composed of the anterior division of the lower trunk (C8–T1), and the posterior divisions of all three trunks form the posterior cord (C5–T1) [Barash et al., 2009; Miller, 2010].

○ **The interscalene block is performed at what level of the brachial plexus?**

Roots.

○ **The function of which nerve is frequently spared after placement of an interscalene brachial plexus block?**

As blockade of the inferior trunk of the brachial plexus is often incomplete with the interscalene approach, function of the ulnar nerve (C8–T1) is frequently spared. These nerves can join the sheath below the level where the block is placed.

○ **Which nerve block(s) is (are) frequently required for supplementation of an interscalene brachial plexus blockade for surgery of the proximal upper extremity?**

The intercostobrachial nerve and the median brachial cutaneous nerve. Thoracic innervation enters the arm, outside of the brachial plexus sheath, especially the skin surface innervated by C2–C4, the medial thorax and the axilla.

○   **What's the major landmark for an interscalene block?**

The major landmark involves identification of the interscalene groove, lying between the anterior and middle scalene muscles at the level of the cricoid cartilage. A line is drawn laterally from the cricoid cartilage to intersect the interscalene grove, indicating the level of the transverse process of C6 [Miller, 2010].

○   **What frequently marks the level of the cricoid cartilage in the interscalene groove?**

The external jugular vein traversing the anterior triangle of the neck. At the level of the cricoid cartilage it intersects with the posterior border of the sternocleidomastoid muscle, overlying the interscalene groove. However, this is not always the case, and therefore not a reliable landmark [Miller, 2010].

○   **What important blood vessel runs in the interscalene groove, just below the brachial plexus?**

The subclavian artery runs in the interscalene groove, forming the notch on the superior surface of the first rib.

○   **How does an interscalene brachial plexus block progress, proximal to distal or vice versa?**

Proximal to distal.

○   **A patient with COPD complains of severe dyspnea after interscalene brachial plexus blockade. What is your differential diagnosis?**

Phrenic nerve blockade almost always occurs with interscalene anesthesia resulting in diaphragmatic paresis and an elevated hemidiaphragm. This is associated with a 25% reduction in pulmonary function. (This is usually of no clinical significance in otherwise healthy patients and may cause subjective feelings of dyspnea only.)

Other possibilities include pneumothorax, which is rare, and epidural or intrathecal injection causing dyspnea with hypotension or local anesthetic toxicity.

○   **What are the potential complications of an interscalene block in a patient having outpatient shoulder surgery?**

Pneumothorax, intravascular injection into the vertebral artery (immediate CNS signs: seizures), Horner syndrome (miosis, ptosis, and enophthalmos), recurrent laryngeal nerve block (hoarseness), subarachnoid and epidural injection, 100% incidence of paralysis of the ipsilateral diaphragm (phrenic nerve blockade), and neuropathy from intraneural injection or direct needle trauma.

○   **Is an interscalene brachial plexus block ideal for hand surgery?**

No. Interscalene brachial plexus blocks provide consistent anesthesia of the shoulder, arm, and elbow. With this approach there is frequently ulnar nerve sparing (a branch of the lower trunk). More distal approaches to the plexus such as infraclavicular or axillary are more appropriate for hand surgery.

○   **Most shoulder surgeries are performed on an outpatient basis. Discuss postoperative pain management.**

Regional anesthesia as a sole anesthetic or used in combination with general anesthesia is ideal. Blocks may be performed preoperatively or postoperatively using either a single-shot, continuous infusion or patient-controlled pain pumps. The addition of clonidine or the mixed agonist–antagonist opioid compounds to local anesthetic has been shown to prolong analgesia for brachial plexus blocks. Adjuvant therapy includes oral, IV, IM, and IV PCA opioids, NSAIDs, acetaminophen, agonist–antagonist analgesics, and ice to minimize pain and swelling.

○ **What are complications reported with a supraclavicular approach to brachial plexus blockade?**

Pneumothorax is the most common complication, with an incidence of at least 1% if sought by x-ray (incidence is less if clinical signs are used for detection). Intravascular injection into the subclavian artery or vein is possible. Injury to the thoracic duct (left-sided block) and nerves of the brachial plexus is possible. Phrenic nerve paresis has been reported to occur in 28–80% of cases [Jen et al., 2010. See reference on page 529].

○ **What are the indications for a supraclavicular block?**

Supraclavicular blocks can be done for surgeries of the distal shoulder, elbow, forearm, and hand. The brachial plexus is blocked at the distal trunks or proximal divisions depending on individual anatomy. The supraclavicular block targets the brachial plexus at the area when it is most compact, requiring less local anesthetic. Although technically more difficult, it can provide a dense, predictable block with rapid onset [Miller, 2010; www.nysora.com].

○ **What are the landmarks for a supraclavicular block?**

The midpoint of the clavicle is identified and a mark is made in the interscalene groove approximately 1.5–2.0 cm posterior to the midpoint of the clavicle. The subclavian artery should be palpated at this site and a needle should be inserted posterolateral to the artery. A small ("hockey stick") ultrasound can also be used [Miller, 2010].

○ **Which block has the highest risk of pneumothorax?**

Supraclavicular. The incidence varies based on operator experience and can range from 0.5% up to 6%. Other complications of a supraclavicular block include phrenic nerve block in 40–60% of patients and Horner syndrome [Miller, 2010].

○ **What are the indications for an infraclavicular block?**

An infraclavicular block can be done for elbow, forearm, wrist, and hand surgery. It also provides analgesia for upper arm tourniquets. The brachial plexus is blocked below the clavicle at the level of the cords.

○ **What are the landmarks for performing an infraclavicular block?**

There are two techniques used. The classic approach involves needle insertion 3 cm caudal to the midpoint of a line connecting the medial clavicular head and the coracoid process. The coracoid technique involves needle insertion 2 cm medial and 2 cm caudal to the coracoid process with the arm abducted and flexed at the elbow. This lateral approach, while decreasing the risk of pneumothorax, may miss the musculocutaneous nerve [Miller, 2010; www.nysora.com].

○ **What are the indications for an axillary block?**

An axillary block is indicated for surgery on the elbow, forearm, and hand. The brachial plexus is blocked at the level of the terminal nerve branches. The patient must be able to abduct the arm [Miller, 2010].

○ **What are the landmarks for an axillary block?**

The surface landmarks include the axillary artery, coracobrachialis muscle, and the pectoralis major muscle. The axillary artery should be palpated and marked as high in the axilla as possible. The median nerve is located superior to the artery and the ulnar nerve is found inferior to the artery. The radial nerve is found posterolateral to the axillary artery. At this level in the axilla, the musculocutaneous nerve has left the axillary sheath and can be found in the coracobrachialis muscle. Blockade of all four nerves can be done using a nerve stimulator and/or ultrasound. A transarterial technique can be done but increases the risk of intravascular injection and has fallen out of favor [Miller, 2010; www.nysora.com].

○ **Of the approaches to blockade of the brachial plexus, which technique is most likely to result in inadvertent, intravenous injection of local anesthetic?**

The axillary approach to brachial plexus blockade is most likely to result in intravenous injection of local anesthetic because a major vein is underlying the nerves, and within the brachial plexus sheath at this level. The transarterial technique (high volume of local anesthetic injected posterior to the axillary artery) requires use of epinephrine for a vascular marker and injection in incremental doses, as the risk of intra-arterial injection is high.

○ **After an interscalene block is performed, it is noted that the patient developed anesthesia in the shoulder earlier than in the fingers. Why?**

Peripheral nerve blockade proceeds from a proximal to a distal distribution. The nerve mantle contains fibers to distal areas in the core and fibers to proximal areas along the outer edge of the mantle.

○ **What is the mantle effect?**

When a peripheral nerve block is performed, a high concentration of local anesthetic surrounds the mantle of the nerve. Diffusion of local anesthetic into the bundle proceeds from the periphery, where the concentration is high, toward the "core," where the concentration will rise more slowly. Fibers located on the outside of the nerve bundle are anesthetized first, followed by fibers located at the "core" of the mantle. As peripherally located fibers innervate proximal structures in a limb, and centrally located fibers innervate more distal structures, anesthesia of the thigh, for example, will precede anesthesia of the foot. This phenomenon has been termed the "mantle effect."

○ **Why should an interscalene approach to brachial plexus blockade not be considered the ideal choice in a 62-year-old patient with moderate to severe COPD, who is to undergo left shoulder replacement?**

An interscalene block is associated with unilateral phrenic nerve paralysis in virtually all cases causing an approximate 25% decrease in FEV_1 and FVC. Patients with pulmonary disease may not tolerate either the subjective dyspnea or the loss of functional residual capacity when respiratory function is driven by only one side of the diaphragm. Other complications include pneumothorax, high subarachnoid or epidural block, and an increased risk of dyspnea, hypoxia, and respiratory arrest.

○ **What complications can be seen with axillary blocks?**

The most significant complications include systemic local anesthetic toxicity and nerve injury. If large volumes of local anesthetic are used, particularly when using the transarterial approach, the risk of systemic toxicity is increased. Other rare complications include hematoma and infection [Miller, 2010].

○ **With an axillary block of the brachial plexus what nerves are frequently missed?**

Nerves that are no longer encased within the sheath.

Frequently the musculocutaneous nerve, the median cutaneous nerve, and the intercostobrachial nerve will be missed.

○ **A 44-year-old construction worker is about to undergo an open reduction and internal fixation of a fracture of the distal left radius. Brachial plexus anesthesia is provided via an axillary approach, using 40 cm³ of a 1.5% lidocaine solution with epinephrine 1:200,000. The patient's hand and fingers are numb to pinprick. On incision over the distal radius, however, the patient reports pain. Which peripheral nerve requires supplemental anesthesia?**

The musculocutaneous nerve.

○ **How would you test motor block of the musculocutaneous nerve?**

Flexion of the elbow (biceps, brachialis, and coracobrachialis) and supination of the forearm.

○ **How can the musculocutaneous nerve be blocked to augment an axillary brachial plexus block?**

An injection into the coracobrachialis muscle will often block the musculocutaneous nerve. Forearm flexion (biceps) in response to peripheral nerve stimulation can be used to locate the nerve.

○ **The axillary block of the brachial plexus is best for procedures located where relative to the elbow?**

It's best for procedures distal to the elbow, innervated by the terminal nerves of the plexus.

○ **How can you prevent upper extremity tourniquet pain?**

Blockage of the intercostobrachial nerve (branch of T2 intercostal nerve) and medial antebrachial cutaneous nerves can be achieved by subcutaneous injections deposited in a fan-like distribution over the medial midhumerus, extending from the biceps to the triceps. Usually 5–10 mL of local anesthetic is used [Barash et al., 2009].

○ **What are the significant anatomical landmarks for a median nerve block at the elbow?**

The median nerve can be blocked at its location just medial to the brachial artery on a line connecting the medial and lateral epicondyles of the humerus (intercondylar line) at a depth of about 5 cm.

○ **What are the significant anatomical landmarks for a radial nerve block at the elbow?**

Lateral epicondyle of humerus, brachioradialis muscle, and tendon of biceps.

○ **How do you perform a radial nerve block at the elbow?**

Insert the needle in the intermuscular groove between the brachioradialis and the long head of the biceps tendon 2 cm proximal to the flexor skin crease. Using an insulated needle and nerve stimulator, advance the needle in the direction of the radial nerve until initial muscle contractions become visible. Reduce current and optimize needle position until visible muscle contractions occur at lower current levels (<0.5 mA). Following needle aspiration for blood, inject the local anesthetic drug in incremental doses. The patient should be fully monitored and receive sedation and supplemental oxygen with resuscitation equipment and suction immediately available.

○ **How do you test motor block of the median nerve?**

Opposition of the thumb (opponens pollicis).

○ **Is the brachial artery medial or lateral to the median nerve at the elbow?**

The brachial artery is lateral to the median nerve at the elbow.

○ **How can the median nerve be rescued if it does not get blocked adequately from an axillary block?**

Depending on the location of the surgery, the median nerve can be blocked at several places. It can be blocked at the midhumeral level, where it runs lateral to the brachial artery. At the elbow, the median nerve has moved to a position medial to the brachial artery (which runs medial to the biceps tendon at the intercondylar line). In the forearm, the median nerve can be found lateral to both the ulnar nerve and the ulnar artery and is more easily found with ultrasound in this location by first visualizing the ulnar nerve and artery. At the wrist, the median nerve runs between the flexor carpi radialis and palmaris longus tendons and can be blocked 2–3 cm proximal to the wrist crease [Barash et al., 2009; Miller, 2010; www.nysora.com].

○ **What symptoms are seen a with medial nerve injury?**

Patients with a medial nerve injury will exhibit decreased sensation over the palmar surface of the lateral three fingers and will have difficulty opposing the first and fifth digits. Anesthetic causes are uncommon and usually attributed to insertion of peripheral intravenous needles into the antecubital fossa or forced elbow extension in an anesthetized patient [Miller, 2010].

○ **What regional block can be used for hand surgery?**

The hand is innervated by the median, ulnar, and radial nerves. Both axillary and wrist blocks can provide complete analgesia. Wrist blocks are effective and easy to perform and complications are rare. Individual digit blocks can also be used.

○ **What nerves must be blocked to provide lower limb anesthesia?**

The lower limb is supplied by both the lumbar plexus and the sacral plexus. While a single central neuraxial injection (epidural or spinal) can result in anesthesia, no single peripheral nerve block can reliably block both nerve plexuses.

○ **What are the major branches of the lumbar plexus?**

The lumbar plexus arises from the ventral rami of T12–L4 and has six main nerves. The three important branches for lower limb anesthesia/analgesia are the femoral nerve (and its saphenous nerve branch which continues below the knee), lateral femoral cutaneous, and the obturator nerve. The other three nerves are the iliohypogastric, ilioinguinal, and genitofemoral nerves.

○ **What is the largest branch of the lumbar plexus?**

The femoral nerve.

○ **What is the relation of the femoral nerve to the femoral artery at the inguinal ligament?**

The femoral nerve is approximately 1 cm lateral to the femoral artery (sometimes posterolateral to the artery), invested within its own fascia and deep to the fascia lata.

○ **What muscle does the lateral femoral cutaneous nerve (LFCN) supply?**

None. It is purely a sensory nerve of L2–3. It emerges from under the inguinal ligament, medial to the anterior superior iliac spine (ASIS). It courses anteriorly over the sartorius muscle before dividing into anterior and posterior terminal branches. The anterior branch provides sensory innervations to the anterolateral thigh down to the knee. The posterior branch supplies the lateral thigh from the hip to midthigh [Miller, 2010; Barash et al., 2009].

○ **What is meralgia paresthetica?**

Meralgia paresthetica is an entrapment syndrome of the LFCN of the thigh, usually resulting from impingement as it courses under the inguinal ligament. Patients exhibit pain and paresthesias of the anterolateral thigh [Hui and Peng, 2011. See reference on page 529].

○ **How is the LFCN blocked?**

A fascia illiaca block can be performed by inserting a needle 2 cm medial and 2 cm caudal to the ASIS. Penetration of the two fascial layers (fascia lata and iliaca) is discerned as distinct "pops" when using a blunt needle. This block is commonly utilized to provide analgesia after hip surgeries and over skin graft harvest sites [Miller, 2010].

○ **What is a "3-in-1" block?**

A large volume of local anesthetic (20–30 mL) is injected at the site of the femoral nerve block and proximal (retrograde) spread within the fascial sheath blocks the femoral, lateral femoral cutaneous, and obturator nerves within the psoas muscle. In practice, while femoral nerve blockade is reliable, actual blockade of all three nerves occurs less frequently.

○ **Which nerve is most likely to be missed in a "3-in-1" block?**

The lateral cutaneous nerve. It is often invested in its own fascial sheath, whereas the femoral and obturator nerves often share a common sheath.

○ **A bed-ridden, 83-year-old male with severe peripheral vascular disease, coronary artery disease, and history of congestive heart failure is to undergo a left above-the-knee amputation. What are the important anatomical landmarks for block of the obturator nerve as part of the peripheral nerve blocks adequate to provide regional anesthesia?**

Important landmarks for an obturator nerve block include the area 2 cm lateral and inferior to the pubic tubercle, and the horizontal ramus of the pubis. Alternatively, a 3-in-1 femoral block (inguinal ligament, femoral artery pulsation as landmarks) can also work.

○ **Can blockade of the obturator nerve be assessed by checking sensation on the medial aspect of the thigh?**

In many people the obturator nerve has no cutaneous nerve supply to the thigh.

○ **Which peripheral nerve blocks are required to provide regional anesthesia for a total knee replacement?**

Both blockade of the lumbar plexus and sciatic nerve are required. A posterior approach to the lumbar plexus more reliably blocks the three nerves (femoral, lateral femoral cutaneous, and obturator nerves) compared with the femoral "3-in-1" approach. The sciatic nerve must be blocked separately.

○ **What are the major branches of the sacral plexus?**

The sacral plexus arises from the ventral rami of L4–S4. The main branches are the sciatic nerve (tibial and common peroneal components), the pudendal nerve, posterior femoral cutaneous nerve, and the superior and inferior gluteal nerves. When a proximal sciatic nerve block is performed, both the sciatic and the posterior femoral cutaneous nerves are blocked.

○ **The sciatic nerve divides distally at the popliteal fossa into what two nerves?**

The sciatic nerve (L4–5 and S1–2) is the largest peripheral nerve of the lower extremity. It provides sensation to the posterior thigh and most of the lower leg below the knee. It divides into tibial and common peroneal (common fibular) nerves. These two nerves diverge about 7 cm proximal to the popliteal crease.

○ **The common peroneal nerve encircles the head of the fibula laterally and divides into what two nerves?**

Deep and superficial peroneal nerves.

○ **What is the nerve supply of the knee joint?**

The articular nerves are branches of the obturator, femoral, tibial, and common fibular (peroneal) nerves (L3–5, S1–2).

○   **Which peripheral nerves must be blocked to provide adequate regional anesthesia for arthroscopic knee surgery with the use of a tourniquet?**

The femoral, lateral femoral cutaneous, sciatic, and obturator nerves.

○   **The sural nerve arises from branches of what two nerves?**

Tibial (medial sural cutaneous nerve) and common peroneal (communicating branch of the common peroneal nerve) nerves.

○   **How is a popliteal block performed?**

There are two common techniques utilized, both of which seek to localize the sciatic nerve prior to its bifurcation. Both ultrasound and nerve stimulation can be used. In the posterior approach, the borders of the popliteal fossa form a triangle that can be identified with flexion of the knee. The triangle borders are formed by the skin crease of the popliteal fossa, the semimembranosus tendon medially and biceps femoris tendon laterally. The needle should be inserted 7–10 cm above the skin crease. Using the lateral approach, the patient is positioned supine. The needle is inserted in the grove between the biceps femoris and vastus lateralis about 8 cm above the popliteal fossa crease. With both techniques, a tibial response is sought.

○   **Does blockade of the sciatic nerve in the popliteal fossa result in complete distal extremity anesthesia?**

No. Cutaneous innervation of the medial leg below the knee is provided by the saphenous nerve, a superficial terminal extension of the femoral nerve.

○   **A 62-year-old veteran male with long-standing insulin-dependent diabetes and chronic obstructive pulmonary disease requires amputation of the right leg below the knee. If peripheral nerve blockade of the lower extremity is considered as the sole anesthetic, which nerves must be blocked to provide adequate regional anesthesia for this procedure?**

The femoral nerve and the sciatic nerve.

○   **What are the important landmarks for peripheral nerve block for an amputation of the leg below the knee?**

• **Femoral nerve:** ASIS, pubic tubercle, and lateral to the femoral artery.
• **Sciatic nerve:**
  ○ **Classic approach of Labat (posterior approach):** posterior superior iliac spine, greater trochanter of the femur, and the sacral hiatus.
  ○ **Anterior approach:** ASIS, pubic tubercle, and greater and lesser trochanter of the femur.
  ○ **Popliteal block:** Sciatic nerve blocked at the level of the popliteal fossa (tibial and common peroneal nerve).
    ▪ **Posterior approach:** Popliteal fossa crease, tendon of biceps femoris (laterally), and tendons of semitendinosus and semimembranosus muscles (medially).
    ▪ **Lateral approach:** Horizontal plane 7 cm cephalad from the most prominent point of the lateral femoral epicondyle, in the groove between the biceps femoris and the vastus lateralis muscles. Ultrasound guided: snowman sign.

○   **What stimulus will be typically elicited by stimulation of the tibial nerve in the popliteal fossa?**

Planter flexion and inversion of the foot. While common peroneal nerve stimulation results in dorsiflexion (extension) and eversion.

○ **Does performing an ankle block include blocking a branch of the lumbar plexus?**

Yes. The saphenous nerve is a sensory branch of the femoral nerve. Except for this branch, an ankle block largely involves blockade of the terminal branches of the sciatic nerve (posterior tibial, sural, deep peroneal, and superficial peroneal nerves).

○ **What are the signs of saphenous nerve damage?**

Decreased sensation or paresthesias of the medial leg below the knee [Miller, 2010].

○ **Which five nerve blocks are required for a complete ankle block?**

Tibial nerve, deep peroneal nerve, superficial peroneal nerve, sural nerve, and saphenous nerve.

○ **What are the landmarks for an ankle block?**

An ankle block requires blockade of five terminal nerve branches. The posterior tibial nerve is identified behind the medial malleolus posterior to the posterior tibial artery. The sural nerve, providing sensation to the lateral foot and sole, can be found superficially between the lateral malleolus and Achilles tendon. The deep peroneal nerve is found lateral to the extensor hallucis longus tendon, immediately lateral to the dorsalis pedis pulse. The superficial peroneal, deep peroneal, and saphenous nerves are found in the subcutaneous tissue extending along the dorsum of the foot between the malleoli. These nerves can be blocked by a band-like deposition of local anesthetic along this path [Miller, 2010; www.nysora.com].

○ **A 23-year-old football player sustained fractures of the fourth and fifth metatarsal bones and presents for open reduction and fixation. An ankle block is performed. On incision over the fifth toe, the patient complains of pain. Which nerve is most likely to be inadequately blocked?**

The sural nerve (lateral dorsal cutaneous nerve) innervates the lateral edge of the foot to the fifth toe.

○ **What is Hilton law?**

Hilton law states that a nerve supplying motor innervation to a muscle responsible for joint movement will also supply sensory innervation to that joint and the skin overlying the joint. In general, any nerve traversing a joint will also supply it. For example, the hip joint is innervated by the femoral, sciatic, and obturator (mixed function), as well as lateral cutaneous (sensory only), nerves.

○ **The retrobulbar block ablates sensation of the eye by blocking what nerve?**

The nasociliary nerve (via the short ciliary nerves), a branch of the ophthalmic nerve.

○ **The retrobulbar block prevents movement of the globe by blocking what nerves?**

Cranial nerves II, III, and VI (cranial nerve IV lies outside the muscle cone).

○ **What is the purpose of blocking the facial nerve in conjunction with a retrobulbar block?**

To prevent movement of the orbicularis oculi muscle.

○ **What are the potential clinical manifestations of retrobulbar hemorrhage?**

Retrobulbar hemorrhage usually manifests as motor block of the globe with proptosis, closing of the upper lid, and increased intraocular pressure. Subconjunctival hemorrhage and eyelid ecchymosis develop as the hemorrhage extends anteriorly.

○   **List at least five potential problems with a retrobulbar block.**

Retrobulbar hemorrhage, central retinal artery occlusion, stimulation of oculocardiac reflex, retinal detachment, puncture of the posterior globe, and intraocular injection (especially in highly myopic patient), seizures secondary to intra-arterial injection, brain stem anesthesia, optic nerve penetration causing optic atrophy and permanent loss of vision.

○   **List the relative contraindications to ocular regional anesthesia.**

Penetrating eye injury

Inability to lie flat

Severe tremors, chronic coughing, or convulsive disorder

Claustrophobia and excessive anxiety

Inability to communicate (disoriented, mental impairment, language barrier, deafness)

Coagulation or bleeding abnormality

Patient refusal (absolute contraindication)

Age less than 15 years

○   **What are the goals of regional anesthesia for cataract extraction with intraocular lens implantation?**

Goals include globe and conjunctival analgesia; globe, lid, and periorbital muscle akinesia; and orbit and globe hypotension.

○   **What is the difference between a retrobulbar and peribulbar block?**

These blocks differ by the depth, degree of angulation, and position of the needle tip in relation to the cone formed by the extraocular muscles. Retrobulbar blocks involve deeper penetration and needle angulation to instill local anesthetic inside the orbital cone. These blocks require smaller volumes and result in rapid onset. Peribulbar blocks involve depositing local anesthetic outside the cone and have a slower onset of action. Since the needle tip remains further from intraorbital structures, periorbital blocks are considered safer [Barash et al., 2009].

○   **A retrobulbar block is performed for cataract surgery. Shortly after injection, the patient has a respiratory arrest. What should you do?**

The optic nerve is usually a brain tract, and it is possible to have an intrathecal injection via the optic nerve sheath with this nerve block. Treatment is supportive and the patient usually recovers promptly. If the patient has good analgesia on recovery, it is possible to proceed with surgery.

○   **What is the most common complication of retrobulbar block?**

Hematoma formation, especially in the vicinity of the point at which the ophthalmic artery crosses the optic nerve. The risk can be minimized by using needles shorter than 35 mm. Other complications include intravascular and subarachnoid injections, optic atrophy, optic nerve injury, globe penetration, and ocular muscle paresis.

○   **What is the occulocardiac reflex?**

Traction on the eye or ocular muscles resulting in bradycardia, asystole, or arrhythmias.

The afferent pathway involves transmission via the ciliary ganglion to the ophthalmic division of the trigeminal nerve while the efferent pathway is the vagus nerve.

○ **What methods can be utilized for pain management with rib fractures?**

Epidural anesthesia: A diluted local anesthetic solution (usually bupivacaine 0.1%) combined with fentanyl can be infused through an appropriately placed thoracic epidural catheter.

Intercostal nerve blockade: The 6th to 11th ribs are easily identified and their accompanying nerves can be reliably blocked by injections along the easily palpated sharp posterior angulation of the ribs – occurs between 5 and 7 cm from the middle of the back.

Paravertebral blockade: The upper five ribs are difficult to palpate because of the overlying scapula and paraspinous muscles. Therefore, blockade of their intercostal nerves is best performed with a paravertebral injection.

Intrapleural anesthesia: The anesthetic appears to diffuse through the parietal pleura onto the intercostal nerves. This method produces anesthesia similar to that produced by multiple intercostal blocks and an epidural catheter can be inserted for administration of local anesthetic infusions.

○ **What are the anatomical landmarks for performing an intercostal block?**

At the posterior angle of the rib, intercostal nerves travel in a neurovascular bundle with their respective artery and vein. They course in the intercostal grove along the caudal surface of each rib. The intercostal nerve can be blocked at the angle of the rib lateral to the sacrospinalis muscle with the patient in the prone position. The needle is walked off the lower edge of the rib 6–8 cm from the midline and is inserted 3–5 mm deep.

The block can also be performed in the supine position at the midaxillary line. This technique may miss the lateral cutaneous branch; however, due to anesthetic spread, blockage is usually achieved [Miller, 2010; www.nysora.com].

○ **What are the landmarks of superficial cervical plexus block?**

Superficial cervical plexus is formed from primary rami of the first four cervical nerves.

Superficial branches supply the skin over the neck from mandible to clavical anteriorly and laterally. They pierce deep cervical fascia just posterior to sternocleidomastoid as four distinct branches. In order to perform the block, at the midpoint along the posterior border of the sternocleidomastoid local anesthetic solution is injected immediately deep and posterior to the muscle.

○ **When using a peripheral nerve stimulator, how should the leads be configured?**

The positive lead connected to the patient (ground electrode) and the negative to the needle.

○ **What is the relationship between needle–nerve distance and current intensity?**

This relationship between stimulus intensity and distance from the nerve is governed by Coulomb's law: $I = K(Q/r^2)$, where I is the current, K is a constant, Q is the minimal current, and r is the distance.

The inverse square indicates that a current of higher intensity is required as the needle travels further from the nerve [www.nysora.com].

○ **What is an acceptable current when using a peripheral nerve stimulator?**

A clear motor response at 0.2–0.5 mA indicates a close needle-to-nerve relationship; these currents are associated with high success rates in neuronal blockade. However, a current of less than 0.2 mA has been associated with intraneural placement of the needle and should be avoided. If a motor response is achieved at less than 0.2 mA, the needle should be slightly withdrawn.

Pulsed, synchronous movement at a current around 0.5 mA when using an insulated needle usually indicates that the tip of the needle is 2–3 mm away from the nerve [Bigeleisen et al., 2009. See reference on page 529].

○ **Explain the principles of Doppler ultrasonography.**

Ultrasound is mechanical sound energy that propagates through a conducting medium as a sinusoidal wave. The frequency of an ultrasound wave is >20,000 Hz, which is above the audible range for humans. Medical imaging utilizes frequencies in the 2–20 MHz range. The velocity of a sound wave is the product of frequency multiplied by wavelength. An ultrasound wave is generated when an electric field is created across a transducer surface consisting of piezoelectric crystals. Mechanical distortion of each crystal by electrical stimulation leads to the conversion of electrical energy to sound energy and produces an ultrasound wave. The summation of waves created by the array of crystals produces an ultrasound beam [Miller, 2010; Marhofer and Chan, 2007. See reference on page 529].

○ **Describe characteristics involved in ultrasound imaging.**

Attenuation (energy loss) occurs as the ultrasound beam travels through tissue layers and increases as depth of penetration increases. This is due to absorption, reflection, and scattering. The degree of attenuation also varies directly with frequency; a higher frequency wave is associated with more attenuation, thereby limiting tissue penetration.

Image resolution is the ability to distinguish between two structures. It is influenced by the transducer characteristics: number of crystals, frequency of transducer, and linear versus curvilinear probe.

○ **What are the two types of ultrasound probes used?**

Linear and curvilinear probes are used. Linear probes have a high scan line density, producing a better imaging quality which is displayed in rectangular format. Linear transducers are generally used for peripheral nerve blocks and central line placement.

Curvilinear transducers produce images in sector format and provide a broader view. These probes are used for neuraxial imaging. Lower frequencies are used for deeper penetration; however, image resolution will be decreased [Miller, 2010; Marhofer and Chan, 2007].

○ **What are the differences in tissue echogenicity?**

On returning to the transducer, an image's amplitude is represented by the degree of brightness on the display, referred to as echogenicity. Reflections in biologic tissues differ in their echogenicity. Smooth, flat interfaces allow for transmission of waves in a single direction, giving rise to bright images (hyperechoic). Bones, tendons, fascial sheaths, the diaphragm, and pericardium are examples of hyperechoic images, as are block needles.

Solid organs produce diffuse reflection, known as scattering and appear hypoechoic. Fluid and blood-filled structures allow easy passage of ultrasound beams without reflection; they appear anechoic. Deeper structures may appear hypoechoic due to enhanced attenuation. Fat is mostly hypoechoic with streaks of irregular hyperechoic lines. Muscle displays a mixture of hyperechoic lines and fascial sheaths within a hypoechoic background [Miller, 2010; Marhofer and Chan, 2007].

○ **What is acoustic impedance?**

Sound travels through materials under the influence of sound pressure.

The **acoustic impedance** (Z) of a material is defined as the product of its density (p) and acoustic velocity (V):

$$Z = pV$$

Acoustic impedance is important in:

1. The determination of acoustic transmission and reflection at the boundary of two materials having different acoustic impedances
2. The design of ultrasonic transducers
3. Assessing absorption of sound in a medium

○ **A patient is concerned about nerve damage with peripheral nerve block. What can you do to minimize these problems?**

Use preservative-free local anesthetic solutions and small short-beveled block needles, avoid the use of epinephrine, and do not intentionally elicit paresthesias, although this is not supported by available data. Avoid heavy sedation to make the presence of paresthesias evident, and prevent accidental injection into a nerve.

○ **How are nerve injuries classified?**

Classically, there are three groups representing the degree of neuronal disruption: neurapraxia (local myelin injury), axonotmesis (axonal disruption with endoneurial preservation), and neurotmesis (complete severing of the entire nerve). Neurapraxia has the greatest chance of functional recovery.

○ **Following neurologic injury to peripheral nerves, how much time must elapse before the nerve conduction study (NCS) demonstrates an abnormality?**

The process of degeneration may take 10–14 days to be completed. NCS performed during this period may be interpreted as normal, despite significant injury.

○ **Does the degree of systemic absorption vary with different regional techniques?**

The extent of systemic absorption is determined by several factors: pharmacokinetic properties of the local anesthetic, dosage, volume, site of injection, and addition of a vasoconstrictor. Local anesthetics deposited into vessel-rich tissues lead to higher peak plasma concentrations at a faster rate. Absorption is highest after intercostal blockade, followed in decreasing order by caudal, epidural, brachial plexus, femoral, and sciatic blockade [Barash et al., 2009].

○ **What's the toxic dose of lidocaine in peripheral nerve blocks?**

Approximately 7–8 mg/kg is considered the maximum dose of lidocaine with epinephrine (plain lidocaine 5 mg/kg). Recommendations are based on subcutaneous administration and apply only to single-shot injections.

Key Terms

Anatomy: upper extremity nerves
Anesthetic absorption: regional anesthetic techniques
Ankle block: anatomy
Axillary block: complications/limitations
Axillary block: median nerve rescue block
Axillary block: supplement
Axillary nerve block: anatomy
Deep peroneal nerve block
Doppler ultrasonography: principles
Femoral nerve block anatomy
Hand surgery: regional anesthesia
Intercostal block: anatomy
Interscalene block: anatomy/side effects
Landmark: superficial cervical plexus block

Lateral femoral cutaneous nerve block: anatomy/landmarks
Local anesthetics: transneural: symptoms
Lower extremity block: anatomy
Lower extremity nerves: sensory distribution
Lumbar nerve roots: innervation
Lumbar plexus block: anatomy
Median nerve injury: symptoms
Meralgia paresthetica
Nerve block: landmarks
Nerve block: plasma lidocaine
Nerve block: stimulating current versus distance
Peribulbar block: oculocardiac reflex in elderly
Popliteal fossa block: innervation

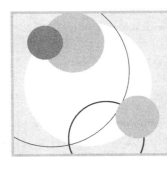

Pharmacogenetics

*Education without values, as useful as it is, seems rather
to make man a more clever devil.*
C. S. Lewis

○ **Characteristics of familial dysautonomia (Riley–Day syndrome) include generalized diminished sensation, emotional lability, and sympathetic denervation. What are the best drug choices for these patients?**

Diazepam or midazolam are used to treat a dysautonomic crisis triggered by stress (hypertension, tachycardia, abdominal pain, diaphoresis, and vomiting). Fluids and direct-acting vasopressors (phenylephrine) are indicated for hypotension, as these patients may elicit denervation hypersensitivity with unpredictable responses to sympathomimetic drugs. Most patients are chronically hypovolemic, so vasodilatory or cardiodepressant drugs may cause profound hypotension. Spinal and epidural anesthesia may be poorly tolerated.

○ **What type of IV fluids should be avoided in patients with the hypokalemic variant of familial periodic paralysis?**

Paralysis can be precipitated by high sodium or carbohydrate loads and exposure to cold temperatures. Glucose-containing solutions should be avoided as they may exacerbate the hypokalemia and muscle weakness.

○ **Which muscle relaxant should be avoided in the hyperkalemic variant of familial periodic paralysis?**

Succinylcholine (myotonia and hyperkalemia).

○ **What are the anesthetic concerns in patients with myotonia congenita?**

Anesthetic management is complicated by the abnormal response to depolarizing relaxants, troublesome intraoperative myotonic contraction, and the need to avoid hypothermia. Nondepolarizing muscle relaxants seem to behave normally. Ideally, short-acting nondepolarizers should be used because myotonia may be precipitated by the nicotinic effects of neostigmine.

○ **What is myotonic dystrophy?**

Myotonic dystrophy is a multisystemic disease with involvement of skeletal as well as cardiac and smooth muscles. Deterioration of skeletal, cardiac, and smooth muscle function is progressive. There is a high mortality from cardiopulmonary complications.

○ **Why do patients with myotonic dystrophy have increased aspiration risk compared with the normal population?**

They have increased aspiration risk due to slowed gastric emptying and weak pharyngeal and thoracic muscles.

○ **Is the response to muscle relaxants different in patients with myotonic dystrophy?**

Yes. Succinylcholine may produce sustained muscle contraction causing trismus and respiratory muscle rigidity, which may make ventilation of the lungs and tracheal intubation difficult or impossible. Hyperkalemia is also possible. The contractions are not relieved by regional anesthetics, nondepolarizing muscle relaxants, or deep anesthesia. Response to nondepolarizing muscle relaxants is usually normal.

○ **Duchenne muscular dystrophy is the most common and severe form of muscular dystrophy. This is a sex-linked recessive disease with an incidence of 3 in 10,000 births. Which muscle relaxant is contraindicated and why?**

Succinylcholine. Patients with Duchenne muscular dystrophy have increased extrajunctional acetylcholine receptors. Succinylcholine may cause massive rhabdomyolysis, hyperkalemia, dysrhythmias, and cardiac asystole.

○ **What are the major clinical features of muscular dystrophy?**

1. Degeneration of cardiac muscle, which may lead to reduced contractility or mitral regurgitation
2. Restrictive lung disease due to degeneration of ventilatory muscles
3. Degeneration and atrophy of skeletal muscle
4. Gastrointestinal tract hypomotility, gastroparesis, and impaired swallowing resulting in an increased aspiration risk

Death is due to congestive heart failure or pneumonia.

○ **What genetic disorders are of concern when succinylcholine is used?**

Pseudocholinesterase deficiency (prolonged apnea), muscular dystrophy (especially unrecognized Duchenne muscular dystrophy causing hyperkalemia), and myotonic dystrophy (muscle contracture).

○ **Esmolol and remifentanil are metabolized by esterases. Does pseudocholinesterase deficiency affect dosing?**

No. Esmolol is hydrolyzed by RBC esterases with an elimination half-life of 9 minutes. Remifentanil is hydrolyzed by blood- and tissue-nonspecific esterases with a $t_{1/2}\,\beta$ of 5–8 minutes.

○ **What percentage of normal children develop myoglobinemia after a single dose of intravenous succinylcholine?**

Approximately 40% [Ryan et al., 1971. See reference on page 529].

○ **What are the drugs that can precipitate hemolysis in patients with glucose-6-phosphate dehydrogenase deficiency?**

Analgesics: phenacetin, acetaminophen, and aspirin in large doses

Antibiotics: nitrofurantoin, streptomycin, chloramphenicol, isoniazid, and sulfa drugs

Antimalarials

Local anesthetics: prilocaine and lidocaine

Miscellaneous: probenecid, quinidine, vitamin K analogues, methylene blue, and nitroprusside

○ **What is the basis of hemolysis in G6PD deficiency?**

This is the most common inherited RBC enzyme disorder. It is seen in about 10% of the African American males in the United States [Beutler, 1991. See reference on page 529]. Chronic hemolysis is the most common presentation. DIC may accompany drug-induced hemolysis.

The common denominator is metabolism to a compound requiring G6PD for detoxification.

Drugs that form peroxidase by interaction with oxyhemoglobin can trigger hemolysis in these patients. Normally, the peroxides are inactivated by metabolic process that depends on G6PD enzyme activity. Oxidant stressors include methemoglobin, glutathione, and hydrogen peroxide.

○ **What are the anesthetic implications of G6PD deficiency?**

The general anesthetic drugs have not been incriminated as triggering agents. However, hemolysis and jaundice during early postoperative period, especially in African American males, require consideration of this diagnosis.

○ **What is the usual time course for drug-induced hemolytic anemia?**

Drug-induced hemolytic anemia is immune-mediated. Therefore, a crisis usually begins 2–5 days after drug administration and generally ceases when drug therapy ends.

○ **Discuss CATCH-22 syndrome (DiGeorge sequence).**

CATCH-22 syndrome occurs with an incidence of 1 in 5,000, and is highly pleiotropic involving cardiac, metabolic, and airway effects. The primary defect alters structures derived from the third and fourth pharyngeal pouches and the fourth branchial arch. Hypocalcemia is the primary metabolic defect. Sterility for intravenous catheters and invasive monitors must be maintained, because these patients may have thymic hypoplasia with low T-lymphocyte counts and relative immunodeficiency.

○ **List the hepatic porphyrias that can cause life-threatening neurologic abnormalities.**

Acute intermittent porphyria, variegate porphyria, and hereditary coproporphyria. Porphyria cutanea tarda causes photosensitivity and liver disease, and does not incur neurologic sequelae.

○ **What are the symptoms of an acute porphyria crisis?**

Severe colicky abdominal pain and neurotoxicity (autonomic instability, psychiatric disorders, and lesions of the lower motor neuron that can progress to bulbar paralysis).

○ **In patients with hepatic porphyria, what should the preanesthesia physical examination specifically document?**

A complete neurologic exam indicating peripheral neuropathies, autonomic dysfunction, and cranial nerve involvement with impaired swallowing and respiratory muscle weakness.

○ **What are "safe" drugs for administration to a patient with acute intermittent porphyria?**

Anticholinergics, anticholinesterases, depolarizing and nondepolarizing muscle relaxants, droperidol, opioids, nitrous oxide, volatile anesthetics, and propofol.

Those of questionable safety include etomidate and ketamine.

Drugs considered "unsafe" induce the enzyme ALA synthetase and exacerbate the disease process. These include barbiturates, diazepam, phenytoin, corticosteroids, and pentazocine.

○ **Which synthetic process and enzyme activity is involved in an acute intermittent porphyria crisis?**

Heme synthesis pathway with a block at the conversion of porphobilinogen to uroporphyrinogen I and III with aminolevulinic acid and porphobilinogen present in the urine.

○ **What is the mechanism by which barbiturates precipitate a porphyria crisis?**

Barbiturates induce the enzyme ALA synthetase that stimulates heme production and in the presence of a functional enzyme deficit results in the overproduction of porphyria compounds and their precursors.

○ **What is the pharmacologic treatment for an acute porphyria crisis?**

The acute attack should be treated with glucose infusion, opioids (pain), beta antagonist (autonomic dysfunction: hypertension and tachycardia), intubation and mechanical ventilatory support (oxygenation and ventilation, prevent aspiration), and nasogastric suctioning (ileus and gastroparesis). Hyponatremia, hypokalemia, and hypomagnesemia should be treated. Pyridoxine and hematin have been valuable in some cases. Prevention includes avoiding starvation, dehydration, sepsis, and triggering drugs.

○ **What species of hemoglobin are contained in adult blood?**

Oxyhemoglobin, reduced hemoglobin, methemoglobin, and carboxyhemoglobin.

○ **What is the definition of methemoglobinemia?**

Greater than 1% methemoglobin.

○ **A 32-year-old male with oral carcinoma was brought to the OR for surgery. A fiber-optic intubation was planned and topical 20% benzocaine spray was administered to achieve oropharyngeal anesthesia. During the procedure, the patient's oxygen saturation fell to 86% on pulse oximetry and he became cyanotic. He is agitated and tachycardic with frequent PVCs. The supplemental oxygen was increased to 6 L/min by nasal cannula without improvement. What is the most likely cause and what is the treatment?**

Methemoglobin is a dark pigment that causes blood to appear chocolate in color. Severe cyanosis out of proportion to the degree of respiratory distress and dark arterial blood suggest methemoglobinemia.

The metabolites of prilocaine (O-toluidine) are a potent oxidant. At doses greater than 600 mg cyanosis may develop.

Various chemicals and drugs also can accelerate the formation of methemoglobin – for example, antimalarials (chloroquine, primaquine), nitrites or nitrates, inhaled nitric oxide, nitroprusside, sulfonamides, metoclopramide, phenacetin, and phenytoin.

The half-life of methemoglobin is 55 minutes. The onset of methemoglobinemia is usually within 20–60 minutes of drug administration. Normally, 5 g/dL of deoxyhemoglobin produces noticeable cyanosis.

Treatment is to administer 100% oxygen, if necessary, with assisted ventilation, send a blood gas sample for methemoglobin level, and rule out other causes. If the methemoglobin level is elevated, the treatment is methylene blue, 1–2 mg/kg intravenously over 5 minutes. The same dose may be repeated within 1 hour if necessary. Less successfully you may also use ascorbic acid, 2 mg/kg.

Methylene blue acts as a reducing agent via the NADPH methemoglobin reductase pathway. (However, when given in high doses, methylene blue oxidizes the ferrous iron of hemoglobin to ferric iron, resulting in methemoglobin production.)

○ **What topical anesthetics have been known to induce methemoglobinemia?**

Prilocaine (500–600 mg), benzocaine, lidocaine, and procaine.

○ **At what methemoglobin levels are patients usually symptomatic?**

Although cyanosis may appear with methemoglobin levels as low as 15%, acquired methemoglobinemia is rarely symptomatic when levels are below 20%.

○ **How does methemoglobin interfere with oxygenation?**

Normal hemoglobin contains an iron molecule that exists in the divalent ferrous state. Methemoglobin results from the conversion of the iron to a trivalent ferric state. Methemoglobin reductase converts methemoglobin back to hemoglobin. Methemoglobin is unable to bind and carry oxygen. The directly measured PO_2 level is usually normal, because the arterial PO_2 measures dissolved oxygen in blood.

High levels of methemoglobin result in functional anemia and disrupt oxygenation by two mechanisms:

1. Methemoglobin reduces the oxygen-carrying capacity of blood.
2. The presence of oxidized iron changes the heme tetramer in a way that reduces oxygen release in the tissues, thus shifting the oxyhemoglobin dissociation curve to the left, as in alkalosis.

Under normal physiologic circumstances, the methemoglobin level is below 2%.

○ **What effect does methemoglobin have on the pulse oximeter reading (SpO$_2$)?**

In the presence of methemoglobin, SpO_2 overestimates arterial oxygen saturation (SaO_2) (i.e., at low levels of SaO_2 the SpO_2 is falsely high) and the pulse oximeter becomes less sensitive to SaO_2 as the levels of metHb increase with SpO_2 approaching 80–85%.

○ **Which classes of drugs are implicated in causing methemoglobinemia?**

- Local anesthetics: prilocaine, benzocaine, and lidocaine (questionable)
- Nitrates, nitrites, sodium nitroprusside, nitroglycerin, amyl nitrite, and silver nitrite
- Antimalarials: chloroquine
- Antileprosy: dapsone
- Miscellaneous: phenacetin, sulfonamides, aniline dyes, chlorates, and nitrobenzenes

○ **How do you diagnose acute drug-induced methemoglobinemia?**

Central cyanosis unresponsive to O_2 therapy without a cardiac or pulmonary explanation. A reddish brown venous blood sample, unchanged in color when exposed to air, is diagnostic.

○ **What is the drug treatment for inherited methemoglobinemia?**

Methylene blue 1 mg/kg IV. Ascorbic acid is given mainly for cosmetic reasons. Homozygous patients are able to tolerate higher methemoglobin levels, although high levels of methemoglobin may cause symptoms due to diminished oxygen-carrying capacity as well as a shift in the oxyhemoglobin dissociation curve.

Avoidance of drugs known to induce methemoglobinemia is prudent.

○ **What causes thalassemia?**

Thalassemia is a hemoglobinopathy where there is a defect in the globin chains of hemoglobin. There are alpha and beta thalassemias, depending on which globin chain is affected. The main problem is excessive hemolysis leading to anemia. (There is no defect in the oxygen-carrying capacity of hemoglobin.)

Thalassemia is an inherited disease that may be inherited as an autosomal recessive or dominant trait. Most thalassemias are inherited as recessive traits. Thalassemia is autosomal dominant in a very small percentage of beta thalassemia cases. A person who has only one mutated or defective gene typically does not experience symptoms and is called a carrier (thalassemia trait or thalassemia minor).

○ **What are the manifestations of beta thalassemia major (Cooley's anemia)?**

This is the most severe form of beta thalassemia and fatal in most cases. Manifestations include frontal bossing, overgrowth of the maxilla, splenomegaly, congestive heart failure, possible pericarditis, and SVT. Multiple transfusions may cause iron overload, diabetes, hypothyroidism, adrenal insufficiency, liver failure, and/or myocardial damage.

Beta thalassemia minor produces a mild hemolytic anemia and iron deficiency.

Alpha thalassemia produces a mild hemolytic anemia in most patients.

○ **What is the main treatment for beta thalassemia major?**

Chronic transfusion therapy, to keep the Hgb over 9 g/dL.

○ **What are the anesthetic considerations of thalassemia?**

Evaluate hepatic and cardiac function (cardiomyopathy) and anemia. Extramedullary hematopoiesis can produce hyperplasia of facial bones.

○ **What is the cause of sickling in HbSS disease?**

Hemoglobin S is a variant of hemoglobin produced by substitution of valine for glutamic acid in the sixth position of the beta chain. When hemoglobin S deoxygenates, a gel structure is formed and deforms red blood cell.

Therefore, low oxygen tension and acidosis exaggerate sickle cell formation.

○ **At what oxygen tension does sickling occur in HbSS?**

Sickling begins at oxygen tensions less than 50 mm Hg and becomes most pronounced when the arterial oxygen tension decreases to 20 mm Hg. If sickling occurs, increasing systemic oxygenation may not reverse the sickling process if arteries supplying the area are occluded. Therefore, better to prevent sickling than to treat it.

The likelihood of sickling is directly related to the amount of hemoglobin S in the blood.

○ **How is sickle cell disease diagnosed?**

The definitive diagnosis of sickle cell disease is made with hemoglobin electrophoresis.

In sickle cell anemia, 70–98% of the hemoglobin is S, and the remainder is hemoglobin F (fetal).

In patients with sickle trait (SA), 10–40% of the hemoglobin is hemoglobin S.

The clinical severity of the disorder is also related to the amount of hemoglobin S.

○ **What are the clinical manifestations of sickle cell disease?**

1. Chronic anemia.
2. Chronic hemolysis.

3. Infarction of multiple organs is produced by occlusion of vessels with deformed erythrocytes.

4. Generalized pulmonary fibrosis – ultimately, cor pulmonale.

5. Cardiac dysfunction, decreased ventricular filling, and reduced EF.

6. Papillary necrosis secondary to medullary ischemia occurs frequently. There is often an inability to concentrate urine.

7. Spleen is virtually nonexistent because of repeated infarctions. The absence of splenic function increases the patient's vulnerability to bacterial infection.

8. Chronic hemolysis – high incidence of cholelithiasis in patients with SS.

○   **Describe different forms of crisis seen in HbSS disease.**

There are three forms of clinical crisis in patients with sickle cell anemia: vaso-occlusive (painful) crisis, aplastic crisis, and splenic sequestration crisis.

○   **What are anesthetic considerations in HbSS?**

Arterial hypoxemia and vascular stasis are powerful stimuli for sickling.

- Minimize during anesthesia and the postoperative period.
- Circulatory stasis prevented with adequate hydration and anticipation of intraoperative volume loss to avoid acute hypovolemia.
- Use of extremity tourniquets is controversial [Fischer and Roberts, 2010. See reference on page 529] – some say we may use it if it is critical to the success of the operation.
- Normothermia: fever increases the rate of gel formation by S hemoglobin. Although hypothermia retards gel formation, the decreased temperature also produces peripheral vasoconstriction. Normothermia is desirable.
- Preoperative transfusion is also controversial

○   **What is the incidence of malignant hyperthermia (MH)?**

The incidence of MH is about 1 in 50,000 when inhaled anesthetics and succinylcholine are considered. For reasons that are not well understood, MH is 5–10 times more common in children than in adults [Rosenberg, 2007. See reference on page 529].

MH is rare in infants, and the incidence decreases after 50 years of age with up to a 5-fold greater incidence in males. Fifty percent of MH-susceptible individuals have had a previous triggering anesthetic without developing MH.

○   **What disorders have been associated with MH?**

MH has been clearly associated with central core disease. Other disorders such as neuroleptic malignant syndrome (NMS), Duchenne muscular dystrophy, myotonia congenita, King syndrome, osteogenesis imperfecta, sudden infant death syndrome, and sudden death in adults are controversial.

○   **What is the genetic transmission of MH?**

Autosomal dominant with highly variable expression.

○   **Which drugs are considered triggering agents in MH?**

Succinylcholine, all volatile anesthetics, and potassium (possible retriggering agent).

○ **What are the clinical signs of MH?**

The earliest signs of MH include tachycardia, tachypnea (in an unparalyzed patient), and increased end-tidal CO_2 levels, all reflecting a fulminant state of increased metabolic activity. MH has been reported to occur as late as 24 hours postoperatively.

Whole-body muscle rigidity, rhabdomyolysis, increased temperature (may be delayed onset), metabolic and respiratory acidosis, and increased sympathetic activity (tachycardia, arrhythmias, sweating, and hypertension) are seen. Masseter spasm causing trismus following inhalation induction and succinylcholine may be associated with an incidence of MH of approximately 50% [Rosenberg, 1987. See reference on page 529].

○ **Which receptor is defective in MH?**

The ryanodine receptor (calcium release channel) on the terminal cisternae of skeletal muscle sarcoplasmic reticulum.

○ **What is the cellular pathophysiology in MH?**

The ryanodine receptor allows free unbound ionized calcium to be released from the sarcoplasmic reticulum. The calcium pumps attempt to restore homeostasis, which results in ATP utilization, increased aerobic and anaerobic metabolism, and finally acidosis and cellular death. Rigidity occurs when unbound myofibrillar calcium approaches the contractile threshold.

○ **Is cerebral palsy predictive of MH?**

No.

○ **What medications are considered safe in MH and how do you prepare an anesthesia machine?**

Safe drugs include barbiturates, narcotics, local anesthetics, benzodiazepines, nitrous oxide, and nondepolarizing muscle relaxants (all of the drug components necessary for total intravenous anesthesia).

Remember that the anesthesia machine is safe when the vaporizers have been removed, the soda lime and circle system with reservoir bag changed, and the system flushed with high-flow oxygen for 10 minutes to prevent patient exposure to trace gas contamination.

○ **What test is diagnostic for MH and what are the two positive phenotypes?**

Muscle biopsy halothane–caffeine contracture testing.

The H-type phenotype develops hypercontracture to either caffeine and halothane alone; they are definitely susceptible to MH. The K-type phenotype exhibits only hypercontracture to halothane and caffeine combined. The degree of susceptibility to MH of these patients is unclear.

○ **A healthy baby presents with increased temperature during hernia repair. He was induced with halothane, nitrous oxide, and O_2. Intubation was facilitated by atropine and succinylcholine and was maintained on halothane, N_2O, and O_2. Most likely diagnosis?**

MH until proven otherwise. Looking for an increase in CO_2 is appropriate as the first sign. In the face of normocarbia, the rise in temperature is most likely due to the anticholinergic effect of atropine on sweat glands or overbundling.

○ **What is the treatment for an acute MH episode?**

- Discontinue volatile anesthetics and triggers.
- Hyperventilate; use 100% O_2 with portable tank.
- Give dantrolene 2.5 mg/kg every 5 minutes (maximum 10 mg/kg).
- Cool patient with packed ice, cold IV fluids, and gastric lavage.
- Maintain adequate volume with diuretics (mannitol and furosemide).
- Monitor arrhythmias.
- Initiate continuous electrolyte monitoring: treat hypocalcemia, hyperkalemia (insulin and glucose), and metabolic acidosis.

After successful treatment, dantrolene is continued at 1 mg/kg IV every 6 hours for 24–48 hours to prevent recrudescence of symptoms. The Malignant Hyperthermia Association of the United States should be notified.

○ **How does dantrolene ameliorate acute MH?**

It inhibits the sarcoplasmic reticulum from releasing calcium.

○ **How is dantrolene prepared?**

Dantrolene is prepared by mixing 20 mg of dantrolene with at least 60 mL of sterile water. Sodium chloride as the diluent will cause precipitation. Preparation is tedious as dantrolene dissolves slowly into solution. Therefore, you will need to call for help.

○ **What treatment is indicated for supraventricular tachycardia after dantrolene?**

With preserved heart function, benzodiazepines, selective β_1-blockers, and mixed β_1- and β_2-blockers can be used. Calcium channel blockers should *not* be used in the treatment of dysrhythmias in combination with dantrolene.

Dantrolene sodium has been shown to have antiarrhythmic potential in animal models.

○ **What is the interaction between dantrolene and verapamil?**

Cardiovascular collapse in patients treated simultaneously with verapamil and dantrolene is a rare but reported finding. The mechanism of action is unknown, but thought to be a synergistic effect on calcium release. Pigs and dogs show cardiovascular collapse and hyperkalemia when given the two drugs concurrently.

○ **What are the essential features of NMS?**

The essential features include:

- History of psychotropic drug within the preceding 24–72 hours (haloperidol, fluphenazine, perphenazine, thioridazine)
- Hyperthermia, tachycardia, and cyanosis
- Autonomic lability
- Extrapyramidal signs (akinesia and muscle rigidity)
- Elevated levels of creatinine kinase
- Mortality rate of 10%

○ **How do NMS and MH differ clinically?**

Unlike NMS, the onset of MH occurs within hours following exposure to the known triggers (volatile anesthetic agent and/or succinylcholine). NMS occurs within 24–72 hours of exposure to a psychotropic drug. MH also originates in skeletal muscle, whereas NMS involves dopamine receptor blockade in the hypothalamus and basal ganglia. Patients with NMS are not prone to MH. Treatment of NMS is with dantrolene or bromocriptine.

○ **Epidermolysis bullosa is a rare hereditary disorder of the skin characterized by bullae formation, especially when lateral shearing forces are applied to the skin. What factors contribute to drug selection for anesthesia?**

Drug selection may be influenced by an increased incidence of porphyria. Succinylcholine is acceptable.

○ **Regional plexus and conduction anesthesia for extremity procedures in epidermolysis bullosa patients is an acceptable technique. What modifications in the regional technique are recommended for these patients?**

• Skin should be prepared by pouring antibacterial solution onto the surface.
• Scrubbing should be avoided.
• When testing for level of blockade, avoid trauma to the skin and mucous membranes.
• Tracheal intubation with minimal frictional trauma to oropharynx.
• Avoid tape when securing the endotracheal tube.
• Supplemental O_2 may be given with nasal prongs or face mask lubricated with steroid ointment.
• Catheters should be sutured or held in place with gauze wrap.

○ **What are the anesthetic considerations in polycythemia vera (PV)?**

PV is a stem cell disorder and diagnosed by elevated hematocrit or RBC mass, and splenomegaly.

1. Increased risk of perioperative thrombosis (baseline hypercoagulability augmented by surgical stress)

2. Potential for bleeding diathesis: often attributable to an acquired von Willebrand disease

Aggressive phlebotomy and avoidance of extreme dehydration lower the above risks during perioperative period.

Key Terms

Complications of HbSS disease
Dantrolene pharmacology
Glucose-6-phosphate deficiency: anesthetic implications
HbSS cause of sickling
Hemoglobin and hemoglobinopathy
Local anesthetic: methemoglobinemia: diagnosis/treatment
Malignant hyperthermia: anesthetic choices
Malignant hyperthermia (MH): dantrolene, repeat dose indication

Methemoglobinemia: laboratory signs
Methemoglobinemia post-benzocaine: diagnosis
MH: associated disorders
Myotonic dystrophy: abnormal drug response
Myotonic dystrophy: aspiration risk
Myotonic dystrophy: NMB/preoperative evaluation
Polycythemia vera: anesthetic management
Treatment of SVT after dantrolene
Verapamil dantrolene interaction

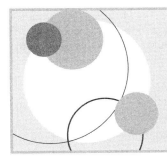

Postoperative Recovery and Outcome

I have learned that success is to be measured not so much by the position that one has reached in life as by the obstacles which he has had to overcome while trying to succeed.
Booker T. Washington

○ **Why are IM injections of opioids a poor choice for postoperative analgesia?**

Variable blood levels often falling under the analgesic threshold, unpredictable absorption, delayed onset, lag to peak analgesic effect, pain, and inadequate analgesia. PCA administration eliminates these problems.

○ **What are the mechanisms of action of the nonsteroidal anti-inflammatory drugs (NSAIDs)?**

Inhibition of the cyclooxygenase and lipoxygenase pathways of prostaglandin synthesis, as well as possible CNS analgesic effects.

NSAIDs act primarily through peripheral inhibition of prostaglandin synthesis. The cyclooxygenase enzyme is inhibited, reducing the conversion of arachidonic acid to cyclic endoperoxide, a prostaglandin and thromboxane precursor. Decreased production of arachidonic metabolites limits inflammation and perceived pain while avoiding opioid chemoreceptor stimulation and attendant side effects.

○ **Where are the proposed sites of action of the NSAIDs?**

They work peripherally to block the cyclooxygenase pathway and centrally to facilitate the descending neural pathways of pain modulation. There are also proposed cellular mechanisms involving release of inflammatory mediators. NSAIDs provide analgesic, anti-inflammatory, and antipyretic effects.

○ **What are the major contraindications to the use of NSAIDs in the postoperative period?**

Peptic ulceration, GI bleeding, renal impairment, concurrent use of nephrotoxic drugs or prerenal acute tubular necrosis conditions (renal artery stenosis and hypovolemia), and coagulopathy or abnormal platelet function. Allergy to aspirin and aspirin-induced asthma (nasal polyps) contraindicate the use of NSAIDs. There are a host of relative contraindications to the use of NSAIDs but they must be weighed against the benefit of their use on an individual basis.

○ **What is the advantage of using NSAIDs as adjunctive analgesics in the postoperative period?**

Less overall incidence of side effects, improved overall postoperative outcomes, and an additive analgesic effect.

○ **How long do NSAID drugs inhibit platelet function?**

Aspirin *irreversibly* inhibits platelet function for the lifetime of the platelet (about 7 days). Many other drugs such as indomethacin or ibuprofen cause *reversible* inhibition of platelet aggregation, but only at significant serum drug levels and only for 1–2 days.

○ **What are the side effects of ketorolac?**

The primary issue is the reversible inhibition of platelet aggregation by inhibition of thromboxane production.

Life-threatening bronchospasm may also occur in patients with nasal polyposis, asthma, and aspirin sensitivity.

Other side effects include a modest increase in liver transaminase plasma levels, nausea, GI irritation, and peripheral edema.

○ **What are the contraindications to the use of ketorolac?**

Cerebrovascular bleeding (suspected or confirmed), hemophilia or other bleeding problems including coagulation or platelet function disorders, gastrointestinal bleeding (active, recent) or a history of gastrointestinal perforation, peptic ulceration, ulcerative colitis, or other ulcerative gastrointestinal disease, nasal polyps associated with bronchospasm (aspirin-induced), angioedema, anaphylaxis, and impairment of renal function.

○ **Can ketorolac be given to patients with renal dysfunction?**

Ketorolac, like other NSAIDs, is contraindicated in patients with impaired renal function. NSAIDs may cause a dose-dependent reduction in prostaglandin formation, resulting in decreased renal blood flow, which may precipitate overt renal decompensation.

○ **What surgical procedures are generally thought to warrant avoidance of ketorolac perioperatively?**

There are several case reports of bleeding following administration of a single dose of ketorolac after cosmetic surgery. It is prudent to avoid in any case where significant surgical or medical bleeding may occur, as ketorolac causes reversible inhibition of platelet aggregation. Other surgical procedures include GI bleeding or peptic ulceration and urological procedures where the risk of nephropathy (especially in patients with a creatinine greater than or equal to 1.3) is increased [White et al., 2012. See reference on page 530].

○ **What is the recommended length of use of ketorolac in the postoperative period?**

Ketorolac has been extensively used in varying doses for analgesia in the postoperative setting with moderate success. A 30 mg IV dose every 6 hours for 48 hours is now recommended in patients who have a normal creatinine clearance and a 15 mg dose for the elderly or those in whom a lower dose would be more prudent. The maximum daily dose is 150 mg on the first day and 120 mg on subsequent days for a limit of 5 days.

○ **What is the estimated potency of ketorolac compared with narcotic medications?**

It has been shown that ketorolac 30 mg has a potency similar to about 5–10 mg of parenteral morphine. The oral form is limited to 10–20 mg because of GI toxicity. It has 50 times the analgesic effect of naproxen and 20 times the antipyretic effect of aspirin.

○ **Are there any NSAIDs that have been shown to reduce the incidence of NSAID gastropathy?**

Misoprostol has been shown to reduce the incidence of peptic mucosal damage (ulceration and bleeding) when taken four times daily. Due to its cost and side effect profile (diarrhea), its clinical use is reserved for this indication.

○ **Is there an increased incidence of perioperative complications in patients taking NSAIDs?**

All NSAIDs produce reversible inhibition of platelet aggregation, which potentially increases the risk of perioperative bleeding, especially if the patient has a preexisting coagulopathy or abnormal platelet function. Aspirin produces irreversible platelet dysfunction. Concurrent use of other NSAIDs, nephrotoxic drugs, or acetaminophen increases the risk of nephropathy or GI side effects.

○ **What is the advantage of using acetaminophen over acetylsalicylic acid (aspirin) postoperatively?**

Although agranulocytosis and thrombocytopenia are possible, platelet dysfunction is not a side effect, as seen with aspirin. GI effects include nausea and vomiting and hepatotoxicity in overdose with fewer incidences of peptic ulceration and bleeding. There is no significant peripheral prostaglandin synthetase inhibition with acetaminophen, although it is equipotent in inhibiting central prostaglandin synthesis. The major risk of nephropathy is administration in combination with NSAIDs.

○ **In what ways can local anesthetics be used for postoperative analgesia?**

Local anesthetics can be combined in the epidural space with epidural narcotics to reduce overall dose requirements and improve analgesia. They can also be used alone. Pain control can be achieved with local infiltration, regional blockade, intravenous infusion, or topical (gel, patch) application of local anesthetics.

○ **What are the most common adverse reactions with local anesthetics in the postoperative period?**

Hypotension, respiratory depression, tinnitus, excessive somnolence, bradycardia, and nausea are most commonly reported.

○ **Is there any benefit to using local anesthetics for postoperative epidural analgesia versus IV PCA narcotics?**

It has been shown that patients who have postoperative epidural analgesia with local anesthetics demonstrate improved lower extremity blood flow, better postoperative pulmonary and cardiac function, less ileus, earlier ambulation and hospital discharge, and overall better pain control, when compared with IV PCA modes of analgesia. A reduced incidence of phantom limb pain is also seen in amputations.

○ **When might it be advantageous to use epidural over IV PCA narcotics for postoperative analgesia?**

Upper abdominal, vascular, and thoracic surgery, especially in patients with significant lung disease.

○ **Is there any evidence that preemptive analgesia works?**

The evidence is contentious that it works for acute postoperative pain. Many experts feel that blocking pathways involved in pain transmission before surgical stimulation reduces postoperative pain. Local infiltration along the planned surgical incision for inguinal hernia repair with general anesthesia is beneficial, if the injection is made prior to skin incision. Intravenous or epidural opiates in patients having thoracotomy and hysterectomy have shown a preemptive effect.

There is stronger evidence for a beneficial effect of preemptive analgesia in preventing the development of chronic postoperative pain.

○ **What combination techniques have been most extensively advocated for preemptive analgesia?**

Epidural or intrathecal local anesthetics and opioids are most studied. Single-shot or continuous regional blocks have also been used. Additionally clonidine and NMDA antagonists have been successfully reported to reduce postoperative narcotic requirements.

○   **What are the appropriate conversions from IV to epidural opioids?**

IV to epidural = 10:1.

○   **What are the appropriate conversions from IV to intrathecal opioids?**

IV to intrathecal = 100:1.

○   **What are the relative IM and p.o. potencies of the opioids?**

Drug	IM	Oral
Morphine	10	30
Hydromorphone	1.5	7.5
Meperidine	75	300
Methadone	10	20
Codeine	130	200

○   **A patient requires 90 mg of IV morphine in 24 hours after surgery and you are asked to convert him or her to oral morphine for discharge home. What is the appropriate dose?**

Due to the first-pass effect of agents taken orally, the conversion from IV to oral opioids is generally 1:3. Therefore, this patient would require about 270 mg of oral morphine in 24 hours. Rarely is this large dose prescribed due to the high incidence of side effects.

○   **What is the appropriate breakthrough dose of oral opioid medication in a patient taking controlled-release opioids for postoperative pain?**

Normally patients should be given one fourth to one third the dose of the scheduled controlled-release preparation every 3–4 hours for breakthrough pain. Therefore, if a patient is taking 30 mg of controlled-release morphine sulfate every 12 hours, a dose of 10 mg immediate-release morphine would be sufficient.

○   **What are the advantages of IV PCA?**

Intravenous patient-controlled analgesia allows the patient to be in control of his or her pain. There is more controlled and steady analgesia, with less adverse side effects. There is less total amount of medication required for analgesia, less fluctuation in plasma opioid levels, less demand on nursing time, less delay from time of request for analgesia to delivery of the medication, and less cost.

○   **What are the advantages of patient-controlled epidural analgesia?**

The ability to titrate analgesic doses in proportion to individual levels of pain intensity, lower total dose requirements compared with other systems, decreased sedation, and increased patient satisfaction.

○   **What are the important terms associated with patient-controlled analgesia?**

Dose: The incremental amount of narcotic (age-dependent, renal function, body habitus) prescribed that the patient self-administers with each push.

Bolus: The loading dose of narcotic given when the patient first begins PCA, generally two to three times the incremental dose.

Lockout: The time between actual delivery of narcotic doses, usually a range of 6–10 minutes.

Basal: The continuous background infusion prescribed in addition to each dose made available to the patient. Generally avoided in opioid naïve patients, especially with associated sleep apnea, renal, or hepatic disease.

○ **A patient receives 60 mg of IV PCA morphine in 24 hours but has intolerable nausea and vomiting and needs to be converted to hydromorphone. What is the conversion dose?**

One milligram of morphine is equal to about 0.2 mg of hydromorphone (five times more potent than morphine), so the equivalent dose of hydromorphone in this patient would be 12 mg in 24 hours. The PCA pump would be set to provide a bolus dose of 0.2–0.4 mg and lockout at 6–10 minutes.

○ **A patient receives 300 mg of IV PCA meperidine in a 24-hour period. The internist is worried about accumulation of normeperidine and seizure activity, so he requests that you change to morphine. What would be the equivalent analgesic dose?**

This is a reasonable request as meperidine is a poor analgesic with only 1/10th the potency of morphine and has substantial risks including negative inotropic effect on the heart, allergic reactions, and normeperidine-induced seizures. The appropriate 24-hour dose equivalent of morphine would be 30 mg.

○ **A patient receives a total of 60 mg of IV morphine each day in hospital. In readiness for discharge, the surgeon requests that you make recommendations for the equivalent dosing of oral hydromorphone.**

IV morphine must first be converted to the PO morphine equivalent dose. Due to the first-pass effect and oral morphine's relatively poor bioavailability, the oral dose of morphine is three times the IV dose, or 180 mg. Hydromorphone is about five times more potent than morphine; therefore, the appropriate total dose in 24 hours would be 36 mg.

○ **What is the purpose of a naloxone infusion in patients receiving epidural opioids?**

Naloxone is an antagonist to opioids and can be used as a single bolus injection to reverse narcotic-induced respiratory depression. Opioid antagonists can reduce or reverse opioid-induced nausea and vomiting, pruritus, urinary retention, rigidity, and biliary spasm associated with neuraxial analgesic techniques.

Naloxone 0.25 µg/kg/h via continuous infusion has been reported to reduce adverse effects associated with PCA analgesia with morphine and enhance analgesia with reduced morphine requirements. The mechanism may be enhanced release of endogenous opiates and opioid receptor upregulation.

○ **What dose of IV naloxone is normally required to reverse the adverse side effects of epidural opioids?**

Generally infusions of 1–5 µg/kg/h are adequate to reverse side effects. At rates above 10 µg/kg/h analgesic effects are reversed.

○ **What are alternative measures to manage postoperative upper extremity/lower extremity pain in patients intolerant to opioids?**

Central axis or peripheral nerve block with a single injection or continuous catheter technique.

Epidural catheter placement for lower extremity surgery with dilute concentrations of local anesthetics is beneficial. In upper and lower extremity surgery, an axillary or femoral/sciatic catheter with a continuous infusion of local anesthetic solution is efficacious.

○ **What are commonly encountered side effects of epidurally administered local anesthetic infusions?**

In large quantities or high concentrations, a partial sympathetic blockade may occur precipitating hypotension, particularly orthostatic hypotension. With more dilute concentrations of, for example, 1/8th to 1/16th bupivacaine, this is avoided. Mild motor and/or sensory loss may occur. Urinary retention, particularly in the very young patient and the elderly male, may occur.

○ **What are the signs and symptoms of an epidural hematoma?**

Severe back pain and new-onset radicular pain of the lower extremities followed quickly by weakness, paralysis, and sensory losses are ominous signs. Loss of bowel and bladder function is a later sign. All of these findings require immediate evaluation.

○ **What is the workup for a suspected epidural hematoma?**

Immediate history and thorough neurological evaluation.

The catheter should be left in place.

Stat consultation among the surgical, neurosurgery, and anesthesia attendings.

MRI evaluation of the epidural space is mandatory (upper cut above the catheter tip).

Surgical evacuation (discontinue heparin and administer steroids) may be required.

○ **What are some common causes of postoperative hypertension?**

Hypertension is due to an increase in preload, contractility, afterload, or rate. With the exception of preexisting essential hypertension, these effects are mediated via sympathetic stimulation from a variety of causes.

Preexisting hypertensive disease (see complete listing above): >90% have essential hypertension.

Surgical procedure: CEA, CABG, and aortic cross-clamping.

Anesthesia-induced: hypervolemia, pain, hypoxia, hypercarbia, malignant hypertension, shivering, and artifacts.

Drugs: rebound hypertension from drug withdrawal and pressors.

Common PACU problems: bladder distension, hypothermia, pain, and hypoglycemia.

○ **What is the role of an NMDA antagonist in postoperative pain management?**

NMDA antagonists (ketamine and dextromethorphan) have been shown to have supplemental analgesic properties when used in combination with opioids. They may decrease the amount of opioid required to control postoperative pain, and may reduce the development of hyperalgesia and chronic postoperative pain syndromes that sometimes occurs secondary to perioperative opioid exposure.

○ **What are nonpharmacological approaches to managing postoperative pain?**

Transcutaneous electrical nerve stimulation (T.E.N.S.), hypnosis and biofeedback, heat/cold therapy, acupuncture, and massage are also advocated and possibly efficacious.

○ **What are the primary nerve fibers that play predominant roles in acute pain?**

The A-delta and the C fibers play the most significant role.

○ **How is acute pain assessed?**

Verbal scales (McGill Pain Questionnaire), visual analogue scale (Numerical, 10-cm line, Faces or Color Pain Intensity Scales), or verbal descriptors or functional ability are used, as pain is a subjective experience. Changes in vital signs (blood pressure, heart rate, respiratory rate) correlate poorly with the degree of pain control. Measuring pain during activity may be a better indicator of efficacy of pain control.

○ **What are the reasons to aggressively treat postoperative pain?**

Physiologic, psychologic, economic, and legal reasons all exist to justify aggressive management. However, compassion and empathy are the greatest reasons.

○ **What are the major physiologic adverse effects of uncontrolled postoperative pain?**

System	Adverse Effect
Gastrointestinal	Ileus
Cardiovascular	Increased sympathetic effect (BP, pulse), angina
Pulmonary	Atelectasis, hypoxia, shunting, CO_2 retention
CNS	Altered mental status, stress, anxiety, and depression
Immunologic	Impaired wound healing

○ **A nurse administers meperidine 25 mg to a patient for control of postoperative shivering. The treatment is ineffective. What are your alternate choices?**

In most patients administration of meperidine 25 mg, clonidine 150 μg, or doxapram 100 mg is efficacious in stopping shivering within 5 minutes compared with placebo. Other drugs that have been described include ketanserin 10 mg, alfentanil 250 μg, physostigmine, fentanyl, morphine, nalbuphine, lidocaine, magnesium, methylphenidate, nefopam, pentazocine, and tramadol.

○ **What are the mechanisms and physiologic effects of postoperative shivering?**

Postoperative shivering usually occurs as a thermoregulatory response to hypothermia secondary to disruption of temperature homeostasis due to anesthesia and surgery. Anesthetic agents inhibit thermoregulation by lowering the threshold for shivering by 2–4°C, so shivering is not seen intraoperatively. As these agents wear off, postoperatively, these reflexes return and the patient will start to shiver. The neurotransmitter pathways are complex and poorly understood. There is evidence that opioid, alpha-2 adrenergic, serotonergic, and anticholinergic systems play a role.

The physiologic effects of shivering include increase in mean total-body oxygen consumption (40%), catecholamine release, cardiac output, heart rate, blood pressure, and intraocular pressure. Oxygen consumption is directly proportional to mean body temperature. Despite similar core temperatures, men have a greater incidence of clinically significant shivering and greater total-body oxygen consumption than women.

Shivering may also occur in PACU patients who are hyperthermic, (as part of postoperative sepsis), and in normothermic patients as a side effect of volatile agents [Horn, 1999. See reference on page 529; Reynolds et al., 2008. See reference on page 530].

○ **What is the treatment for corneal abrasions?**

Time heals corneal abrasions. Following general anesthesia the incidence may be as high as 44%, if the eye is left partly opened. Simple precautions, such as instilling a bland ointment (possible chemical keratitis) or taping closed the lids of the inoperative eye, may prevent surface trauma produced by the surgical drape, anesthetic mask, or exposure. Decreased tear production under general anesthesia and proptosis may worsen corneal exposure, requiring eyelid suturing in some susceptible patients. Treatment includes topical antibiotics or fluoroquinolones, ice compresses for 24–48 hours and then warm compresses, pain management with NSAID drops to the eye, or narcotics for severe pain. A soft bandage may be applied to the eye.

○ **What is the incidence of postoperative delirium in elderly patients?**

The reported incidence of postoperative delirium varies from 5.1% to 61.3%. Elderly patients usually manifest delirium following a lucid interval of first postoperative day or more, a condition known as interval delirium. Fortunately, the postoperative cognitive dysfunction is a reversible condition in the majority of elderly surgical patients. Only 1% of elderly surgical patients have persistent cognitive dysfunction at 1–2 years after the surgery. Preoperative risk factors predisposing to delirium include aging, lack of education, reoperation, polypharmacy and drug interaction, alcohol and sedative–hypnotic withdrawal, endocrine and metabolic compromise, impaired vision and hearing, sleep deficiency, anxiety, depression, and dementia [Lepousé et al., 2006. See reference on page 530; Sharma et al., 2005. See reference on page 530].

○ **Is general anesthesia associated with a higher postoperative rate of infection?**

Total hip or knee replacement under general anesthesia is shown to be associated with higher risk of surgical site infection compared with epidural or spinal anesthesia. Neuraxial anesthesia by increasing peripheral perfusion might reduce surgical site infection [Chang et al., 2010. See reference on page 529]. General anesthesia has been identified as a major "stand-alone" risk factor for postoperative surgical site infection.

○ **A patient expresses concern about postoperative nausea and vomiting (PONV). What would be your advice?**

PONV is multifactorial in origin. The risk of PONV with general anesthesia is between 20% and 50%. It is much less common with regional anesthesia, approximately 15%, especially if one avoids narcotics. Propofol-based anesthetic regimens have an inherent antiemetic effect. Prophylactic administration of 5-HT3 blockers such as 12.5 mg dolasetron or 4 mg ondansetron works equally well as the much cheaper 1.25 mg of droperidol. In addition, one may avoid nitrous oxide, administer antiemetics, adequately hydrate, remove gastric contents with suctioning, limit mask ventilation (especially avoiding high pressures or inexperienced operators), avoid opioid-based anesthesia, and administer a bolus dose of steroids [Gan et al., 2007. See reference on page 529].

○ **What are the risk factors for PONV [Apfel et al., 2002. See reference on page 529]?**

The incidence of nausea and vomiting in patients undergoing general anesthesia is reported as 37% and 20%, respectively. Risk factors for PONV can be divided into patient, procedural, anesthetic, and postoperative risk factors:

Patient: women > men, surgery during menstruation and ovulation, children 6–16 years > adults, obesity, migraine history, emergency surgery, excessive starvation, history of PONV or motion sickness, and gastroparesis

Surgery: type (gynecological, gastrointestinal, laparoscopic, ear nose and throat, middle ear, T &A, strabismus) and longer duration

Anesthetic: choice of premedication, opioids, nitrous oxide, inhalation agents, bag and mask ventilation (inexperienced operator), longer procedures, and greater depth of anesthesia

Postoperative: pain, opioid analgesics, dizziness, early ambulation, hypotension, and premature oral intake

○ **Does PONV prophylaxis need to be given to all patients going for GA?**

Patients should be stratified for their risk of having PONV based on characteristics categorized as above. Interventions to prevent PONV are not needed in the majority of patients. If needed, prophylaxis is most commonly a serotonin receptor antagonist. Other agents are added for higher risk patients, such as dexamethasone, phenothiazines, haloperidol, and scopolamine. Nonpharmacological alternatives are acupuncture and acupressure.

○ **Between ondansetron, droperidol, and metoclopramide, which is the best antiemetic prophylaxis for a 22-year-old healthy female scheduled for a therapeutic abortion?**

Eight milligrams of intravenous ondansetron appears to be superior to 10 mg of metoclopramide or 1.25 mg of droperidol in preventing postoperative vomiting after general anesthesia for minor gynecological surgery. 1.25 mg of droperidol is as efficacious as 4 mg of ondansetron with a similar incidence of side effects. However, in 2001 December FDA issued a black box warning about droperidol. This is in relation to the deaths associated with cardiac rhythm abnormalities in patients treated with droperidol (QT prolongation). The warning states that droperidol should be reserved for those who fail to show response to other adequate treatments, and monitoring should be used for a period of one hour after administration of droperidol. Currently, droperidol is rarely used in the anesthesiology community.

○ **What is the presumed mechanism of action of the perioperative antiemetic effect of ephedrine?**

Ephedrine increases sympathetic tone, and therefore is thought to minimize PONV that is secondary to a high degree of vagal tone. Intestinal motility may decrease as an adrenergic side effect. Ephedrine corrects hypotension-induced nausea and vomiting seen with spinal anesthesia.

○ **What type of patients would you not give ephedrine to as an antiemetic?**

Any patient who would be adversely affected by the hypertension and tachycardia associated with the use of ephedrine, as well as patients taking MAO inhibitors.

○ **How are extrapyramidal reactions to droperidol classified?**

Extrapyramidal reactions to droperidol are mediated via central dopaminergic receptor blockade involved in motor function. Three major categories include: (1) *acute dystonic reactions* that involve spasm of muscles of the tongue, face, neck, and back (this can also include oculogyric crisis and episodes including sweating, tachypnea, and vasodilation); (2) *parkinsonian signs* and symptoms, which include bradykinesia, rigidity, mask-like facies, drooling, cogwheel rigidity, and tremor; and (3) *akathisia*, which are feelings of motor restlessness.

○ **Describe some life-threatening side effects of droperidol.**

QT interval prolongation, torsade de pointes, cardiac arrest, and ventricular tachycardia have been reported in patients treated with droperidol. Some of these cases were associated with death.

○ **What is the antiemetic of choice for patients with Parkinson disease?**

Diphenhydramine, which has the additional benefit of reducing tremor by modifying a chemical imbalance of decreased dopamine relative to acetylcholine in the striatum. Propofol may unpredictably reduce tremor.

○ **What are the relative contraindications of metoclopramide?**

Metoclopramide is relatively contraindicated in patients who can't tolerate an increase in GI motility (GI hemorrhage, obstruction, or perforation); pheochromocytoma (may cause hypertensive crisis due to release of catecholamines); sensitive to metoclopramide, procaine, and procainamide; seizure disorders; at risk for extrapyramidal side effects (epilepsy, renal failure, Parkinson disease) or bronchospasm.

○ **What are the effects of metoclopramide on a patient with Parkinson disease?**

Since metoclopramide is a dopamine antagonist, it can potentially worsen the symptoms of Parkinson disease. Case reports suggest that it might also lead to the development of prolonged encephalopathy in these patients.

○ **What is the association between antiemetic drugs and QT prolongation?**

Most antiemetic drugs are known to result in QT prolongation, although the clinical significance of this is debatable. Droperidol, the agent most associated with this phenomenon, has been given a black box warning by the FDA based on a small number of case reports. Other antiemetic classes of drugs such as 5-HT3 antagonists (e.g., ondansetron) and antipsychotics (e.g., haloperidol) are also linked to QT interval lengthening.

○ **List some causes of QT prolongation?**

Electrolyte imbalances: hypokalemia, hypomagnesemia, and hypocalcemia.

Antiarrhythmic drugs: quinidine, procainamide, sotalol, and amiodarone.

CNS disorders: subarachnoid or IC hemorrhage, closed head injury, and tumor.

Cardiac: myocarditis and ischemia.

Drugs: phenothiazines, TCAs, lithium, and droperidol.

Congenital form (Jervell and Lange-Nielsen syndrome).

○ **Describe perioperative management of a patient with history of long QT syndrome (LQTS).**

Obtain preoperative ECG as baseline and to rule out LQTS if there is a family history of sudden death or syncope. LQTS is defined as a prolongation of the QTc to more than 460–480 milliseconds.

LQTS can be congenital or acquired. Acquired form is more common.

1. Avoid drugs that prolong QTc:

   Anesthetic drugs – Although currently there is insufficient information, isoflurane and sevoflurane have been shown to prolong QTc.

   Droperidol and other antiemetics.

2. Events that prolong QTc should be avoided:

   Correction of electrolyte abnormalities (magnesium and potassium)

   Sympathetic stimulation with anxiety and intraoperative noxious stimuli

   Acute hypokalemia due to hyperventilation

3. Establish patient on beta-blockers preoperatively (prevent ventricular dysrhythmias) if believed to be at high risk. Cardiac pacing and ICD implantation may be required to treat arrhythmias.

4. Defibrillator should be available.

○ **What are the causes of respiratory difficulty and/or hypoxemia in the PACU?**

1. Even 0.1 MAC of volatile agents blunts the ventilatory response to hypoxia, and the response is abolished at 1 MAC.

2. Atelectasis due to anesthetic and surgical effects on the respiratory system (decreased FRC and V/Q mismatch).

3. Residual neuromuscular blockade.

4. Diffusion hypoxia: first 5–10 minutes when the patients are allowed to inhale room air at the conclusion of N_2O anesthetic.

5. Opioids affect the ventilatory pattern. The ventilatory response to hypoxia is blunted and there is a dose-related depression of ventilatory response to CO_2.

6. Secretions and airway obstruction.

7. Fluid overload.

8. Postextubation stridor and obstructive pulmonary edema.

○ **What is the rationale for PACU bypass or fast-tracking?**

In PACU bypass, or fast-tracking, ambulatory surgery patients are discharged from the operating room directly to the second-stage recovery unit, without an intermediary stay in PACU. The PACU is a labor-intensive area, with a high ratio of specialist trained recovery nurses to patients. The SSRU by contrast has a lower nursing ratio, and may have less specialized nurses. By reducing usage of the PACU, significant savings in nursing costs may be achieved.

○ **Do fast-tracked patients have the same recovery criteria before arrival to the second stage recovery as patients who are not fast-tracked?**

The criteria for admission to the SSRU are based on the Aldrete scoring system, and are the same whether the patient is admitted directly from the OR or whether he or she is admitted from the PACU. By careful selection of appropriate patients (ASA 1–3, no sleep apnea), use of short-acting agents, and increased utilization of regional blocks, these criteria are achieved in fast-tracked patients before they leave the operating room [ASA Practice Guidelines for postanesthesia Care, 2002. See reference on page 529].

○ **Is a chest radiograph required for diagnosis of a tension pneumothorax?**

Tension pneumothorax should be suspected in a patient with surgery/trauma/central line placement involving the neck or chest who develops respiratory distress. It may also develop as a complication of mechanical ventilation or upper abdominal surgery. The awake patient appears anxious and in pain, and the trachea may be deviated. However, the unconscious patient manifests tachycardia, hypotension, and hypoxemia. The chest x-ray shows translucence of the affected hemithorax, with a depressed hemidiaphragm, and may show tracheal and mediastinal deviation. If untreated, tension pneumothorax may lead to circulatory collapse. For this reason diagnosis should not be delayed for radiologic confirmation. Treatment is immediate decompression by needle thoracostomy, followed by placement of a chest drain.

○ **What is the differential diagnosis of delayed awakening in the PACU?**

The causes of delayed emergence fall into three categories: *drugs* (residual narcotics, sedatives, muscle relaxants, phenothiazines, anticholinergics), *metabolic* (hypothermia, hypoglycemia, hyperglycemia, hypercarbia, hypothyroidism), and *neurological* (cerebral hypoperfusion, cerebral hemorrhage, cerebral edema, seizure). Psychiatric disorder is a rare cause of delayed awakening.

○   **What are the causes of postoperative pulmonary edema?**

Aside from negative pressure pulmonary edema, other causes are aspiration pneumonitis, cardiac failure, fluid overload, sepsis, transfusion-associated lung injury, and anaphylaxis

Key Terms

Antiemetic: QT interval effects
Antiemetics: Parkinson
Congenital long QT: management
Delayed emergence: differential diagnosis
Droperidol: side effects
Intestinal motility: drug effects
Ketorolac: contraindications
Metoclopramide: contraindications
Metoclopramide: esophageal sphincter tone/gastric effects
Negative pressure pulmonary edema: causes/management

PACU bypass: rationale
PACU stage 1 bypass criteria
Parkinson disease: metoclopramide effects
Pneumothorax: x-ray findings
PONV prophylaxis
Respiratory difficulty in PACU
Risk factors: PONV
Tension pneumothorax: diagnosis and treatment
Treatment: shivering

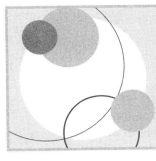

Preoperative Evaluation

It is no measure of health to be well adjusted to a profoundly sick society.
Jiddu Krishnamurti

○ **What is the American Society of Anesthesiologists (ASA) physical status classification?**

The ASA physical status classification system was initially created in 1941 by the American Society of Anesthetists, an organization that later became the ASA. The purpose of the grading system is to assess the patient's physical state prior to selecting an anesthetic plan. The system is used for recordkeeping, for communicating between colleagues, and to create a uniform system for statistical analysis. It is not intended for use as a measure to predict operative risk. The current system is as follows:

ASA Physical Status 1 – A normal healthy patient
ASA Physical Status 2 – A patient with mild systemic disease
ASA Physical Status 3 – A patient with severe systemic disease
ASA Physical Status 4 – A patient with severe systemic disease that is a constant threat to life
ASA Physical Status 5 – A moribund patient who is not expected to survive without the operation
ASA Physical Status 6 – A declared brain-dead patient whose organs are being removed for donor purposes

In all cases, an "E" after the classification indicates a procedure being done on an emergency basis.

○ **Preoperative lab results are valid for what length of time [ASA Practice Advisory for PreAnesthetic Evaluation, 2012. See reference on page 530]?**

The *ASA Task Force on Preanesthesia Evaluation* states that test results obtained from the medical record within 6 months of surgery are generally acceptable, if the patient's medical history has not changed substantially. More recent test results are necessary when the medical history has changed or when a test result may play a role in the selection of a specific anesthetic technique (e.g., regional anesthesia in the setting of anticoagulation therapy).

○ **An 18-year-old healthy white male is scheduled for knee surgery. What types of preoperative testing are mandatory for this type of patient and surgery?**

None. For male patients with no significant past medical history who are scheduled for minor surgical procedures there is no "mandatory" preoperative testing.

○ **What are the recommended indications for preoperative hemoglobin testing?**

Any procedure commonly associated with major blood loss, pregnancy, any suspicion of anemia, renal disease, malignancy, patients older than 75 years, neonates, smoking history of greater than 20 packs per year, and patients with cardiovascular disease.

○ **At what age would an otherwise healthy patient need a preoperative screening chest x-ray?**

ASA task force does not believe that extremes of age, smoking, stable COPD, stable cardiac disease, or resolved recent URI should be considered unequivocal indications for chest radiograph.

○ **At what diastolic blood pressure would it be reasonable to delay an elective surgical case?**

The answer to this question is dictated by the patient, surgical procedure, and surgeon's and anesthesiologist's preference. A reasonable cutoff would be a diastolic pressure of greater than 110 mm Hg, in a patient previously undiagnosed or not well medically managed. Old studies suggest an increased risk of severe cardiopulmonary complications.

If the patient is normally well controlled but suffering from "white coat anxiety," treatment may be as simple as IV anxiolytics and reevaluation. Checking several serial blood pressures is appropriate. Clonidine will reduce lability of intraoperative blood pressure and anesthetic requirements. Weksler et al., evaluate the efficacy and complications of immediate preoperative reduction of arterial BP (using intranasal nifedipine 10 mg) in patients with well-controlled hypertension but with DBP of 110–130 on arrival at the operating room. They reported that immediate preoperative reduction of DBP is safe and avoids unnecessary surgery postponement and associated costs [Weksler et al., 2003. See reference on page 530].

Diastolic hypertension is associated with an increase in SVR and is thought to be the major contributor to hypertensive morbidity (coronary artery disease, intracranial hemorrhage, and renal failure). Cardiac complications include myocardial ischemia, congestive heart failure (CHF), intraoperative lability in blood pressure, and death.

○ **What is Bayes' theorem, and how does it apply to perioperative testing?**

Bayes' theorem is a theorem of probability that examines how new information affects the original hypothesis. For instance, if you randomly draw a playing card out of a well-shuffled deck, the chance that the card is a jack is 4/52, since there are 4 jacks in the deck. Now if you tell me that the card you drew is a face card, the chance that it is a jack is modified to 4/12, since there are 12 face cards in the deck. With respect to perioperative testing, Bayes' theorem allows us to better understand the sensitivity and specificity of a test given the incidence of an abnormal test in that specific population. In essence, Bayes' theorem tells us that a test is most useful in a population with a moderate incidence of the disease for which the test is designed to detect.

○ **In the review of systems of a 70-year-old male with multiple cardiac risk factors, what pieces of information are particularly important in deciding whether the patient requires further cardiac evaluation or can proceed with noncardiac surgery, according to the American Heart Association/American College of Cardiology recommendations?**

Presence of active cardiac conditions or clinical risk factors, high-risk surgery, and poor functional capacity.

○ **What factors increase the cardiac risk (cardiac death, MI) during noncardiac surgery?**

Important factors to consider are the presence of active cardiac conditions and the surgical severity. The presence of any active cardiac conditions warrants postponement for all except life-saving emergencies and mandates intensive management.

As far as the surgical severity is concerned, vascular surgery has reported cardiac risk of >5%. Intermediate-risk surgery has a cardiac risk of 1–5%. Low-risk surgery has a cardiac risk of <1% [ACC AHA guidelines on perioperative cardiovascular evaluation and care for noncardiac surgery, 2007. See reference on page 530].

Clinical risk factors become important in patients with poor or unknown functional capacity when scheduled for vascular, intermediate-, or high-risk procedures. If no clinical risk factors, proceed with the planned surgery

If the patient has one or two clinical risk factors it is reasonable to proceed with planned surgery. If appropriate, one may use heart rate control with beta blockers. Consider preoperative testing only if it will change the management. In patients with three or more clinical risk factors, *surgery-specific cardiac risk is important. Consider testing if it will change the management.* One should also consider the urgency of the noncardiac surgery (cancer), the life expectancy of the individual, and the potential long-term benefit of medical management versus revascularization.

○ **What surgeries are considered high risk (>5%) for perioperative myocardial infarction?**

Aortic and other major vascular surgery

Peripheral vascular surgery

○ **What surgeries are considered intermediate risk?**

These are intrathoracic or intraperitoneal surgery, carotid endarterectomy, head and neck surgery, orthopedic surgery, and prostate surgery.

○ **What surgeries are considered low risk?**

These are endoscopic procedures, superficial procedures, cataract surgery, breast surgery, and ambulatory surgery.

○ **How is poor functional capacity defined?**

The inability to exercise at 4 METs (metabolic equivalents), which is equivalent to walking up one flight of stairs.

○ **What are the active cardiac conditions?**

Unstable coronary syndrome, decompensated heart failure, significant arrhythmias, or severe valvular disease.

○ **What are the clinical risk factors?**

The clinical risk factors are history of ischemic heart disease, history of compensated or prior heart failure, history of cerebrovascular disease, diabetes mellitus, and renal insufficiency.

○ **What is unstable coronary syndrome?**

This includes unstable or severe angina (Canadian Cardiovascular Society [CCS] class III or IV) or recent MI. (This may include stable angina in patients who are unusually sedentary.)

○ **What is considered recent MI?**

Recent MI means an acute MI within the past 7 days or recent MI within the past 8–30 days with evidence of myocardium at risk (because of persistent symptoms or the results of stress testing).

○ **What are the significant dysrhythmias?**

High-grade AV block, Morbitz II AV block, third-degree AV heart block, symptomatic ventricular arrhythmias, supraventricular arrhythmias (including AF) with uncontrolled ventricular rate (HR >100), symptomatic bradycardia, and newly recognized ventricular tachycardia.

○ **What is considered severe valvular disease?**

Severe AS (mean pressure gradient >40 mm Hg, aortic valve area <1 cm^2, or symptomatic) and symptomatic mitral stenosis (progressive dyspnea on exertion, exertional presyncope, or HF).

○ **What is the most common significant cardiac valvular lesion found in the noncardiac patient planned for surgery?**

Aortic valve stenosis (AS) affect ~40% of the population over the age of 80 [Ngo et al., 2012. See reference on page 530]. The prevalence of mitral-valve prolapse in the general population is shown to be about 2–3% [Freed et al., 1999. See referenc on page 530].

○ **What is the leading cause of postoperative morbidity in patients undergoing surgery for peripheral vascular disease?**

The major cause of postoperative death is cardiac, primarily myocardial infarction.

Comorbid risk factors are present in a large number of patients with peripheral vascular disease. These include hypertension (51%), hypercholesterolaemia (45%), concurrent CAD (41.1%), and disease in all three vascular beds (cerbrovascular, coronary, and periphreal) seen in 8.6% patients [Ouriel, 2001. See reference on page 530]. In addition, many are heavy smokers (40–50%) with COPD, chronic bronchitis, and bronchospasm.

○ **A 75-year-old man who has severe claudication and is unable to ambulate freely is scheduled for a femoral–popliteal bypass. He had an episode of severe chest pain 1 month ago. A preoperative ECG shows left ventricular hypertrophy with left bundle branch block; no prior ECG is available for comparison. Does he need further cardiac evaluation?**

Step 1: Is this emergency surgery?

No. (He is scheduled to undergo high-risk surgery.)

Step 2: Does the patient have one of the active cardiac conditions?

Yes, acute coronary syndrome.

These conditions warrant postponement for all except life-serving emergencies and mandate intensive management.

This patient should be evaluated and treated prior to surgery according to 2007 ACC/AHA guidelines.

○ **What is the goal of the perioperative history and physical, and selected noninvasive testing?**

It is to clarify:

1. What is the amount of myocardium in jeopardy?
2. What is the ischemic threshold (amount of stress → ischemia)?
3. What is the patient's ventricular function?
4. Is the patient on his or her optimal medical regimen?

○ **What is the goal of further preoperative cardiac evaluation and testing?**

These are done to identify patients who would benefit from the following:

1. Myocardial revascularization or angioplasty prior
2. Intensive intraoperative and postoperative measures to reduce operative risks
3. More limited surgical approach
4. Canceling surgery altogether

○ **What advantage does exercise thallium imaging offer over exercise electrocardiography?**

Exercise thallium imaging is another noninvasive test that can be used in patients who have abnormal electrocardiograms suggestive of ischemic heart disease. It increases the sensitivity and specificity of the exercise ECG. Thallium is taken up by the coronary circulation and distributed to the myocardium. Fixed perfusion defects include infarcted myocardium and poorly perfused areas. The poorly perfused areas later refill and indicate areas at risk for ischemia.

○ **To lessen the risk and severity of perioperative cardiac events in high-risk patients what therapeutic options are available before noncardiac surgery?**

1. Revascularization by surgery
2. Revascularization by percutaneous coronary intervention (PCI)
3. Optimal medical management: antiplatelet drugs, beta-blockers, calcium channel blockers, nitrates, and ACE inhibitors

○ **Beta-blockers should be titrated to what heart rate in order to maximize protection from perioperative ischemia?**

At present most agree that beta-blockers should be administered to high-risk patients (high-risk surgery, major clinical risk factors, or positive ischemia on preoperative stress testing) and titrated to an HR of 60 bpm. For ease of dosing and consistency of effect, longer acting beta-blockers such as atenolol or bisoprolol may be more efficacious.

Initiation of beta-blockers in low-risk group requires careful consideration (risk/benefit ratio). Initiate well before a planned procedure and titrate. Routine perioperative use, particularly high fixed dose on the day of surgery, is not recommended.

Beta-blocker withdrawal has been associated with increased risk of MI. Continuation in the perioperative period in patients already taking the drug is a class I indication (should be performed) [ACCF/AHA Focused Update on Perioperative Beta Blockade, 2009. See reference on page 530].

○ **Why is it not recommended to administer perioperative high-dose beta-blockade routinely?**

The PeriOperative ISchemic Evaluation (POISE) – a large, randomized, controlled trial of fixed higher-dose beta-blockade trial [POISE Study Group, 2008. See reference on page 530] confirmed a reduction in primary cardiac events such as cardiovascular death, MI (30% reduction), and cardiac arrest with perioperative beta-blockade therapy. However, the benefit was offset by an increased risk of 30-day all-cause mortality and stroke, suggesting routine administration of high-dose beta-blockers in the absence of dose titration is not useful and may be harmful to beta-blocker-naïve patients undergoing surgery.

○ **How long after placement of a coronary artery stent is it safe to perform surgery?**

Six weeks minimum, as surgical stress may precipitate occlusion of the stent. Generally, patients with drug-eluting stents (DES) should be on clopidogrel for 1 year. Risk/benefit of individual cases may favor shorter periods. At the time of surgery, the patient may need to have discontinued clopidogrel for 7 days (although most surgeries can be performed while on clopidogrel, except perhaps closed space surgery such as neurosurgery). It is recommended that patients should be continued on aspirin during the perioperative period. High-risk patients with comorbidities, who present for urgent surgery with less than 12 months of DES, should be considered for bridging therapy, if the surgical procedure requires discontinuation of clopidogrel and aspirin.

In summary, elective surgery should be postponed for >6 weeks with bare metal stents and >12 months with DES [ACC/ACH recommendation for perioperative revascularization and antiplatelet therapy, 2007. See reference on page 530].

○ **What is the risk of perioperative stent thrombosis and what causes it?**

Abrupt withdrawal of antiplatelet medications preoperatively has a rebound effect. This leads to significantly increased inflammatory prothrombotic state, increased platelet adhesion/aggregation, and excessive thromboxane A_2 activity. Surgical interventions also increase inflammatory prothrombotic state. This state when combines with partially endothelialized stent(s) can cause stent thrombosis, MI, and death.

○ **What is the difference between hypertensive urgency and a hypertensive emergency?**

Both are defined as a BP >180/120 mm Hg. A hypertensive *emergency* exists when this severe elevation of BP is associated *with* target organ dysfunction such as hypertensive encephalopathy, intracerebral hemorrhage, acute myocardial infarction, acute left ventricular failure with pulmonary edema, unstable angina pectoris, dissecting aortic aneurysm, or eclampsia. It requires immediate BP reduction (not necessarily to normal) to prevent or limit target organ damage.

Hypertensive *urgency* exists when there is severe elevation in BP *without* progressive target organ dysfunction. It should be treated with oral agents over days and follow-up care. There is actually no evidence that failure to treat hypertensive urgency aggressively is associated with any increased short-term risk, while aggressive reduction of BP does have risks [Cherney and Straus, 2001. See reference on page 530].

○ **Which two classes of hypertensive medications cause withdrawal hypertension and should not be stopped prior to a patient having surgery?**

β-Blockers and clonidine.

Withdrawal of both is associated with rebound hypertension and myocardial ischemia. All antihypertensive medications should be continued until the day of surgery with the possible exception of diuretics (depletion of intravascular volume) and ACE inhibitors (hypotension with induction; avoid in unstable patients and during immediate perioperative period).

Note that withdrawal hypertension may occur with many different antihypertensive drugs including reserpine, hydralazine, guanethidine, methyldopa, and hydrochlorothiazide.

○ **What is the definition of moderate COPD?**

The Global Initiative for Chronic Obstructive Lung Disease (GOLD) Workshop summary defines COPD as *moderate* when airflow restriction of FEV_1 is <80% of predicted. A patient with FEV_1 <30% of predicted is defined as having *severe* disease [GOLD Scientific Committee, 2001. See reference on page 530].

○ **Are there any therapies that will reduce the perioperative pulmonary risk in a patient with COPD?**

Yes. A decades-old study showed addressing the reversible component of obstructive disease improved outcomes. There is evidence that aggressive preoperative treatment of COPD may reduce the risk of perioperative pulmonary complications. This includes cessation of smoking, optimizing pharmacologic therapy (bronchodilators, steroids, antibiotics), detection and treatment of acute pulmonary infection and maximizing nutrition, hydration, and chest physiotherapy.

○ **When should clinicians obtain preoperative spirometry in patients scheduled for nonthoracic surgery?**

If a patient has poorly characterized dyspnea or exercise intolerance and diagnostic uncertainty exists between a cardiac and a pulmonary limitation. In addition, spirometry might be useful in patients who have established obstructive lung disease if it is not clear from the clinical evaluation that patients' chronic therapy has maximally improved function.

○ **Can the FEV₁ value on preoperative pulmonary function tests indicate whether or not a patient has obstructive lung disease?**

No. The FEV_1 may be reduced in both obstructive and restrictive lung disease. It is necessary to know the FVC as well to determine if the pattern is obstructive by calculating the FEV_1/FVC ratio.

○ **Is COPD a contraindication to prescribing beta-blockers?**

Generally not. In carefully selected patients with COPD, the use of cardioselective β-blockers appears to be safe and associated with reduced mortality. [Van Gestel et al., 2008. See reference on page 530]. Hawkins et al., showed that Initiation of bisoprolol in patients with heart failure and concomitant moderate or severe COPD resulted in a reduction in FEV_1. However, symptoms and quality of life were not impaired. [Hawkins et al., 2009. See reference on page 530].

○ **Is asthma a contraindication to the use of beta-blockers?**

Cardioselective β-blockers do not seem to produce clinically significant adverse respiratory effects in patients with mild-to-moderate asthma, similar to the patients with chronic obstructive airway disease. Because of the benefit of these drugs in conditions such as heart failure, cardiac arrhythmias, and hypertension, cardioselective β-blockers should not be withheld from patients with mild-to-moderate asthma. [Salpeter et al., 2002. See reference on page 530].

○ **Should elective surgery be delayed in an asthmatic patient who is wheezing?**

Yes, if the patient has not been absolutely optimized. History, physical examination, temperature, WBC, chest x-ray, and response to aerosolized bronchodilator therapy should be assessed. Wheezing may be caused by bronchoconstriction, inspissated secretions, aspiration, vocal cord dysfunction, pulmonary edema, or pneumothorax. If a patient with severe persistent asthma is compliant with optimal drug therapy and, although still wheezing, is considered to be stable and optimized, it may be reasonable to proceed, employing minimal instrumentation of the airway, and maximizing drugs that are bronchodilating. If, however, the etiology of the wheezing is not firmly established, or therapy could be improved, surgery should be delayed.

○ **What is the association between smoking and postoperative complications?**

Increased risk of pulmonary, cardiac, and wound complications.

○ **How long does a patient need to stop smoking prior to elective surgery to reduce the risk of postoperative pulmonary complications?**

Smoking cessation results in improvement in some parameters such as a decrease in carboxyhemoglobin levels (with resultant increased tissue oxygen availability) within days. However, evidence on the optimal regime for preoperative smoking cessation is less clear. Limited prospective data suggest that cessation for at least 6–8 weeks preoperatively is necessary to decrease the incidence of pulmonary complication, improve ciliary function and pulmonary mechanics, and reduce sputum production. There is evidence to suggest that smoking cessation a few days prior to surgery may increase airway reactivity and anxiety [Warner, 2005. See reference on page 530].

○ **T/F: The ASA Task Force on Preanesthesia Evaluation recommends the routine use of drug therapy to reduce the risk of pulmonary aspiration.**

False [ASA Practice Guidelines for Preoperative Fasting, 2011. See reference on page 530].

○ **Sildenafil (Viagra) is useful for what problem an anesthesiologist might encounter (aside from the obvious one)?**

Phosphodiesterase inhibitors such as sildenafil show promise in the management of pulmonary hypertension through pulmonary vasodilation.

○ **In patients with Parkinson disease, should levodopa/carbidopa be discontinued prior to surgery?**

No, except for neurosurgical procedures for tremor ablation.

Even brief interruptions in scheduled Parkinson medications may unmask tremors, dysphagia, and/or ventilatory inadequacy secondary to chest wall rigidity. Levodopa/carbidopa should be given immediately prior to surgery. The half life of levodopa is short (1–3 h) and interruption of therapy can result in severe skeletal muscle rigidity that interferes with ventilation. If a prolonged postoperative NPO course is anticipated, placement of a duodenal feeding tube should be considered. Prior to thalamotomy, pallidotomy, and placement of deep brain stimulators, Parkinson medications are deliberately held in order to maximize tremor [Nicholson et al., 2002. See reference on page 530].

○ **What can be done to reduce the risk of acute alcohol withdrawal in surgical patients?**

Prophylactic benzodiazepines, haloperidol, carbamazepine, beta-blockers, and/or clonidine may be useful for both prophylactic and acute treatment of alcohol withdrawal.

○ **What are the anesthetic implications of acute alcohol intoxication?**

In contrast to chronic alcoholic patient, intoxicated patient requires less anesthetic due to depressant effect of alcohol.

Alcohol may decrease the tolerance of the brain to hypoxia.

Alcohol delays gastric emptying and decreases lower esophageal sphincter tone. The patient is therefore more vulnerable to aspiration.

Surgical bleeding may be increased – may reflect interference with platelet aggregation (due to alcohol).

○ **What are the recommended indications for preoperative liver function testing?**

Patients with liver disease, a remote history of hepatitis or exposure to hepatitis, and known metastatic malignancy.

○ **How is the creatinine level affected by age?**

Serum creatinine levels slowly rise with age after 40 years.

○ **According to the American Society of Regional Anesthesia and Pain Medicine Consensus Statement, how long before neuraxial anesthesia do NSAIDs need to be stopped?**

NSAIDs do not need to be discontinued. The use of NSAIDs alone does not create a level of risk that will interfere with the performance of neuraxial blocks. There are little data concerning extremely high-dose therapy however.

○ **How long before neuraxial anesthesia does clopidogrel (Plavix) need to be stopped?**

Seven to 10 days.

○ **How long before neuraxial anesthesia does coumadin need to be stopped?**

Four to 5 days, with documented normalization of the PT.

○ **Why would a preoperative hematocrit in a pregnant woman be low?**

Pregnant women have a relative anemia. While the red blood cell volume increases 20%, the plasma volume increases 45%, resulting in a dilutional decrease in the hematocrit.

○ **What is SLUDGE syndrome?**

Signs and symptoms of muscarinic overstimulation in a patient with myasthenia gravis.

Salivation

Lacrimation

Urinary incontinence

Diarrhea

GI upset and hypermotility

Eyes: miosis and blurred vision (paralysis of accommodation)

Key Terms

Acute alcohol intoxication: anesthetic implications
ASA physical status classification
Cardiac evaluation for noncardiac surgery
Cardiac morbidity: preoperative factors
Congestive heart failure (CHF) and anesthesia risk
Guidelines: preoperative cardiac testing

Old myocardial infarction: preoperative risk assessment
Parkinson disease: anesthetic implications
Perioperative antihypertensive drug management
Perioperative cardiac risk
Perioperative ischemia/beta-blockers
Preoperative testing: Bayes' theorem

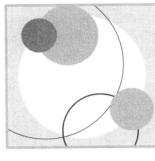

Respiratory Physiology and Anesthesia

*To laugh often and much: to win the respect of intelligent people and the affection of children,
to earn the appreciation of honest critics and endure the betrayal of false friends;
to appreciate beauty, to find the best in others, to leave the world a bit better
whether by a healthy child, a garden patch, or redeemed social
condition; to know even one life has breathed easier because
you have lived. This is to have succeeded.*
Ralph Waldo Emerson

○ **What constitutes anatomic dead space?**

Volume of the regions of the airway that histologically cannot participate in gas exchange: upper airways (oral cavity, nasopharynx, larynx) and cartilagenous airways (trachea, bronchi, membranous bronchioles). Dead space can be calculated from the single-breath nitrogen washout test (Fowler's method). It is approximately 2 mL/kg, ideal body weight.

○ **What is physiologic dead space?**

Physiologic dead space = anatomic + alveolar dead space.

Anatomic dead space accounts for the majority of physiologic dead space and is approximately 2 mL/kg ideal body weight in the upright position in most adults.

○ **What causes an increase in dead space?**

Increase in anatomic dead space: neck extension and anticholinergic drugs.

Increase in alveolar dead space (West Zone I) due to decreased perfusion: upright position, positive pressure ventilation, PEEP, hypotension, low cardiac output, and pulmonary embolism.

Increase in V/Q mismatch: ARDS, general anesthesia and age, emphysema, COPD, pulmonary fibrosis, smoking, and increased gas density.

○ **How do you derive V_D/V_T?**

V_D/V_T is normally 33% and can be derived using the Bohr equation:

$$\frac{V_D}{V_T} = \frac{P_A CO_2 - P_E CO_2}{P_A CO_2}$$

where $P_A CO_2$ is the alveolar CO_2 tension and $P_E CO_2$ is the mixed expired CO_2 tension.

Assume alveolar CO_2 partial pressure is equal to arterial CO_2 partial pressure.

○ **What causes a decrease in end-tidal CO_2?**

Hyperventilation, decrease in CO_2 production (e.g., hypothermia), decrease in alveolar CO_2 due to higher fraction of second alveolar gas (increased alveolar nitrous oxide or oxygen), pulmonary hypoperfusion due to hypotension, pulmonary (air) embolus, low cardiac output, cardiac arrest, sampling error, esophageal intubation, circuit disconnection, kinked endotracheal tube, or air leak around endotracheal tube.

○ **What is the etiology of the alveolar to end-tidal PCO_2 gradient?**

Mixing of exhaled gases from the physiologic dead space with gases from the alveoli causes a dilution of alveolar (equal to arterial) PCO_2. The alveolar fraction of CO_2 is exhaled last and represented in peak end-tidal CO_2 with complete exhalation. With incomplete exhalation, alveolar CO_2 is not represented on the expiratory CO_2 trace.

○ **List causes of increased end-tidal to arterial PCO_2 gradient.**

Usually, $ETCO_2$ is less than arterial PCO_2 due to increased alveolar to arterial gradient and/or increased end-tidal to alveolar gradient. Pulmonary hypoperfusion due to hypotension, pulmonary (air) embolus, low cardiac output, hypoventilation, sampling error due to esophageal intubation, circuit disconnection, kinked endotracheal tube, or air leak around endotracheal tube. During heavy exercise $ETCO_2$ can overestimate arterial PCO_2.

○ **List causes of increased end-tidal to alveolar PCO_2 gradient.**

$ETCO_2$ less than alveolar PCO_2 is caused by increased dead space fraction, incomplete exhalation with $ETCO_2$ not representative of alveolar PCO_2, leakage of alveolar gas prior to sampling site (ETT leak, obstruction, circuit disconnect), and artifact through high sampling rate of side stream capnograph in the face of elevated fresh gas flow.

○ **What conditions extend the volume of Zone I of the pulmonary circulation?**

Decreased perfusion: upright position, hypotension, low cardiac output, and pulmonary embolism.

Increased alveolar pressure: positive pressure ventilation and PEEP.

Decreased vasculature: age, emphysema, COPD, pulmonary fibrosis, and smoking.

○ **What is the relationship between asthma and PEEP?**

Patients with bronchospasm can develop intrinsic auto-PEEP due to incomplete expiration. Addition of extrinsic PEEP may exacerbate this effect with resultant hemodynamic compromise and no improvement in respiratory function.

○ **How do you diagnose auto-PEEP?**

Observe the end-expiratory pressure on the airway pressure gauge (some ventilators have an expiratory hold feature for this purpose). If this value is greater than the external PEEP you set, the difference is auto-PEEP.

○ **What is the cause and treatment of auto-PEEP?**

"Breath stacking" causes auto-PEEP. This happens when inspiration begins before completion of expiration. During mechanical ventilation this is caused by a fast respiratory rate or a short expiratory time. During spontaneous ventilation this is caused by an airway obstruction that makes it difficult to exhale.

Treatment consists of bronchodilator therapy and adjustment of the ventilator settings to allow for full exhalation. If this is not sufficient, interrupt ventilation periodically to allow for complete exhalation.

○ **List signs of intraoperative asthma.**

Wheezing, prolonged exhalation, incomplete exhalation with developing auto-PEEP, upward slope on the end-tidal CO_2 trace, hypotension due to decreased venous return with increasing intrathoracic gas volume, and hypoventilation.

Changes in arterial blood gases: progressive hypoxemia; initial normocarbia and then respiratory alkalosis deteriorating to respiratory acidosis.

○ **How would you treat intraoperative bronchospasm due to asthma?**

Intraoperative bronchospasm usually manifests as increasing peak inspiratory pressure (unchanged plateau pressure), rising waveform on the capnograph, and decreasing expired tidal volumes.

1. Deepen anesthetic with a volatile agent such as sevoflurane or isoflurane with 100% oxygen.

2. If there is no response, other causes of mechanical obstruction in the breathing circuit, airway, or endotracheal tube (kinking, secretions, bronchial intubation) should be excluded.

3. The bronchospasm should be treated with beta-adrenergic agonists (albuterol) delivered as aerosol or a metered dose inhaler into the inspiratory limb of the breathing circuit. Or use terbutaline subcutaneous.

4. Intravenous corticosteroid can be administered. However, it may take several hours before the therapeutic effect of steroid is apparent.

5. Ventilation should be adjusted to provide small to moderate tidal volumes and slow respiratory rates with long expiratory time to avoid air trapping.

6. Avoid nitrous oxide.

7. Measurement of arterial blood gases may be necessary to detect intrapulmonary shunting or increased dead space (widen arterial to end-tidal CO_2 gradient). And guide ventilation.

8. At the end of the case, lidocaine intravenous bolus (1.5 mg/kg) may help prevent recurrence of bronchospasm on emergence by obtunding the airway reflexes.

○ **Is there a role for intravenous epinephrine in severe bronchospasm?**

Yes. (Infused to effect, not CPR dose.)

Other mild bronchodilators include magnesium sulfate and atropine.

○ **What is the best ventilation strategy for asthmatics?**

Providing adequate expiratory time to avoid incomplete exhalation and auto-PEEP: low respiratory rate and low I:E ratio. Permissive hypercapnia.

○ **List differential diagnosis for wheezing during anesthesia.**

The machine, the endotracheal tube, or the patient.

Examples: endobronchial intubation, pulmonary embolism, bronchospasm, pulmonary edema, mucus secretions, cuff herniation, bronchial flow disturbance by tumor, infection, swelling, and foreign body aspiration.

○   **What are the signs of endobronchial intubation?**

The clues to the diagnosis of endobronchial intubation include:

1. Unilateral breath sounds.
2. Unexpected hypoxia with pulse oximetry.
3. Inability to palpate the ETT cuff in the sternal notch during cuff inflation.
4. Decreased breathing bag compliance. The earliest manifestation of endobronchial intubation is an increase in peak inspiratory pressure.

Neck extension or lateral rotation moves an ETT away from the carina, while neck flexion moves the tube toward the carina.

○   **What information is obtained from spirometry?**

A spirogram illustrates expiration of a vital capacity (VC) breath recorded over 4 or 5 seconds. The most clinically useful measurements are forced vital capacity (FVC), forced expiratory volume in 1 second (FEV_1), and flow between 25% and 75% of the FVC ($MMMF_{25-75}$). Calculation of the FEV_1/FVC ratio is an indicator of the severity of obstructive airway disease. Spirometry does not provide information about lung volumes and capacities or indicate the cause of airway obstruction.

○   **How can pulmonary function testing distinguish between obstructive disease states?**

Decreased FEV 25–75% for midsize airways obstruction (effort independent), FEV_1/FVC ratio response with and without bronchodilators for distinguishing between reactive airways disease (i.e., asthma), and structural airways disease (i.e., emphysema).

○   **What are the findings of pulmonary function tests in restrictive versus obstructive lung disease?**

A reduction in VC to less than 80% predicted with normal FEV_1/FVC ratio (both FEV_1 and FVC are decreased) is indicative of restrictive lung disease. VC-normal = 70 mL/kg; if <15 mL/kg, indicates severe dysfunction.

Diffusion capacity of lungs (DLCO) may be decreased <30–50% in severe restrictive diseases such as pulmonary fibrosis or sarcoidosis.

A reduction in FEV_1/FVC ratio to less than 70% indicates mild, less than 60% moderate, and less than 50% severe obstructive disease.

○   **Give examples of diseases that cause restrictive pattern on spirometry.**

Scoliosis, pulmonary fibrosis, sarcoidosis, obesity, and ascites.

○   **What arterial blood gas changes are seen in patients with COPD?**

The patients with COPD can be categorized as "pink puffers" or "blue bloaters" depending on the arterial blood gases.

The "pink puffers" usually have PaO_2 higher than 60 mm Hg and normal PCO_2. They have features of severe emphysema such as severe dyspnea due to loss of elastic recoil of the lung and decreased diffusion capacity.

The "blue bloaters" have PaO_2 usually less than 60 mm Hg and chronically increased PCO_2 to more than 45 mm Hg. They have features of chronic bronchitis. This includes moderate dyspnea and cough due to decreased airway diameter from mucus and inflammation, recurrent respiratory tract infection, and cor pulmonale.

○ **Can supplemental oxygen slow the progression of disease in "blue bloaters?"**

The goal of chronic oxygen administration is to increase and maintain PaO_2 between 60 and 80 mm Hg in order to decrease pulmonary vascular resistance and prevent excessive erythrocytosis. The relief of hypoxemia with oxygen is more effective than any drugs in decreasing pulmonary vascular resistance. Therefore, home oxygen therapy is recommended if the PaO_2 is <55 mm Hg, hematocrit is >55%, or there is evidence of cor pulmonale.

○ **Is there a change in the carbon monoxide (CO) diffusing capacity in patients with COPD?**

Yes, it is decreased in proportion to the severity of the emphysema and is the best functional predictor for the severity of the disease. However, it is not a sensitive test for young smokers or mild emphysema.

○ **How do you calculate the chest wall compliance?**

Compliance is defined as the change in volume for a given change in pressure. The clinical units are L/cm H_2O. Normal values are chest wall compliance = 0.2 L/cm H_2O, lung compliance = 0.2 L/cm H_2O, and total compliance = 0.1 L/cm H_2O. The total compliance is calculated as follows:

$$\frac{1}{C(\text{total})} = \frac{1}{C(\text{chest wall})} + \frac{1}{C(\text{lung})}.$$

A simple way to measure the lung compliance is to have the subject breath in and out of a spirometer at different lung volumes and measure esophageal pressure simultaneously to obtain a pressure volume curve.

The compliance varies with the lung volume and therefore should be interpreted in relation to lung volume. Usually report the slope of the compliance curve over a liter above the functional residual capacity (FRC) during deflation.

Chest wall compliance is decreased in kyphoscoliosis, abdominal disorders, which elevate the diaphragm, and also marked obesity.

○ **A 78-year-old female with severe, long-standing kyphoscoliosis is to undergo triple arthrodesis of the right foot under general anesthesia. What physiologic changes are suspected in this patient?**

Scoliosis impacts primarily the pulmonary and cardiovascular systems.

Pulmonary:

• Restrictive disease of the lungs with an associated reduction in lung volumes
• Pulmonary hypertension (reactive and fixed)
• Limited pulmonary reserve or respiratory failure; increase in normal postoperative pulmonary dysfunction that may require postoperative ventilatory support

Cardiovascular:

• Right ventricular dysfunction from chronic hypoxemia and pulmonary hypertension
• Polycythemia (chronic hypoxemia)
• Restrictive pericarditis and possible secondary pericardial effusion

○ **Describe the lung volume, blood gas, and hematological changes seen in scoliosis.**

Scoliosis is defined as a lateral curvature of the spine greater than 10 degrees accompanied by vertebral rotation. The degree of respiratory dysfunction is related to the type and severity of the scoliosis (measured by the Cobb method), age of onset, age of the patient, and the associated disease process.

In the early stages, thoracic cavity deformity causes decreased lung volumes, elasticity, and compliance. Increased work of breathing imposed by these changes leads to rapid shallow breathing pattern, alveolar hypoventilation, abnormal V/Q ratio, hypoxemia with increased A–a DO_2, and increased V_D/V_T.

In advanced stages of the disease, hypoxemia leads to polycythemia, hypoxic pulmonary vasoconstriction, and pulmonary hypertension. At this stage the arterial blood gases show an increase in the $PaCO_2$ levels.

In the late stages, pulmonary hypertension leads to right ventricular hypertrophy, cor pulmonale, and finally congestive heart failure and death.

○ **List causes and effects of surfactant deficiency.**

Pulmonary surfactant deficiency can result from destruction of type II pneumatocytes or from the destruction or inactivation of surfactant. Genetic deficiencies have been described. Surfactant lines the alveolus to provide a host defense barrier and reduces alveolar surface tension preventing collapse (adhesive atelectasis). Deficiency produces diffuse loss of lung volume, shunt, and the influx of interstitial fluid resulting in impaired gas exchange. ARDS, hyaline membrane disease, pneumonia, interstitial lung diseases, alveolar proteinosis, obstructive lung disease, smoke inhalation, coronary artery bypass graft surgery, uremia, and prolonged shallow breathing are conditions that frequently produce generalized surfactant deficiency. Pulmonary embolism and radiation pneumonitis have a similar effect localized to the affected segment of lung.

○ **Which patients are at risk of developing postoperative pulmonary complications (PPC) (atelectasis and pneumonia) following abdominal surgery?**

The risk factors are cigarette smoking (risk of PPC doubled), underlying chronic respiratory disease, emergency surgery, anesthetic time >180 minutes, age >70 years, and operative site, the most important determinant. The highest risk is seen with upper abdominal (nonlaparoscopic) followed by lower abdominal and intrathoracic.

○ **Does cessation of smoking reduce the perioperative pulmonary risk?**

Yes.

PPC are 2-fold more common in current smokers versus those who have never smoked.

Cessation of smoking for 12–24 hours decreases CO levels and nicotine levels. After 48–72 hours cessation, carboxyhemoglobin levels normalize and ciliary function improves. Decreased sputum production requires 1–2 weeks of cessation. Acute stopping of smoking for 1–2 days may cause a hypersecretory state and increase airway irritability.

After 4–6 weeks of cessation PFTs improve.

Smokers have delayed wound healing probably secondary to peripheral vascular effects and decreased immune function. They also show abnormal bone metabolism and this may cause delayed fracture healing. After 6–8 weeks of cessation, immune function and metabolism normalizes.

The maximal benefit of smoking cessation is seen only after 8–12 weeks, with improvement in closing volume, increase in maximum voluntary ventilation, and reduction in sputum.

There is decreased overall postoperative morbidity and mortality [Warner, 2005. See reference on page 531].

○ **What is the etiology of hypoxemia?**

Hypoxemia results from decreased delivery of O_2 from the atmosphere to the arterial blood.

Causes are:

Decreased inspired O_2 – for example, high altitude

Hypoventilation – for example, respiratory center depression and neuromuscular disease

Shunts – for example, pulmonary shunts such as atelectasis and pneumonia, and cardiac shunts such as ASD and VSD

V_A/Q mismatch – for example, bronchospasm

Diffusion defect – for example, pulmonary edema

○ **What is the etiology of hypoxia?**

Hypoxia refers to decreased delivery of O_2 to the tissues.

Causes of hypoxia:

Hypoxemic hypoxia (inadequate pulmonary function)

Anemic hypoxia (decrease in hemoglobin)

Histotoxic hypoxia (cyanide poisoning)

Circulatory hypoxia (inadequate cardiac output)

○ **What are the physiologic effects of hypoxemia/hypoxia?**

Cardiovascular effects: catecholamine and renin–angiotensin release cause excitatory and vasoconstrictive effects mediated via aortic and carotid chemoreceptor, baroreceptor, and central cerebral stimulation. Direct local hypoxemic effects are inhibitory and vasodilatory and occur late. The response depends on the degree of hypoxemia:

SaO_2 decrease up to 80%: increased heart rate, stroke volume, cardiac output, and inotropy.

SaO_2 60–80%: decrease in blood pressure and SVR with vasodilation.

SaO_2 <60%: slow pulse, low blood pressure, shock, and cardiac dysrhythmia. Also, increased cerebral blood flow due to cerebral vasodilation, increased ventilatory drive, increased pulmonary artery pressure, and increased hemoglobin in chronic hypoxemia with right-shifted oxyhemoglobin dissociation curve.

○ **What is the definition of hypoventilation?**

Reduced alveolar ventilation resulting in an increase in arterial PCO_2.

○ **If a patient becomes cyanotic, what is the likely hemoglobin saturation and PaO_2?**

The hemoglobin saturation is less than 70% and the PaO_2 is about 40 mm Hg, assuming arterial concentration of desaturated blood is 5 g/dL, at hemoglobin of 16 g/dL.

○ **What is the maximum FiO_2 that can be given through a nasal cannula?**

When using nasal cannula, the inspired O_2 concentration is determined by the O_2 flow rate, nasopharyngeal volume, and the patient's inspiratory flow rate (which depends on both TV and RR).

Oxygen from the cannula fills the nasopharynx in between breaths. During each inspiration, O_2 is entrained from the nasopharynx into the trachea. Mouth breathing does not appreciably affect the inspired concentration as long as the passage between the nasopharynx and the oropharynx is patent.

The inspired O_2 concentration increases by approximately 3–4%/L of O_2 given through nasal cannula in most adults. However, inspired O_2 concentrations greater than 40–50% cannot be reliably achieved with nasal cannula. Flow rates greater than 4–6 L/min for prolonged periods are poorly tolerated because of drying and crusting of the nasal mucosa.

○ **What is the status of PaO_2 and $PaCO_2$ when V_A/Q is 0.01?**

As V/Q ratio decreases (increased right-to-left shunting), PaO_2 decreases rapidly and progressively. $PaCO_2$ increases gradually at first and then quite rapidly.

$V_A/Q = 0.01$ indicates a large shunt. The shunt alveolus is not ventilated, so it will equilibrate with mixed venous blood, that is, $PaO_2 = 45$ mm Hg and $SaO_2 = 70\%$.

○ **What is the status of PaO_2 and $PaCO_2$ when V_A/Q is 100?**

$V_A/Q = 100$ indicates a large dead space. The alveolus does not participate in gas exchange, so it will equilibrate with inspired gases.

○ **What are the effects of increased V/Q mismatch?**

Increased dead space ventilation and increased shunt fraction. Thus, arterial hypoxemia and increased carbon dioxide levels. Also, change in the rate of uptake of anesthetic gases with the effect depending on the mismatch and solubility of the agent.

Increase in dead space ventilation primarily affects CO_2 elimination and has little influence on arterial oxygenation until dead space ventilation exceeds 80–90% of minute ventilation.

Physiologic shunt primarily affects arterial oxygenation with little effect on CO_2 elimination until the physiologic shunt function exceeds 75–80% of the cardiac output.

With no shunt, a linear increase in FiO_2 results in a linear increase in PaO_2. As the shunt is increased, PaO_2 increases with increased FiO_2 becoming progressively flatter.

○ **What are the causes of atelectasis?**

Obstruction of major airways and bronchioles (secretions or tumor), compression of the lung from fluid or air in the pleural space, infection, surfactant deficiency (adhesive atelectasis), high alveolar PO_2 (absorption atelectasis), or hypoventilation especially in areas with low V/Q.

○ **What is closing capacity? How is it measured?**

Closing volume is the volume at which the small airways (basal dependent areas) begin to close.

Closing capacity, which is closing volume + residual volume (RV), is usually well below FRC. When closing capacity is increased well above the FRC, atelectasis occurs (as with increasing age or morbid obesity), and intrapulmonary shunting leads to decline in arterial oxygen tension.

Closing volume is measured using tracer gas xenon-133.

○ **What are the components of FRC?**

Expiratory reserve volume (ERV) and RV. FRC is the lung volume remaining at the end of normal exhalation.

○ **What type of lung diseases will alter the FRC?**

Decreased compliance of the lung or chest as seen in restrictive pulmonary disease is associated with low FRC. Obstructive disease such as emphysema elevates both FRC and compliance.

○ **How can one measure the FRC?**

FRC can be measured by nitrogen washout or helium wash-in technique or by body plethysmography.

○ **How does FRC affect airway resistance?**

Airway resistance decreases with increased lung volumes. The reduction in FRC associated with changing from upright to supine position and general anesthesia would be expected to increase airway resistance.

○ **How can you increase the FRC?**

Intermittent positive pressure ventilation does not increase the FRC. In patients with decreased lung volumes (e.g., obesity), adding PEEP increases the FRC and tidal ventilation above closing capacity leading to improved arterial oxygenation.

○ **Describe the physiologic effect of continuous positive airway pressure (CPAP).**

When positive pressure is applied during both inspiration and expiration with spontaneous breathing, this is referred to as CPAP. When the patient is not intubated, a tightly fitting full face mask can be used to apply CPAP. In patients with decreased lung volumes, CPAP (similar to PEEP) increases FRC and tidal ventilation above closing capacity allowing some oxygen uptake to occur in these alveoli, and improves pulmonary compliance. Reexpansion of collapsed alveoli corrects ventilation/perfusion abnormalities, decreases intrapulmonary shunting, and improves arterial oxygenation.

○ **What is the significance of increased A–a gradient?**

The magnitude of difference indicates the degree of oxygen exchange abnormality.

In healthy individuals there is an A–a gradient of <10 mm Hg.

Abnormal A–a gradient occurs due to:

1. Diffusion limitations:
    a. The pressure head driving O_2 diffusion across the blood–gas barrier (P_AO_2) is too low, for example, high altitude.
    b. The diffusion capacity of lung for O_2 (DLco) is not sufficient for the O_2 demands of the body, for example, interstitial lung disease.
2. Pulmonary blood flow shunts (right-to-left shunts; collapsed or fluid-filled alveoli, R to L intracardiac shunts).
3. Mismatching of ventilation and blood flow in different parts of the lung. This is the most common cause of increased A–a gradient (when breathing 100% O_2, hypoxia from V/Q mismatch should get corrected).

○ **What causes decreased P_AO_2 (alvolar partial pressure of oxygen)?**

$P_AO_2 = FiO_2(PB - PH_2O) - (PaCO_2/R)$, where R is the respiratory quotient (=CO_2 production/O_2 consumption).

Decreased P_AO_2 occurs with decreased FiO_2, decreased barometric pressure (e.g., high altitude), and increased $PaCO_2$ (e.g., hypoventilation).

○ **What are the normal values for PaO_2 in newborns?**

Neonatal PaO_2 50–70 mm Hg, as a result of an (A–a) DO_2 gradient mostly due to shunting.

○ **How do you diagnose intrathoracic airway obstruction?**

Utilizing direct bronchoscopy, radiographic imaging, CT, flow–volume loops, and pulmonary function tests.

○ **What is a flow–volume loop and how do you interpret the information?**

This is most helpful in the anatomic localization of airway obstruction. Lung volume is plotted on the x-axis; expiratory (above) and inspiratory flow (below) are plotted on the y-axis as the subject inhales fully to total lung capacity (negative flow), performs an FVC maneuver (positive flow), and then inhales back to TLC. The curves are highly effort dependent. A fixed obstruction decreases inspiratory and expiratory flow creating a plateau effect; a variable extrathoracic obstruction above the sternal notch decreases flow that flattens the inspiratory loop; a variable intrathoracic obstruction decreases flow and flattens the expiratory loop.

○ **What information is provided by flow–volume loops but not spirometry?**

Flow–volume loops aid in the anatomic localization of airway obstruction and indicate if the obstructive component is variable or fixed/intrathoracic or extrathoracic.

Lung volume is plotted on the x-axis; expiratory (above) and inspiratory flow (below) are plotted on the y-axis as the subject inhales fully to total lung capacity (negative flow) and performs an FVC maneuver (positive flow) and then inhales back to TLC. The curves are highly effort dependent.

The ratio of FEF_{50}, or mid-VC ratio (forced expiratory flow at 50% of FVC), to forced inspiratory flow at 50% FVC (FIF_{50}) determines the nature of the obstruction:

$FEF_{50}/FIF_{50} < 1$: variable intrathoracic obstruction decreases flow and flattens the expiratory loop.

$FEF_{50}/FIF_{50} = 1$: fixed airway obstruction decreases inspiratory and expiratory flow creating a plateau effect.

$FEF_{50}/FIF_{50} > 1$: variable extrathoracic obstruction above the sternal notch decreases flow that flattens the inspiratory loop.

With a variable intrathoracic obstruction, forced exhalation causes the thoracic volume to decrease, which allows for the mass to only go into the airway, and forced inhalation causes the thoracic volume to increase that allows for the airways to prop open.

With a variable extrathoracic obstruction, forced exhalation causes the airway pressure to increase, which effectively pushes the extrathoracic mass out of the way, and forced inhalation causes the airway pressure to decrease that effectively sucks the extrathoracic mass into the airway.

○ **Which pharmacologic agents worsen hypoxemia?**

Agents that decrease ventilation, increase pulmonary shunt, inhibit HPV, inhibit oxygenation of hemoglobin by causing methemoglobinemia, and increase oxygen consumption. Examples: opiates, hypnotics, neuromuscular blocking agents, nitrates, nitroglycerin, sodium nitroprusside, inhaled anesthetic agents, prilocaine, antimalarials, sulfonamides, and catecholamines.

○ **How is ventilation regulated to maintain optimal levels of pH, O_2, and CO_2?**

The ventilation is regulated via the respiratory center. There is neural and chemical control of respiration.

Neural control:

Respiratory center consists of group of nuclei within the medulla and pons.

Inspiratory center is located dorsally in the medulla and controls inspiration. This is the site of basic respiratory drive and has an intrinsic automaticity.

Expiratory center is located ventrally in the medulla and controls expiration.

Pneumotaxic center is located in the pons and assists in regulation of inspiration.

Chemical control:

Central chemoreceptors are located bilaterally in the medulla. This area is very sensitive to hydrogen ions. However, hydrogen ions cross the blood brain barrier poorly and PCO_2 indirectly influences the level of hydrogen ions in CSF.

$$CO_2 + H_2O \rightarrow H_2CO_3 \rightarrow H^+ + HCO_3.$$

Peripheral chemoreceptors are located in the carotid bodies and are sensitive to O_2, CO_2, and pH.

Haldane effect: The Haldane effect states that deoxygenated Hb has a greater affinity for CO_2 than does oxyHb. Thus, O_2 release at the tissues facilitates CO_2 pickup while O_2 pickup at the lungs facilitates CO_2 release. Likewise, CO_2 pickup at the tissues facilitates O_2 release while CO_2 release at the lungs promotes O_2 pickup.

○ **Describe how carbon dioxide is carried by blood.**

Carbon dioxide is carried by blood in three forms:

1. Soluble in plasma – 20 times more soluble in blood than O_2. Still dissolved CO_2 is only 5% of total CO_2 in arterial blood.

2. Carbamino compound – CO_2 combines with terminal amine group in blood proteins, especially globin of Hb. Comprises only 5% of the total CO_2 in arterial blood.

3. Bicarbonate ion (HCO_3) – the most important form (90%). $CO_2 + H_2O \rightarrow H_2CO_3 \rightarrow H^+ + HCO_3$. (Carbonic anhydrase in RBC catalyzes the reaction.)

○ **What is the distribution of pulmonary blood flow in the upright lung?**

Pulmonary blood flow is distributed according to gravity with the lowest flow in the apical aspects of the lung and maximal flow in the basilar regions.

○ **What are the effects of gravity on respiratory physiology?**

Pulmonary blood flow is gravity dependent, leading to the definition of West Zones I, II, and III. Pulmonary ventilation is higher in the dependent alveoli in an awake spontaneously breathing person because the basal alveoli are in the steeper portion of the compliance curve of the alveoli to the increase in pleural pressure. Due to increase in pleural pressure, basal alveoli are one fourth the volume of the apical alveoli and therefore more compliant. Apical alveoli are maximally inflated and relatively noncompliant. The V/Q ratio decreases rapidly at first and then more slowly into the dependent lung regions.

○ **What distinguishes the basilar regions of the lungs?**

Highest rate of perfusion, least distended alveoli at end-expiration, majority of tidal volume generation, lowest V/Q ratio, regional hypoxemia, and hypercarbia.

○ **What is the difference in work of breathing for infants versus adults?**

The work of breathing is increased for infants due to reduced lung compliance and increased airway resistance. Therefore, in pediatric patients the work of breathing can account for up to 40% of the cardiac output, particularly in stressed conditions.

The components of work of breathing include elastic work (lung elastic recoil, chest wall compliance), frictional work (airflow resistance), and inertial work (tissue frictional resistance which is negligible in healthy subjects).

In a healthy adult, the metabolic cost of the work of breathing at rest constitutes only 1–3% of the total O_2 consumption, but may increase considerably (up to 50%) in patients with pulmonary disease.

Key Terms

ABG: COPD
Air trapping: ventilator mgmt
Alveolar–arterial O_2 gradient (A–a O_2): factors affecting
Alveolar gas equation
Anatomic dead space
Anesthetic implications of COPD
Ascites: PFTs
Asthma, intraoperative bronchospasm: treatment
Atelectasis: anesthesia induced

Bronchodilation: anesthetic drugs
Bronchospasm: acute treatment
Bronchospasm: mechanical ventilation diagnosis
Bronchospasm triggers: ETT
Carbon dioxide: transport/bicarbonate
Carbon monoxide (CO) diffusion capacity: abnormal differential diagnosis
Carbon monoxide (CO) diffusion capacity – COPD
Cardiovascular response to hypoxemia

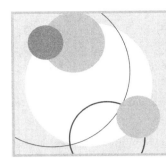

Statistics

The energy of the mind is the essence of life.
Aristotle

○ **What is meant by descriptive statistics? How does it differ from inferential statistics?**

There are two distinct steps in the process of analyzing study data. The first step is to describe the study sample or data using standard methods to determine the average value, the range of data around the average, and other characteristics. For example, in a study comparing the incidence of postdural puncture headache after two different types of spinal needles, if one reports that 55% of patients are under 40 years and the average BMI is 32, one is describing the study sample and thus is engaging in descriptive statistics.

The second step in most studies is to derive a conclusion from facts or premises. Inferential statistics are used to draw conclusions about a population based on a random sample selected from that population.

○ **What are variables?**

Variables are anything that is measurable or manipulated in a study.

○ **Variables have different levels of measurements. What are they?**

Variables are typically measured at one of four different levels of measurements. Ordered from low to high, the levels of measurement are nominal (e.g., sex, eye color), ordinal (e.g., upper middle, lower social class), interval (e.g., shoe size, temperature in Fahrenheit), and ratio (e.g., height, weight, distance).

○ **Explain the four different variables.**

1. Nominal variables: These are data that cannot be ordered or ranked. Dichotomous data allow only two possible variables (e.g., male vs. females).

2. Ordinal variables: These data can be ordered or measured without a constant scale interval, for example, social class – upper, middle, and lower or pain rating.

3. Interval variables: For example, shoe size and temperature in Fahrenheit. Interval variables may be discrete or continuous.

   Discrete interval data can only have integer values such as number of children per family, parity, and number of teeth.

   Continuous interval data can be decimal fractions, for example, temperature, heights, and blood pressure.

4. Ratio variables: For example, height, weight, and distance.

○ **Can you use mode, median, and mean with variables at all levels of measurement?**

No, only mode may be used with variables at all levels.

The median may only be used when the level of measurement is ordinal or interval/ratio (because one has to order values from low to high and nominal values cannot be ordered).

The mean requires interval/ratio measurements. These values may be classified, ordered, and measured.

○ **Describe parametric and nonparametric tests. When do you use parametric versus nonparametric tests?**

Interval and ratio variables assume that the data follow a bell curve and therefore use so-called parametric statistics, such as Student *t* tests, ANOVA, and ANCOVA. Student *t* test is used in two-sample test and ANOVA used in multiple-sample test (multiple comparisons).

First two types of variables (nominal and ordinal) consist of counts of people or things in different categories. For example, you cannot put a bell curve through a histogram displaying percentage of students who are males versus females. Therefore, these two variables use different classes of statistics – called nonparametric statistics, which do not make assumptions about the way in which data are distributed in the population. Examples of nonparametric statistics are chi-square, Fisher exact test, Mann–Whitney *U* test, and Wilcoxon rank-sum test.

Chi-square test is used in two- or multiple-sample test.

○ **When do you use Fisher exact test?**

If any of the expected values is less than 5, the chi-square test is not valid. In this case Fisher exact test should be used instead.

○ **Consider the values 5, 8, 5, 10, 9, 11, and 43. These numbers represent the accumulated central line insertion experience of each of the seven members of the CA-1 class. Regarding these values, what are the mode, median, and mean?**

Mode, median, and mean are measures of central tendency in descriptive statistical procedures.

The mode is the most commonly occurring value. In this example, the mode is 5 because it occurs twice, more than any other value.

The median is the value with the same number of values higher than and lower than it.

To determine the median, order the values from low to high: 5, 5, 8, 9, 10, 11, 43. The median is 9 as there are three lower values and an equal number (three) of higher values.

The mean is the sum of all cases divided by the number of cases. The mean is 13: (5 + 8 + 5 + 10 + 9 + 11 + 43)/7 = 13.

○ **Describe symmetrical and skewed distribution.**

Symmetrical distribution – mean, median, and mode all occur at the same point on the curve.

Skewed distribution – the curve has one tail longer than the other.

○ **Once again let's consider the values 5, 8, 5, 10, 9, 11, and 43. What is the range?**

Range is equal to the highest score minus the lowest score = 43 − 5 = 38.

Range is a measure of variability used for interval/ratio variables.

○ **What is variability?**

Variability refers to the degree to which values are dispersed or "spread out" around some central value (mean, median).

○ **List three measures of variability for interval/ratio-level variables.**

Range, standard deviation (SD), and the variance.

○ **What is the definition of SD?**

SD is the square root of the variance. Variance can be of the population, or of the sample.

The sample variance is the sum of squares of each individual value minus the sample mean divided by the number of samples minus 1, or mathematically, $s^2 = \Sigma(X_i - X)^2/(n - 1)$.

○ **What is the difference between the SD and the standard error (SE)?**

SE or SE of the mean is the SD divided by square root of the sample size. The SD is always larger.

They quantify different things.

SD is descriptive statistics and describes the dispersion of the observation.

SE is an inferential statistics, which describes the precision with which a sample mean estimates the true population mean.

○ **What is confidence interval?**

Confidence interval indicates that there is roughly 95% chance that the true mean of the population from which the sample was drawn lies within 2 SEM of the sample mean.

○ **List some basic rules and steps in the procedure of statistical inference.**

1. (a) The starting point is almost always to assume that there is no difference between groups (null hypothesis – Ho). (b) They are all samples drawn at random from the same statistical population.
2. The next step is to determine the likelihood that the observed differences could be caused by chance variation alone.
3. If this probability is sufficiently small (<1 in 20 or <0.05), one "rejects" the null hypothesis (accepts "alternative hypothesis – H1) and concludes that there is some true difference between the groups.

○ **What is a Type I error?**

Type I error (alpha) is the probability of incorrectly rejecting the null hypothesis when the null is true. Most statistical analyses use an alpha level of 0.05 (5% significance level). This is the risk (out of 100 null hypotheses that we reject, 5 will be incorrectly rejected) you are willing to take in making a Type I error. If the *P*-value is less than the risk you are willing to take ($P < .05$), then you reject the null and state with a 95% level of confidence that the two parameters are not the same.

○ **What is a Type II error?**

Type II error (beta) is the probability of failing to reject the null when the null is not true; it's the probability of saying there is no significant effect when there really is one. If you reject the null, you cannot make a Type II error.

○ **What is "power?"**

Power is the probability of rejecting the null hypothesis given that the null is incorrect (correctly rejecting the null). Some people also refer to power as precision or sensitivity. *Power is equal to 1 – beta.* To calculate the power you need the population means under both the null and the alternative, the SE, and alpha. Power is generally recommended at levels of at least 0.8 (therefore, Type II is 0.2).

○ **What factors increase the statistical power of a study?**

A larger alpha, directional hypotheses, one-tailed test, larger sample size, little measurement error, and a larger effect size.

○ **What is the relationship between Type I, Type II, and Power?**

	Truth of Null	
Decision	True	Not true
Reject null	Type I	Power
FTR null	Correct	Type II

○ **What is a biased sample?**

A sample is biased if its characteristics differ systematically from those of the population about which one seeks to make inferences.

○ **When would you be concerned about the possibility of bias?**

Whenever nonrandom sampling methods have been used.

○ **Define sensitivity and specificity.**

Sensitivity is the percentage of patients with disease in whom test is positive (percent positive in disease) or the ability of the test to identify correctly those who truly have the disease.

Specificity is the percentage of persons without disease in whom test is negative (percent negative in health) or the ability of the test to identify correctly persons who do not have the disease.

○ **What is positive predictive value?**

This is the percentage of patients with positive results, who actually do have the disease.

○ **What is negative predictive value?**

This is the percentage of patients with negative test results, who really do not have the disease.

○ **What is an odds ratio?**

The odds ratio is a way of comparing whether the probability of a certain event is the same for two groups.

Suppose that in a sample of 100 men, 90 have drunk wine in the previous week, while in a sample of 100 women only 20 have drunk wine in the same period. The odds of a man drinking wine are 90 to 10, or 9:1, while the odds of a woman drinking wine are only 20 to 80, or 1:4 = 0.25:1. The odds ratio is thus 9/0.25, or 36, showing that men are much more likely to drink wine than women.

○ **Describe relative risk.**

The relative risk is the ratio of the probabilities of two events; if p is the probability of the first event and q is the probability of the second, then the relative risk is p/q.

○ **Define *sensitivity* of a test.**

This is the percentage of patients with a disease who have a positive test (positivity in disease).

Sensitivity = (true positives)/(true positives and false negatives); see table below.

○ **Define *specificity*.**

This is the percentage of healthy patients with a normal test (negativity in health).

Specificity = (true negatives)/(true negatives + false positives); see table below.

○ **Define the *predictive value* of a positive test.**

The predictive value of a positive test is the percentage of positive results that are true positives.

Predictive value = (true positives)/(true positives + false positives); see table below.

	Disease +	Disease −
Test +	a (TP)	b (FP)
Test −	c (FN)	d (TN)

In the above table, TP is the true positive, FP is the false positive, FN is the false negative, and TN is the true negative.

Sensitivity = $a/(a + c)$.

Specificity = $d/(b + d)$.

Positive predictive value = $a/(a + b)$.

Key Terms

ANOVA indications
Categorical data: chi-square
Chi-square test – application
Clinical trial: study power
Descriptive statistics
Experimental design
Experimental statistical analysis
Factors affecting statistical power
Odds ratio calculation
Paired versus unpaired *t* test
Parametric statistical tests
Power analysis for sample size
Power analysis: study design

Standard error (SE) versus standard deviation (SD)
Statistical differences: interpretation
Statistical power analysis: use
Statistical test: choice
Statistics: analysis of variance
Statistics: chi-square/appropriate data
Statistics: confidence level
Statistics: Fisher exact test
Statistics: median
Student *t* test: application
Study design: blinding
Type I statistics error/definition
Variability of sample

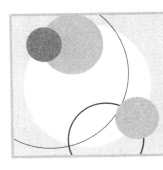

Thoracic Surgery

A wise man is he who knows how much is enough.
Chinese Proverb

○ **What preoperative pulmonary function tests (PFTs) are needed in patients for thoracic surgery?**

Arterial blood gas, spirometry, and chest x-ray. A bronchoscopy, flow–volume loops, and computed tomography (CT) of the chest may be indicated. Occasionally, split lung function studies are appropriate if the first-line tests suggest resection may leave a patient ventilator-dependent. However, since split function test do not seem to have sufficient predictive value, it has been replaced by objective measures of pulmonary function tests [Datta and Lahiri, 2003. See reference on page 531].

○ **Are there any contraindications to lung resection?**

A predicted residual FEV_1 of less than 800 mL in a 70-kg patient.

○ **What additional information is useful when interpreting an FEV_1/FVC ratio of 60%?**

Response to bronchodilators and apparent effort.

○ **How can you predict the postoperative FEV_1?**

The ratio of the number of lung segments resected to the total number can be used to calculate the expected decline in FEV_1 following lung resection. This may overestimate the decline. A radioisotope perfusion scan will delineate the contribution of the diseased lung to overall ventilation/perfusion.

○ **How do you assess the operative risk of pneumonectomy?**

   a. Start with a detailed history of the patient's quality of life.

   b. All patients should have baseline simple spirometry.

   c. Objective measures of pulmonary function: think in three related areas (the "three-legged" stool of prethoracotomy respiratory assessment):

      1. Respiratory mechanics

      2. Gas exchange

      3. Cardiorespiratory interaction

○ **What is included in respiratory mechanics?**

These include FEV_1, FVC, MVV, and RV/TLC ratio. The tests should be expressed as a percent of predicted volume corrected for age, sex, and height. Of these, the most important test is the predicted postoperative FEV_1 ($ppoFEV_1\%$):

$$ppoFEV_1\% = \text{preoperative } FEV_1\% \times \left(\frac{1 - \text{functional lung tissue removed [\%]}}{100}\right).$$

The percentage of functional lung tissue removed is estimated by calculating the number of functioning subsegments of the lung removed.

○ **How is the gas exchange capacity measured?**

The most useful test of gas exchange capacity is DL_{CO}.

Postresection DL_{CO} is calculated using the same calculation as for FEV_1.

$ppoDL_{CO}$ <40% predicted correlates with increased respiratory and cardiac complications.

It has been shown that preoperative FEV_1 or DL_{CO} <20% has high perioperative mortality rate.

○ **How is cardiorespiratory interaction measured?**

Maximal oxygen consumption (VO_2 max) is the most useful predictor of postthoracotomy outcome.

Preoperative VO_2 max <15 mL/kg/min means high risk of morbidity and mortality.

Stair climbing is the test used to calculate VO_2 max. The ability to climb five flights correlates with a VO_2 max >20 mL/kg/min and climbing two flights correlates to a VO_2 max 12 mL/kg/min (high-risk patient).

Patients with a decrease of SpO_2 >4% during stair climbing also have increased risk of morbidity and mortality.

Postresection exercise capacity can be estimated using the same calculation as for FEV_1 based on the amount of lung tissue removed. If this estimate ($ppoVO_2$ max) is <10 mL/kg/min, this may be an absolute contraindication to pulmonary resection.

Postresection pulmonary function prediction can be further refined using ventilation–perfusion (V/Q) lung scanning. If the area to be resected is nonfunctional, prediction can be modified.

○ **What is the predictive value of split function studies?**

Split function studies do not seem to have sufficient predictive value and therefore have been replaced by the above objective measures in most centers [Miller, 2010].

○ **Which PFTs have been related to increased perioperative pulmonary complications following abdominal or thoracic surgery?**

	Abdominal	Thoracic
FVC	<70% predicted	<70% predicted or <1.7 L
FEV_1	<70% predicted	<2 L (pneumonectomy) <1 L (lobectomy) <0.8 L (segmentectomy)
FEV_1/FVC	<65%	<35%
MVV	<50% predicted	<50% predicted or 28 L/min
RV		<50% predicted
DL_{CO}		<50%
VO_2		<15 mL/kg/min

○ **A patient with COPD is to have a right lung resection for carcinoma. How do you interpret preoperative PFTs?**

PFTs suggestive of increased operative risk for pneumonectomy and prolonged postoperative ventilatory support include FVC <50% predicted, FEV_1 <2 L, FEV_1/FVC <50%, maximum breathing capacity (MBC, or maximum minute ventilation) <50% predicted, RV/TLC >50%, diffusing capacity <50% predicted, hypercapnia on room air, ppoFEV_1 <0.85 L, and >70% blood flow to the diseased lung.

○ **Which methods are used for lung separation?**

Endobronchial intubation with a double-lumen tube

Endobronchial blocker deployed through a single-lumen tube to occlude one of the mainstem bronchi

○ **What are the absolute indications for double-lumen tubes or one-lung ventilation?**

Patient-related:

1. Protection of a healthy lung from a contaminated lung due to infection or massive hemoptysis
2. Separate ventilation of each lung (bronchopleural fistula, tracheobronchial disruption, cyst, or bulla)
3. Severe hypoxemia due to unilateral lung disease

Procedure-related:

1. Surgical opening of major airways, disruption of bronchial system, or unilateral cyst or bullae
2. Repair of thoracic aortic aneurysm
3. Esophageal surgery
4. Bronchoalveolar lavage of one lung
5. Anterior approach to the thoracic spine

○ **What are the relative indications for double-lumen tubes or one-lung ventilation?**

Surgical exposure requiring the collapse of one lung:

Thoracoscopy

Pleural surgery

Lobectomy

Pneumonectomy

Bullectomy

Lung volume reduction

Surgeries on the descending thoracic aorta

Pulmonary endarterectomy

○ **Which methods are available in children?**

Endobronchial intubation with a single-lumen tube

Endobronchial blocker

There is no double-lumen tube small enough for a child less than about 10 years of age.

○ **How can one-lung ventilation be accomplished in a patient with a tracheostomy or stoma?**

A shorter double-lumen tube (Sheridan), an endobronchial blocker, or endobronchial intubation may be used. Unless a laryngectomy has been performed, it may be possible to intubate with the usual equipment via the larynx.

○ **For one-lung ventilation is a right- or left-sided tube more commonly used, and why?**

A left-sided tube is more common. The distance between the right upper lobe bronchus and the right mainstem bronchus is 2.1 cm in females and 2.3 cm in males. The distance between the left upper lobe bronchus and the left mainstem bronchus is 5 cm in females and 5.3 cm in males. Therefore, it is less likely one will inadvertently obstruct the left upper lobe with the bronchial cuff of a left-sided tube than the possibility that one will inadvertently obstruct the right upper lobe with the bronchial cuff of a right-sided tube.

○ **What are the advantages of double-lumen tubes?**

Ability to ventilate or collapse either lung sequentially

Access to both lungs for endotracheal suction or application of continuous positive airway pressure (CPAP)

○ **What are the disadvantages of double-lumen tubes?**

Misplacement

Laryngeal trauma

Bronchial trauma from low-volume, high-pressure cuff

Tracheal cuff easily torn on teeth

Difficult to insert if the larynx is not easily visualized

Need to change to single lumen if postoperative ventilation is required

○ **What are the advantages of endobronchial blockers?**

Can be used in patients too small for double-lumen tubes, such as children

Can be used in an emergency in a patient with an existing ETT

Can be used for selective blockade of a specific lobe

Safer for patients with a difficult airway

No need to change to a different ETT if using postoperative mechanical ventilation

○ **What are the disadvantages of endobronchial blockers?**

Require fiber-optic bronchoscopy for positioning

Not able to suction the bronchus containing the blocker without deflating the balloon

More likely to become dislodged during patient positioning and surgical manipulation

○ **What is the major complication of a double-lumen tube for independent lung ventilation?**

Malpositioning. The tube may be too deep or not deep enough, or have entered the wrong side resulting in loss of lung separation and potentially hypoxemia.

○ **What percentage of double-lumen tubes are placed incorrectly and not detected by auscultation?**

About 30% [Campos et al., 2006. See reference on page 531]: less common for nondisposable tubes (Robertshaw) and more common for disposable tubes (Mallinckrodt). This is why confirmation of placement with a fiber-optic bronchoscope, especially after turning to the lateral position, is mandatory.

○ **How do you check the placement of a double-lumen tube?**

Advance the double-lumen tube through the larynx under direct visualization (tip anterior and then rotated counterclockwise after passing through the cords) with blind advancement until the resistance of the carina is felt, and then pull back slightly and inflate the tracheal cuff. Confirm tracheal placement with auscultation of bilateral breath sounds and the presence of CO_2 on capnography.

Placement of the double-lumen tube should be confirmed after the patient is turned to the lateral position. Inflate the (left) bronchial cuff, clamp the tracheal lumen, and check for unilateral left-sided breath sounds. The tube should be advanced if you still hear air entry on the right side. Right-sided air entry without left-sided air entry indicates that the tube is in the right bronchus. Unclamp the tracheal lumen, clamp the bronchial lumen, and check for unilateral right-sided breath sounds. A diminution of breath sounds may be heard if the bronchial cuff is partially occluding the distal trachea; the tube needs to be advanced.

The best test for proper placement is fiber-optic visualization. With the fiber-optic bronchoscope in the tracheal lumen, one should see the opening of tracheal lumen above the carina, the bronchial lumen in the left mainstem bronchus, and, slightly, the edge of the blue bronchial balloon.

Ultimately, proper placement should be verified by looking at the surgical field and observing the appropriate one-lung ventilation.

○ **What size fiber-optic bronchoscope should be used when placing a standard single-lumen endotracheal tube?**

The standard adult fiber-optic bronchoscope will pass through an ETT 7.0 mm or greater, but because of decreased cross-sectional area available for ventilation, a pediatric fiber-optic bronchoscope should be used for ETT <8.0 mm.

○ **What uses can be made of the suction port on a fiber-optic bronchoscope?**

Oxygen insufflation and limited suctioning, depending on the size.

Oxygen insufflation can be effective at clearing secretions.

○ **How can jet ventilation be accomplished through a fiber-optic bronchoscope?**

The Luer lock connection of a handheld jet ventilation device attaches to the biopsy port of a fiber-optic bronchoscope. The tip of the fiber-optic bronchoscope must be in the trachea and the glottis must be open to avoid barotrauma. Driving pressure, inspiratory time, and ventilatory rate are dictated by the operator. A driving pressure of 50 psi results in a tracheal pressure of 6–8 mm Hg, FiO_2 of 88–93%, and PaO_2 of 340–478 mm Hg.

○ **What are the positioning complications of a left-sided double-lumen tube?**

A left-sided DLT placed into the right mainstem bronchus can result in obstruction of the right upper lobe and unexpected ventilation of the contralateral lung. If the tube is not advanced far enough into the left mainstem bronchus, the cuff may still be in the trachea, resulting in normal ventilation when deflated, but resulting in partial to complete tracheal obstruction when inflated. A right-sided tube commonly obstructs the right upper lobe. It is less likely for a left-sided tube to obstruct the left upper lobe unless advanced way too far, at which point there will also be impingement of the tracheal lumen on the carina, resulting not only in collapse of the left upper lobe but also in failure to ventilate the right lung.

○   **What serious complications could occur with malpositioning?**

Complete obstruction of the trachea with the inability to ventilate.

Inadvertent ventilation of the lung intended for isolation, resulting in barotrauma and cardiac arrest if pneumothorax or bullae are present.

Blood and purulent secretions may be disseminated to the contralateral, healthy lung.

○   **What complications can occur with one-lung ventilation despite correct tube placement?**

Hypoxemia, hypercapnia, increasing airway pressure, air trapping, pneumothorax, arrhythmias, and hypotension.

○   **Are the decreases in PaO_2 the same when comparing right and left one-lung ventilation?**

Theoretically, collapse of the right lung involves more lung segments than the left, resulting in a greater decrease in Pao_2. In practice, the collapsed lung may well be diseased and have minimal contribution to ventilation and oxygenation. Patients with normal lungs requiring one-lung ventilation often develop more hypoxia.

○   **What effect does the lateral decubitus position have during two-lung ventilation?**

Increased V/Q mismatch.

There is relatively good ventilation but poor perfusion to the nondependent lung and relatively poor ventilation but good perfusion to the dependent lung. West's zones of the lung are with respect to gravity, so zone 1 is in the lateral portion of the nondependent lung and zone 4 is in the lateral portion of the dependent lung (rotated 90° when compared with a standing patient). The fractional blood flow is 40% to the nondependent lung and 60% to the dependent lung. The shunt fraction is normal.

○   **Is there a difference between right and left lateral decubitus positioning?**

Yes. If the left lung is nondependent (right lateral decubitus position), it gets 35% of the blood flow.

If the right lung is nondependent (left lateral decubitus position), it gets 45% of the blood flow.

○   **What effect does lateral decubitus positioning have on one-lung ventilation?**

Shunt. The nonventilated lung still receives blood flow, although gravity causes this to be less pronounced. Fractional blood flow is 22.5% to the nondependent lung and 77.5% to the dependent lung. The resulting shunt fraction is 27.5%. This causes a significant decrease in PaO_2, which may continue to decrease for 45 minutes.

○   **What other factors will affect blood flow to the nondependent lung?**

Gravity (vertical gradient), surgical interference (lung stroking or compression), preexisting lung disease (of either the nondependent or dependent lung), pneumothorax (dependent lung), vascular clamping of the opposite pulmonary artery, or positive airway pressure.

○   **What is hypoxic pulmonary vasoconstriction (HPV)?**

HPV is an important local physiologic response of the lung to areas of alveolar hypoxia (and to a much lesser extent mixed venous desaturation) resulting in pulmonary vasoconstriction. The mechanism involves an effect of hypoxia on the pulmonary vasculature either directly or mediated by the release of leukotrienes. Local vasoconstriction causes a local increase in pulmonary vascular resistance, which diverts blood to more oxygenated alveoli, thereby reducing V/Q mismatch and preventing hypoxemia.

○ **What conditions activate HPV?**

Alveolar PO_2 less than 100 mm Hg and maximal response at PO_2 30 mm Hg. Elevations in arterial hydrogen ion concentration or alveolar PCO_2 may augment pulmonary vasoconstriction.

○ **What conditions inhibit HPV?**

Inhaled anesthetic agents (only high concentration of newer agents) including nitrous oxide, direct vasodilating drugs (NTG, SNP, isoproterenol), and hypocapnia directly decrease HPV. Conditions that increase pulmonary arterial pressure will decrease HPV: mitral stenosis, volume overload, a progressive increase in the amount of diseased lung, thromboembolism, hypothermia, and vasoactive drugs. Selective application of positive end-expiratory pressure (PEEP) to nondiseased lung can divert flow back to diseased lung.

○ **Does HPV work with one-lung ventilation?**

Yes. HPV in the nonventilated lung shifts blood flow to the ventilated lung. HPV is typically preserved when using less than 1 MAC of volatile agents.

○ **What physiologic effect does HPV have on one-lung ventilation?**

Improvement in oxygenation due to a decrease in V/Q mismatch.

○ **What other factors will affect blood flow to either lung?**

Surgical stimulation, vascular clamping, the application of PEEP, preexisting lung disease, and gravity.

○ **How much shunt is created when one-lung ventilation is instituted in a healthy lung? What will be the PaO_2 on 100% oxygen?**

If HPV is intact, the shunt is usually 25–30%.
PaO_2 150–210 mm Hg.

○ **What is the normal shunt fraction?**

Five to 10%.

○ **What factors contribute to a decrease in arterial oxygenation during one-lung ventilation when the patient is in the lateral decubitus position (improper positioning of the double-lumen tube, hemodynamic instability excluded)?**

The major cause of hypoxemia is the pulmonary arteriovenous shunting of deoxygenated blood through the nonventilated lung. An increased V/Q mismatch in the ventilated dependent lung accounts for one third of the 35–40% shunt that occurs during one-lung anesthesia. HPV in the nonventilated lung is the most important variable determining PaO_2. Other contributory factors: gravity, application of PEEP, use of very small tidal volumes, atelectasis, secretions, and increased interstitial fluid in the dependent lung.

○ **Once the treatable causes of hypoxemia are ruled out, what are your options during one-lung ventilation?**

After reinflating the alveoli in the nonventilated lung, add oxygen insufflation or CPAP (5 cm H_2O) to the nonventilated lung. Increase CPAP until further lung expansion would compromise surgical exposure. Then, apply PEEP (5 cm H_2O) to the ventilated lung. Incrementally increase the CPAP and PEEP in alternate lungs until the optimal balance is achieved, permitting maximum PaO_2. Intermittent inflation of the collapsed lung, high-frequency jet ventilation to the collapsed lung, and differential lung ventilation are other options. Finally, returning to two-lung ventilation, even temporarily, may be necessary. For pneumonectomy, the surgeon can clamp the pulmonary artery to the nondependent lung, eliminating shunt from this source.

Treatable causes include inadequate FiO_2, tidal volume, and respiratory rate; improper positioning of the ETT; and obstruction (secretions, kinking).

○ **How does CPAP work during one-lung ventilation?**

During one-lung ventilation, it works best if a tidal volume is delivered to the collapsed lung before initiating CPAP. If CPAP is applied to a collapsed lung, it could take 45 minutes to have its full effect. The amount of CPAP applied must be balanced with encroachment of the lung into the surgical field. CPAP is unacceptable for video-assisted thoracoscopic surgery as it obstructs the surgical field.

○ **How does PEEP work?**

PEEP is applied during mechanical ventilation to maintain the end-expiratory airway pressure above ambient pressure. If FRC is inadequate, PEEP improves PaO_2 by increasing lung volumes, resulting in an increase in FRC, which lowers pulmonary vascular resistance, improves V/Q mismatch, and limits atelectasis. If FRC is adequate and PaO_2 >80 mm Hg, PEEP may have a negative effect due to redistribution of blood flow from the ventilated lung to the nonventilated lung and due to a reduction of cardiac output.

○ **What are the causes of increasing peak airway pressures during one-lung ventilation?**

Problems can be related to the anesthetic machine, the double-lumen endotracheal tube, or the patient.

Switching to manual ventilation will exclude ventilator dysfunction.

Endotracheal tube factors:

Occlusion (kink, secretions, debris, cuff herniation)

Malposition (too far with the tracheal lumen against the carina, not far enough with both lumens in the trachea and the bronchial cuff occluding the trachea)

Loss of lung isolation with soiling into the dependent lung

Patient factors (affecting the dependent hemithorax or lung):

Tension pneumothorax

Bronchospasm

Overinflation of the lung

Pulmonary edema

ARDS

Positioning (i.e., Trendelenburg)

Chest wall issues (closed chest, chest wall rigidity due to opioids, surgeon leaning on the chest wall, and light anesthesia/paralysis)

○ **What amount of FiO₂ is recommended with one-lung ventilation?**

One hundred percent for the highest safety margin, but this should be limited to the shortest period possible and weaned as tolerated. Accept an SaO₂ of 90% or lower in patients who have received chemotherapeutic agents (especially bleomycin). The presence of nitrogen in inspired air splints open alveoli and decreases atelectasis [Grocott, 2008. See reference on page 531].

○ **What complications can be associated with a high inspired oxygen concentration?**

Absorption atelectasis

Oxygen toxicity, especially in patients with a history of bleomycin therapy (ARDS and pulmonary fibrosis)

○ **What percentage of inspired oxygen cause pulmonary toxicity?**

Alveolar rather than arterial oxygen tension is more important and 100% O₂ for up to 10–20 hours is generally considered safe.

However, exposure to high oxygen tension clearly causes pulmonary damage.

Dose–time curves indicate:

One hundred percent O₂ should not be administered for >12 hours.

Eighty percent O₂ not for >24 hours.

Sixty percent O₂ not for >36 hours.

No measurable changes in pulmonary function or blood-gas exchange occur in humans during <50% O₂, even for longer periods.

○ **Which tidal volumes should be used for one-lung ventilation?**

Relatively large tidal volumes (10 mL/kg and greater) have been used to improve oxygenation during one lung ventilation (OLV). However, the use of larger tidal volumes during OLV has been shown to be associated with lung injury. Kozian et al., showed that combination of alveolar recruitment maneuvers (ARM) and low tidal volumes achieved improved oxygenation with improved tissue stretching during OLV. By applying ARM, the atelectatic areas of the lungs are expanded. Therefore, the subsequent tidal volumes and ventilatory stresses are more uniformly distributed. However, the experiments were done in healthy pigs, not in humans with various lung diseases [Kozian et al., 2011. See reference on 531].

○ **What is the ideal respiratory rate?**

As low as is required to avoid air trapping.

Permissive hypercapnia is well tolerated during general anesthesia in most patients. The major risk is for those patients with right ventricular dysfunction who will not tolerate the pulmonary hypertension associated with high PaCO₂ and acidosis.

○ **Can the choice of anesthetic technique influence postoperative lung function?**

Patients undergoing upper abdominal and thoracic procedures under general anesthesia exhibit a reduction in lung volumes (VC and FRC) that may take 7–14 days to normalize. The ideal plan comprises complete reversal of neuromuscular blockade, minimal residual sedation, minimal narcosis, effective thoracic epidural analgesia, and incentive spirometry. It is crucial to be able to cough effectively and clear secretions [Xu et al., 2010. See reference on page 531].

○ **What must you take into consideration when using inhalation agents on these patients?**

Inhaled anesthetic agents are dose-dependent vasodilators that affect HPV above 0.5MAC, thereby increasing blood flow to the nonventilated lung.

○ **Is nitrous oxide an appropriate anesthetic agent for thoracic surgery?**

No. An FiO_2 of 100% is ideal, which nitrous oxide would limit. With nitrous oxide, there is the chance of air expansion in air-filled spaces (bulla, air trapping, pneumothorax). Nitrous oxide increases pulmonary vascular resistance and depresses HPV (reported in a dog model at MAC equivalent >0.5).

○ **What about opioids and intravenous anesthetics?**

They have no effect on HPV, and oxygenation is well preserved. Many thoracic patients rely on hypoxic pulmonary drive. However, with long-acting opioids there is a propensity to respiratory depression. Avoid drugs that cause histamine release.

○ **Which drugs are known to cause histamine release?**

Morphine, meperidine, atracurium, D-tubocurarine, mivacurium, and doxacurium.

○ **What should the peak inspiratory pressure be after lobectomy, pneumonectomy, or lung transplant? Why?**

Ideally, the peak inspiratory pressure should not exceed 30 mm Hg, so as to prevent possible damage to the bronchial stump or new suture line. For such patients, volume-targeted pressure-controlled ventilatory modes are typically used to limit the potential for barotrauma. Permissive hypercapnia is tolerated if required.

○ **How do you test for integrity of the suture line on the bronchial stump?**

Before closing the chest, the surgeon will submerse the bronchial stump in saline and then check for air bubbles as you apply a "PEEP maneuver" of 35–40 mm Hg to the surgical lung.

○ **What factors contribute to arrhythmias and hypotension?**

The most important causes are hypoxemia, hypercapnia, and myocardial ischemia. Another cause is pericardial manipulation, especially with a left thoracotomy and pulling of the great vessels. Always check tube position and evaluate for air trapping and pneumothorax.

○ **Are there any special considerations when extubating patients with a double-lumen tube or an endobronchial blocker?**

Stimulation of the carina may cause laryngospasm or bronchospasm. Accidental suturing of the endobronchial tube or endobronchial blocker to the bronchial wall may cause hemorrhage or bronchopleural fistulae.

○ **What if the patient needs postoperative ventilation?**

If the patient has a DLT, it is best to change it to a single-lumen ETT. If the patient has been given a large amount of fluid and the airway is edematous, or the patient was a difficult intubation and there is a potential for losing the airway, the DLT should be changed over a tube exchange catheter (Sheridan or Cook). The risks of leaving the DLT in place include tracheal or bronchial trauma, increased airway resistance, and difficulty clearing secretions.

○ **Are there any indications for leaving a double-lumen tube in place?**

If the patient requires postoperative ventilation, the double-lumen ETT is usually removed and replaced with a conventional single-lumen ETT.

Indications for leaving the DLT in place are history of difficult intubation, intolerance of hypoxemia, requirement for uninterrupted PEEP, need for continued differential ventilation of the lungs, presence of a residual bronchopleural fistula, and concern for cross-contamination of the lungs.

○ **What is the anesthesiologist's concern with an anterior mediastinal mass?**

The potential for the mass to compress vital structures on induction of anesthesia.

Potentially catastrophic situations include airway obstruction, compression of the superior vena cava (SVC) syndrome, and compression of the pulmonary vessels or heart.

○ **How can the airway be assessed preoperatively in a patient with a mediastinal mass?**

Ask the patient if he or she is able to breathe without difficulty when supine (or if there is difficulty with any particular position), review the chest x-ray and CT scan of the chest (tracheal deviation, compression, or obstruction distal to the carina), and evaluate the flow–volume loops in the upright and supine positions (airway obstruction). In adults, lack of symptoms, including cough or hemoptysis, usually indicates that an airway obstruction will not occur. In children, however, lack of symptoms is *not* an indication that the airway will not obstruct. This is because a child's cartilaginous rib cage is more compliant than an adult's bony rib cage, and thus it is not as able to support the thorax.

○ **How can cardiac involvement of a mediastinal mass be assessed preoperatively?**

CT evaluation of the mass and its involvement of surrounding structures, echocardiogram upright and supine (cardiac function, direct myocardial invasion, pericardial fluid), EKG, and arterial pressure tracing during a Valsalva maneuver.

○ **What should you do before induction of a patient with a mediastinal mass?**

Place an arterial catheter and have the patient perform a Valsalva maneuver. If the patient has hypotension, the mediastinal mass may be impeding venous return.

○ **What are your anesthetic options in a patient with a symptomatic anterior mediastinal mass found on preoperative evaluation?**

Local anesthesia for cervical or scalene node biopsy, preoperative radiation or chemotherapy for mass reduction, and prophylactic cannulation of the femoral vessels with cardiopulmonary bypass on standby.

A rigid bronchoscope should be immediately available so that the mass can be lifted off the airway. Multiple individuals should be immediately available so that the patient can be repositioned (often to the prone position) to move the mass off critical structures.

○ **What options are available for general anesthesia?**

Awake fiber-optic intubation with an armored ETT passed distal to the potential obstruction, 100% oxygen, volume loading, IV access in lower extremities, determining the ability to ventilate before paralysis, standby rigid bronchoscope, and standby cardiopulmonary bypass. If it is not possible to perform an awake fiber-optic intubation with placement of the ETT distal to the obstruction, then strongly consider an inhalation or slow ketamine induction with spontaneous respiration.

○ **What is the primary disease associated with thymectomy?**

Myasthenia gravis is associated with abnormalities of the thymus gland (anterior mediastinal mass).

○ **What causes myasthenia gravis?**

It is an autoimmune disorder caused by decrease in ACh receptors at the neuromuscular junction due to their destruction by circulating antibodies. The disease is marked by exacerbations and remissions. Ptosis and diplopia are the most common initial symptoms, finally leading to weakness of pharyngeal and laryngeal (bulbar) muscles.

○ **What preoperative factors are suggestive of the need for postoperative ventilation following transsternal thymectomy in myasthenia gravis patient?**

   a. Disease duration of more than 6 years
   b. Concomitant pulmonary disease such as COPD
   c. Vital capacity less than 40 mL/kg (<2.9 L) Preoperative forced vital capacity (FVC) and forced mid-expiratory flow rate between 25 and 75% of FVC (FEF25–75%) were noted to have large discrimination coefficient value to predict the need for postoperative ventilation [Naguib et al., 1996. See reference on 531].
   d. Pyridostigmine more than 750 mg per day

○ **Are patients with myasthenia gravis at increased risk for aspiration pneumonitis?**

Yes. Myasthenics are at increased risk for aspiration pneumonitis, as more than 60% will have a history of bulbar symptoms such as difficulty swallowing and clearing secretions during the course of their disease.

○ **What are the perioperative considerations for patients with myasthenia gravis?**

Clinical presentation: ocular, bulbar, or skeletal muscle involvement (aspiration risk and respiratory insufficiency requiring postoperative ventilation)

Associated syndromes: anterior mediastinal mass, autoimmune diseases (hypothyroidism, diabetes mellitus, rheumatoid arthritis, and collagen vascular disease), arrhythmia, and cardiomyopathy

Drug therapy: immunosuppressants (steroids, azathioprine, cyclophosphamide), anticholinesterases (myasthenic vs. cholinergic crises leading to weakness), and plasmapheresis

Drug interactions or side effects: altered response to neuromuscular blockers, adrenal insufficiency with chronic steroid use, and medications that may exacerbate myasthenic symptoms

○ **What are the effects of neuromuscular blocking drugs in myasthenic patients?**

They are sensitive to nondepolarizing neuromuscular blockers and theoretically resistant to depolarizing neuromuscular blockers. There is also a resistance to the effects of succinylcholine probably due to decreased number of acetylcholine receptors. However, this has not been shown to be clinically relevant.

Other considerations are: pyridostigmine will modify the response to relaxants and the sensitivity to nondepolarizers will be diminished. The response to succinylcholine may be lengthened due to inhibition of pseudocholinesterase.

The reversal may be ineffective because much acetylcholinesterase inhibition already exists. Therefore, it is probably safer to allow spontaneous recovery postoperatively while continuing mechanical ventilation.

Monitoring neuromuscular blockade at the orbicularis oculi may overestimate the degree of blockade but helps to avoid persistent blockade.

Therefore, it is preferable to avoid all neuromuscular blockers. If a nondepolarizing neuromuscular blocker is needed, start with one tenth of the usual dose and select one of short or intermediate action.

○ **What is myasthenic syndrome?**

Myasthenic syndrome is also known as Eaton–Lambert syndrome and is often seen in patients with small cell carcinoma of the lung. It is an acquired autoimmune disease. It predominantly affects men and presents with proximal limb weakness (legs > arms), which improves with exercise. Muscle pain is common. Reflexes are absent or decreased. Patients are sensitive to both depolarizing and nondepolarizing neuromuscular blockers. Therapeutic response is poor with anticholinesterase drugs.

○ **What causes Eaton-Lambert syndrome?**

In this syndrome there is decreased function of the calcium channels due to antibodies against the channels. This leads to a decreased release of transmitter resulting in muscle weakness. Patients are sensitive to depolarizing and nondepolarizing relaxants. Presynaptic release of acetylcholine is triggered by the influx of calcium. There are several types of calcium channels. P channels are only found in the nerve terminals and probably the most important one for normal release of acetylcholine.

○ **Does a mediastinoscopy require one-lung ventilation?**

No.

○ **What are the complications with a mediastinoscopy?**

Most common is hemorrhage because of the proximity of major blood vessels and the vascularity of certain tumors. The second most common complication is a pneumothorax, usually right-sided. Recurrent nerve damage is the third most common complication and is permanent in 50% of cases. Autonomic reflexes can be stimulated due to manipulation of the trachea or the aortic arch. Obstruction of the innominate artery may occur that will result in decreased cerebral blood flow. Less common complications may include tracheal collapse, tension pneumomediastinum, mediastinitis, hemithorax, and chylothorax.

○ **Which vessels are more likely to be injured during a mediastinoscopy?**

SVC, pulmonary artery, and azygos vein are the most commonly injured. The right radial arterial line will indicate compression of the innominate artery by the mediastinoscope, but it is rarely injured.

○ **What are the anesthetic implications of thoracic lymphoma?**

Thoracic lymphoma primarily involves anterior mediastinal lymph nodes, possibly producing a mass effect on the trachea, bronchi, SVC, and heart chambers (typically right atrium as it is anterior and compressible). It can also lead to a pericardial effusion that may present with tamponade physiology.

○ **When is rigid bronchoscopy indicated?**

Foreign bodies, massive hemoptysis, vascular tumors, small children, endobronchial resection, and mediastinal tumors causing compression of the airway.

○ **How is ventilation accomplished with a rigid bronchoscope?**

Apneic oxygenation, jet ventilation, or apnea with intermittent ventilation when the eyepiece is closed.

○ **What are the choices for pain control after thoracic surgery?**

IV opioids, patient-controlled analgesia, thoracic epidural with opioids and/or local anesthetics, intrathecal opioids (single dose), and paravertebral intercostal nerve blocks.

○ **What nerve damage can occur during thoracic surgery?**

Intercostal nerve damage is the most common. Branches of the brachial plexus, recurrent laryngeal nerve, and the phrenic nerve may be injured. The brachial plexus is easily damaged during lung transplantation with the "clam shell" incision and retraction.

○ **What nerve damage can occur specifically during thoracic *aortic* surgery?**

The left recurrent laryngeal nerve courses around the aorta, and injury may lead to vocal cord paralysis. The left vagus nerve lies in the esophagoaortic groove but due to bilateral innervation, injury would be clinically asymptomatic. Phrenic nerve injury is also possible either from direct surgical trauma or from ice in the pericardium (incidence 1.7–11%). The left phrenic nerve courses along the posterior pericardium before dividing and penetrating the diaphragm lateral to the left border of the heart [Kunlyoshi, et al., 2004. See reference on page 531].

○ **What steps are taken in diagnosing an intraoperative pneumothorax in an intubated and ventilated patient?**

Initial signs of absent breath sounds, wheezing, reduced SpO_2, hypercarbia, and increased airway pressure. Hemodynamic instability (tachycardia, hypotension) is a late sign. Tension pneumothorax is far more likely during intermittent positive-pressure ventilation and nitrous oxide administration. A CXR provides a definitive diagnosis. Needle and tube thoracostomy will be accompanied by a distinctive hiss with relief of the tension pneumothorax.

○ **What are the possible complications of needle thoracostomy?**

Although needle thoracostomy can be a lifesaving procedure in a patient with tension pneumothorax, it may cause several complications. Usually, it is performed by inserting a 16 or 14 G Angiocath through the second intercostal place in the midclavicular line. The needle is directed over the superior surface of the rib in order to avoid damage to the neurovascular bundle.

Possible complications are damage to the lung, hematoma, and laceration of internal mammary artery or vein. Incorrect insertion may damage the neurovascular bundle.

○ **Describe important features of the design of chest tube drainage systems.**

Underwater seal

Drainage chambers for up to 2,000 mL fluid

Ability to apply suction up to −40 cm H_2O

Parallel chambers to allow grading of an air leak

An underwater seal involves a balanced system that prevents volume and pressure changes in the thoracic cavity. This prevents mediastinal shift and hemodynamic compromise. There is no option to inadvertently apply suction to these systems.

○ **What are the major considerations for providing safe anesthesia for lung volume reduction surgery in patients with severe bullous emphysema?**

The patient may be difficult to ventilate, and selective ventilation of bullae will result in ineffective gas exchange and distension of the bullae with potential hemodynamic effects similar to a tension pneumothorax. The treatment for overdistension is to temporarily disconnect the ventilator to allow deflation. Pressure-controlled ventilation with a low respiratory rate (6–10 breaths/min) is mandatory. Permissive hypercapnia is tolerated. Short-acting opiates may be used at induction, and the volatile agent must be totally cleared before extubation. Using TIVA or propofol toward the end of the case is effective in allowing time for excretion of the volatile agent. The patient needs to have minimal sedation but good analgesia at the end of the case. This involves the use of thoracic epidural analgesia with local anesthetics and as little epidural opiate as required. Continuous epidural analgesia should be maintained for at least 72 hours. Postoperative intensive care is required. Early mobilization is important.

○ **What are the causes of bronchopleural fistulae?**

Rupture into the pleural space: lung abscess, bronchus (typically traumatic), bulla, cyst, or parenchymal tissue (barotrauma).

Erosion of the airway or lung parenchyma: carcinoma, chronic inflammation, or breakdown of a bronchial suture line.

○ **How is a bronchopleural fistulae diagnosed?**

Failure to reinflate the lung despite chest tube drainage, or continued air leak 24 hours after a pneumothorax.

○ **What are the anesthetic considerations for bronchopleural fistula?**

Achieve adequate ventilation (intubate awake), avoid a pneumothorax (insert a chest tube), and prevent contamination of the healthy lung (use a double-lumen tube). This is one of the best clinical indications for using high-frequency ventilation because it allows for a reduction in peak airway pressures and a reduction of gas flow across the fistula. It is particularly good when applied via a double-lumen tube to the side with the fistula, while applying normal ventilation to the unaffected side.

○ **What heart chambers are usually injured following blunt cardiac trauma?**

The right ventricle is most commonly injured followed by the ventricular septum, the left ventricle, and the right atrium. Injuries to the valves and coronary arteries are also reported.

○ **What are the major complications associated with cardiac trauma?**

Exsanguination typically occurs in the field. For survivors, compensated cardiac tamponade may be revealed on induction of anesthesia. Sternotomy or pericardiotomy can result in exsanguination; cardiopulmonary bypass should be on standby. Femoral cannulation should be planned if there is radiological or echocardiographical evidence of intracardiac or aortic injury. Myocardial infarction can result from coronary artery injury. A ventricular septal defect can result from septal injury.

○ **How is the thoracic duct injured and what are the possible sequelae?**

Thoracic duct injury may occur during attempted insertion of a left internal jugular or subclavian catheters (it enters the left SC vein just before IJ insertion), although sequelae are rare if injury is limited to needle puncture. Avulsion or rupture causing chylothorax can occur with hyperextension injury at the time of spinal trauma, with surgical mobilization or injury to the aortic arch, esophagus, or left subclavian artery, and rarely spontaneously with coughing or vomiting. Chylothoraces are reported to have a high mortality, but this may be due to the fact that 50% of chylothoraces are associated with tumor infiltration.

Key Terms

Anesthetic management: anterior mediastinal mass
Anterior mediastinal mass: effects
Bronchial blocker: advantages
Bronchopleural fistula: diagnosis
Bronchopleural fistula: ventilatory management
Bronchoscopic anatomy
Cardiac trauma, signs of arterial injury
DLT misplacement: auscultation diagnosis
Double-lumen tube placement
Flow–volume loop: mediastinal mass
Hypoxemia during pneumonectomy: treatment
Lateral position: lung function
Lung resection outcome: pulmonary function tests (PFTs)
Mediastinal mass: evaluation and management
Mediastinal tumor: airway obstruction
Mediastinoscopy

Mediastinoscopy: BP monitoring
Mediastinoscopy complications
Mediastinoscopy: vascular compression
Myasthenia gravis: drug responses
Myasthenia gravis: postoperative management
Myasthenia: muscle relaxant effect
Myasthenia: physiology/preoperative risk evaluation
Needle thoracostomy: complications
Nitroprusside effects on oxygenation (HPV)
One-lung ventilation: indication
One-lung ventilation: oxygen desaturation treatment
Oxygenation during one-lung ventilation
PDA repair recurrent laryngeal nerve injury
Pneumonectomy mortality: high RV/TLV
Thoracoscopy: hypoxemia treatment
Thoracic lymphoma: complications

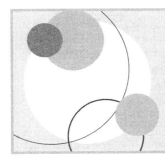

Transplant Surgery

Live as if you were to die tomorrow. Learn as if you were to live forever.
M. K. Gandhi

○ **Management of organ donors involves stabilization of a brain-dead patient. List common physiologic sequelae of brain death.**

Hypotension, arrhythmias, electrolyte abnormalities (hypernatremia, hypokalemia, hypomagnesemia, and hypocalcemia), hypothermia, anemia, coagulopathies, hypoxemia, and endocrine abnormalities (adrenal insufficiency, hypothyroidism, diabetes insipidus).

○ **What are the fluid management goals for the donor?**

Aggressive restoration and maintenance of the intravascular volume and the temporary use of vasoactive drugs, as needed.

The specific organ(s) to be retrieved determines fluid management (colloid, crystalloid, or blood products), ideal CVP, and the choice of allowable maximum doses for pressor drug support (dopamine first, and then phenylephrine, epinephrine, or norepinephrine).

Targeted hemodynamic goals are described as the "rule of 100s." This includes maintaining a minimum systolic blood pressure of 90–100 mm Hg (mean arterial pressure of 65 mm Hg), CVP <10 mm Hg, PCWP <10 mm Hg, SVR <1,000 dyne s/cm^5, and heart rate <100 beats/min, with a urine output >100 mL/h.

○ **What is the treatment of bradycardia in the organ donor?**

Clinically significant bradycardia in brain-dead patients may not respond to atropine, so a direct-acting chronotrope such as dobutamine, epinephrine, or dopamine should be available. External transcutaneous pacing (or transvenous) may be necessary if drug therapy fails.

○ **What is the treatment of diabetes insipidus in the organ donor?**

Vasopressin bolus and infusion: hypotonic IV fluids to match urine output; monitor serum sodium, 24-hour urine volumes, and specific gravity.

○ **List the diagnostic criteria for brain death determination in the adult patient.**

- Coma or unresponsiveness.
- No movement (spontaneous, elicited to pain, seizures, or posturing).
- Absence of brain stem reflexes.
- Apnea with an arterial PCO_2 of 60 mm Hg or greater.

"Brain death" is defined as irreversible cessation of all functions of the entire brain, including the brain stem. In patients with coma of undetermined origin, the patient must meet the clinical criteria, have an observation period >24 hours, have no cerebral blood flow, and have neuroimaging evidence of an acute CNS catastrophe that is compatible with brain death in the absence of confounding factors (hypothermia, sedation, shock, neuromuscular blocking agents, drug intoxication or poisoning, and no severe electrolyte, acid–base, or endocrine disorder).

○ **What are the confirmatory tests of brain death [Wijdicks et al., 2010. See reference on page 531]?**

These confirm loss of bioelectrical activity of the brain. These are optional for adults but strongly recommended for children, especially <1 year.

1. *Lack of EEG activity*: isoelectric EEG is a reliable confirmatory test; however, may also occur after drug intoxication such as barbiturates.

2. *Evoked responses*: brain stem auditory evoked responses (BAEP) and median nerve SSEP are used. Previous deafness or severe auditory system damage should be checked.

3. *Measurement of blood flow*: absence of intracranial circulation indicates irreversible damage to the brain. Advantage of angiography (contrast, radionuclide) is that it is not influenced by CNS depressant drugs or hypothermia. CT, MRI, MR angiography, transcranial Doppler, and positron emission tomography also have been used.

○ **List the most common immunosuppressive protocol drugs.**

Cyclosporine, azathioprine, prednisone, OKT_3, mycophenolate mofetil, sirolimus, and FK506.

○ **What is the current US Food and Drug Administration recommendation for prevention of transfusion-associated graft-versus-host disease in immunosuppressed patients?**

Controlled irradiation of blood products, which eliminates the proliferative capacity of lymphocytes present in red cell, platelet, and freshly collected plasma components. The penetrated photons of radiation beam into blood components cause the formation of electrically charged particles or secondary electrons. These electrons damage the DNA of lymphocytes either by direct interaction or by reacting initially with cell water to form free radicals. The damaged lymphocytes are unable to proliferate in the host and therefore cannot mediate transfusion-associated GVHD.

○ **Describe the causes of encephalopathy in liver transplant recipients.**

Portal–systemic encephalopathy (PSE) is the most common form and usually seen in patients with cirrhosis and portal hypertension. Arterial or CSF ammonia concentration or CSF glutamine levels correlate with the degree of CNS suppression. PSE is usually precipitated by ingestion of protein (meal or GI bleed), infection (spontaneous bacterial peritonitis), or dehydration due to overdiuresis.

Pseudo-PSE is difficult to distinguish clinically. It is caused by decreased clearance of sedatives, analgesics, and tranquilizing drugs or metabolic abnormalities (alkalosis, acidosis, or hypoglycemia).

○ **Describe the types of renal insufficiency seen in the liver transplant patient.**

- Preexisting from the underlying process causing liver disease: hepatitis B, hepatitis C, analgesic overdose, amyloidosis, and autoimmune disease.
- Preexisting from other systemic illness: diabetes or hypertension.
- Functional renal impairment from liver failure: mild sodium retention to hepatorenal syndrome.
- Management of encephalopathy and ascites: prerenal secondary to hypovolemia from diuretic therapy.
- Immunosuppression-related complication: cyclosporine and FK506 nephrotoxicity.

○ **Why is adequate venous access so critical in liver transplantation anesthesia?**

    a. Potential for major blood loss (liver surgery, clamping portal vein and vena cava, coagulopathy) and for transfusion

    b. Maintain preload to the heart during caval clamping

    c. Allow venovenous bypass (VVB) during anhepatic period

    d. Route for administration of vasopressors/dilators

    e. Access for invasive monitoring and PA catheter insertion

○ **Describe the hemodynamic changes associated with hepatic vascular occlusion.**

Pringle maneuver: inflow vascular occlusion with clamping of the portal vein and hepatic artery in the hepatic pedicle. No interruption of caval flow, 10% decrease in cardiac index with compensatory increase in systemic vascular resistance, and MAP is maintained or increased 10%.

Total hepatic vascular occlusion (HVE) combines portal triad clamping and occlusion of the inferior vena cava. The hemodynamic response to HVE is characterized by a 50% decrease in cardiac output, decrease in pulmonary artery pressure, and increase in heart rate and systemic vascular resistance.

○ **Define liver transplant terms: VVB, piggyback technique, and reperfusion syndrome.**

VVB: An extracorporeal circulatory assistance device that improves venous return during the anhepatic stage. Nonheparinized blood flowing through cannulae inserted into the portal and/or femoral veins is returned to the right atrium via the axillary or subclavian vein through a centripetal pump.

Piggyback technique: Hepatectomy in the recipient with preservation of the full length of the vena cava. The donor liver is then "piggybacked" to the recipient IVC with the outflow venous anastomosis made end-to-side (donor IVC to recipient hepatic vein cuff) or side-to-side (donor IVC to recipient IVC).

Reperfusion syndrome: Hypotension (decrease in MAP >30%) for at least 1 minute, within 5 minutes of reperfusion of the donor liver. Often accompanied by bradycardia, arrhythmias, and, occasionally, cardiac arrest. Incidence: 30%. Etiology: unclear but likely systemic vasodilation and possibly myocardial depression from vasoactive substances, volume overload, and transient hyperkalemia.

○ **What are the major problems associated with reperfusion of the new liver?**

    1. Postreperfusion syndrome.

    2. Hyperkalemia (bradycardia, asystole, cardiac arrest, malignant ventricular arrhythmias).

    3. Pulmonary embolism.

    4. Pulmonary hypertension (precipitating right ventricular failure).

    5. Volume overload.

    6. Hypothermia.

    7. Hypotension (active bleeding, air or thrombus embolism, hyperkalemia, acidosis, hypocalcemia).

    8. Hyperglycemia.

    9. Coagulopathy (especially primary fibrinolysis, donor heparin, low fibrinogen, factor deficiency, dilutional thrombocytopenia).

    10. Primary nonfunction or delayed primary graft function.

○ **Discuss intraoperative management of liver transplant patients with pulmonary hypertension.**

Following insertion of a PA catheter and establishing an adequate level of anesthesia, if the mean pulmonary artery pressure exceeds 35 mm Hg, this is potentially a huge problem requiring management decisions (including canceling the case: normal MPAP <25 mm Hg, normal pulmonary vascular resistance [PVR] <120 dyne s/cm^5). Evidence of response of PA pressures to therapy and preserved right ventricular function is essential. Pre-liver transplant combination of MPAP greater than 35 mm Hg and PVR greater than 250 dyne s/cm^5 has been associated with a perioperative mortality rate of nearly 50%. Therapies for reduction of PA pressures include nitric oxide 10–60 ppm (inhaled); IV: flolan (epoprostenol 2 μg/kg/min, increasing in increments of 2 μg/kg/min every 15 minutes), nitroglycerine 0.1-7 μg/kg/min, milrinone (0.375–0.75 μg/kg/min, bolus 50 μg/kg), and fenoldopam 0.01–1.6 μg/kg/min; PO: Viagra®.

○ **On induction of anesthesia for lung transplantation, patients with severe COPD are often hemodynamically unstable. Why?**

This represents a transition from spontaneous breathing to controlled positive-pressure ventilation and loss of sympathetic tone.

Hemodynamic instability is due to a reduction in venous return and cardiac output from volume depletion, auto-PEEP secondary to air trapping, hyperinflation with "breath stacking," increase in intrathoracic pressure, and possibly right ventricular dysfunction from increased PVR. These patients should be preloaded with 1 L of crystalloid and ventilation adjusted to allow shallow tidal volumes and a long expiratory time (avoid high peak pressures, PEEP, auto-PEEP). In addition, chronotropic agents (to increase heart rate) and inotropic support (maintain systemic pressure for coronary perfusion) with pulmonary vasodilator drugs may be necessary.

○ **Explain why "permissive hypercapnia" is frequently unavoidable during lung transplant surgery [Lucangelo et al., 2012. See reference on page 531].**

Permissive hypercapnia is a technique of deliberate hypoventilation in which conventional positive-pressure ventilation is limited and the arterial PCO$_2$ is allowed to rise. Maintaining hemodynamic stability and normal ventilation are often mutually exclusive, as positive-pressure ventilation and air trapping may lead to pulmonary tamponade and circulatory arrest. Elevated PaCO$_2$ values are accepted as long as the pH is maintained above 7.1. Intraoperative PaCO$_2$ values of 120 mm Hg may be tolerated with adequate oxygenation.

○ **What clinically significant changes in physiology occur post-lung transplant?**

1. Airway hyperresponsiveness from denervation hypersensitivity of airway smooth muscle muscarinic receptors.

2. Interruption of the afferent limb of the cough reflex and impairment of mucociliary clearance.

3. Reduced gastroesophageal motility, most likely from vagal nerve injury.

○ **What are the anesthetic considerations for induction of anesthesia in the cardiac transplant recipient?**

1. Rapid sequence induction due to aspiration risk (full stomach or gastroparesis due to gut hypoperfusion).

2. Low cardiac output state requires placement of invasive monitoring in the awake patient and adjustment of drug dosages for a prolonged circulation time and reduced volume of distribution.

3. Unpredictable responses to sympathomimetic agents.

4. Vasoactive drugs are continued and adjusted accordingly to maintain adequate CO, and coronary and cerebral perfusion pressures.

5. Avoid drugs and ventilatory maneuvers that will increase PVR.

◯ **What are the primary indications for heart–lung transplantation?**

Congenital heart disease and primary pulmonary hypertension.

◯ **Describe methods for minimizing increases in PVR in the heart–lung transplant recipient during induction and the pre-bypass period.**

Preoxygenation is critical. Induction is generally accomplished with a high-dose opiate and a small dose of a cardiostable induction agent such as etomidate or midazolam. Ketamine is relatively contraindicated because of its deleterious effects on PVR. Vasoactive drugs are frequently required. Useful combination therapies include prostaglandin E1, milrinone, or nitroglycerine for PVR reduction combined with norepinephrine for increased systemic blood pressure and cardiac contractility. Nitric oxide may also be useful for selective pulmonary vasodilation. Avoid hypercarbia, hypoxemia, and hypothermia.

◯ **What are the most important considerations in the preoperative assessment of the heart transplant patient scheduled for laparoscopic cholecystectomy?**

1. Functional evaluation of the graft:
   - Early: detection of infection or rejection
   - Late: ischemia risk or the failing transplanted heart (diminished left ventricular ejection fraction or diastolic dysfunction)
2. Patient factors:
   - Residual physiologic alterations
   - Coexisting systemic disease
   - Transplant surgery-related complications
   - Functional status
3. Immunosuppressive therapy:
   - Pharmacology of cyclosporine, prednisone, mycophenolate mofetil, and tacrolimus
   - Complications, toxicities, and adverse effects

◯ **Describe the physiology of the denervated transplanted human heart.**

- Preload-dependent
- Afterload:
  - a. Drug-induced systemic hypertension
  - b. Delayed or blunted blood pressure response (altered response to exercise)
- Heart rates and intrinsic rate of donor SA node (sinus tachycardia)
  - a. Delayed and attenuated heart rate response
  - b. Beta-adrenergic and cholinergic supersensitivity
- Dysrhythmias and SA node dysfunction
- Normal cardiac output and contractility
- Normal PAP and PCWP
- Potential for coronary artery disease (silent ischemia), diastolic dysfunction, and chronic hypertension

◯ **Describe the physiologic consequences of acute denervation of the heart.**

Afferent denervation results in the lack of angina pectoris, alterations of peripheral autonomic responses (Valsalva, carotid sinus massage, body position changes, heart rate variability, and drug responses), and changes in sodium and water balance. Loss of efferent fibers results in an increase in the resting heart rate to 90–110 bpm (intrinsic rate of the donor heart) and a blunted chronotropic response to stresses such as exercise.

○ **Describe the unique features of the SA node in a transplanted heart.**

The native SA node is isolated from the myocardium by the suture line, and does not influence the heart rate, although its P-wave may be visible on the EKG. The SA node from the donor heart controls the heart rate, with an intrinsic rate of 90–110 bpm due to denervation from sympathetic and parasympathetic modulation. Direct-acting chronotropic agents are preferred to increase heart rate. Heart rate responses are delayed and attenuated, with possible beta-adrenergic and cholinergic supersensitivity. There is evidence supporting autonomic reinnervation of the transplanted heart. Neostigmine may induce bradycardia or sinus arrest.

○ **In a patient undergoing renal transplantation, is succinylcholine contraindicated?**

No, if the baseline serum potassium is normal and the patient has no other condition that would suggest increased risk of an exaggerated hyperkalemic response with IV succinylcholine (any disorder in which there is proliferation of extrajunctional receptors, i.e., burns, muscular dystrophies, spinal cord injuries, upper and lower motor neuron disease). Case reports describe an exaggerated hyperkalemic response in patients with chronic renal insufficiency secondary to diabetes mellitus, with evidence of significant peripheral neuropathy and muscle wasting in the hands. Succinylcholine is a known trigger for malignant hyperthermia.

○ **What effect does heart transplantation have on the sympathetic and parasympathetic innvervation of the heart?**

The heart becomes unavoidably denervated at the time of transplantation. That means that the immediate adaptation to increases in workload of an increase in heart rate that the heart must do during exercise is not available. Over time the heart may become partially innervated again but in many cases this never occurs and instead increases in heart rate occur gradually via humoral mediators, such as catecholamines. The heart adapts to the increased workload of exercise by increasing stroke volume. Therefore maintaining adequate preload is vital in a transplanted patient.

○ **What are the pharmacological implications of this new state?**

The pharmacological implication of this new state is that drugs that increase heart through modification of sympathetic and parasympathetic output are not as potent or simply do not work at all. Drugs such as ephedrine, atropine, and glycopyrrolate have little to no effect on heart rate. Instead, drugs that modulate heart rate via receptors on the heart are preferred such as epinephrine, isoproterenol, and glucagon. Also, the modulation of heart rate through the changes in blood pressure will not be possible (the baroreceptor reflex). The carotid body, which is innervated by the sinus nerve of Hering, a branch of glossopharyngeal nerve (cranial nerve IX), is connected to the nucleus tractus solitaries, which modulates the sympathetic and parasympathetic neurons in the medulla. The sympathetic and parasympathetic fiber connections to the donated heart are nonexistent in the immediate posttransplant period and may only partially return after some time.

○ **In a patient undergoing renal transplantation are any of the nondepolarizing muscle relaxants absolutely contraindicated?**

No. Theoretically it would be best to avoid muscle relaxants with significant renal excretion (pancuronium, metocurine, doxacurium, tubocurarine).

○ **In a patient undergoing renal transplantation, in theory, which inhalational agent(s) should be avoided?**

Enflurane and sevoflurane. Methoxyflurane is no longer available.

Inorganic fluoride is a potentially nephrotoxic product of anesthetic metabolism. Fluoride-associated renal dysfunction may be a risk with methoxyflurane >> enflurane and sevoflurane. Sevoflurane on contact with the soda lime in a rebreathing apparatus, especially at higher temperatures and when the soda lime is desiccated, undergoes degradation producing compound A (PIFE). Compound A has been shown to cause nephrotoxicity in rats. In humans, direct histological evidence of renal toxicity has not been demonstrated, although there are dose-related proteinuria, glycosuria, and enzymuria. During low-flow anesthesia, compound A may build up to clinically significant levels, although there have never been any reports of adverse events in humans even under low flow rates of < 2 L/min.

○ **Should Ringer's lactate (RL) be avoided in all patients with chronic renal failure due to the risk of hyperkalemia?**

No. The potassium level has been shown to increase more with normal saline than with RL, due to the hyperchloremic acidosis causing an extracellular shift of potassium. The amount of potassium in RL (4 mmol/L) is not enough to cause a dangerous rise in potassium, and RL should be considered safe to use in chronic renal failure.

○ **Should mannitol be given prior to vessel clamping to protect the transplanted kidney?**

The use of mannitol as a protective agent during renal transplantation stems from its ability to increase renal blood flow. Evidence is limited with one small study showing a decrease in ATN in the transplanted kidney. Despite no evidence of an outcome benefit, it has become common practice to give 12.5–25 g of mannitol to the living donor, alongside intravascular expansion with crystalloid prior to vessel clamping.

○ **What are some common systemic manifestations of end-stage renal disease that are important in the preoperative anesthetic assessment of the kidney transplant patient?**

Neurologic:

- Central: seizures and lethargy
- Peripheral: sensory and motor neuropathy, and autonomic dysfunction

Respiratory:

- Hypocarbia
- Pleural effusion, edema, pneumonitis, and infection

Cardiovascular:

- Indeterminate volume status, susceptible to fluid overload
- High cardiac output
- Hypertension and LVH
- Accelerated peripheral and coronary atherosclerosis
- Tachycardia, arrhythmias, and conduction disorders
- Attenuated reactivity of the sympathetic nervous system
- Reduced oxygen-carrying capacity and increased peripheral extraction of O_2
- Pericarditis and cardiac tamponade

Endocrine:

- Electrolyte disorders (hyperkalemia, hyponatremia, hypermagnesemia, hypocalcemia)
- Metabolic acidosis
- Secondary hyperparathyroidism
- Glucose intolerance

Gastrointestinal:

- Delayed gastric emptying and increased volume and acidity of gastric contents, and aspiration risk

Musculoskeletal: osteodystrophy and muscle wasting

Hematologic:

- Chronic anemia and right shift of hemoglobin dissociation curve
- Platelet dysfunction and coagulopathy
- Increased susceptibility to infection and carrier state for hepatitis B antigen and HIV

○ **Why is the hemoglobin level low in a renal transplant patient?**

Chronic anemia with hemoglobin levels of 5–7 g/dL is a result of decreased production of erythropoietin and diminished red cell survival time. Iron absorption from the gastrointestinal tract may also be decreased in patients with ESRD leading to iron deficiency. Following kidney transplantation, immunosuppressive therapy (steroids, azathioprine, and cyclosporine) may cause bone marrow depression resulting in various degrees of anemia, thrombocytopenia, and lymphopenia. Hemoglobin levels may be normal in chronic renal failure patients treated with Procrit® (epoetin alfa).

○ **Is the renal transplant recipient at risk for pseudocholinesterase deficiency?**

Not due to chronic renal insufficiency. Plasma cholinesterase is produced in the liver.

○ **What are the commonest causes of chronic kidney disease (CKD)?**

Diabetes mellitus and hypertension account for two thirds of cases. Additional risk factors include a family history of chronic renal disease, advanced age, and populations with a high incidence of diabetes and hypertension (African Americans, Hispanic Americans, Asian, Pacific Islanders, and American Indians).

○ **In a patient with end-stage renal disease is platelet function normal? Is there any treatment?**

The platelet count is often low and platelet function is abnormal (prolonged bleeding time, decreased platelet adhesiveness, and inhibition of secondary platelet aggregation from an increased plasma level of guanidine-succinic acid which causes a decline in platelet factor 3). Platelet function improves with dialysis and IV desmopressin 0.3 μg/kg.

○ **What are the causes of the bleeding diathesis seen in a patient with end-stage renal disease?**

Multifactorial. Platelet dysfunction, thrombocytopenia, decreased antithrombin III, excess heparin from dialysis, and increased factor VIII and fibrinogen.

○ **What are some of the immediate postoperative complications following kidney transplantation?**

1. Residual neuromuscular blockade requiring continued mechanical ventilation.
2. Hypertension (myocardial ischemia, LV failure, pulmonary edema, hemorrhage at the vascular anastomosis, or direct injury to the graft) and hypotension with fluid depletion.
3. Delayed primary function of the transplanted kidney (oliguria with adequate CVP), acute tubular necrosis, or rejection.
4. Hyperglycemia and electrolyte disorders, and persistent metabolic acidosis.
5. Complications of IV immunosuppressive therapy.
6. Pneumothorax from central line insertion.
7. Anemia requiring transfusion.
8. Surgical: arterial thrombosis, venous occlusion, graft hematoma or rupture, wound infection, urologic complications (urine leak or obstruction to flow), or loss of the graft.

○ **What are the hallmarks of clinical rejection in the transplanted kidney?**

- Fever
- Diminishing urine output
- Fluid retention

- Hypertension
- Worsening renal function (increased BUN, creatinine, beta-2 microglobulins)
- Enlargement and tenderness of the ectopic kidney

Diagnosis of rejection is difficult, requiring definitive renal biopsy. Causes of functional impairment of the transplanted kidney include accelerated progression of an underlying disease process, cyclosporine nephrotoxicity, rejection (acute or chronic), and hypertension.

○ **What would be your choice for monitoring during renal transplantation, and why?**

Standard ASA monitors: EKG, noninvasive blood pressure, temperature, pulse oximetry, and capnography. Urine output.

Invasive: central venous pressure catheter to measure central filling pressure for volume loading, and to sample for hematocrit, glucose, and electrolytes. Intra-arterial blood pressure monitoring should be considered based on cardiovascular morbidity.

○ **What is the primary indication for isolated pancreas transplantation?**

Diabetes mellitus with severe neuropathy and labile diabetes (HbA1c levels persistently >10% despite insulin therapy or frequent hypoglycemia without attempts at strict control of glucose levels). Selected patients have been transplanted in an attempt to halt the progression of diabetic nephropathy.

○ **What are the intraoperative anesthetic considerations for pancreatic transplantation?**

1. Physiologic alterations and systemic manifestations of diabetes mellitus, most importantly assessment of cardiovascular and renal function, with predictable end-organ dysfunction.
2. Patients are at risk for aspiration requiring rapid sequence induction and intubation.
3. Maintain hemodynamic stability.
4. Strict perioperative control of glucose levels (70–100 mg/dL) with the administration of insulin. Hyperglycemia on reperfusion of the pancreatic graft should be anticipated.

○ **How does pancreatic islet transplantation differ from pancreas transplantation?**

Pancreatic islet transplantation is a form of selective transplantation since only the cells required by the recipient are transplanted. When only the islet cells are transplanted, complications related to the exocrine portion of the pancreas and immunologic reactivity are minimized.

Key Terms

Carotid sinus stimulation: post-heart transplant
Denervated heart: exercise physiology
Heart transplant: autonomic effect
Heart transplant: autonomic pharmacology
Hyperkalemia treatment in renal transplant
Liver transhepatic phase: transfusion
Liver transplant – anhepatic phase
Liver transplant: electrolyte disturbances
Liver transplant: management

Organ donor: bradycardia treatment
Organ donor: treatment of diabetes insipidus
Perfusion during renal transplant: treatment
Postcardiac transplant patient
Postcardiac transplant: physiology
Renal replacement: treatment selection
Renal transplant: mannitol
Respiratory physiology: post-lung transplant

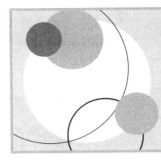

Vascular Surgery

I have the body of an eighteen year old. I keep it in the fridge.
Spike Milligan

○ **What is the most common site of aortic aneurysm?**

The abdominal aorta. About 75% of all arteriosclerotic aneurysms are confined to the abdominal aorta, usually below the renal arteries. The other 25% are in the thoracic aorta, most commonly the arch over the descending portion [Swensson and Rodriguez. See reference on page 531].

○ **What are the most common sites of aortic dissection?**

Over 85% arise in one of the following two locations: (1) the ascending aorta within several centimeters of the aortic valve and (2) the descending thoracic aorta distal to the origin of the subclavian artery at the site of the ligamentum arteriosum.

○ **What are the classification schemes for aortic dissection?**

There are two major classification schemes:

DeBakey classification.

Stanford classification: type A that denotes any involvement of the ascending with variable involvement of the descending aorta and type B in which the dissection is confined to the descending aorta.

○ **What is the DeBakey classification of aortic dissections?**

DeBakey and his colleagues classified aortic dissections into four categories, depending on the anatomy of the dissection:

- Type I dissections, the most severe, begin at the proximal ascending aorta and extend caudally to the common iliac arteries.
- Type II dissections, the rarest form, are limited to the ascending aorta.
- Type IIIa dissections begin in the descending aorta, distal to the takeoff of the left subclavian artery. They are fully contained within the thorax.
- Type IIIb dissections have the same origin as Type IIIa, but they extend to the abdominal aorta.

Daily and Stanford later simplified the nomenclature as Type A dissections (including I and II) and Type B dissections (including IIIa and IIIb) [Swensson, 2008. See reference on page 531].

○ **Which hereditary disorders are associated with aortic dissection?**

Marfan syndrome and Ehlers–Danlos syndrome.

○   **What is the most common presenting symptom of aortic dissection?**

Severe pain located in the anterior chest (ascending and arch dissections) and midscapular in the back for descending. This symptom is found in more than 90% of patients, typically abrupt and severe in onset, described as tearing in nature.

○   **How does the pain of a ruptured thoracic aneurysm differ from typical angina?**

Angina is classically described as a gradually worsening substernal pressure radiating to the left shoulder, neck, and jaw. A ruptured thoracic aortic aneurysm is heralded by the immediate onset of excruciating pain in the center of the chest that may radiate to the back. The pain begins instantly and reaches its peak intensity within seconds.

○   **Which tests are used to diagnose an aortic aneurysm?**

Chest x-ray is often the first sign of the pathology; the aortic aneurysm typically presents as a widened mediastinum. CT, MRI, or transesophageal echocardiography (TEE) will reveal an aorta with a false lumen (created by the dissection) in addition to the vessel's true lumen.

○   **What is the best imaging study for diagnosis of aortic dissection?**

MRI for hemodynamically stable patients without pacemakers or orthopedic hardware (sensitivity 98.3% and specificity 97.8%), and spiral CT scan and TEE for patients who need a quicker diagnosis (hemodynamic instability and/or impending rupture). A TEE has certain limitations such as difficult visualization of the entire aortic arch and abdominal aorta beyond the level of the stomach. Aortography is the gold standard, but used selectively due to its higher complication rate.

○   **Are aortic dissections managed medically or surgically?**

Dissections that involve the ascending aorta (Type A) are managed surgically, whereas dissections that spare the ascending aorta (Type B) can initially be managed medically. Surgery may be required for Type B dissections when there is evidence of ischemia to the viscera, kidneys, or lower limbs. Medical management includes the administration of an IV antihypertensive agent, as well as a β-blocker to decrease the force of LV contraction.

○   **Describe the medical management of aortic dissection.**

Acute management of all dissections generally involves medical therapy, even if definitive treatment is urgent surgery. The principles of medical management include:

- Oxygenation
- Monitoring (EKG, intra-arterial blood pressure, CVP, PAP, urine output, SpO_2)
- Control of systolic blood pressure to 105–120 mm Hg (vasodilators)
- Decreasing ejection velocity and heart rate (beta-blockers)
- Transfusion as needed
- Pain control

○ **What are the most commonly used drugs for the treatment of aortic dissection?**

Initial management should be directed at decreasing aortic wall stress by controlling HR and BP as follows:

a. In the absence of contraindications, intravenous beta blockers titrated to HR 60 bpm or less.

b. With clear contraindications to beta blockers, nondihydropyridine calcium channel blockers to control HR.

c. If SBP is >120 after adequate heart rate control, ACE inhibitors and /or other vasodilators should be given IV.

d. Beta blockers should be used carefully if acute aortic regurgitation is present because the compensatory tachycardia will be blocked.

e. Vasodilator should not be started before rate control to avoid associated reflex tachycardia that may increase aortic wall stress.

f. Urgent surgical consultation regardless of the anatomic location [2010 ACC/AHA/AATS....Guidelines on management of thoracic aortic disease. See reference on 531].

Nitroglycerin is a relatively weak agent. Nitroprusside is generally very effective. Use of this agent alone, however, can result in increased shear forces associated with increased heart rate; thus, it is generally wise to use a beta-blocker when administering nitroprusside. When nitroprusside is ineffective or contraindicated, labetalol is also an effective agent. This drug, a combination of alpha-blocker and nonselective beta-blocker, depresses shear forces as well as systolic blood pressure. Trimethaphan is a second-line agent for refractory hypertension, but the side effects of tachyphylaxis (develops within the first 24 hours), severe hypotension, somnolence, sympathoplegia, and pupillary dilation render this a seldom-used drug. Nicardipine (Cardene) is an effective vasodilator that works via calcium channel blockade with minimal myocardial effects.

○ **What are the most common side effects of nitroprusside?**

Reflex tachycardia in clinical doses. For overdose/toxicity, nausea, restlessness, somnolence, hypotension, and cyanide toxicity. This generally develops after at least 48 hours of continuous use.

○ **How is perfusion maintained during surgical therapy?**

If the dissection is in the ascending aorta, cardiopulmonary bypass is typically used. Surgery on the arch will require retrograde cerebral perfusion to maintain CBF. Descending arch repair is managed with aortic cross-clamping distal to the left subclavian or left common carotid artery; a shunt is used to relieve the LV and permit perfusion below the diaphragm.

○ **Where would you place the arterial line preoperatively?**

If a descending thoracic aneurysm is being repaired, the a-line should be placed on the right, as the left subclavian artery may be cross-clamped. If an aortic clamp is used, the addition of a right dorsalis pedis arterial line will monitor pressure below the clamp and indicate hypoperfusion to the lower extremities and renal bed.

Ascending aortic surgery calls for a left radial a-line in case the innominate artery is cross-clamped.

○ **Is a double-lumen tube indicated?**

Single-lung ventilation may be useful for resection of a descending aortic aneurysm, as left lung collapse provides better surgical access to the field. Adhesion of the aorta to the left bronchus may result in bleeding into the left bronchus; ventilation in this case is further assisted by single-lung ventilation.

○ **What are the cardiovascular effects of applying a cross-clamp to the descending aorta?**

The primary effect is a significant increase in afterload for the left ventricle. Blood flow is elevated proximal to the clamp (intracranial flow, pulmonary artery pressure, and wedge pressure all increase) and significantly decreased distal to the clamp (spinal cord perfusion, renal blood flow, and lower extremity perfusion all decrease). The increase in afterload, coupled with an increase in preload, may result in systolic and diastolic dysfunction in a patient with a compromised heart.

○ **What are the metabolic effects of applying a cross-clamp to the descending aorta?**

Anaerobic metabolism begins distal to the clamp in the absence of inadequate oxygen delivery. The lactic acidosis that results is aggravated if the aortic clamp reduces hepatic blood flow, as the liver then has a reduced capability to clear the lactate. Application of the clamp also results in the release of many humoral mediators, including renin, angiotensin, prostaglandins, cytokines, and free radicals.

○ **How do you manage hypertension secondary to aortic cross-clamping?**

The first line of defense is to begin lowering the blood pressure before the clamp is applied. If normal autoregulatory mechanisms are in place, the systolic blood pressure should be lowered below 100 mm Hg prior to the placement of the clamp. After cross-clamping, hypertension can be managed in three ways:

- Vasodilation: Drugs such as sodium nitroprusside or intravenous calcium channel blockers can reduce the afterload on the LV. However, they may reduce perfusion to the spinal cord and kidneys, and must be used with care.
- Shunt: Diverting blood from the circulation proximal to the clamp to the distal aorta or femoral arteries will ensure oxygenation to the structures fed from arteries beyond the clamp. Furthermore, blood that is shunted will help reduce afterload and blood pressure.
- Anesthesia: The concentration of the volatile agents can be increased to reduce SVR.

○ **What is the danger of dropping the proximal aortic pressure too low?**

The cerebral and coronary circulations depend on the pressure in the proximal (preclamp) aorta. Blood pressure should be maintained to adequately perfuse the brain and avoid coronary hypoperfusion.

○ **How do you avoid spinal cord ischemia?**

The most reliable way to ensure adequate flow of oxygenated blood to the spinal cord is through the use of a shunt. Surgeons will typically use partial left heart bypass (LHB; left atrium to femoral vein), femoral venoarterial bypass (femoral venous blood is shunted through an oxygenator and pumped into the femoral artery), or a Gott shunt (left ventricle to distal aorta or femoral artery.)

○ **How can spinal cord ischemia be detected clinically?**

The use of somatosensory evoked potential (SSEP) monitoring is an invaluable tool for the clinician. The presence of an increased latency and/or a decrease in amplitude is suggestive of hypoperfusion.

○ **Can volatile anesthetic agents be used when SSEPs are being monitored?**

All of the volatile agents are known to increase the latency and decrease the amplitude of SSEPs, but the effect is limited when the MAC is kept at or below 0.5. However, many clinicians choose to employ a total intravenous anesthetic (TIVA) technique to ensure that there is no misinterpretation of the SSEPs.

○ **How can the spinal cord be protected during aortic cross-clamping?**

The most important measure is to minimize the time of aortic cross-clamping; times above 30 minutes result in a significantly greater incidence of postoperative paraplegia. In addition to maintenance of blood pressure and shunting, as discussed previously, the following measures may also be useful:

- CSF drainage: Removal of CSF to keep CSF pressure at or below 10 mm Hg reduces cord pressure and improves perfusion.
- Hypothermia: Cooling the patient to 33–34°C reduces metabolic rate and may further protect the cord from ischemia.
- Avoidance of hyperglycemia: While data on this have mostly pertained to the brain, many believe that anaerobic metabolism of glucose, and the resultant lactic acidosis, may worsen spinal ischemia too.
- Drugs: The use of agents such as mannitol, steroids, and free radical scavengers may offer CNS protection.

○ **What thoracic aortic surgery typically requires deep hypothermic circulatory arrest (DHCA)?**

Aneurysms or dissections involving the ascending aorta or aortic arch where distal application of the cross-clamp would be needed. Bleeding from arterial sites after congenital heart surgery may also require DHCA for repair. The safe limit of DHCA with interruption of cerebral blood flow is 45–60 minutes.

○ **How is cerebral protection achieved during DHCA?**

Cooling on cardiopulmonary (femoral–femoral) bypass, surface cooling with the head packed in ice, EEG monitoring to maintain isoelectric tracing with thiopental, and retrograde (internal jugular vein) or anterograde (innominate artery) selective cerebral perfusion with cold oxygenated blood (may extend the safe time of DHCA to 90 minutes). Mannitol, furosemide, and steroids are given to limit cerebral edema and ischemic injury following reperfusion.

○ **What is the major determinant of cerebral dysfunction following DHCA?**

Circulatory arrest time and age.

○ **How is distal aortic perfusion achieved?**

LHB with outflow typically from the left atrium and inflow typically into the left femoral artery. Oxygenation is via the lungs.

○ **What are the major complications associated with LHB?**

Right ventricular dysfunction and hypoxemia.

Distal perfusion with extracorporeal support has been shown to reduce the incidence of paraplegia (risk of 10–20% for simple thoracoabdominal repair), but is probably not beneficial if the cross-clamp time is less than 20–30 minutes.

○ **How can the kidneys be protected during aortic cross-clamping?**

Again, a short cross-clamping time (under 30 minutes) in addition to maintenance of blood pressure and the use of a shunt is the best means of defense. Preoperative hydration and intraoperative mannitol may be reasonable strategies for preservation of renal function in open repairs of the descending aorta [2010 guidelines on management of thoracic aortic disease. See reference on 531].

○   **What is the incidence of postoperative paraplegia after thoracic aorta aneurysm resection surgery?**

Spinal cord injury can occur not only during extensive thoracoabdominal aneurysm repair but also postoperatively. Etz et al., reported an overall paraplegia rate of 2.4%. He studied a series of 858 cases of thoracoabdominal aneurysm repair and found total of 20 cases of paraplegia (3 occurred intraoperatively and 7 occurred late postoperatively. In 10 cases spinal cord injury occurred within 48 hours after thoracoabdominal aneurysm repair, despite intact somatosensory evoked potentials at the end of the procedure. He concluded "the study suggests paraplegia can result from inadequate postoperative spinal cord perfusion caused by relatively minor differences from control subjects in perfusion parameters. Delayed paraplegia can perhaps be prevented with better hemodynamic and fluid management" [Etz et al., 2008. See reference on 531].

○   **What are the cardiovascular and metabolic effects of removing the aortic cross-clamp?**

Cross-clamp removal is marked by extreme hypotension, as afterload is suddenly reduced. In addition, metabolic (lactic) acidosis products that result from anaerobic metabolism distal to the clamp can cause myocardial depression, further reducing SVR. Volume expansion prior to release of the clamp, as well as slow release of the cross-clamp (over 2–4 minutes), can attenuate this response. Minute ventilation should be increased to provide a compensatory respiratory alkalosis. If necessary, the aorta may need to be reclamped until the patient is further hydrated and other corrective measures are instituted.

○   **How does the surgical approach to abdominal aortic aneurysm (AAA) repair relate to postoperative pain?**

The classic approach to the abdominal aorta is through a midline vertical abdominal incision. However, this approach causes more postoperative pain and respiratory impairment than a transverse abdominal incision or a retroperitoneal approach.

○   **What is the major cause of perioperative morbidity and mortality in patients undergoing AAA repair?**

Myocardial infarction is by far the greatest cause of postoperative mortality, responsible for 55% of deaths after this surgery. Lesser causes are renal failure, visceral ischemia, and hepatic failure. Schermerhorn et al., reported that when compared with open repair, endovascular repair of abdominal aortic aneurysm is associated with lower short-term rates of death and complications (1.2% vs. 4.8%, $P < 0.001$), for example, myocardial infarction (7.0% vs. 9.4%, $P < 0.001$), pneumonia (9.3% vs. 17.4%, $P < 0.001$), acute renal failure (5.5% vs. 10.9%, $P < 0.001$), and need for dialysis (0.4% vs. 0.5%, $P = 0.047$). Conversion from endovascular repair to open repair occurred in 1.6% of patients. However, the late re-interventions related to abdominal aortic aneurysm are shown to be more common after endovascular repair [Schermerhorn et al., 2008. See reference on page 531].

○   **Which type of anesthesia is safest for this patient: general, regional, or a combination of both?**

There are no well-controlled studies that suggest a greater safety profile for any specific type of anesthetic. The choice must be individualized based on the patient's status and coexisting diseases. The placement of an epidural catheter may be helpful to control postoperative pain and promote postoperative ambulation and pulmonary toilet.

○   **Can an epidural catheter be safely placed if the patient is going to be heparinized intraoperatively?**

It is safe to insert the catheter if the patient's coagulation status is normal at the time of catheter placement. The concern that exists with placing a catheter in an anticoagulated patient is the formation of an epidural hematoma, and the difficulty of diagnosing this postoperatively (vs. cord ischemia from the surgery itself). The epidural catheter should be left in place until the patient's coagulation status has normalized, at which time it can be safely removed.

○ **What are the cardiovascular effects of applying a cross-clamp to the abdominal aorta?**

The physiologic effects of clamping the abdominal aorta mimic those discussed for the thoracic aorta. Afterload is significantly increased, and blood flow to the area above the clamp (coronary arteries, CNS) is augmented at the expense of the circulation below the level of the clamp. Suprarenal clamping will significantly decrease renal blood flow and GFR, but even clamping distal to the renal arteries has been shown to decrease flow to the kidneys. As is the case with thoracic aneurysm repair, renal-dose dopamine may have a protective effect.

○ **What is the mechanism for ischemia during aortic cross-clamping?**

There are several pathways that lead to ischemia. The most obvious is the reduction of blood flow distal to the clamp site, with a resultant increase in anaerobic metabolism. The release of mediators and free radicals may also worsen ischemia. The heart, despite an increase in coronary blood flow, may suffer ischemia secondary to working against an enhanced afterload.

○ **What are the hemodynamic effects of cross-clamp removal from the abdominal aorta?**

The "declamping shock" seen with thoracic aortic aneurysm clamp release is also seen in this case. Afterload is significantly reduced, and the release of humoral mediators further promotes vasodilation. Volume expansion beginning 30 minutes before cross-clamp removal may attenuate the response; severe and persistent hypotension may require temporary reapplication of the aortic cross-clamp.

○ **A 74-year-old female scheduled for left carotid endarterectomy presents for her preoperative evaluation. What medical conditions is she likely to have?**

Patients with carotid artery atherosclerosis have a high likelihood of having arterial plaques in other vascular beds. Up to 50% of patients have coexisting coronary artery disease, and hypertension is present in up to 80% of patients. Other conditions, such as diabetes and chronic renal insufficiency, are also correlated to carotid disease.

○ **What are the different methods of ensuring adequate cerebral perfusion during carotid endarterectomy?**

The best measure of adequate cerebral perfusion is to perform repeated neurologic tests on the patient during the procedure. The ability to count backwards or repeat a series of objects is a good indicator of adequate perfusion. Obviously, this can only be done when the case is performed under local or regional anesthesia. If general anesthesia is used, methods to assess cerebral perfusion include EEG monitoring, SSEP monitoring, internal carotid stump pressure, transcranial Doppler, mixed jugular venous O_2 saturation, and transconjunctival O_2 tension.

○ **Is the EEG an effective method to measure cerebral blood flow?**

While the EEG (either processed or unprocessed) is often used during carotid endarterectomy, the EEG itself is not a direct monitor of cerebral blood flow. It acts as a functional monitor and indicates that specific intracerebral areas may be at risk for infarction. Unfortunately it suffers from low specificity; conditions such as hypothermia, hypocarbia, and deep anesthesia mimic the EEG signs of inadequate perfusion.

○ **Is SSEP monitoring an effective method to measure cerebral blood flow?**

While SSEPs are also frequently used, there is mounting evidence that they may in fact overpredict the presence of ischemia, resulting in unnecessary shunting.

○ **Is the internal carotid stump pressure a reliable indicator of cerebral blood flow?**

Proponents of the carotid stump pressure suggest that it is an accurate measure of collateral intracerebral flow. However, it is also marked by a lack of specificity; anesthetic agents have been shown to alter the stump pressure without reducing CBF. In awake patients, changes in the stump pressure do not always correlate with alterations in mental status, which is considered a better indicator of cerebral perfusion.

○ **Is the transcranial Doppler an effective method to measure cerebral blood flow?**

The Doppler is an excellent method of measuring middle cerebral artery flow velocity, and is therefore a good choice to monitor CBF after carotid clamp application. As an added benefit, the Doppler is also sensitive at detecting intra-arterial air or embolic material.

○ **Is the mixed jugular O_2 saturation a reliable indicator of cerebral blood flow?**

The mixed jugular O_2 saturation is an indicator of global CBF; a drop in venous saturation is an indicator of enhanced extraction of oxygen from the arterial blood. This indicates either a reduction in flow or an increased $CMRO_2$ without an accompanying increase in CBF (or both). However, the mixing of venous blood from both hemispheres of the brain gives no indication of the location of the oxygen deficit.

○ **Is the transconjunctival O_2 a reliable indicator of adequate cerebral blood flow?**

There appears to be little or no correlation between transconjunctival O_2 saturation and CBF.

○ **What are the advantages of regional anesthesia for this patient? General anesthesia?**

The primary advantage of regional anesthesia is the ability to constantly ensure adequate CBF by repeatedly performing basic neurologic tests. However, general anesthesia can be safely used if CBF is monitored via an alternative method. Advantages of general anesthesia include a completely still operating field and the ability to reduce $CMRO_2$ (hypothermia, barbiturates, etc.) should hypoperfusion develop. However, 2004 meta-analysis of the seven available randomized trials continues to show no significant difference in outcome between regional and general anesthesia [Rerkasem et al., 2004. See reference on 531].

○ **If regional anesthesia is chosen, which nerves need to be blocked?**

The patient must be blocked from the C2 to the C4 dermatomes ipsilaterally. This can be accomplished with a combination of a superficial and deep cervical plexus block. The anesthesiologist must avoid deep palpation in the vicinity of the carotid artery as this may trigger a bradycardic reflex or dislodge a portion of the atherosclerotic plaque.

○ **Since CO_2 causes arterial vasodilatation, won't hypercapnia have the beneficial effect of increasing CBF?**

While CO_2 does cause arterial vasodilatation, the arteries in the ischemic portion of the brain are already maximally dilated. Raising the CO_2 will therefore vasodilate the arteries in the well-perfused area of the brain, resulting in luxury perfusion there at the expense of intracerebral steal from the hypoperfused areas.

○ **In what range would you aim to maintain the patient's blood pressure during the procedure?**

Initially, the pressure should be maintained in the normal to high-normal range, as this promotes collateral CBF. If necessary, an α-agonist should be used to maintain the blood pressure. After the clamp is removed, the pressure should be allowed to return to normal, or kept slightly below normal, to decrease stress on the carotid suture line.

○ **How would you manage hemodynamic instability during the surgery?**

Patients initially demonstrate hypertension and/or tachycardia secondary to anxiety and pain. Several studies have shown that patients receiving α-receptor agonists (either clonidine or dexmedetomidine) benefit from a smoother hemodynamic course. Manipulation of the carotid sinus may result in a vagal-mediated bradycardia with hypotension; antimuscarinic agents are useful at this stage of the procedure.

○ **Would you expect intraoperative bradycardia during the procedure?**

Bradycardia is typically seen as a result of stimulation of the carotid sinus. The sinus, which is innervated by branches of CN IX, synapses with CN X to modulate the decrease in heart rate. Vagolytic drugs are effective at managing the bradycardia, but the reflex often abates spontaneously when the sinus is not being manipulated.

○ **Is bradycardia also associated with carotid stenting?**

Bradycardia can result from carotid stenting via the same mechanism discussed in the previous question. Parodi et al., reported 16% incidence of bradycardia and 3% asystole without consequence in a series of 100 patients who underwent carotid angioplasty and stent placement. There was 11% incidence of hypotension. [Parodi et al., 2005. See reference on 531].

○ **What physiologic changes would you expect to result from bilateral carotid endarterectomy?**

The physiologic changes seen are the result of diminished function of the carotid bodies and sinuses. The carotid bodies are sensitive to PaO_2, and to a lesser extent pH and $PaCO_2$ (in contrast to the central chemoreceptors, which are more attuned to changes in $PaCO_2$). Alteration in carotid body function results in a decreased hypoxic ventilator drive and an increased resting partial pressure of arterial CO_2. The central chemoreceptors therefore become the primary chemoregulators of ventilation.

○ **Postoperatively, the patient has a delayed emergence from general anesthesia. What would you include in your differential diagnosis?**

In this case, as in any case of delayed emergence from anesthesia, three factors must be considered:

- Metabolic abnormalities: Hypoglycemia, hyponatremia, hypothermia, and hypercarbia.
- Pharmacologic effects: Residual volatile anesthetic and incomplete reversal of paralytic agents.
- Neurologic compromise: In this patient, this must be your primary concern. Conditions such as ischemic CVA must top the list. Reperfusion injury is also a possibility – the arterioles distal to the carotid occlusion, faced with chronic hypoperfusion, may have lost the ability to vasoconstrict. Postoperatively, they may be unable to accommodate the increase in CBF, and may therefore rupture.

○   **You are called to the PACU 20 minutes postoperatively to evaluate respiratory distress in your patient. What conditions are in your differential diagnosis?**

Carotid endarterectomy (especially when performed bilaterally) is associated with a prolonged dysfunction of the carotid body. Patients will therefore lose some of their hypoxemic drive to hyperventilate, and may exist with a baseline elevated $PaCO_2$. Other concerns are hematoma formation (with tracheal impingement), tension pneumothorax (from air escaping from the incision site into the mediastinum), and vocal cord paralysis from intraoperative tension on the laryngeal nerves.

Key Terms

Abdominal aortic cross-clamp: hemodynamics
Aortic clamping: ischemia mechanism
Aortic cross-clamp: cardiovascular complications
Aortic cross-clamp: physiologic changes
Bilateral carotid endarterectomy: physiology
Bradycardia during carotid surgery
Cardiopulmonary bypass: aortic dissection
Carotid endarterectomy: blocking hemodynamic response
Carotid endarterectomy: chemoreceptors

Carotid endarterectomy: CNS monitoring
Carotid endarterectomy: perioperative risks
Carotid stent: bradycardia causes/prevention
Jugular bulb oxygen saturation
Monitoring brainstem ischemia: methods
Symptoms of bilateral carotid endarterectomy
Thoracic aneurysm repair: complications
Transcranial Doppler utility in carotid endarterectomy

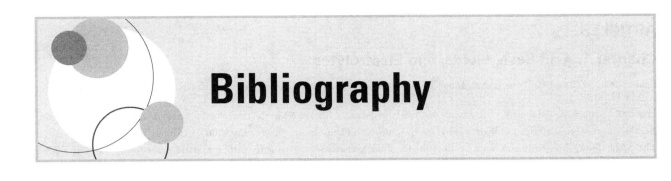

Bibliography

BOOKS

Barash PH, Cullen BF, Stoelting RK, Cahalan MK, Stock MC. *Clinical Anesthesia*. 6th ed. Philadelphia, PA: Lippincott Williams & Wilkins; 2009:644–695.

Benzon H, Raja SN, Fishman SM, Liu S, Cohen SP. *Essentials of Pain Medicine*. 3rd ed. Philadelphia, PA: Elsevier Saunders; 2011.

Chestnut DH, Polley LS, Tsen LC, Wong CA. *Chestnut's Obstetric Anesthesia Principles and Practice*. 4th ed. Philadelphia, PA: Mosby Elsevier; 2009.

Deutschman CS, Neligan PJ. *Evidence-Based Practice of Critical Care*. Philadelphia, PA: Elsevier Saunders; 2010.

DiNardo JA, Zvara DA. *Anesthesia for Cardiac Surgery*. 3rd ed. Oxford: Blackwell Publishing; 2008.

Dorsch JA, Dorsch SE. *Understanding Anesthesia Equipment*. 5th ed. Philadelphia, PA: Lippincott Williams & Wilkins; 2008.

Eisenach JC. Intraspinal analgesia in obstetrics. In: *Shnider and Levinson's Anesthesia for Obstetrics*. 4th ed. Philadelphia, PA: Lippincott Williams and Wilkins; 2002:152–153.

Friedman LM, Furberg CD, DeMets DL. *Fundamentals of Clinical Trials*. New York: Springer; 1998.

Hines RL, Marschall KE. *Stoelting's Anesthesia and Co-Existing Disease*. 5th ed. Philadelphia, PA: Churchill Livingstone Inc; 2008.

Irwin RS, Rippe JM. *Irwin and Rippe's Intensive Care Medicine*. 6th ed. Philadelphia, PA: Lippincott Williams and Wilkins; 2008.

Longnecker DE. *Anesthesiology*. New York: McGraw-Hill, 2008.

Miller RD. *Miller's Anesthesia*. 7th ed. Philadelphia, PA: Churchill Livingstone Inc; 2010.

Morgan GE. *Clinical Anesthesiology*. 4th ed. New York: McGraw-Hill; 2006.

Motoyama E, Davis P. *Smith's Anesthesia for Infants and Children*. 8th ed. Philadelphia, PA: Elsevier Saunders; 2011.

Norman GR, Streiner DL. *PDQ Statistics*. Hamilton: B.C. Decker Inc; 1999.

Sidebotham D. *Practical Perioperative Transesophageal Echocardiography*. 2nd ed. Philadelphia, PA: Elsevier Saunders; 2011.

Spiess BD, Spencer RK, Shander A. *Perioperative Transfusion Medicine*. 2nd ed. Philadelphia, PA: Lippincott Williams & Wilkins; 2006.

Vincent J, Abraham E, Kochanek P, Moore FA. *Textbook of Critical Care*. 6th ed. Philadelphia, PA: Elsevier Saunders; 2011.

COURSES/CONFERENCES

ASA Refresher Course; 2010, 2011.

ASA Workshop on Statistics; 2009.

ARTICLES

Chapter 1. Acid Base, Fluids, and Electrolytes

Brunkhorst FM, Engel C, Bloos F, et al. Intensive insulin therapy and pentastarch resuscitation in severe sepsis. *N Engl J Med.* 2008; 358:125–139.

Hartog CS, Bauer M, Reinhart K. The efficacy and safety of colloid resuscitation in the critically ill. *Anesth Analg.* 2011;112:156–164.

Kozek-Langenecker SA. Effects of hydroxyethyl starch solutions on hemostasis. *Anesthesiology.*2005;103:654.

The SAFE Study Investigators. Saline or albumin for fluid resuscitation in patients with traumatic brain injury. *N Engl J Med.* 2007;357:874–884.

Chapter 2. Airway and Intubation

Brimacombe J, Keller C. The ProSeal laryngeal mask airway. *Anesthesiol Clin North Am.* 2002;20:871–891.

Hung OR, Pytka S, Morris I, et al. Light wand failure rate. *Anesthesiology.* 1995;83:509–514.

Loeser EA, Orr DL 2nd, Bennett GM, Stanley TH. Endotracheal tube cuff design and postoperative sore throat. *Anesthesiology.* 1976; 45:684–687.

Peppard SB, Dickens JH. Laryngeal injury following short term intubation. *Ann Otol Rhinol Laryngol.* 1983;92:327–330.

Perry JJ, Lee J, Wells G. Are intubation conditions using rocuronium equivalent to those using succinylcholine? *Acad Emerg Med.* 2002;9:813–823.

Practice guidelines for management of the difficult airway: an updated report by the American Society of Anesthesiologists Task Force on Management of the Difficult Airway. American Society of Anesthesiologists Task Force on Management of the Difficult Airway. *Anesthesiology.* 2003;98:1269–1277.

Chapter 3. Allergic Reactions

Bochner BS, Lichtenstein LM. Anaphylaxis. *N Engl J Med.* 1991;324:1785–1790.

Delaney A, Carter A, Fisher M. The prevention of anaphylactoid reactions to iodinated radiological contrast media: a systematic review. *BMC Med Imaging.* 2006;6:2.

Chapter 4. Anesthesia Risks/Standards/Billing

Cheney FW, Posner KL, Lee LA, Caplan RA, Domino KB. Trends in anesthesia-related death and brain damage: a closed claims analysis. *Anesthesiology.* 2006;105:1081–1086.

Lagasse RS. Anesthesia safety: model or myth? *Anesthesiology.* 2002;97:1609–1617.

Sebel PS, Bowdle TA, Ghoneim MM, et al. The incidence of awareness during anesthesia: a multicenter United States study. *Anesth Analg.* 2004;99:833–839.

Chapter 5. Anesthesia and the Liver

Landowitz RJ, Currier A. Clinical practice. Postexposure prophylaxis for HIV infection. *N Engl J Med.* 2009;361:1768–1775.

Chapter 6. Aspiration Pneumonitis

Sakai T, Planinsic RM, Quinlan JJ, Handley LJ, Kim TY, Hilmi IA. The incidence and outcome of perioperative pulmonary aspiration in a university hospital: a 4-year retrospective analysis. *Anesth Analg.* 2006;103:941–947.

Chapter 7. Autonomic Pharmacology and Physiology

Colachis SC III, Clinchot DM. Autonomic hyperreflexia associated with recurrent cardiac arrest; case report. *Spinal Cord.* 1997;35: 256–257.

Chapter 8. Blood Therapy

ASA Task Force on Perioperative Blood Transfusion and Adjuvant Therapies. Practice guidelines for perioperative blood transfusion and adjuvant therapies. *Anesthesiology.* 2006;105:198–208.

Boliger D, Görlinger K, Tanaka KA. Pathophysiology and treatment of coagulopathy in massive hemorrhage and hemodilution. *Anesthesiology.* 2010;113:1205–1219.

Dodd RY. Current risk for transfusion transmitted infections. *Curr Opin Hematol.* 2007;14:671–676.

Hendrickson JE, Hillyer CD. Noninfectious serious hazards of transfusion. *Anesth Analg.* 2009;108:759–769.

Chapter 9. Cardiac Physiology and Surgery

American College of Cardiology Foundation/American Heart Association Task Force on Practice Guidelines, American Society of Echocardiography, American Society of Nuclear Cardiology, et al. 2009 ACCF/AHA focused update on perioperative beta blockade. *J Am Coll Cardiol.* 2009;54:2102–2128.

American Society of Anesthesiologists. Practice advisory for the perioperative management of patients with cardiac implantable electronic devices: pacemakers and implantable cardioverter-defibrillators: an updated report by the American Society of Anesthesiologists Task Force on Perioperative Management of Patients with Cardiac Implantable Electronic Devices. *Anesthesiology.* 2011;114:247–261.

Antman EM, Hand M, Armstrong PW, et al. 2007 focused update of the ACC/AHA 2004 guidelines for the management of patients with ST-elevation myocardial infarction. *J Am Coll Cardiol.* 2008;51:210–247.

Fleisher LA, Beckman JA, Brown KA, et al. ACC/AHA 2007 guidelines on perioperative cardiovascular evaluation and care for noncardiac surgery: executive summary: a report of the American College of Cardiology/American Heart Association Task Force on Practice Guidelines (Writing Committee to Revise the 2002 Guidelines on Perioperative Cardiovascular Evaluation for Noncardiac Surgery): developed in collaboration with the American Society of Echocardiography, American Society of Nuclear Cardiology, Heart Rhythm Society, Society of Cardiovascular Anesthesiologists, Society for Cardiovascular Angiography and Interventions, Society for Vascular Medicine and Biology, and Society for Vascular Surgery. *J Am Coll Cardiol.* 2007;50:1707–1732.

Gauthier N, Anselm AH, Haddad H. New therapies in acute decompensated heart failure. *Curr Opin Cardiol.* 2008;23:134–140.

Leuchte HH, Schwaiblmair M, Baumgartner RA, et al. Hemodynamic response to sildenafil, nitric oxide, and iloprost in primary pulmonary hypertension. *Chest.* 2004;125:580–586.

Memtsoudis S, Rosenberger P, Loffler M, et al. The usefulness of transesophageal echocardiography during intraoperative cardiac arrest in noncardiac surgery. *Anesth Analg.* 2006;102:1653–1657.

Newman MF, Wolman R, Kanchuger M, et al. Multicenter preoperative stroke risk index for patients undergoing coronary artery bypass graft surgery. Multicenter Study of Perioperative Ischemia (McSPI) Research Group. *Circulation.* 1996;94:II74–II80.

Porsche R, Brenner ZR. Allergy to protamine sulfate. *Heart Lung.*1999;28:418–428.

Siobal RRT. Pulmonary vasodilators. *Respir Care.* 2007;52:886–899.

Wilson W, Taubert KA, Gewitz M, et al. Prevention of infective endocarditis: guidelines from the American Heart Association: a guideline from the American Heart Association Rheumatic Fever, Endocarditis, and Kawasaki Disease Committee, Council on Cardiovascular Disease in the Young, and the Council on Clinical Cardiology, Council on Cardiovascular Surgery and Anesthesia, and the Quality of Care and Outcomes Research Interdisciplinary Working Group. *Circulation.* 2007;116:1736–1754.

Chapter 10. Cardiopulmonary Resuscitation

Peberdy MA, Callaway CW, Neumar RW, et al. Part 9: post-cardiac arrest care: 2010 American Heart Association guidelines for cardiopulmonary resuscitation and emergency cardiovascular care. *Circulation.* 2010;122:S768–S786.

Chapter 11. Caudal, Epidural and Spinal Anesthesia

Auroy Y, Narchi P, Messiah A, Litt L, Rouvier B, Samii K. Serious complications related to regional anesthesia: results of a prospective survey in France. *Anesthesiology.* 1997;87:479–486.

Crystal GJ, Salem MR. Review article: the Bainbridge and the "reverse" Bainbridge reflexes: history, physiology, and clinical relevance. *Anesth Analg.* 2012;114:520–532.

Hakim SM. Cosyntropin for prophylaxis against postdural puncture headache after accidental dural puncture. *Anesthesiology.* 2010;113:413–420.

Horlocker TT, Wedel DJ, Rowlingson JC, et al. Regional anesthesia in the patient receiving antithrombotic or thrombolytic therapy. American Society of Regional Anesthesia and Pain Medicine evidence-based guidelines (third edition). *Reg Anesth Pain Med.* 2010;35:64–101.

Levine E, Muravchick S, Gold MI. Density of normal human cerebrospinal fluid and tetracaine solutions. *Anesth Analg.* 1981;60:814–817.

Rodgers A, Walker N, Schug S, et al. Reduction of postoperative mortality and morbidity with epidural or spinal anaesthesia: results from overview of randomised trials. *BMJ.* 2000;321:1495.

Sessler DI. Neuraxial anesthesia and surgical site infection. *Anesthesiology.* 2010;113:265–267.

Zaric D, Pace NL. Transient neurologic symptoms (TNS) following spinal anaesthesia with lidocaine versus other local anaesthetics. *Cochrane Database Syst Rev.* 2009;(2):CD003006.

Chapter 12. Chronic Pain Management

Harden RN, Bruehl S, Stanton-Hicks M, Wilson PR. Proposed new diagnostic criteria for complex regional pain syndrome. *Pain Med.* 2007;8:326–331.

Merskey H, Bogduk N. *Classification of Chronic Pain: Descriptions of Chronic Pain Syndromes and Definitions of Pain Terms.* Seattle, WA: IASP Press; 1994.

Oakley JC, Prager JP. Spinal cord stimulation mechanism of action. *Spine.* 2002;27(22):2574–2583.

Polati E, Luzzani A, Schweiger V, Finco G, Ischia S. The role of neurolytic celiac plexus block in the treatment of pancreatic cancer pain. *Transplant Proc.* 2008;40:1200–1204.

Portenoy RK, Hagen NA. Breakthrough pain: definition, prevalence and characteristics. *Pain.* 1990;41:273–281.

Wilson PR, Low PA, Bedder MD, Covington EC, Rauck RL. Diagnostic algorithm for complex regional pain syndromes. In: Janig W, Stanton-Hicks M, eds. *Reflex Sympathetic Dystrophy: A Reappraisal.* Seattle, WA: IASP Press; 1996:93–106.

Chapter 13. Clinical Pharmacology

Canadian Cardiovascular Society, American Academy of Family Physicians, American College of Cardiology, et al. 2007 focused update of the ACC/AHA 2004 guidelines for the management of patients with ST-elevation myocardial infarction: a report of the American College of Cardiology/American Heart Association Task Force on Practice Guidelines. *J Am Coll Cardiol.* 2008;51:210–247.

Jacqueline M, Dzankic S, Manku K, Yuan S. The prevalence and predictors of the use of alternative medicine in presurgical patients in five California hospitals. *Anesth Analg.* 2001;93:1062–1068.

Pfeffer MA, Greaces SC, Arnold JM, et al. Early versus delayed angiotensin-converting enzyme inhibition therapy in acute myocardial infarction. The healing and early afterload reducing therapy trial. *Circulation.* 1997;95:2643–2651.

Salpeter S, Greyber E, Pasternak G, Salpeter E. Risk of fatal and nonfatal lactic acidosis with metformin use in type 2 diabetes mellitus. *Cochrane Database Syst Rev.* 2006;(1):CD002967.

Chapter 14. Critical Care Medicine

Briccard AF. Prone position in ARDS. *Chest.* 2003;123:1334–1335.

Casaer MP, Hermans G, Wilmer A, Van den Berghe G. Impact of early parenteral nutrition completing enteral nutrition in adult critically ill patients (EPaNIC trial): a study protocol and statistical analysis plan for a randomized controlled trial. *Trials.* 2011;12:21.

Jones AE, FochtA, Horton JM, Kline JA. Prospective external validation of the clinical effectiveness of an emergency department based early goal directed therapy protocol for severe sepsis and septic shock. *Chest.* 2001;132:425–432.

Latronico N, Peli E, Botteri M. Critical illness myopathy and neuropathy. *Curr Opin Crit Care.* 2005;11:126–132.

Ventilation with lower tidal volumes as compared with traditional tidal volumes for acute lung injury and the acute respiratory distress syndrome. The acute respiratory distress syndrome network. *N Engl J Med.* 2000;342:1301–1308.

Chapter 16. Endocrine

Preiser JC, Devos P, Ruiz-Santana S, et al. A prospective randomised multi-centre controlled trial on tight glucose control by intensive insulin therapy in adult intensive care units: the Glucontrol study. *Intensive Care Med.* 2009;35:1738–1748.

Sawka AM, Jaeschke R, Singh RJ, Young WF Jr. A comparison of biochemical tests for pheochromocytoma: measurement of fractionated plasma metanephrines compared with the combination of 24-hour urinary metanephrines and catecholamines. *J Clin Endocrinol Metab.* 2003;88:553–558.

Sprung CL, Annane D, Keh D, et al. Hydrocortisone therapy for patients with septic shock. *N Engl J Med.* 2008;358:111–124.

The NICR-SUGAR Study Investigators. Intensive versus conventional glucose control in critically ill patients. *N Engl J Med.* 2009; 360:1283–1297.

Wingert DJ, Freisen SR, Iliopoulos JI, Pierce GE, Thomas JH, Hermreck AS. Post-thyroidectomy hypocalcemia. Incidence and risk factors. *Am J Surg.* 1986;152:606–610.

Chapter 17. ENT Surgery

Dulguerov P, Marchal F, Lehmann W. Postparotidectomy facial nerve paralysis: possible etiologic factors and results with routine facial nerve monitoring. *Laryngoscope.* 1999;109:754–762.

Saifeldeen K, Evans R. Ludwig's angina. *Emerg Med J.* 2004;21:242–243.

Windfuhr JP, Schloendorff G, Sesterhenn AM, Prescher A, Kremer B. A devastating outcome after adenoidectomy and tonsillectomy: ideas for improved prevention and management. *Otolaryngol Head Neck Surg.* 2009;140:191–196.

Chapter 18. Genitourinary and Renal Surgery

Abbott MA, Samuel JR, Webb DR. Anaesthesia for extracorporeal shock wave lithotripsy. *Anaesthesia.* 1985;40:1065–1072.

Hahn RG. Transurethral resection syndrome from extravascular absorption of irrigating fluid. *Scand J Urol Nephrol.* 1993;27:387–394.

Papademetriou V, Doumas M, Tsioufis K. Renal sympathetic denervation for the treatment of difficult-to-control or resistant hypertension. *Int J Hypertens.* 2011;2011:196518 [published online].

Chapter 19. Geriatric Patients

American College of Cardiology Foundation/American Heart Association Task Force on Practice Guidelines, American Society of Echocardiography, American Society of Nuclear Cardiology, et al. 2009 ACCF/AHA focused update on perioperative beta blockade. *J Am Coll Cardiol.* 2009;54:2102–2128.

Fleisher LA, Beckman JA, Brown KA, et al. ACC/AHA 2007 guidelines on perioperative cardiovascular evaluation and care for noncardiac surgery. *J Am Coll Cardiol.* 2007;50:159–242.

Woon VC, Lim KH. Acute myocardial infarction in the elderly—the differences compared with the young. *Singapore Med J.* 2003; 44:414–418.

Zeeh J, Platt D. The aging liver: structure and functional changes and their consequences for drug treatment in old age. *Gerontology.* 2002; 48:121–127.

Chapter 20. GI Disorders and Obesity

Brown CD, Higgins M, Donato KA, et al. Body mass index and the prevalence of hypertension and dyslipidemia. *Obes Res.* 2000;8: 605–619.

Foster NM, McGory ML, Zingmond DS, Ko CY. Small bowel obstruction: a population based appraisal. *J Am Coll Surg.* 2006;203(2):170.

Ingrande J, Lemmens HJM. Dose adjustment of anesthetics in the morbidly obese. *Br J Anaesth.* 2010;105:i16–i23.

Nellgård P. Mechanisms of fluid losses in small-bowel obstruction. *Acta Anaesthesiol Scand.* 1996;40:1253.

Tsueda K, Debrand M, Zeok SS, et al. Obesity supine death syndrome: reports of two morbidly obese patients. *Anesth Analg.* 1979; 58:345–347.

Chapter 21. Hemostasis

Federici AB, Mannucci PM. Management of inherited von Willebrand disease in 2007. *Ann Med.* 2007;39:346–358.

Gogarten W, Vandermuelen E, Van Aken H, et al. Regional anaesthesia and antithrombotic agents: recommendations of the European Society of Anaesthesiology. *Eur J Anaesthesiol.* 2010;27:999–1015.

Koutrouvelis A, Abouleish A, Indrikovs A, Alperin J. Case scenario: emergency reversal of oral anticoagulation. *Anesthesiology.* 2010;113:1192–1197.

Warkentin TE, Greinacher A. Heparin-induced thrombocytopenia: recognition, treatment, and prevention: the seventh ACCP conference on antithrombotic and thrombolytic therapy. *Chest.* 2004;126:311S–337S.

Chapter 22. Hypothermia

Kurtz A, Sessler DI, Lenhardt R. Perioperative normothermia to reduce the incidence of surgical-wound infection and shorten hospitalization. *N Engl J Med.* 1996;334:1209–1215.

Peberdy MA, Callaway CW, Neumar RW, et al. Part 9: post-cardiac arrest care: 2010 American Heart Association guidelines for cardiopulmonary resuscitation and emergency cardiovascular care. *Circulation.* 2010;122:S768–S786.

Chapter 23. Inhalation Agents

Myles PS, Leslie K, Chan MT, et al. Avoidance of nitrous oxide for patients undergoing major surgery: a randomized controlled trial. *Anesthesiology.* 2007;107:221–231.

Nijoku D, Laster MJ, Gong DH, Eger EI 2nd, Reed GF, Martin JL. Biotransformation of halothane, enflurane, isoflurane, and desflurane to trifluoroacetylated liver proteins: association between protein acylation and hepatic injury. *Anesth Analg.* 1997;84:173–178.

Chapter 24. Local Anesthetics

Drasner K. Chloroprocaine spinal anesthesia: back to the future? *Anesth Analg.* 2005;100:549–552.

Hahh I, Hoffman RS, Nelson LS. EMLA-induced methemoglobinemia and systemic topical anesthetic toxicity. *J Emerg Med.* 2004;26:85–88.

Jeng CL, Torillo TM, Rosenblatt MA. Complications of peripheral nerve blocks. *Br J Anaesth.* 2010;105:i97–i107.

Chapter 25. Machines

National Institute for Occupational Safety and Health. *Occupational Exposure to Waste Anesthetic Gases and Vapors: Criteria for a Recommended Standard.* Cincinnati, OH: US Department of Health, Education, and Welfare, Public Health Service, Center for Disease Control, National Institute for Occupational Safety and Health; 1977:77–140. Publication DHEW (NIOSH).

Occupational Safety and Health Administration. *Waste Anesthetic Gases.* Washington, DC: US Department of Labor; 1991. Publication 91–38.

Chapter 26. Muscle Relaxants

Brull SJ, Murphy GS. Residual neuromuscular block: lessons unlearned. Part II: methods to reduce the risk of residual weakness. *Anesth Analg.* 2010;111:129–140.

Hemmerling TM, Donati F. Neuromuscular blockade at the larynx, the diaphragm and the corrugator supercilii muscle: a review. *Can J Anaesth.* 2003;50:779–794.

Hemmerling TM, Schmidt J, Hanusa C, Wolf T, Schmidt H. Simultaneous determination of neuromuscular block at the larynx, diaphragm, adductor pollicis, orbicularis oculi and corrugator supercilii muscles. *Br J Anaesth.* 2000;85:856–860.

Miller RD, Ward TA. Monitoring and pharmacological reversal of a nondepolarizing neuromuscular blockade should be routine [editorial]. *Anesth Analg.* 2010;111:3–5.

Plaud B, Debaene B, Donati F. The corrugator supercilli, not the orbicularis oculli reflects rocuronium neuromuscular blockade at the laryngeal muscles. *Anesthesiology.* 2001;95:96–101.

Srivastava A, Hunter JM. Reversal of neuromuscular block. *Br J Anaesth.* 2009;103:115–129.

Chapter 27. Neonatal Anesthesia

Kattwinkel J, Perlman JM, Aziz K, et al. Part 15: neonatal resuscitation: 2010 American Heart Association guidelines for cardiopulmonary resuscitation and emergency cardiovascular care. *Circulation.* 2010;122:S909–S919.

Stege G, Fenton A, Jaffray B. Nihilism in the 1990s: the true mortality of congenital diaphragmatic hernia. *Pediatrics.* 2003;112:532–535.

Chapter 28. Neurosurgery

Coleman WP, Benzel D, Cahill DW, et al. A critical appraisal of the reporting of the National Acute Spinal Cord Injury Studies (II and III) of methylprednisolone in acute spinal cord injury. *J Spinal Disord.* 2000;13:185–199.

Delbert E, Alyagari V, Diringer MN. Reversible left ventricular dysfunction associated with raised troponin I after subarachnoid haemorrhage does not preclude successful heart transplantation. *Heart.* 2000;84:205–207.

Fraticelli AT, Cholley BP, Losser MR, Saint Maurice JP, Payen D. Milrinone for the treatment of cerebral vasospasm after aneurysmal subarachnoid hemorrhage. *Stroke.* 2008;39:893–898.

Peberdy MA, Callaway CW, Neumar RW, et al. Part 9: post-cardiac arrest care: 2010 American Heart Association guidelines for cardiopulmonary resuscitation and emergency cardiovascular care. *Circulation.* 2010;122:S768–S786.

Rao U, Tetzlaff JE. Perioperative management of patients with chronic spinal cord injury. *Am J Anesthesiol.* 2000;27(6):355–358.

van Middendorp JJ, Hosman AJ, Donders AR, et al. A clinical prediction rule for ambulation outcomes after traumatic spinal cord injury: a longitudinal cohort study. *Lancet.* 2011;377:1004–1010.

Chapter 29. Nonopioid Intravenous Anesthetics

Hepner DL, Castells MC. Anaphylaxis during the perioperative period. *Anesth Analg.* 2003;97:1381–1395.

Kam PCA, Cardone D. Propofol infusion syndrome. *Anaesthesia.* 2007;62:690–701.

Chapter 30. Obstetrics

American College of Obstetricians and Gynecologists Committee on Practice Bulletins-Obstetrics, Society for Maternal-Fetal Medicine, ACOG Joint Editorial Committee. ACOG practice bulletin #56: multiple gestation: complicated twin, triplet, and high-order multifetal pregnancy. *Obstet Gynecol.* 2004;104:869–883.

Barnes EJ, Eben F, Patterson D. Direct current cardioversion during pregnancy should be performed with facilities available for fetal monitoring and emergency caesarean section. *Br J Obstet Gynecol.* 2002;109:1406–1407.

Berg CJ, Callaghan WM, Syverson C, Henderson Z. Pregnancy-related mortality in the United States, 1998 to 2005. *Obstet Gynecol.* 2010;116:1302–1309.

Chen LK, Lin CJ, Huang CH, et al. The effects of continuous epidural analgesia on Doppler velocimetry of uterine arteries during different periods of labour analgesia. *Br J Anaesth.* 2006;96:226–230.

Dyer RA, van Dyke D, Dresner A. The use of utrotonics during CS. *Int J Obstet Anesth.* 2010;19:313–319.

Edwards LE, Hellerstedt WL, Alton IR, et al. Pregnancy complications and birth outcomes in obese and normal-weight women: effects of gestational weight change. *Obstet Gynecol.* 1996;87:389–394.

Jouppila P, Jouppila R, Hollmen A, Koivula A: Lumbar epidural analgesia to improve intervillous blood flow during labor in severe preeclampsia. *Obstet Gynecol.* 1982;52:158.

Karaye KM, Henein MY. Peripartum cardiomyopathy: a review article. *Int J Cardiol.* 2011 Dec 20 [Epub ahead of print].

Kundra P, Khanna S, Habeebullah S, Ravishankar M. Manual displacement of the uterus during caesarean section. *Anaesthesia.* 2007;62:460–465.

Lew TW, Tay DH, Thomas E. Venous air embolism during cesarean section: more common than previously thought. *Anesth Analg.* 1993;77:448–452.

Miller DA, Chollet JA, Goodwin TM. Clinical risk factors for placenta previa-placenta accreta. *Am J Obstet Gynecol.* 1997;177:210–214.

Norris MC. Patient variables and the subarachnoid spread of hyperbaric bupivacaine in the term parturient. *Anesthesiology.* 1990;72:478–482.

Report of the National High Blood Pressure Education Program Working Group on High Blood Pressure in Pregnancy. *Am J Obstet Gynecol.* 2000;183:S1–S22.

Van de Velde M, Van Schoubroeck D, Lewi LE, et al. Remifentanil for fetal immobilization and maternal sedation during fetoscopic surgery. A randomized double blind comparison with diazepam. *Anesth Analg.* 2005;101:251–258.

Wong CA, Scavone BM, Peaceman AM, et al. The risk of cesarean delivery with neuraxial analgesia given early versus late in labor. *N Engl J Med.* 2005;352:655–665.

Chapter 31. Opioids and Substance Abuse

Baldini G, Bagry H, Aprikian A, Carli F. Postoperative urinary retention, anesthetic and perioperative considerations. *Anesthesiology.* 2009; 110:1139–1157.

Bryson EO, Silverstein JH. Addiction and substance abuse in anesthesiology. *Anesthesiology.* 2008;109:905–917.

Carvalho B. Respiratory depression after neuraxial opioids in the obstetric setting. *Anesth Analg.* 2008;107:956–961.

Krantz MJ, Lewkowiez L, Hays H, Woodroffe MA, Robertson AD, Mehler PS. Torsade de pointes associated with very-high-dose methadone. *Ann Intern Med.* 2002;137:501–504.

Chapter 32. Orthopedic Surgery

Buckley N. Regional vs. general anaesthesia in orthopaedics. *Can J Anaesth.* 1993;40:R104–R112.

Chang DJ, Paget SA. Neurologic complications of rheumatoid arthritis. *Rheum Dis Clin North Am.* 1993;19:955.

Deloughry JL, Griffiths R. Arterial tourniquets. *Contin Educ Anaesth Crit Care Pain.* 2009;9:56–60.

Geerts WH, Bergqvist D, Pineo GF, et al. Prevention of venous thromboembolism. American College of Chest Physicians evidence-based clinical practice guidelines (8th edition). *Chest.* 2008;133:381S–453S.

Horlocker TT. Regional anaesthesia in the patient receiving antithrombotic and antiplatelet therapy. *Br J Anaesth.* 2011;107(S1): i96–i106.

Jacob AK, Mantilla CB, Sviggum HP, Schroeder DR, Pagnano MW, Hebl JR. Perioperative nerve injury after total knee arthroplasty: regional anesthesia risk during a 20-year cohort study. *Anesthesiology.* 2011;114:311–317.

Kassim AKJ, Yoon P, Vorlicky LN. Complications of total hip arthroplasty. *Am J Orthop.* 2002;31:485.

Tapson VF. Acute pulmonary embolism. *N Engl J Med.* 2008;358:1037–1052.

Chapter 33. Outpatient Surgery

American Society of Anesthesiologists Committee. Practice guidelines for preoperative fasting and the use of pharmacologic agents to reduce the risk of pulmonary aspiration: application to healthy patients undergoing elective procedures: an updated report by the American Society of Anesthesiologists Committee on Standards and Practice Parameters. *Anesthesiology.* 2011;114:495–511.

Gordley KP, Basu CB. Optimal use of local anesthetics and tumescence. *Semin Plast Surg.* 2006;20:219–224.

Horlocker TT, Wedel DJ, Rowlingson JC, et al. Regional anesthesia in the patient receiving antithrombotic or thrombolytic therapy: American Society of Regional Anesthesia and Pain Medicine evidence-based guidelines (third edition). *Reg Anesth Pain Med.* 2010;35:64–101.

Le Manach Y, Perel A, Coriat P, Godet G, Bertrand M, Riou B. Early and delayed myocardial infarction after abdominal aortic surgery. *Anesthesiology.* 2005;102:885–891.

Rodgers A, Walker N, Schug S, et al. Reduction of postoperative mortality and morbidity with epidural or spinal anaesthesia: results from overview of randomised trials. *BMJ.* 2000;321:1493.

Chapter 34. Patient Monitors

American Society of Anesthesiologists Task Force on Central Venous Access, Rupp SM, Apfelbaum JL, et al. Practice guidelines for central venous access. A report by the American Society of Anesthesiologists Task Force on Central Venous Access. *Anesthesiology.* 2012;116:539–573.

Chapter 35. Patient Positioning

American Society of Anesthesiologists Task Force on Perioperative Visual Loss. Practice advisory for perioperative visual loss associated with spine surgery. An updated report by the American Society of Anesthesiologists Task Force on Perioperative Visual Loss. *Anesthesiology.* 2012;116:274–285.

Canbaz S, Turgut N, Halici U, Sunar H, Balci K, Duran E. Brachial plexus injury during open heart surgery—controlled prospective study. *Thorac Cardiovasc Surg.* 2005;53:295–299.

Cheney FW, Domino KB, Caplan RA, Posner KL. Nerve injury associated with anesthesia: a closed claims analysis. *Anesthesiology.* 1999;90:1062–1069.

Edgcombe H, Carter K, Yarrow S. Anaesthesia in the prone position. *Br J Anaesth*. 2008;100:165–183.

Lee LA. ASA postoperative visual loss registry: preliminary analysis of factors associated with spine operations. *ASA Newsletter*. 2003;67:7–8.

Postoperative Visual Loss Study Group. Risk factors associated with ischemic optic neuropathy after spinal fusion surgery. *Anesthesiology*. 2012;116:15–24.

Roth S. Perioperative visual loss: what do we know, what can we do? *Br J Anaesth*. 2009;103:i31–i40.

Chapter 36. Pediatric Anesthesia

American Society of Anesthesiologists Committee. Practice guidelines for preoperative fasting and the use of pharmacologic agents to reduce the risk of pulmonary aspiration: application to healthy patients undergoing elective procedures: an updated report by the American Society of Anesthesiologists Committee on Standards and Practice Parameters. *Anesthesiology*. 2011;114:495–511.

Freeman SB, Taft LF, Dooley KJ, et al. Population-based study of congenital heart defects in Down syndrome. *Am J Med Genet*. 1998;80:213–217.

Josephson CD, Su LL, Hillyer KL, Hillyer CD. Transfusion in the patient with sickle cell disease: a critical review of the literature and transfusion guidelines. *Transfus Med Rev*. 2007;21:118–133.

Oh AY, Kim JH, Hwang JW, Do SH, Jeon YT. Incidence of postoperative nausea and vomiting after paediatric strabismus surgery with sevoflurane or remifentanil–sevoflurane. *Br J Anaesth*. 2010;104:756–760.

Tait AR, Malviya S. Anesthesia for the child with an upper respiratory tract infection: still a dilemma? *Anesth Analg*. 2005;100:59–65.

Wilson W, Taubert KA, Gewitz M, et al. Prevention of infective endocarditis: guidelines from the American Heart Association: a guideline from the American Heart Association Rheumatic Fever, Endocarditis, and Kawasaki Disease Committee, Council on Cardiovascular Disease in the Young, and the Council on Clinical Cardiology, Council on Cardiovascular Surgery and Anesthesia, and the Quality of Care and Outcomes Research Interdisciplinary Working Group. *Circulation*. 2007;116:1736–1754.

Chapter 37. Peripheral Nerve Blocks

Bigeleisen PE, Moayeri N, Groen GJ. Extraneural versus intraneural stimulation thresholds during ultrasound-guided supraclavicular block. *Anesthesiology*. 2009;110:1235–1243.

Hui GK, Peng PW. Meralgia paresthetica: what an anesthesiologist needs to know. *Reg Anesth Pain Med*. 2011;36:156–161.

Jen CL, Torillo TM, Rosenblatt MA. Complications of peripheral nerve blocks. *Br J Anaesth*. 2010;105:i97–i107.

Marhofer P, Chan VW. Ultrasound-guided regional anesthesia: current concepts and future trends. *Anesth Analg*. 2007;104:1265–1269.

Chapter 38. Pharmacogenetics

Beutler E. Glucose-6-phosphate dehydrogenase deficiency. *N Engl J Med*. 1991;324:169–174.

Fischer B, Roberts CS. Tourniquet use and sickle cell hemoglobinopathy: how should we proceed? *South Med J*. 2010;10:1156–1160.

Rosenberg H. Trismus is not trivial. *Anesthesiology*. 1987;67:453–455.

Rosenberg H, Davis M, James D, Pollock N, Stowell K. Malignant hyperthermia. *Orphanet J Rare Dis*. 2007;2:21.

Ryan JF, Kagen LJ, Hyman Al. Myoglobinemia after a single dose of succinylcholine. *N Engl J Med*. 1971;285:824–827.

Chapter 39. Postoperative Recovery and Outcome

American Society of Anesthesiologists Task Force on Postanesthetic Care. Practice guidelines for postanesthetic care. A report by the American Society of Anesthesiologists Task Force on Postanesthetic Care. *Anesthesiology*. 2002;96:742–752.

Apfel CC, Kranke P, Eberhart LH, et al. Comparison of predictive models for postoperative nausea and vomiting. *Br J Anaesth*. 2002;88:234–240.

Chang CC, Lin HC, Lin HW, Lin HC. Anesthetic management and surgical site infections in total hip or knee replacement: a population-based study. *Anesthesiology*. 2010;113:279–284.

Gan TJ, Meyer TA, Apfel CC, et al. Society for Ambulatory Anesthesia guidelines for the management of postoperative nausea and vomiting. *Anesth Analg*. 2007;105:1615–1628.

Horn EP. Postoperative shivering: aetiology and treatment. *Curr Opin Anaesthesiol*. 1999;12;449–453.

Lepousé C, Lautner CA, Liu L, Gomis P, Leon A. Emergence delirium in adults in the post-anaesthesia care unit. *Br J Anaesth.* 2006;96:747–753.

Reynolds L, Beckmann J, Kurz A. Perioperative complications of hypothermia. *Best Pract Res Clin Anaesthesiol.* 2008;22:645–657.

Sharma P, Sieber F, Zariya KJ, et al. Recovery room delirium predicts postoperative delirium after hip fracture. *Anesth Analg.* 2005; 101:1215–1220.

White PF, Raeder J, Kehlet H. Ketorolac: its role as part of a multimodal analgesic regimen. *Anesth Analg.* 2012;114:250–253.

Chapter 40. Preoperative Evaluation

American College of Cardiology Foundation/American Heart Association Task Force on Practice Guidelines, American Society of Echocardiography, American Society of Nuclear Cardiology, et al. 2009 ACCF/AHA focused update on perioperative beta blockade. *J Am Coll Cardiol.* 2009;54:2102–2128.

American Society of Anesthesiologists Committee. Practice guidelines for preoperative fasting and the use of pharmacologic agents to reduce the risk of pulmonary aspiration: application to healthy patients undergoing elective procedures: an updated report by the American Society of Anesthesiologists Committee on Standards and Practice Parameters. *Anesthesiology.* 2011;114:495–511.

Cherney D, Straus S. Management of patients with hypertensive urgencies and emergencies: a systematic review of the literature. *J Gen Intern Med.* 2001;17:937–945.

Committee on Standards and Practice Parameters, Apfelbaum JL, Connis RT, et al. Practice advisory for preanesthesia evaluation. An updated report by the American Society of Anesthesiologists Task Force on Preanesthesia Evaluation. *Anesthesiology.* 2012;116: 522–538.

Fleisher LA, Beckman JA, Brown KA, et al. ACC/AHA 2007 guidelines on perioperative cardiovascular evaluation and care for noncardiac surgery: executive summary: a report of the American College of Cardiology/American Heart Association Task Force on Practice Guidelines (Writing Committee to Revise the 2002 Guidelines on Perioperative Cardiovascular Evaluation for Noncardiac Surgery) developed in collaboration with the American Society of Echocardiography, American Society of Nuclear Cardiology, Heart Rhythm Society, Society of Cardiovascular Anesthesiologists, Society for Cardiovascular Angiography and Interventions, Society for Vascular Medicine and Biology, and Society for Vascular Surgery. *J Am Coll Cardiol.* 2007;50:1707–1732.

Freed LA, Levy D, Levine RA, et al. Prevalence and clinical outcome of mitral-valve prolapse. *N Engl J Med.* 1999;341:1–7.

Hawkins NM, MacDonald MR, Petrie MC, et al. Bisoprolol in patients with heart failure and moderate to severe chronic obstructive pulmonary disease: a randomized controlled trial. *Eur J Heart Fail.* 2009;11:684–690.

Ngo DT, Sverdlov AL, Horowitz JD. Prevention of aortic valve stenosis: a realistic therapeutic target? *Pharmcol Ther.* 2012 Apr 6 [Epub ahead of print].

Nicholson G, Pereira AC, Hall GM. Parkinson's disease and anaesthesia. *Br J Anaesth.* 2002;89:904–916.

Ouriel K. Peripheral arterial disease. *Lancet.* 2001;358:1257–1264.

Pauwels RA, Buist AS, Calverley PM, Jenkins CR, Hurd SS, GOLD Scientific Committee. Global strategy for the diagnosis, management, and prevention of chronic obstructive pulmonary sisease. NHLBI/WHO global initiative for chronic obstructive lung disease (GOLD) workshop summary. *Am J Respir Crit Care Med.* 2001;163:1256–1276.

POISE Study Group. Effects of extended-release metoprol succinate in patients undergoing non-cardiac surgery (POISE trial): a randomised controlled trial. *Lancet.* 2008;371:1839–1847.

Salpeter SR, Ormiston TM, Salpeter EE. Cardioselective β-blockers in patients with reactive airway disease: a meta-analysis. *Ann Int Med.* 2002;137:715–725.

van Gestel YR, Hoeks SE, Sin DD, et al. Impact of cardioselective β-blockers on mortality in patients with chronic obstructive pulmonary disease and atherosclerosis. *Am J Respir Crit Care Med.* 2008;178:695–700.

Warner DO. Helping surgical patients quit smoking: why, when, and how. *Anesth Analg.* 2005;101:484–487.

Weksler N, Klein M, Szendro G, et al. The dilemma of immediate preoperative hypertension: to treat and operate, or to postpone surgery? *J Clin Anesth.* 2003;15:179–183.

2007 Focused Update of the ACC/AHA/SCAI 2005 Guideline Update for Percutaneous Coronary Intervention A Report of the American College of Cardiology/American Heart Association Task Force on Practice Guidelines. *Circulation.* 2008;117:261–295.

Chapter 41. Respiratory Physiology and Anesthesia

Warner DO. Helping surgical patients quit smoking: why, when, and how. *Anesth Analg.* 2005;101:484–487.

Chapter 43. Thoracic Surgery

Campos JH, Hallam EA, Van Natta T, Kernstine KH. Devices for lung isolation used by anesthesiologists with limited thoracic experience: comparison of double-lumen endotracheal tube, Univent® torque control blocker, and Arndt wire-guided endobronchial blocker. *Anesthesiology.* 2006;104:261–266.

Datta D, Lahiri B. Preoperative evaluation of patients undergoing lung resection surgery. *Chest.* 2003;123;2096–2103.

Grocott HP. Oxygen toxicity during one-lung ventilation: is it time to re-evaluate our practice? *Anesthesiol Clin.* 2008;26:273–280.

Kozian A, Schilling T, Schütze H, Senturk M, Hachenberg T, Hedenstierna G. Protective strategies during thoracic surgery: effects of alveolar recruitment maneuver and low-tidal volume ventilation on lung density distribution. *Anesthesiology.* 2011;114:1025–1035.

Kunlyoshi Y, Koja K, Miyagi K, Uezu T, Yamashiro S, Arakaki K. The prevention of nerve injury in aortic arch aneurysmal surgery. *Asian Cardiovasc Thorac.* 2004;12:374–375.

Naguib M, Dawlatly AA, Ashour M, Bamgboye EA. Multivariate determinants of the need for postoperative ventilation in myasthenia gravis. *Can J Anaesth.* 1996;43:1006–1013.

Xu Y, Tan Z, Wang S, Shao H, Zhu X. Effect of thoracic epidural anesthesia with different concentrations of ropivacaine on arterial oxygenation during one-lung ventilation. *Anesthesiology.* 2010;112(5):1146–1154.

Chapter 44. Transplant Surgery

Lucangelo U, Del Sorbo L, Boffini M, Ranieri VM. Protective ventilation for lung transplantation. *Curr Opin Anesthesiol.* 2012;25:170–174.

Wijdicks EF, Varelas PN, Gronseth GS, Greer DM, American Academy of Neurology. Evidence-based guideline update: determining brain death in adults: report of the Quality Standards Subcommittee of the American Academy of Neurology. *Neurology.* 2010;74;1911.

Chapter 45. Vascular Surgery

Etz CD, Luehr M, Kari FA, et al. Paraplegia after extensive thoracic and thoracoabdominal aortic aneurysm repair: does critical spinal cord ischemia occur postoperatively? *J Thorac Cardiovasc Surg.* 2008;135:324–330.

Hiratzka LF, Bakris GL, Beckman JA, et al. 2010 ACCF/AHA/AATS/ACR/ASA/SCA/SCAI/SIR/STS/SVM guidelines for the diagnosis and management of patients with thoracic aortic disease: a report of the American College of Cardiology Foundation/American Heart Association Task Force on Practice Guidelines, American Association for Thoracic Surgery, American College of Radiology, American Stroke Association, Society of Cardiovascular Anesthesiologists, Society for Cardiovascular Angiography and Interventions, Society of Interventional Radiology, Society of Thoracic Surgeons, and Society for Vascular Medicine. *Circulation.* 2010;121:e266–e369.

Parodi JC, Ferreira LM, Sicard G, La Mura R, Fernandez S. Cerebral protection during carotid stenting using flow reversal. *J Vasc Surg.* 2005;41:416–422.

Rerkasem K, Bond R, Rothwell PM. Local versus general anaesthesia for carotid endarterectomy. *Cochrane Database Syst Rev.* 2004;(2):CD000126.

Schermerhorn ML, O'Malley AJ, Jhaveri A, Cotterill P, Pomposelli F, Landon BE. Endovascular vs. open repair of abdominal aortic aneurysms in the Medicare population. *N Engl J Med.* 2008;358:464–474.

Svensson LG, Rodriguez ER. Aortic organ disease epidemic, and why do balloons pop? *Circulation.* 2005;112:1082–1084.

Swensson LG. Acute aortic syndromes: time to talk of many things. *Cleve Clin J Med.* 2008;75:25–28.

INDEX